PHARMACOLOGY for the EMS PROVIDER

FIFTH EDITION

PHARMACOLOGY for the EMS PROVIDER

FIFTH EDITION

Richard K. Beck, BBA, MS, EMT-P

Education Consultant/Associate
Center for EMS Education
Castries, St. Lucia, West Indies

Formerly: Associate Dean of Academic Affairs/EMS
Broward College
Ft. Lauderdale, FL

Formerly: Director of EMS Education
University of Alabama School of Medicine/Huntsville Campus
Huntsville, Alabama

F.A. Davis Company • Philadelphia

F. A. Davis Company
1915 Arch Street
Philadelphia, PA 19103
www.fadavis.com

Printed in the United States of America

Last digit indicates print number: 10 9 8 7 6 5 4 3 2 1

Publisher: Quincy McDonald
Director of Content Development: George W. Lang
Developmental Editors: Joanna E. Cain and Pamela Speh
Art and Design Manager: Carolyn O'Brien

Library of Congress Cataloging-in-Publication Data

Beck, Richard K., 1947-, author.
Pharmacology for the EMS provider / Richard K. Beck.—Fifth edition.
p. ; cm.
Includes bibliographical references and index.
ISBN 978-0-8036-4364-2—ISBN 0-8036-4364-0
I. Title.
[DNLM: 1. Drug Therapy–Handbooks. 2. Emergencies–Handbooks. 3. Emergency Medical Technicians–Handbooks. 4. Emergency Treatment–Handbooks. QV 39]
RM300
615.1–dc23

2015004986

Working on this book required time and sacrifice. I am blessed to have a home team that understands and supports me. This textbook is dedicated to my team—my wife Suzy (who saved my life) and my children Amanda and Brian. At my feet for most of the writing of this text was my companion Dixie. Dixie didn't make it through this entire writing. However, at my feet now is Emma. Anyone who loves dogs knows how special and supportive they are.

On March 26, 2014 at 6:15 a.m., my heart decided to stop while I was sleeping. Through Suzy's quick thinking, perfect CPR, and the rapid response of Williamson Medical Center EMS in Franklin, TN, I am here today. All involved knew exactly what to do and when to do it. It was not a coincidence that everyone was at the right place at the right time. So, to Suzy, and all the great EMS personnel at Williamson EMS, THANK YOU! This text is also dedicated to you.

RKB

Foreword

Paramedics and emergency responders are called up each day to provide emergency (and nonemergency) care to patients in time of need. Regardless of our geographical location or community populations, paramedic and health providers administer medications in hopes of alleviating pain, discomfort, or life-threatening events. As medications and pharmacologic agents continue to evolve and implement into our arsenal of patient care options, so should our training and knowledge of proper use of these medications.

This comprehensive book will provide the paramedic (or student) with convenient, easy-to-understand, and up-to-date information on drug therapy.

Taking a user-friendly approach, ***Pharmacology for the EMS Provider***, fifth edition was designed with student learning styles in mind and with additional resources to help the students and educator understand the material and have an effective learning experience. Paramedics in the field and students in the classroom can use this book and resources to help strengthen their comprehension of pharmacology and allow them to apply what they've learned to the patient care environment with patient safety in mind.

David L. Sullivan, PhD, NRP, NCEE
Professor
Health Occupations—Emergency Medical Services Program
Pasco-Hernando State College
New Port Richey, Florida

Preface

Emergency Medical Services (EMS) professionals are routinely placed in positions in which quick decisions can mean the difference between life and death—especially when administering drugs. Drug administration carries an enormous responsibility, and the knowledge the EMS professional brings to the out-of-hospital setting can make all the difference in a successful patient outcome.

Pharmacology for the EMS Provider, fifth edition was revised to fulfill the core module for the pharmacology component of the Personnel Licensure Levels within the EMS Educational Standards. These levels include Emergency Medical Responder (EMR), the Emergency Medical Technician (EMT), the Advanced Emergency Medical Technician (AEMT), and Paramedic. All of these licensure levels include some aspect of pharmacology, from the very basic (EMR) to the most advanced (Paramedic). This edition also serves as a comprehensive reference text after graduation for practicing EMS professionals.

Background

This text was originally written to be a resource for both the EMS student and the EMS graduate. Admittedly, this text contains too much information for the entry-level paramedic. However, once a student graduates, this text changes from a textbook to a good pharmacology resource text.

Organization

Chapters 1 through 9 present basic introductory topics. For example, Chapter 1 introduces you to pharmacology. It explains essential drug information about each drug presented. Drug origins, drug preparation, drug testing, and legislation that governs drugs manufactured in the United States are also discussed. An added topic for the fifth edition is professionalism, which is discussed in Chapter 2. When dealing with patients and their families, it is important to present ourselves as professionals and also continue to maintain our professional status through constant learning and updating on changing and new trends within EMS. Chapter 3 provides a review of how drugs travel and respond once in the body. It is not enough to know what drugs a patient is taking; EMS professionals may also need to know how the drug(s) works once in the body and how the body may respond to the drug(s). Pharmacokinetics reviews drug movement including absorption, solubility, distribution, biotransformation, and excretion. Once a drug reaches its destination, pharmacodynamics explains how a drug's mechanism of action affects the patient. Many drugs given in out-of-hospital emergency medicine affect the autonomic nervous system. Chapter 4 gives an overview of the autonomic nervous system and explains how selected drugs interact with its functions. The conditions of the body's pH, fluids, and electrolytes affect the therapeutic effects of drugs. Chapter 5 reviews fluids, electrolytes, and intravenous therapy in an attempt to explain the importance of maintaining these factors within normal limits to enable drugs to produce their therapeutic effects. Chapter 6 presents a discussion on blood and blood product administration. It is becoming more common for EMS professionals to administer blood or to transport patients who are receiving blood or blood products. Therefore, it is important to know the different blood types, who can receive and who can donate the various blood types, and how to recognize the signs and symptoms of blood transfusion reactions. Indications for the various volume expanders and for the use of antihyperlipidemic drugs used to decrease the lipid level in the blood are also included. Some drugs are administered according to body weight, others by a predetermined dosage, and some by being added to intravenous solutions before they are administered. Chapter 7 explains mathematics and illustrates how to calculate drug dosages. Each chapter includes mathematical problems for you to practice your math skills. Chapter 8 presents various routes by which drugs can be administered and gives step-by-step instruction on the procedures for correct drug administration. Chapter 9 explains drug classification and makes it easier for you to rationalize and understand when to use a drug, its contraindications, and precautions for its use.

Drug monographs in Chapters 10 through 19 are presented by body system affected. Chapter 12 presents drugs used to treat disorders of the eyes, ears, nose, and throat, which is an added topic for the fifth edition. Each monograph contains detailed descriptions of the drug's generic and trade names, pregnancy classification, mechanism of action, indications for use, contraindications, precautions, route and dosage, adverse reactions and side effects, and any implications of which EMS professionals should be aware.

Appendices for quick reference include (A) Drugs (Generic and Trade Names) and Their Therapeutic Classifications, (B) Pediatric Normal Values, Dosages, and Infusion Rates, (C) Herbal Remedies, (D) Street Drugs, and (E) Commonly Used Abbreviations and Symbols.

Chapter Features

The following features should help make learning pharmacology less confusing:

- Classifications of Drugs—Each drug discussed in the chapter is listed according to its classification(s).
- Learning Outcomes—List the major content areas to be mastered in the chapter.
- Key Terms—Chapter key terms are in **bold** and defined in the text the first time they are used. There is also a

comprehensive glossary at the end of the book that includes key term definitions.

- Introduction—Each chapter includes an introduction to the topics and drugs presented and their relationship to treating emergencies in that specific body system.
- Drug Monographs—Drug monographs in Chapters 10 through 19 are presented in alphabetical order by generic name. The most common trade name(s) are listed immediately below the generic name.
- Let's Recap—This presents a final statement regarding the topics and drugs contained in each chapter.
- Practice Exercises—There are practice exercises at the end of each chapter for you to review key information presented in the chapter and help you understand the drugs more fully.
- Case Studies—Each chapter includes case studies to help you work through specific EMS scenarios.

Instructor Resources

- Instructor's Guide
- Access to a comprehensive Test Bank of over 400 questions with answers that include rationales, located on Davis*Plus*
- PowerPoint presentations including over 360 slides that outline the important concepts in each chapter

Student Resources

- Animations available on Davis*Plus* that illustrate how drugs work when introduced into the body.
- A Student Quiz for each chapter that allows students to review and practice content

Contributor and Reviewers

Contributor

Gordon M. Smith, D.Ph., M.B.A.
Spring Hill, TN

Reviewers

Kevin D. Barnard, MS, NREMT-P, CCEMTP, EMSI
Assistant Professor
Cuyahoga Community College
Cleveland, Ohio

Alan Benney, NREMT-P, Community Paramedic
EMS Faculty
Hennepin Technical College
Brooklyn Park, Minnesota

David Scott Blevins, BPS, NREMT-P
Director of EMS Programs
Roane State Community College
Knoxville, Tennessee

Steven M. Carlo, BS, NYS C I/C, EMT-I
Department Chair
Erie Community College—North Campus
Williamsville, New York

Noël RJ Dunn, Advanced Care Paramedic/Paramedic Instructor
Instructor
Saskatchewan Institute of Applied Science and Technology
Saskatoon, SK
Canada

Jerry S. Findley, BS, MA, LP
Program Director
South Plains College
Lubbock, Texas

Fidel O. Garcia, EMT-Paramedic
President/Owner
Professional EMS Education
Grand Junction, Colorado

David Frank Garmon, BS, MA Ed, NRP
Executive Director, Alabama Gulf EMS System
University of South Alabama
Mobile, Alabama

Grant Blackstone Goold, BA, MPA/HSA, PhD
Program Director and Department Chair
American River College
Sacramento, California

John Gosford, MS, NREMT-P
EMS Program Coordinator
College of Southern Maryland
La Plata, Maryland

Wesley Hutchins, BS, MPA
Dean of Health and Emergency Services Programs
Forsyth Technical Community College
Winston-Salem, North Carolina

Kevin Johnson, AS, BS, NREMT-P
EMS Faculty
Inver Hills Community College
Inver Grove Heights, Minnesota

Kenneth W. Kirkland, Jr., RN, BSN, NREMT-P
EMS Faculty
Calhoun Community College
Decatur, Alabama

Joanne Moss, Advanced Care Paramedic
Instructor
Saskatchewan Institute of Applied Science and Technology
Saskatoon, SK
Canada

Jeannine Thomas, EMS Educator
PA-C
San Antonio College
San Antonio, Texas

Adriana Laura Torrez, LP
EMS Education Coordinator
Methodist Health System
Dallas, Texas

Ailsa R. Vogelsang, BTAS, NREMT-P
EMS/Fire Coordinator
Belmont College
St. Clairsville, Ohio

Acknowledgments

Many people were involved in producing this text. My name is on the cover, but this book exists because of the contributions of many talented people. Some of these folks are listed at the front of this book. I could attempt to list everyone responsible in the making of this book, but I just know that I will forget someone. So, to everyone responsible—thank you!

The author and F. A. Davis would like to thank Dr. Gianluca Ghiselli of the Università degli Studi di Torino for providing us with a thorough technical review. And, finally, if it were not for Don Weiss, formerly of F. A. Davis, this text would have never been a reality. Back in 1990, Don guided me to the right people at F. A. Davis and educated me on the publishing business, launching the first edition of *Pharmacology for Prehospital Emergency Care*.

The reviewers of a manuscript tell it like it is. Their expertise, honest criticism, and suggestions provided valuable recommendations for improvement. And, finally, I want to thank my wife Suzy. She read the manuscript and also made an enormous number of recommendations on how to make improvements. This book would not be a reality without her support.

I am hopeful that *Pharmacology for the EMS Provider*, fifth edition will be of value in the classroom and an aid for practicing EMS professionals.

Richard K. Beck

Abbreviations

Resp	respiratory
CV	cardiovascular
CNS	central nervous system
EENT	eye, ear, nose, and throat
GI	gastrointestinal
GU	genitourinary
Derm	dermatologic
Endo	endocrinologic
F and E	fluid and electrolyte
Hemat	hematologic
Local	local
Metab	metabolic
MS	musculoskeletal
Neuro	neurological
Misc	miscellaneous

Contents in Brief

Contents

Appendices

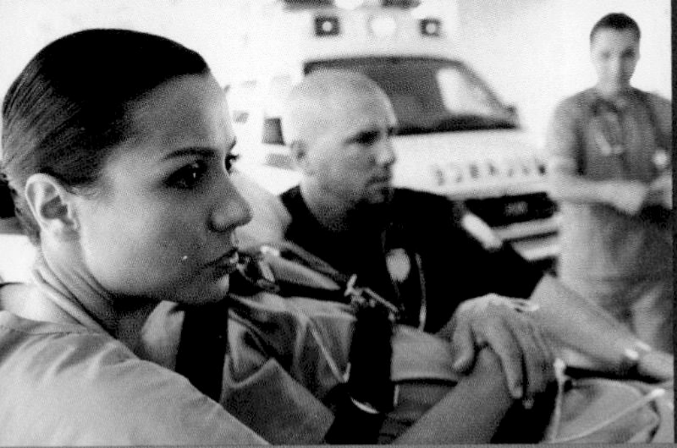

CHAPTER 1

Introduction to Pharmacology

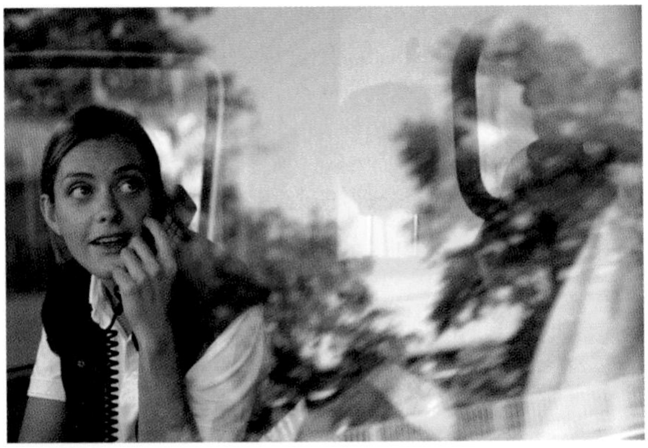

Paramedics checking equipment prior to beginning their shift. *(Photograph © Thinkstock)*

LEARNING OUTCOMES

- Differentiate between the laws, regulations, and standards regarding infection control.
- Explain the importance of performing a thorough patient medication assessment.
- Describe historical trends in pharmacology.
- Differentiate between the chemical, generic (nonproprietary), trade (proprietary), and official names of drugs.
- List the five main sources of drugs.
- Describe how drugs are classified.
- Describe the three phases of drug development.
- List and describe the components of a drug profile.
- List the sources of drug information.
- List the legislative acts controlling the use of drugs in the United States.
- Describe the standardization of drugs.
- Describe investigational drugs, including the approval process and the U.S. Food and Drug Administration classifications for newly approved drugs.
- Describe special considerations of drugs as they relate to the pregnant, pediatric, and geriatric patient.

KEY TERMS

Assay
Bioassay
Black box warning
Body substance isolation
Chemical name
Drug
U.S. Food and Drug Administration (FDA)
Generic name
Official name
Parenteral
Pharmacodynamics
Pharmacogenetics
Pharmacokinetics
Pharmacology
Pharmacotherapy
Physicians' Desk Reference (PDR)
Standard Precautions
Therapeutic index
Therapeutic
Toxicity
Toxicology
Trade name
United States Pharmacopoeia (USP)

SCENARIO OPENING

You are assigned to Rescue 6 in a busy district of the city. Your preceptors, Rick and Phil, have just completed inspecting the unit but now will go through the inspection again to show you the importance of the daily inspection of both the vehicle and the medical equipment. First, Phil instructs you on some of the important aspects of the vehicle inspection. For example, Rescue 6 must have a full tank of fuel and the correct amount of oil. The tires must be inflated properly and have sufficient tread life. All lights must be operable and the siren in proper working order.

After the vehicle inspection is complete, you and Rick check all medical equipment. Some of the important aspects of this inspection include the ECG monitor/defibrillator operation, oxygen levels, airway equipment, and the drug box. Rick explains that every drug must be inspected to make sure that each drug is in date, labeled properly, has not been tampered with, and is stored appropriately. If there is any question concerning a drug, that drug must be replaced. The entire inspection process must be appropriately documented by the crew preforming the inspection. As soon as your inspection is complete, a call comes in for "an unconscious woman."

effective **Communication**

It is important that EMS crew members discuss all components of the vehicle and equipment inspection/evaluation process, making sure everything is in good working order. All drugs must be stored appropriately and any out-of-date drugs immediately replaced. Any missing drugs must be accounted for and replaced.

Introduction

If you like solving puzzles, then EMS and especially pharmacology is for you. One of the most important aspects of EMS is a thorough patient assessment. The patient assessment in itself is a puzzle. For example, when you arrive at an emergency scene, you must attempt to determine the following: scene safety, chief complaint, what occurred prior to the chief complaint, airway and circulatory status, level of consciousness, pain level, and so on.

As a paramedic, you must also put together a second puzzle—the medication assessment. For example, you must attempt to determine medications the patient is currently taking, the last time any medications were taken, the conditions those medications are treating, and so on.

Before you administer any medications to your patient, you must know what the patient is currently taking so serious drug-drug interactions do not occur. For example, you do not want to administer nitroglycerin to a patient who has recently taken sildenafil. This combination of drugs may lead to fatal hypotension.

Check the **Evidence**

Nitroglycerin and medications that are used to treat erectile dysfunction (sildenafil, tadalafil, and vardenafil) are potent vasodilators. If nitroglycerin is taken concurrently with any of these mediations, cardiovascular (CV) collapse can occur, causing sudden death.

If EMS professionals fail to obtain patient medication information while on scene or during transport, the receiving facility will have to begin its own medication assessment, which may delay treatment and cause serious consequences.

Precautions Against Blood-Borne Pathogens and Infectious Diseases

By just looking at a patient, it is not possible to tell if he or she has a blood-borne infection such as hepatitis, tuberculosis (TB), or HIV, which can lead to AIDS. Therefore, the Centers for Disease Control and Prevention (CDC) in Atlanta, Georgia, recommend certain body substance isolation precautions. **Body substance isolation** precautions, known as **Standard Precautions,** are infection-control precautions that health-care professionals should apply with *all* patients in *all* situations. Figure 1-1 provides a comprehensive review of Standard Precautions.

Transmission-based precautions are intended for patients diagnosed with or suspected of specific highly transmissible diseases. These precautions condense the seven existing categories of isolation precautions developed by the CDC in 1970 into three sets of precautions based on routes of infection. Updated in 2007 to complement Standard Precautions, transmission-based precautions (Figs. 1-2, 1-3, and 1-4) reduce the risk of airborne, droplet, and contact transmission of pathogens and are always to be used in addition to Standard Precautions.

Health-care professionals should wear gloves whenever touching a patient. This is especially important for health-care professionals in contact with blood or any body fluid. Health-care professionals should also wear gloves when performing procedures such as starting IV lines, drawing blood, giving injections, or inserting an endotracheal tube. After each patient contact, carefully remove the gloves and immediately properly dispose of them. If blood or body fluids come in contact with the skin, thoroughly wash all exposed areas.

If there is a chance that patient blood or body fluids may come in contact with face or clothing, wear protective masks and gowns. Once contact with the patient is completed, carefully remove the mask and gown and properly dispose of them.

Whenever possible, health-care professionals should use disposable equipment. Once used, properly dispose of the equipment. Do not re-cap, bend, break, or remove needles from the syringe. Discard needles and disposable syringes in designated puncture-resistant containers immediately after use.

To protect yourself against TB infection, you should have a *high-efficiency particulate air (HEPA) respirator* approved by

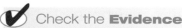

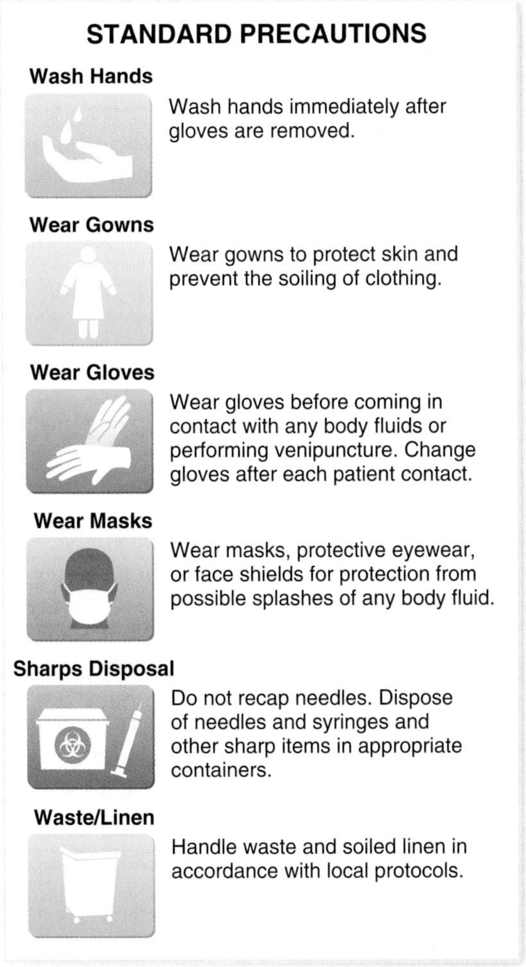
STANDARD PRECAUTIONS
Wash Hands
Wash hands immediately after gloves are removed.
Wear Gowns
Wear gowns to protect skin and prevent the soiling of clothing.
Wear Gloves
Wear gloves before coming in contact with any body fluids or performing venipuncture. Change gloves after each patient contact.
Wear Masks
Wear masks, protective eyewear, or face shields for protection from possible splashes of any body fluid.
Sharps Disposal
Do not recap needles. Dispose of needles and syringes and other sharp items in appropriate containers.
Waste/Linen
Handle waste and soiled linen in accordance with local protocols.

Figure 1-1 Standard precautions.

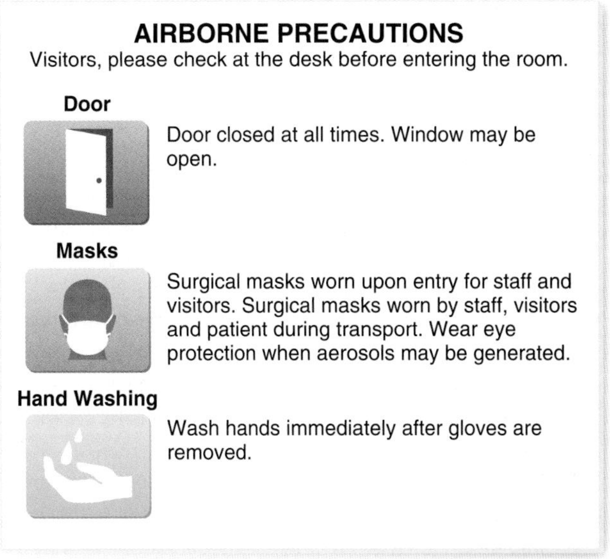
AIRBORNE PRECAUTIONS
Visitors, please check at the desk before entering the room.
Door
Door closed at all times. Window may be open.
Masks
Surgical masks worn upon entry for staff and visitors. Surgical masks worn by staff, visitors and patient during transport. Wear eye protection when aerosols may be generated.
Hand Washing
Wash hands immediately after gloves are removed.

Figure 1-2 Airborne precautions.

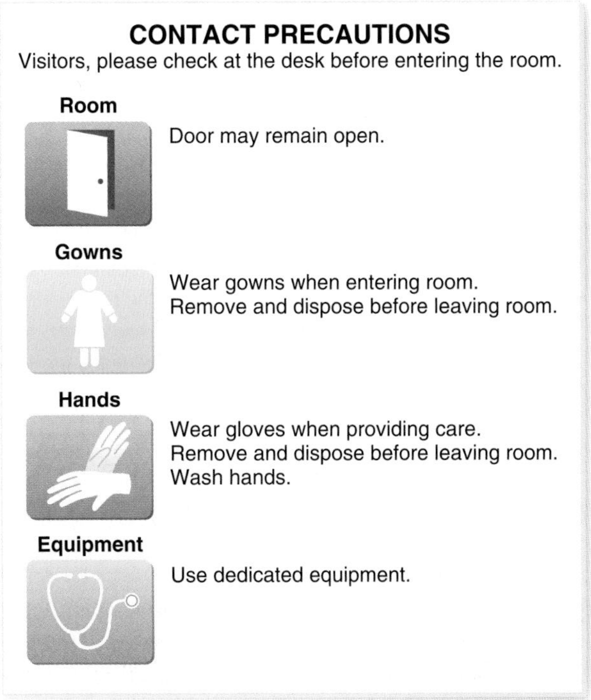
CONTACT PRECAUTIONS
Visitors, please check at the desk before entering the room.
Room
Door may remain open.
Gowns
Wear gowns when entering room. Remove and dispose before leaving room.
Hands
Wear gloves when providing care. Remove and dispose before leaving room. Wash hands.
Equipment
Use dedicated equipment.

Figure 1-3 Contact precautions.

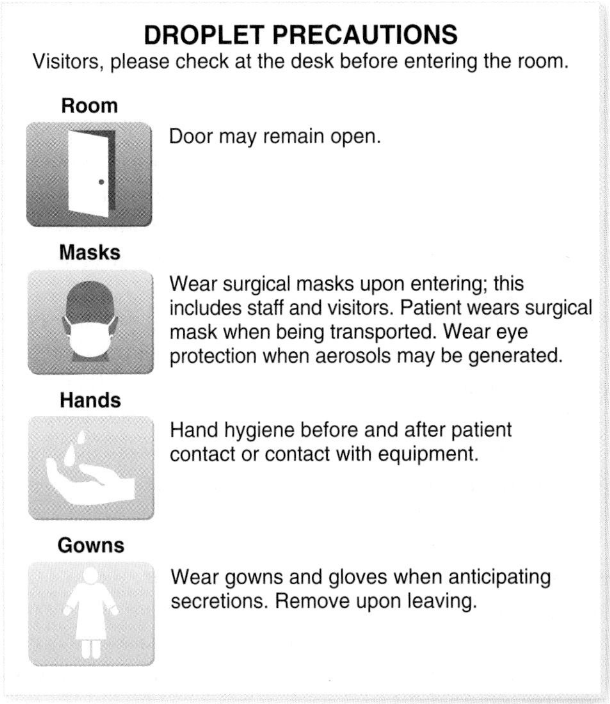
DROPLET PRECAUTIONS
Visitors, please check at the desk before entering the room.
Room
Door may remain open.
Masks
Wear surgical masks upon entering; this includes staff and visitors. Patient wears surgical mask when being transported. Wear eye protection when aerosols may be generated.
Hands
Hand hygiene before and after patient contact or contact with equipment.
Gowns
Wear gowns and gloves when anticipating secretions. Remove upon leaving.

Figure 1-4 Droplet precautions.

the National Institute of Occupational Safety and Health. This should be worn whenever coming in contact with a confirmed or suspected TB-infected patient.

All routes for transmission of blood-borne infections have yet to be identified. Therefore, it is extremely important for health-care professionals to take all appropriate precautions against contact with such infections while treating patients. Remember:

- Always wear protective equipment when handling contaminated equipment or coming in contact with the patient.
- Place all contaminated equipment and supplies in properly marked biological hazard bags and dispose of them properly.
- Ensure that all used sharps are properly secured in a puncture-resistant and clearly marked container. Do not re-cap needles after use or leave them at the scene.
- Properly clean all reusable equipment as soon after use as possible.
- If exposed to an infectious disease, contact medical control and the receiving facility immediately.

For complete information on the *2007 Guideline for Isolation Precautions: Preventing Transmission of Infectious Agents in Healthcare Settings,* go to http://www.cdc.gov/hicpac/2007ip/2007isolationprecautions.html.

effective **Communication**

Remember, first, do no harm. Sometimes we have a tendency to work too fast, which can cause mistakes and place us at risk for exposure. In many instances, accuracy can save more lives than speed.

The Patient Medication Assessment

All health-care professionals know the importance of a thorough patient assessment. A medication assessment should be part of every patient assessment. Information gained from the medication assessment can provide important information not only for EMS personnel but for hospital personnel as well.

Information gained from the medication assessment can be used to design a treatment plan for EMS personnel and alerts personnel at the receiving facility what treatment was done and what may need to be done upon arrival. Knowing what medications the patient is taking will aid in preventing drug interactions or overdoses, which might occur from administration of drugs in the out-of-hospital setting as well as at the receiving facility.

As discussed previously, if EMS personnel fail to obtain patient medication information while on scene, the receiving facility will have to begin its own medication assessment, which may delay treatment and cause serious consequences.

Patient medication information may be obtained in several ways. Usually, the patient is the best source. However, in some cases, patients may not know what medications they are taking. They may know why they are taking a medication but not its name. In other cases, patients may not know what medications they are taking or why. If patients are unable to communicate for a medication assessment, other sources include a family member, friend, Vial of Life, or a home-health aide. Questions that may be asked in a medication assessment include:

- Are you currently taking any medications (drugs) prescribed by a doctor?
- What are the names of these medications (drugs)? Some patients may not know the actual names of the drugs they are taking. If this is the case, EMS personnel should also ask: Do you have some of the medication(s) (drugs) to show me? We must take it (them) to the hospital.
- Why are you taking the medications (drugs)? If the patient does not know the name of the medications, they may know the reason for taking the drugs.
- When did you last take your medication(s)?
- Have you been taking your medications according to the prescribed directions? If not, how have you been taking them?
- Are you taking any over-the-counter medications (drugs purchased without a prescription at the store)? If so, what are these medications and when did you last take them?
- Are you taking any herbal preparations?
- Are you taking any medications that were prescribed for someone else?
- Have you recently completed your prescription or stopped taking your medications? If so, what were they and why were you taking them?
- Have you experienced any side effects or illness from your medications? If so, have you reported these to your doctor?

Depending on the circumstances, the medication assessment can be adjusted to address special situations. Additional questions may have to be asked. It is generally useful to bring any patient medications to the receiving facility with the patient.

effective **Communication**

The most common places patients keep medications include the bathroom, bedroom, and kitchen (do not forget to look in the refrigerator). To save time, EMS dispatch may have instructed the caller to have any medications ready for EMS personnel when they arrive.

EMS professionals should be familiar with medication labels and the information on them. Figure 1-5 outlines the elements of a prescription.

Also, be aware that many medication containers have additional secondary labels that include additional information, such as: *"Swallow whole. DO NOT crush or chew," "Take on an empty stomach," "Important: take or use exactly as directed; do not discontinue or skip doses unless directed by your doctor,"* and *"may cause drowsiness."*

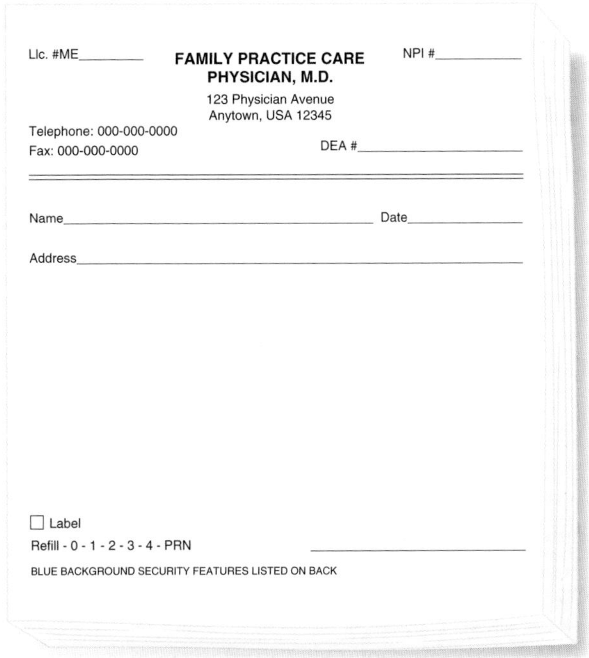
Llc. #ME________ FAMILY PRACTICE CARE PHYSICIAN, M.D. NPI #__________
123 Physician Avenue
Anytown, USA 12345
Telephone: 000-000-0000
Fax: 000-000-0000
DEA #__________

Name__________ Date__________

Address__________

☐ Label
Refill - 0 - 1 - 2 - 3 - 4 - PRN __________
BLUE BACKGROUND SECURITY FEATURES LISTED ON BACK

Figure 1-5 Elements of a prescription.

Medication Assessment Scenarios

Knowledge of the medications each patient is taking often provides a basis for determining treatment. Medications may be one of your most useful assessment tools, especially if the patient is unresponsive or incoherent. The three scenarios that follow illustrate the importance of your medication assessment.

SCENARIO ONE

You respond to a 72-year-old male who states he has been feeling weak for the past 4 hours. While performing your initial assessment, you notice some medication containers on the kitchen table. These include Lanoxin, Cardizem, and glyburide. What information do these medications tell you about this patient?

- **Lanoxin** is the trade name for digoxin, an antiarrhythmic. Digoxin increases both the force and velocity of ventricular contractions while simultaneously slowing conduction through the atrioventricular (AV) node of the heart.
- **Cardizem** is the trade name for diltiazem, a calcium channel blocker that decreases conduction velocity and ventricular rate.
- **Glyburide** is an oral antidiabetic agent used to treat type 2 diabetes.

Knowledge of the use of these medications or having access to a resource to research the drugs tells us that this patient is a diabetic with underlying CV problems.

SCENARIO TWO

You are called to a 59-year-old female patient who is complaining of dizziness and feeling weak. Her pulse rate is 44 beats/minute and regular. Upon questioning her about medications, she tells you that she is on blood pressure medicine but cannot remember its name. She finds the bottle, and the drug name is atenolol. When questioned further, she admits not taking her medicine for "about a couple of days." Further questioning reveals that she had taken three tablets today to make up for not taking any over the last couple of days.

- **Atenolol** is a beta-adrenergic blocking agent used for hypertension and angina pectoris caused by hypertension. It causes slowing of the heart rate and can mask or hide any other problems that might induce tachycardia.

Check the **Evidence**

Atenolol is a beta$_1$- (myocardial) adrenergic blocker that can cause severe bradycardia if an overdosing occurs. Severe bradycardia can contribute to severe hypotension, congestive heart failure (CHF), or pulmonary edema, all of which can be fatal.

By taking a multiple dose, this patient most likely is experiencing side effects caused by overdosing. Overdosing on prescribed medications is a common problem with patients who forget to take their medications and try to "catch up" or who just do not understand the instructions on the container.

SCENARIO THREE

You respond to a 69-year-old male who states "my heart feels like a runaway train." His pulse is 128 beats/minute and regular. During your assessment, you find out that he has chronic obstructive pulmonary disease (COPD) and has just been prescribed Ventolin. The patient used the Ventolin approximately 30 minutes before he began to feel his heart racing.

- **Ventolin** is a trade name for albuterol, a bronchodilator used to treat reversible airway obstruction caused by asthma or COPD. CV side effects of albuterol include hypertension, chest pain, and arrhythmias, including tachycardia. Unfortunately, the elderly, in whom COPD is most common, are more prone to developing adverse reactions and side effects.

It is very important for EMS professionals to perform a thorough patient assessment, including a medication assessment. Medication interactions are sometimes difficult to assess in the out-of-hospital setting. However, any information gathered will benefit the patient when planning a treatment plan, whether in or out of the hospital.

Historical Trends in Pharmacology

Primitive civilizations once believed that evil spirits could inhabit the body and cause disease. This belief continued until 460 B.C. when Hippocrates, known as the Father of Medicine, concluded that disease resulted from natural causes and could only be understood through the study of natural laws. Hippocrates believed that the physician's role in healing was to assist the body's recuperative powers.

The roots of pharmacology date back to the ancient civilizations that used plants and plant extracts to treat illness and cure disease. For example, opium and morphine were used for pain relief and foxglove extracts (digitalis) for treating symptoms of heart disease. Jesuits' bark was used to treat malaria, willow bark for treating fever, and extracts of the poppy plant (opium) for treating dysentery. Pharmacology continues to make advances based on knowledge gained from ancient civilizations. The oldest known prescriptions were found around 3000 B.C. on papyrus tablets.

After the fall of the Roman Empire, Christian orders built monasteries. These monasteries became major sites for learning, including the science of pharmacology. Additionally, the monasteries aided the sick with medicines that were grown in their gardens. In 1240, Emperor Frederic II declared that pharmacy was to be a separate science from medicine. However, it was not until the 16th century that Valerius Cordus authored the first pharmacopoeia, or drug reference book.

Some of the most significant pharmacologic discoveries that have taken place throughout history include:

- 17th century: opium, coca, and ipecac, which are still used today
- 1785: digitalis used as a cardiac medication
- 19th century: the beginning of large-scale drug manufacturing plants
- 1815: morphine used to treat severe pain
- Early 1800s: ether and chloroform used as first general anesthetics, allowing development of surgical treatment of disease
- 1922: insulin used to treat diabetes mellitus
- Mid-1940s: the introduction of antibiotics such as penicillin for treating infections
- 1955: polio vaccine introduced
- Mid-1970s: antivirals for treating viral diseases
- 1983: Orphan Drug Act signed into law to aid in the research of new treatments to prevent and cure disease
- 1997: Food and Drug Administration Modernization Act

Each of these, along with many other advances, significantly enhanced the progress of medical treatment of disease.

Today more than ever, modern health care is experiencing rapid change. Consumer health education has motivated members of the public to take more responsibility for their health and disease prevention. For example, more people are now on regular exercise programs and are paying more attention to what they eat. Many people are using Internet sites such as WebMD and Medline for personal disease self-research. Communities are regulating where people can and cannot use tobacco products. Pharmaceutical companies are advertising directly to consumers, encouraging them to ask their physicians about specific medications.

Pharmacology has become multidisciplinary in scope and now includes such subjects as chemistry, genetics, immunology, microbiology, pathology, and physiology.

During the last few decades, there has been remarkable progress in developing new drugs and understanding how they act on the body. However, continuous research will raise discoveries in this century. Research is directed toward new treatments, cures, or methods to prevent disease. For example, the Orphan Drug Act was signed into law January 4, 1983. The term "orphan drug" refers to a product that treats a disease that affects fewer than 200,000 Americans. The intent of the act is to stimulate research, development, and approval of products that treat rare diseases. Since the Orphan Drug Act was passed, more than 353 orphan drugs and biological products have been brought to market. In contrast, in the decade prior to 1983, fewer than 10 such products were brought to market.

There are also social questions to be addressed. Many of the questions involve responsibility issues such as ensuring that basic drugs are available to the public. For example, the sudden withdrawal of Compazine without warning and the bretylium manufacturing problem caused health concerns for millions of patients. There are also large-scale efforts to preserve the South American Amazonian rain forest, which is rich in diversity of plant life and thus is a large source for new medication development.

Drug Names

A **drug** is any substance that, when taken into the body, changes one or more of the body's functions. Drugs are most commonly used in medicine to diagnose, treat, or prevent disease, which has resulted in an improved quality of life. **Pharmacology** is the science of drugs, including the study of their origin ingredients, uses, and actions on the body. Branches of pharmacology include:

- **Pharmacokinetics:** The movement of a drug in the body, with particular emphasis on its distribution, duration of action, and method of excretion
- **Pharmacodynamics:** The study of drugs and their actions on the body
- **Pharmacotherapy:** The use of drugs in the treatment of disease
- **Toxicology:** The study of poisons and adverse drug effects
- **Pharmacogenetics:** The study of the influence of hereditary factors on the response of drugs

From the time a drug is initially tested in the laboratory until it is approved and marketed, it can acquire up to four names. A drug's **chemical name** is the exact description of the drug's structure and composition. For example, $C_{18}H_{23}NO_3$.*HCl,1,2-benzenediol,4-[2-[[3-(4-hydroxyphenyl)-1-methylpropyl]-,hydrochloride,()-* is the chemical name for a drug used in treating low cardiac output. The same drug's **generic** (or nonproprietary) **name** is dobutamine hydrochloride. The manufacturer that first formulates the drug usually gives it the generic name. Third, the manufacturer registers a drug using a **trade** (or proprietary) **name.** A trade name is often designated in print by its initial capital letter and the raised registered symbol ® following the name. For example, a trade name of dobutamine hydrochloride is Dobutrex®. Finally, the **United States Pharmacopeia (USP)** and the National Formulary (NF) give a drug its **official name** after it has met specific standards for quality, strength, purity, packaging, and labeling. The letters USP following their name designates drugs meeting these standards. The official name for dobutamine hydrochloride is dobutamine hydrochloride, USP. Table 1-1 illustrates examples of the chemical, generic, trade, and official names of some common EMS drugs as well as some common over-the-counter (OTC) and prescription drugs.

Sources of Drugs

Drugs originate from five main sources: plants, animals/humans, minerals or mineral products, chemicals made in the laboratory, and DNA (Table 1-2).

Plant Sources

Leaves, roots, seeds, and other plant parts may be processed for use as a medicine and are known as *crude drugs*. Some of

Table 1-1 Drug Nomenclature

Chemical Name	Generic Name	Trade Name*	Official Name
Common Out-of-Hospital Drugs			
2-(diethylacono)-N-(2,6-dimethylphenyl) acetamide momchydrochloride	lidocaine hydrochloride	Xylocaine®	lidocaine hydrochloride, USP
1,2-benzenediol, 4-(2-aminoethyl)-,hydrochloride	dopamine hydrochloride	Intropin®	dopamine hydrochloride, USP
Common Home Prescription Drugs			
Card-20(22)-enolide,3[(0,2,dideoxy-β-D-ribohexopyranosyl-(1→4)-02,6-dideozy-D-ribo-hexopyransoyl)oxy]-12, 14-dihydroxy-,(3β, 5β, 12β)-	digoxin	Lanoxin®	digoxin, USP
Benzoic acid, 5-(aminosulfonyl)-4-chloro-2-[(2-furanylmethyl) amino]-	furosemide	Lasix®	furosemide, USP
2-propanol, l-[1-methylethyl) amino]-3-(1-naphthalenyloxy)-,hydrochloride	propranolol hydrochloride	Inderal®	propranolol hydrochloride, USP
Common Over-the-Counter Drugs			
Benzoic acid, 2-(acetyloxy)-	aspirin	Ecotrin®	aspirin, USP
Ethanamine, 2-(diphenylmethyoxy)-N, N-dimethyl-,hydrochloride	diphenhydramine hydrochloride	Benadryl®	diphenhydramine hydrochloride, USP
Acetemide, N-(4-hydroxy-phenyl)-	acetaminophen	Tylenol®	acetaminophen, USP

* A single drug may have several different trade names.

Table 1-2 Drug Sources

Sources	Examples	Drug Name	Classification
Plants	Cinchona bark Purple foxglove	Quinidine Digoxin	Antiarrhythmic Digitalis glycoside
Minerals	Magnesium Gold	Milk of Magnesia Solganal; auranolin	Antacid, laxative Anti-inflammatory used to treat rheumatoid arthritis
Animals	Pancreas of cow, hog Thyroid gland of animals	Insulin Thyroid, USP	Antidiabetic hormone Hormone
Synthetic	Meperidine Diphenoxylate	Demerol Lomotil	Analgesic Antidiarrheal
DNA	Oxytocin Insulins	Pitocin Humulin R	Hormone Antidiabetic

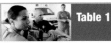

the types of pharmacologically active compounds found in plants are alkaloids, glycosides, gums, and oils. *Alkaloids* are a group of organic alkaline substances found in plants that react with acids to form salts. Examples of alkaloids include morphine and atropine. *Glycosides* are plant substances that, on hydrolysis, produce a sugar in addition to one or more other active substances. A common cardiac glycoside used in medicine is digoxin. *Gums* are plant exudates. When water is added, some gums form gelatinous masses, while others remain unchanged in the gastrointestinal tract. Examples of the uses of gums include their use as a natural laxative or topical preparations used to soothe irritated skin and mucous membranes. *Oils* are viscous liquids that are generally one of two kinds: volatile or fixed. A volatile oil emits a pleasant odor and taste and is usually used as a flavoring agent, for example, peppermint. Fixed oils are generally greasy. An example of a fixed oil medicine is castor oil.

Animal and Human Sources

Some of the most powerful drugs are extracted from animal and human tissue. These drugs are often used to replace insufficient glandular secretions. Examples of drugs derived from animal and human sources include epinephrine, insulin, and adrenocorticotropic hormone.

Minerals or Mineral Products

Materials such as iron and iodine and mineral salts are commonly used to manufacture drugs. Common drugs made from mineral sources include sodium bicarbonate, which is used to treat metabolic acidosis, and calcium chloride, which is used to treat acute hyperkalemia and acute hypocalcemia.

Laboratory-Produced Chemicals

Synthetic drugs are produced by chemical processes in the laboratory. Today, most drugs are synthetic. Two common emergency drugs produced in the laboratory are lidocaine, which is used to treat cardiac dysrhythmias, and diazepam, which is used to treat seizures, anxiety, and other neurological disorders.

DNA-Produced Drugs

Drugs that are produced through DNA engineering have revolutionized medicine. One example of how DNA engineering has developed is insulin. Insulin controls the metabolism and uptake of sugar in our bodies. It is secreted by the beta cells of the pancreas. In the past, insulin came mainly from beef or pork pancreas. When given to patients, beef or pork insulin occasionally caused drug resistance. Today, insulin for injection made from DNA engineering is equivalent to human insulin.

Check the Evidence

Researchers are using DNA engineering to develop therapies and drugs to treat diseases such as cancer, Alzheimer disease, HIV, diabetes, and cystic fibrosis.

Drug Classifications

Drugs are generally classified into categories according to the body tissues that they affect and their therapeutic and physiological effects. For example, adenosine is therapeutically classified as an antiarrhythmic, which is used to slow conduction through the AV node of the heart. It may also interrupt reentry pathways through the AV node. Therapeutically, adenosine can restore normal sinus rhythm in patients experiencing paroxysmal supraventricular tachycardia. Understanding drug classifications will help you understand why a particular drug is prescribed and how that drug affects the body.

Drugs can have more than one therapeutic classification. For example, epinephrine can be therapeutically classified as a bronchodilator, cardiac stimulator, or peripheral vasoconstrictor. You should be familiar with the following therapeutic drug classifications:

- **Adrenocorticoids:** Adrenocorticoids are one of a group of hormones secreted by the adrenal cortex.
- **Alkylating agents:** Alkylating agents donate an alkyl group of biological macromolecules. They are commonly used to fight cancer.
- **Alpha$_1$-adrenergic blocking agents:** Alpha$_1$-adrenergic blocking agents selectively block postsynaptic alpha$_1$-adrenergic receptors, resulting in dilation of both arterioles and veins, leading to a decrease in blood pressure.
- **Aminoglycosides:** Aminoglycosides are broad-spectrum antibiotics believed to inhibit protein synthesis.
- **Amphetamines** and derivatives: Amphetamines and their derivatives are thought to act on the cerebral cortex and reticular activating system (including medullary, respiratory, and vasomotor centers) by releasing norepinephrine from central adrenergic neurons.
- **Analgesics:** Analgesics include all drugs that relieve pain.
- **Angiotensin-converting enzyme (ACE) inhibitors:** ACE inhibitors are believed to act by suppressing the renin-angiotensin-aldosterone system, subsequently lowering blood pressure. They are also used to treat CHF.
- **Antianginal drugs—nitrates/nitrites:** Antianginals are drugs that relieve the pain of angina pectoris. Nitrates relax vascular smooth muscle, especially in coronary vessels.
- **Antiarrhythmic drugs:** Antiarrhythmics correct cardiac arrhythmias. They are classified as follows:
  - *Group I:* decrease the rate of entry of sodium during cardiac membrane depolarization and decrease the rate of the rise of phase 0 of the cardiac membrane action potential (Fig. 1-6).
    - Group IA: Depress phase 0 and prolong the duration of the action potential.
    - Group IB: Slightly depress phase 0 and are thought to shorten the action potential.
    - Group IC: Have a slight effect on repolarization but marked depression of phase 0 of the action potential.

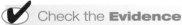

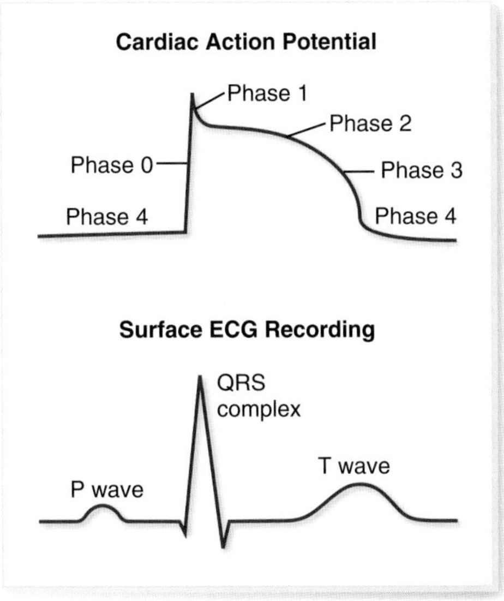

Figure 1-6 Cardiac action potential.

Examples of drugs classified as group I include phenytoin, disopyramide, procainamide, and lidocaine.

- *Group II:* competitively block beta-adrenergic receptors and depress phase 4 depolarization. Examples of some of these beta-blockers include propranolol, metoprolol tartrate, and atenolol.
- *Group III:* prolong the duration of the membrane action potential (relative refractory period) without changing the phase of depolarization of the resting membrane potential. Examples of group III drugs include amiodarone, ibutilide, and sotalol.
- *Group IV:* includes calcium channel blockers and cardiac glycosides. A calcium channel blocker inhibits the influx of calcium through the cell membrane, resulting in a depression of automaticity and conduction velocity in both smooth and cardiac muscle. Cardiac glycosides increase the force and velocity of myocardial contraction by increasing the refractory period of the AV node and increasing total peripheral resistance. An example of a calcium channel blocker is verapamil. Verapamil slows conduction velocity and increases the refractoriness of the AV node. An example of a cardiac glycoside is digoxin. Digoxin causes a decrease in maximal diastolic potential and increases the slope of phase 4 depolarization. Digoxin is used to treat CHF.

- **Anticoagulant agents:** Anticoagulants are drugs that affect blood clotting and can be divided into three classes:
  - *Anticoagulants:* drugs that prevent or slow coagulation
  - *Thrombolytic agents:* drugs that increase the rate at which an existing blood clot dissolves
  - *Hemostatics:* drugs that prevent or stop internal bleeding
- **Anticonvulsants:** Anticonvulsants depress abnormal neuronal discharges in the central nervous system (CNS) that may cause seizures.
- **Antidepressants:** All antidepressants cause adaptive changes in the serotonin and norepinephrine receptor systems, resulting in changes in the sensitivities of both presynaptic and postsynaptic receptor sites.
- **Antidiabetic agents:** Antidiabetic agents are drugs that control diabetes.
- **Antidotes:** Antidotes are drugs that neutralize poisons or alter their effects on the body.
- **Antiemetic:** An agent that is effective in treating nausea and vomiting.
- **Antihistamines (H_1 blockers):** An antihistamine is a drug that blocks the effects of histamine, relieving the symptoms associated with allergic reactions. H_2 blockers block production of gastric acid secretion.
- **Antihypertensive agents:** An antihypertensive drug lowers blood pressure.
- **Antipsychotic agents:** An antipsychotic is a drug that blocks dopamine receptors in the brain. These drugs help relieve the despondency of the severely depressed, making some patients more accessible to psychotherapy.
- **Antitussives:** Antitussives are drugs that suppress coughing.
- **Beta-adrenergic blocking agents:** Beta-adrenergic blocking agents combine reversibly with beta-adrenergic receptors to block the response of sympathetic nerve impulses, circulating catecholamines, or beta-adrenergic drugs.
- **Bronchodilators:** Bronchodilators are drugs used to treat airway obstruction caused by asthma or COPD. They also reverse bronchospasm.
- **Calcium channel blocking agents:** Calcium channel blocking agents inhibit the influx of calcium through the cell membrane, resulting in a depression of automaticity and conduction velocity in both smooth and cardiac muscle.
- **Calcium salts:** Calcium salts return to normal values the calcium levels essential for maintaining optimal function of nerves, muscles, and the skeletal system as well as the permeability of cell membranes and capillaries.
- **Cardiac glycosides:** Cardiac glycosides increase the force and velocity of myocardial contraction (positive inotropic effect) by increasing the refractory period of the AV node and increasing total peripheral resistance.
- **Cholinergic agonists:** Cholinergic agonists strengthen, prolong, or prevent the breakdown of the neurotransmitter acetylcholine.
- **Cholinergic blocking agents:** Cholinergic blocking agents prevent the neurotransmitter acetylcholine from combining with receptors on the post-ganglionic parasympathetic nerve terminal.
- **Coronary vasodilators:** Coronary vasodilators are drugs that increase the diameter of the coronary blood vessels.
- **Corticosteroids:** Corticosteroids basically have two functions: 1) the regulation of metabolic pathways involving protein, carbohydrates, and fat; and 2) electrolyte and water balance.

- **Diuretics:** Diuretics act to inhibit reabsorption of sodium and chloride in the proximal and distal tubules and the loop of Henle.
- **Emetics:** Emetics are agents that cause vomiting.
- **Histamine H_2 antagonists:** Histamine H_2 antagonists are competitive blockers of histamine.
- **Hydrogen ion buffers:** Hydrogen ion buffers are used to bring the hydrogen ion concentration of the blood within normal limits.
- **Hyperglycemics:** Hyperglycemics are drugs used to treat hypoglycemia by restoring blood sugar levels to normal.
- **Inotropics:** Inotropic drugs increase cardiac output. They are used for short-term management of CHF or poor cardiac output.
- **Medicinal gases:** The most common uses for medicinal gases in the out-of-hospital setting are to increase or maintain the partial pressure of oxygen (P_aO_2) in the arterial blood, provide pain relief, and help bronchodilation.
- **Narcotic analgesics:** Narcotic analgesics competitively block the action of previously given narcotics from their receptor sites or by preventing narcotics from attaching to the opiate receptors.
- **Neuromuscular blocking agents:** Neuromuscular blocking agents are categorized as competitive (nondepolarizing) and depolarizing drugs, both of which act peripherally. These drugs prevent muscle contraction or muscle spasm.
- **Skeletal muscle relaxants:** Skeletal muscle relaxants decrease muscle tone and involuntary movement. Many of these drugs *may* relieve anxiety and tension as well.
- **Succinimide anticonvulsants:** Succinimide anticonvulsants act by depressing the motor cortex and by raising the threshold of the CNS to convulsive stimuli.
- **Sympathomimetic drugs:** Sympathomimetic drugs are adrenergic drugs that act by mimicking the action of norepinephrine or epinephrine by combining with alpha and/or beta receptors or by causing or regulating the release of the natural neurohormones from their storage sites at the nerve terminals.
- **Theophylline derivatives:** Theophyllines stimulate the CNS, directly relax the smooth muscles of the bronchi and pulmonary blood vessels, produce diuresis, inhibit uterine contractions, stimulate gastric acid secretion, and increase the rate and force of contractions of the heart.
- **Tranquilizers/hypnotics:** These drugs are thought to affect the limbic system and reticular formation to reduce anxiety by increasing or facilitating the inhibitory neurotransmitter activity.
- **Vasodilators:** Vasodilators are drugs that relax the blood vessels.
- **Vasopressors:** Vasopressors are drugs that cause contractions of the muscles of the capillaries and arteries, thus increasing peripheral vascular resistance.

Drug Preparations

Drugs generally come in three types of preparations: solid, liquid, or gas. A drug preparation may produce either local or systemic effects.

Drugs taken orally have the advantage of being easy to take; generally, this is the safest way to take medicines. The disadvantages of oral medications are: 1) the drug absorption process generally takes longer; 2) the eventual concentrations of the drug in the bloodstream are often unpredictable; and 3) some drugs may be destroyed or altered by gastric acids.

Drugs administered directly into the bloodstream have the advantage of bypassing the absorption process, which enables the drug to produce its desired therapeutic effect much sooner. However, this type of drug administration has the disadvantage of being more difficult and much more dangerous.

A local drug effect is confined to one specific area of the body. For example, a medicated lotion may be applied to an irritated area of the skin for the relief of a rash. A systemic effect occurs when a drug enters into the bloodstream, affecting all body tissues.

You should become familiar with the common drug preparations that follow.

Drug Preparations for Local Effects

Topical Use

- **Aerosol:** An aerosol is a colloid or glue-like substance finely subdivided into liquid or solid particles that are dispensed in the form of a mist.
- **Colloid:** A colloid is a glue-like substance, such as a protein or starch, whose particles, when dispersed in a solvent to the greatest possible degree, remain uniformly distributed and fail to form a true solution.
- **Cream:** A cream is a smooth, thick liquid or a semisolid emulsion for external application.
- **Liniment:** A liniment is a liquid containing a medication in oil, alcohol, or water.
- **Lotion:** A lotion is a liquid suspension for external application.
- **Ointment:** An ointment is a semisolid preparation for external application of a drug or medicine.
- **Paste:** A paste is a semisolid gelatinous substance for external application that may contain specific active ingredients or simple materials such as oils, waxes, and starch.
- **Plaster:** Although rarely used, a plaster is an external medicinal preparation formed into a mass harder than an ointment and spread over muslin, linen, skin, or paper.

Drug Preparations for Systemic Effects

Oral Use (Liquids)

- **Aqueous solution:** An aqueous solution is a substance dissolved in water.
- **Elixir:** An elixir is a sweetened hydroalcoholic liquid used alone or as a vehicle for active drugs.

- **Extract:** An extract is the active ingredient of a vegetable or animal drug obtained by distillation or other chemical process. There are three forms of extracts: semisolid, solid, or powdered.
- **Fluidextract:** A fluidextract is a solution of the dissolved component part of vegetable drugs such that each milliliter equals 1.0 gram of the drug. Fluidextracts contain alcohol as a solvent or preservative or both.

Understand the Numbers

How many milligrams (mg) are contained in a 5 milliliter (mL) bottle of a fluidextract?

5 mL = 5 g of fluidextract in the bottle. To convert grams to milligrams, multiply grams by 1,000 or move the decimal point 3 spaces to the right. Therefore, 5 g × 1,000 = 5,000 mg.

- **Tincture:** A tincture is an alcoholic solution of vegetable or chemical material.

Oral Use (Solids)

- **Capsule:** A capsule is a gelatin container used for a single-dose drug administration.
- **Pill:** A pill is a medication in the form of a small solid mass or pellet.
- **Powder:** A powder consists of fine particles of a medicine.
- **Tablet:** A tablet is a small solid mass of medicinal powder. Tablets may be round, oblong, or triangular.
- **Troche or lozenge:** A troche is a solid disk or cylindrical mass of a medication in a flavored base.

Parenteral Use

A **parenteral** route is defined as any route other than the alimentary canal. IV, transtracheal, intraosseous, subcutaneous, or intramuscular routes are all parenteral routes.

- **Ampule:** An ampule is a small, sealed single-dose glass container that holds a liquid injectable drug.
- **IV infusion:** An IV infusion is a sterile liquid preparation with or without added drugs.
- **Prefilled syringe:** A prefilled syringe is usually a single-dose glass cartridge containing a liquid drug.
- **Vial:** A vial is a small glass bottle that contains more than one dose of a drug.

Other Preparations for Systemic Effect

- **Inhalants:** An inhalant is a gas, a mixture of gases, or water vapors that transport a drug to the body via the lungs.
- **Suppositories:** A suppository is a semisolid cylinder or cone-shaped mass that provides a drug via the mucous membrane of the rectum, vagina, or urethra.

Investigational Drugs

Before a potential drug comes to market, it must go through a screening process that may take years of research and testing and require large amounts of financial investment. The **U.S. Food and Drug Administration (FDA)** requires the following testing sequence:

- **Animal studies** to help determine the following:
  - *Toxicity*
    - Acute toxicity: the medial lethal dose; that is, the dose that is lethal to 50 percent of the laboratory animals tested (LD_{50}). Acute toxicity generally develops rapidly.
    - Subacute and chronic toxicity: the terms subacute and chronic refer to the speed at which toxicity develops. For example, chronic shows little change or slow progression over time. Subacute shows moderate change or progression over time.
  - *Therapeutic index:* the ratio of the LD_{50} to the median effective dose
    - Modes of absorption, distribution, biotransformation, and excretion
- **Human studies:**
  - Initial pharmacologic evaluation (phase I)
  - Limited controlled evaluation (phase II)
  - Extended clinical evaluation (phase III)
  - Post-marketing evaluation (phase IV)

Drug Development/FDA Approval Process

After the data on the safety and effectiveness of a proposed drug have been reviewed, the FDA will approve an application for an Investigational New Drug (IND). The investigation covered under IND is divided into four phases:

- **Phase I**: *Initial pharmacologic evaluation.* Phase I involves small groups of healthy subjects. The goals of phase I are to prove the drug's safety and to identify tolerable dosages. The investigators determine the pharmacokinetics of the drug (absorption, distribution, biotransformation, and excretion). If phase I testing shows that the drug is safe to give in expected therapeutic doses, the study continues to phase II.
- **Phase II:** *Limited controlled evaluation.* Phase II consists of controlled evaluations designed to test the drug's effect on the specific illness for which it was designed. Phase II testing also helps to establish dosage and other pharmacokinetic information. Individuals are closely monitored for drug effectiveness and for side effects. After phase II is complete, investigators submit all collected data to the FDA. At this point, the FDA may approve or reject a New Drug Application (NDA). If the NDA is approved, the drug can be marketed for the selected indication in the dosing schedules as studied, and phase III is begun.
- **Phase III:** *Extended clinical evaluation.* Phase III consists of the full-scale or extended clinical evaluations. Phase III evaluations are performed on a large number of subjects to determine therapeutic effect and possible side effects and to decide if the side effects are low

enough to be acceptable. Phase III has three objectives: determine clinical effectiveness, determine safety, and establish tolerable dosage ranges.

Once a drug is placed on the market, it is inevitable that it will be reported to produce additional effects. These effects can be therapeutic or adverse and may not have been noted during the trial studies. Therefore, phase IV drug testing is a postmarketing evaluation designed to update safety and product results. This phase clarifies incidence or adverse drug reactions and long-term effects. Phases I through III are almost always required. Although phase IV is not required of all drugs, the FDA prefers that all drugs go through all four phases.

Orphan Drugs

The Office of Orphan Products Development (OOPD) was created in 1982. The OOPD is dedicated to promoting the development of products that demonstrate promise for the diagnosis and/or treatment of rare diseases. It administers the major provision of the Orphan Drug Act, which provides incentives for sponsors to develop drugs for rare diseases. Approximately 200 drugs for rare diseases have been brought to market since 1983. The OOPD also administers the Orphan Products Grants Program, which provides funding for clinical research in rare diseases.

Black Box Warnings

A **black box warning,** also known as a "black label warning" or "boxed warning," is named for the black border surrounding the text of the warning that appears on the package insert, label, and other literature describing the medication. A black box warning is the strongest warning the FDA can give to a medication while it still remains on the market in the United States.

The FDA requires a black box warning for one of the following situations:

- The medication can cause serious undesirable effects (such as a fatal, life-threatening, or permanently disabling adverse reaction) compared with the potential benefit from the drug.
- A serious adverse reaction can be prevented, reduced in frequency, or reduced in severity by proper use of the drug.

"Off-Label" Uses of Medications

"Off-label" means that a particular medication is being used in a manner not specified in the FDA's approved packaging label, or insert. Every prescription drug marketed in the United States carries an individual FDA-approved label. This label is a written report that provides detailed instructions regarding the approved uses and doses, which are based on the results of clinical studies that the drug maker submitted to the FDA.

The FDA regulates drug approval, not drug prescribing. Physicians are free to prescribe a drug for any reason that they think is medically beneficial and appropriate. Off-label prescribing of beta-blockers is a good example of this. Beta-blockers are FDA approved for the treatment of high blood pressure but are widely recognized by cardiologists as a standard of care for patients with heart failure. In fact, some beta-blockers are now formally approved to treat heart failure. It is not uncommon for off-label uses to eventually get approved by the FDA. Another example is the drug glucagon. Glucagon is approved for the acute management of severe hypoglycemia when administration of glucose is not feasible. However, some protocols include glucagon for the off-label use of treating beta-blocker or calcium channel blocker overdose. Off-label use of medications has become common practice. Therefore, it is extremely important that, whenever possible, all patient medications should be transported to the receiving facility with the patient.

Components of a Drug Profile

Administering drugs carries an enormous responsibility. Without question, EMS professionals are placed in a position that may save many lives through proper drug administration. Drugs produce a variety of physiological responses, including raising or lowering blood pressure, increasing or decreasing heart rate, and sedating or stimulating the patient. If the wrong drug or the incorrect dose of the appropriate drug is given, the results could be fatal. Therefore, it is essential that you be thoroughly familiar with the following components of a drug profile:

- **Classification:** Each drug can be placed in a group that indicates how the drug works. A drug can have more than one classification. For example, epinephrine can be classified as a bronchodilator, cardiac stimulator, and peripheral vasoconstrictor.
- **Pregnancy class:** A drug's pregnancy class weighs the degree to which available information has ruled out risk to the fetus against the drug's potential benefit to the mother. For example, epinephrine is classed as "C," which means risk cannot be ruled out.
- **Mechanism of action:** A drug's mechanism of action describes how the drug produces its desired therapeutic effects (pharmacodynamics). For example, epinephrine works by affecting both alpha- and beta-adrenergic receptors.
- **Pharmacokinetics:** Once given, the drug must move to its site of action before it can produce its therapeutic effects. Drug movement also includes how the drug is absorbed, distributed, and eliminated. For example, epinephrine is rapidly absorbed and does not cross the blood-brain barrier, and its action is rapidly terminated by metabolism and uptake by nerve endings.
- **Indications:** The indications for a drug's use include the most common uses for that drug in the out-of-hospital setting. Common uses for epinephrine include the management of reversible airway disease and severe allergic reactions as well as the treatment of cardiac arrest.
- **Contraindications:** A drug's contraindications are the circumstances under which it should not be used or when alternative drugs should be considered. A contraindication to the use of epinephrine is in patients who are hypersensitive to adrenergic amines.

- **Precautions:** Precautions describe situations in which drug use may be dangerous to the patient or when dosage or administration techniques may have to be modified. For example, epinephrine should be used with caution in patients with cardiac disease or hypertension.
- **Route and dosage:** The route of a drug describes how the drug is given. Examples of routes include IV, endotracheal, intraosseous, intramuscular, and so forth. The dosage is how much of the drug should be given, depending on the route used. For example, the route and dosage of epinephrine for asthma in the adult patient is 0.1 to 0.5 mg either by subcutaneous or intramuscular injection.
- **How supplied:** This includes each drug's common concentration and packaging information. Epinephrine can come supplied for injection in 0.1 mg/mL (1:10,000 solution).

Understand the Numbers

You are ordered to give 0.4 mg of epinephrine to your patient via IV bolus. The epinephrine comes packaged as 1 mg in 10 mL of solution. How much volume of the epinephrine do you administer to give your patient 0.4 mg?

Concentration = amount of drug (1 mg) ÷ amount of volume (10 mL) = 0.1 mg/mL

Volume = dosage (0.4 mg) ÷ concentration (0.1 mg/mL) = 4 mL

- **Adverse reactions and side effects:** A drug's adverse reactions and side effects are any actions or effects other than those desired. However, some side effects of a drug are predictable and may occur in addition to the expected therapeutic effects. For example, a common CNS side effect of epinephrine is restlessness. However, an adverse CV reaction of epinephrine may include chest pain.
- **Drug interactions:** Before giving a drug to a patient, you must know what other drugs he or she is taking in an attempt to avoid causing inappropriate drug-drug reactions. For example, giving epinephrine to patients taking monoamine oxidase inhibitors may cause a hypertensive crisis. Concurrent use of beta-blockers may negate the therapeutic effects of epinephrine.
- **EMS considerations:** EMS considerations explain special information that may be helpful when giving a specific drug. For example, lung sounds should be assessed before giving epinephrine to a patient with an airway emergency, and they should be assessed after administration as well. Also, if a 1:1,000 solution of epinephrine is inadvertently given via IV bolus, sudden hypertension or cerebral edema may develop.

Sources of Drug Information

There are numerous sources where health-care professionals can obtain information on drugs. For example, drug manufacturers, package inserts, pharmacists, medical journals, and the Internet are just a few sources where you can obtain information on drugs. Because no one reference is a complete source of drug information, EMS professionals should be familiar with the following primary drug reference sources:

- American Hospital Formulary Service's *AHFS Drug Information,* (Bethesda, MD: American Society of Hospital Pharmacists, Inc.)
- *Drug Facts and Comparisons* (St. Louis, MO: Wolters Kluwer)
- *Handbook of Nonprescription Drugs* (Washington, DC: American Pharmaceutical Association)
- ***Physicians' Desk Reference* (PDR),** (Montvale, NJ: PDR Networks)
- **United States Pharmacopeia, (USP),** DI (Rockville, MD: U.S. Pharmacopeial Convention)
- *PDR Nurse's Drug Handbook* (Montvale, NJ: PDR Networks)

U.S. Drug Legislation

At the beginning of the 20th century, no federal laws controlled drug distribution. However, during the first 10 years of that century, the use of chemicals in medicine increased rapidly. This increase brought with it an increased use of dangerous ingredients and complex formulas. Some drug companies used poor quality control and made unproven claims for their products. This made it necessary to develop national standards and government regulations to guarantee that drugs sold to the public were accurately identified and of uniform strength and purity. For these reasons, Congress enacted several laws.

Food and Drug Act (Pure Food Act of 1906)

In 1906, Congress enacted the Pure Food Act as the first U.S. law to protect the public from mislabeled, poisonous, or harmful food and drugs. This legislation named the *United States Pharmacopoeia (USP)* and the *National Formulary (NF)* as official drug standards and established the FDA. The Pure Food Act authorized the FDA to determine whether drugs were safe and effective and to enforce these standards.

Harrison Narcotics Act of 1914

The Harrison Narcotics Act was the first federal legislation designed to stop drug addiction or dependence. It established federal control over the importation, manufacture, and sale of opium and coca plants and all their compounds and derivatives. The Harrison Narcotics Act established the word *narcotic* as a legal term.

Federal Food, Drug, and Cosmetic Act of 1938

The Federal Food, Drug, and Cosmetic Act updated the Pure Food Act. This legislation required that labels list the possible habit-forming properties and side effects of drugs. It also authorized the FDA to determine the safety of drugs before marketing and required that dangerous drugs be issued only by prescription of a physician, dentist, or veterinarian. This act was amended in 1951 by the Durham-Humphrey amendment, which classified certain drugs as "legend" drugs and restricted pharmacists from distributing legend drugs without a prescription. Legend drugs are those that must be labeled "Caution: Federal Law prohibits dispensing without a prescription." In 1962, the Federal Food, Drug, and Cosmetic Act was amended again by the Kefauver-Harris amendment. The Kefauver-Harris amendment authorized the FDA to establish official names for drugs and required drug manufacturers to prove a drug's ability to produce therapeutic results.

Other Drug Laws and Regulations

The Harrison Narcotics Act and all further drug abuse amendments were superseded by the Controlled Substances Act of 1970. The Controlled Substances Act classifies drugs with abuse potential into five schedules by weighing a drug's potential for abuse against its medical usefulness (Table 1-3). For example, a Schedule I drug has a high potential for abuse and no accepted medical usefulness, whereas a Schedule V drug has little potential for abuse and recognized medical use.

The Food and Drug Administration Modernization Act (FDAMA) of 1997 amended the Federal Food, Drug, and Cosmetic Act relating to the regulation of food, drugs, devices, and biological products for the 21st century characterized by increasing technological, trade, and public health complexities.

Other federal agencies involved in regulating drugs include the Drug Enforcement Administration (DEA), the Public Health Service, and the Federal Trade Commission (FTC). The DEA is empowered to enforce the Controlled Substances Act. The Public Health Service, part of the U.S. Department of Health and Human Services, regulates biological products such as vaccines. The FTC regulates drug advertising. It has the power to prevent false or misleading advertising of food, drugs, and cosmetics to the public. The FTC also regulates prescription drug advertising to the medical profession for those drugs regulated by the FDA. The FTC relies on the FDA to regulate the claims of nonprescription drug advertisements.

Table 1-3 Schedule of Controlled Substances

Drug Schedule	Description	Example Drugs
I	Schedule I drugs are not considered to be legitimate for medical use in the United States. They are used for research only, and they cannot be prescribed, since they have a high risk for abuse.	Lysergic acid diethylamide (LSD), Heroin
II	Schedule II drugs have accepted medical use but have a high potential for abuse or addiction. These drugs must be ordered by written prescription and cannot be refilled without a new written prescription.	Morphine, Cocaine, Codeine, Demerol, Dilaudid
III	Schedule III drugs have moderate potential for abuse or addiction and low potential for physical dependence. These drugs may be ordered by written prescription or by telephone order. Prescription expires in 6 months. They may not be refilled more than five times in a 6-month period.	Tylenol with codeine, Butisol, Hycodan
IV	Schedule IV drugs have less potential for abuse or addiction than those of Schedule III, with limited physical dependence. These drugs may be ordered by written prescription or by telephone order. They may be refilled up to five times over a 6-month period. Prescription expires in 6 months.	Librium, Valium, Darvon, Equanil
V	Schedule V drugs have a small potential for abuse or addiction. These drugs may be ordered by written prescription or by telephone order, and there is no limit on prescription refills. Some of these drugs may not need a prescription.	Robitussin A-C, Donnagel-PG, Lomotil

Drug Standardization

The strength and activity of drugs may vary considerably. For example, drugs obtained from plants can vary in strength because of where the plants were grown and the plants' age when they were harvested. Additionally, the type of preservation process used after harvesting can affect the potency of the drug. Drugs must be of uniform strength and purity when offered on the market, which means standardization is essential. The federal government establishes and enforces drug standards.

A note of caution about herbal supplements should be observed. Herbal supplements are plant derivatives over which the FDA does not have regulatory control, or has only limited control, regarding potency and purity. Herbal preparations can be of varying quality and have the potential to interact with many drugs.

Drug standardization techniques can either be chemical or biological. Chemical processing, known as a chemical **assay,** determines the ingredients present in the drug and their amounts. For example, opium contains certain alkaloids, which may vary in different preparations. The U.S. official standard states that opium must contain no less than 9.5 percent and no more than 10.5 percent of anhydrous morphine.

In some drugs, either the active ingredients are unknown or there are not methods of chemically analyzing and standardizing them. In these cases, the drug must be standardized by biological methods. The **bioassay** determines the amount of a preparation required to produce a predetermined effect on a laboratory animal. For example, the potency of a sample of insulin is measured by its ability to lower the glucose level of rabbits.

The only official book of drug standards in the United States is the *United States Pharmacopeia (USP)*. When a drug is added to the USP, it has met high standards of quality, purity, and strength. The USP after the official name can identify drugs meeting these high standards.

Special Considerations

Administering drugs can be further complicated by the added factors of patient age, pregnancy, and lactation. For example, the very young and the elderly are generally more susceptible to the adverse effects of drugs. Therefore, drug dosages may have to be modified for these age-groups. Additionally, some drugs can cross the placental barrier and reach the fetus, causing adverse effects. Once the baby is born, certain drugs can also be transferred to the child via breast milk.

Pregnancy and Lactation

There are two potential problems that may occur when giving drugs to pregnant patients. First, drugs have the potential to cross the placental barrier and affect the fetus. When giving drugs to pregnant patients, the potential benefits must always be weighed against the risks. The FDA categorizes drugs based on potential risk during pregnancy (Table 1-4).

Second, pregnancy causes several anatomical and physiological changes that must be considered prior to administering drugs. These changes include a(n):

- Increase in heart rate
- Increase in cardiac output
- Up to 45 percent increase in blood volume
- Decrease in blood pressure
- Decrease in protein binding
- Decrease in hepatic biotransformation

Another concern may develop after the baby is born. If the mother must begin a medication for any reason and is also breastfeeding, many drugs can be excreted into the breast milk and ingested by the baby.

Pediatric Patients

Neonates pose a particular concern during drug administration. The major organ for biotransformation is the liver. However, the neonate's liver is not fully developed, impairing biotransformation. Drug excretion through the neonate's kidney may be impaired as well. Therefore, drug dosages to the neonate have to be modified to account for these factors.

In most cases, drug dosages for the pediatric patient are reduced from that of the adult. Drug dosages for the pediatric patient are generally based on body weight and body surface area. Therefore, EMS professionals must determine the body weight of the pediatric patient before administering drugs.

There are several devices available to aid paramedics in determining pediatric drug dosages. Each EMS system should determine the best and most appropriate device for them when determining pediatric medication dosages.

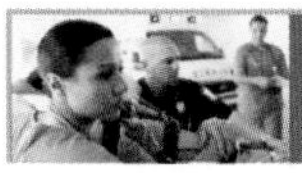

Table 1-4 Pregnancy Categories: FDA Assigned

The U.S. FDA's use-in-pregnancy rating system weighs the degree to which available information has ruled out risk to the fetus against the drug's potential benefit to the patient. The ratings, and their interpretation, are as follows:

Category	Interpretation
A	**CONTROLLED STUDIES SHOW NO RISK.** Adequate, well-controlled studies in pregnant women have failed to demonstrate a risk to the fetus in any trimester of pregnancy.
B	**NO EVIDENCE OF RISK IN HUMANS.** Adequate, well-controlled studies in pregnant women have not shown increased risk of fetal abnormalities despite adverse findings in animals, or, in the absence of adequate human studies, animal studies show no fetal risk. The chance of fetal harm is remote but remains a possibility.
C	**RISK CANNOT BE RULED OUT.** Adequate, well-controlled human studies are lacking, and animal studies have shown a risk to the fetus or are lacking as well. There is a chance of fetal harm if the drug is administered during pregnancy, but the potential benefits may outweigh the potential risk.
D	**POSITIVE EVIDENCE OF RISK.** Studies in humans, or investigational or post-marketing data, have demonstrated fetal risk. Nevertheless, potential benefits from the use of the drug may outweigh the potential risk. For example, the drug may be acceptable if needed in a life-threatening situation or serious disease for which safer drugs cannot be used or are ineffective.
X	**CONTRAINDICATED IN PREGNANCY.** Studies in animals or humans, or investigational or post-marketing reports, have demonstrated positive evidence of fetal abnormalities or risk that clearly outweighs any possible benefit to the patient.

Geriatric Patients

As the baby boomers age, there will be an increased use of the EMS system by this particular age-group. As patients become older, they are more likely to develop more than one disease process at a time. When this occurs, generally an increased use of medications must become a part of their daily lives. Body systems will respond to these medications differently than they would in younger years. Common physiological effects of aging include a decrease in:

- Cardiac output
- Brain mass
- Renal function
- Respiratory capacity
- Serum albumin
- Body fat

- Total body water
- Biotransformation
- Excretion

These changes that occur with age may also cause changes in pharmacokinetics and pharmacodynamics. Therefore, the dosages of many drugs may have to be reduced when given to the elderly.

Pharmacologic Abbreviations

Abbreviations are common in medicine. Using abbreviations appropriately can make you more efficient, especially in your never-ending battle with paperwork. Standard pharmacologic and other medical abbreviations and symbols with which you should be familiar are listed in Appendix F in the back of this book.

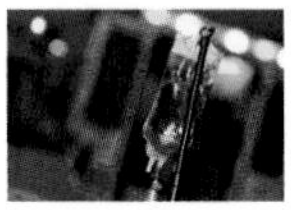

SCENARIO REVISITED

As you recall, after you completed your inspection of Rescue 6, an emergency call came in for "an unconscious woman." Upon arrival, you are met by the patient's brother, George, who states that when he arrived to visit his sister, Genevieve, he found her unconscious on the bathroom floor. George states that he has no idea how long his sister has been unconscious, because he has not spoken with her for a couple of days. She did not answer the phone when he called about an hour ago. George did remember that his sister had a stroke about 10 years ago, when she was 55 years old. She fully recovered. To George's knowledge, Genevieve has never been diagnosed as a diabetic.

Patient assessment reveals the following:

- LOC: unresponsive and no reaction to painful stimuli
- Respirations: 10 respirations/minute and shallow
- ECG: sinus bradycardia with occasional PVCs
- Blood pressure: 160/94
- Skin: warm and dry
- Blood glucose level: 200 mg/dL

Rick and Phil explain to you that the treatment protocol will follow "unconscious with unknown origin." However, it is essential that the hospital know that Genevieve has a previous history of stroke.

Check the Evidence

An elevation in blood glucose is common in the early phase of stroke. Many of these patients are likely to have *stress hyperglycemia,* partly due to the release of cortisol and norepinephrine. This form of hyperglycemia is associated with poor outcomes.

Let's Recap

Administering drugs is a part of complete EMS patient care that carries an enormous responsibility. EMS professionals are held responsible for safe and therapeutically effective drug administration. Each EMS professional is personally responsible legally, morally, and ethically for each drug administered.

Understanding pharmacology is more than knowing which drug to administer and when to administer it. Each EMS professional administering drugs must be familiar with the drugs used in the local EMS system. Knowledge of each drug's actions, indications, contraindications, precautions, side effects, and correct dosage, as well as the route in which the drug should be given and any pertinent drug interactions, is essential. Giving the correct drug appropriately can save a life. Giving the same drug inappropriately can prove deadly.

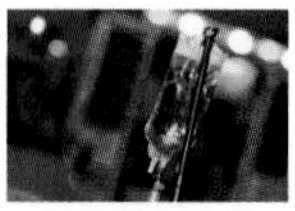

SCENARIO CONCLUSION

Genevieve may have had another stroke. However, this cannot be determined until further examination at the receiving facility, which in this case will be a hospital with a stroke team. En route, treatment consisted of administering 100 percent humidified oxygen via non-rebreather mask and an IV of normal saline, continuous monitoring of the ECG and vital signs, and rapid transport to a receiving facility with a stroke team.

After the call is complete, Rick and Phil explain that possible drugs, if indicated, could include thiamine and/or naloxone if alcoholism or other drug abuse had been suspected, $D_{50}W$ if blood glucose levels had been low, or intramuscular glucagon if an IV was unable to be started.

PRACTICE EXERCISES

1. The *primary* reason for drug legislation (such as the Federal Food, Drug, and Cosmetic Act) is to:
   a. Keep health-care professionals from abusing drugs
   b. Ensure the safety of the drug manufactured
   c. Ensure the sterility of manufactured goods
   d. Control narcotic drugs

2. In most cases, drug dosages for the pediatric patient are based on patient:
   a. Age
   b. Height
   c. Weight
   d. Gender

3. The initials "USP" after a drug's name indicate the drug's _____ name.
   a. Generic (nonproprietary)
   b. Trade (proprietary)
   c. Chemical
   d. Official

4. Body substance isolation precautions are also known as _____ precautions:
   a. Droplet
   b. Contact
   c. Airborne
   d. Standard

5. The use of drugs in the treatment of disease is called:
   a. Toxicology
   b. Pharmacology
   c. Pharmacotherapy
   d. Pharmacogenetics

6. The proprietary name of a drug is also known as its _____ name.
   a. Trade
   b. Generic
   c. Official
   d. Chemical

7. Drugs are assigned to one of five pregnancy categories assigned by the FDA. The definition of a drug assigned to category "C" is:
   a. Positive evidence of risk
   b. Risk cannot be ruled out
   c. No evidence of risk in humans
   d. Contraindicated in pregnancy

8. An example of a drug assigned to Drug Schedule III is:
   a. Tylenol with codeine
   b. Valium
   c. Lomotil
   d. LSD

9. How a drug produces its desired therapeutic effects is called:
   a. Therapeutic classification
   b. Mechanism of action
   c. Therapeutic benefits
   d. Pharmacokinetics

10. Most drugs go through four phases of evaluation during the FDA approval process. Phase IV is the drug's:
   a. Extended clinical evaluation
   b. Limited controlled evaluation
   c. Initial pharmacologic evaluation
   d. Postmarketing evaluation

CASE STUDY

You respond to the home of a woman "having chest pain." Upon arrival, you find a 30-year-old female (Karin) who states that she is 7-months pregnant. Karin also states that she has had a headache for the past 2 days and today has developed chest pain. Further history and assessment identify the chest pain as epigastric pain. Your assessment reveals the following:

LOC: alert, oriented
Respirations: 18 breaths/minute and clear lungs bilaterally
Pulse: 94 beats/minute and regular
Blood pressure: 164/110
Skin: pale and edematous

Karin says that this is her first pregnancy. She has no history of high blood pressure or any other illness.

All signs and symptoms indicate that Karin is preeclamptic. Preeclampsia can lead to true eclampsia. Therefore, Karin should be transported to the hospital without delay. Headache and epigastric pain in this situation could be signs of impending seizure activity. The drug of choice for the prevention of seizure activity in the preeclamptic patient is:

- Diazepam
- Oxytocin
- Mannitol
- Magnesium sulfate

Before administration of a drug to a pregnant patient, you must ask "Do the benefits from the use of the drug outweigh the potential risk?" All drugs are given pregnancy categories assigned by the FDA. Mannitol is a Class C drug and is indicated for patients who require treatment for edema. Class C suggests that risk cannot be ruled out but that there is little chance of fetal harm. However, this patient needs a drug that will prevent seizure activity, which now is the more serious developing situation. Oxytocin is a class X drug used for induction of labor at term or postpartum control of bleeding after expulsion of the placenta. A class X drug is contraindicated in pregnancy.

Diazepam is a class D drug used in the treatment of status epilepticus/uncontrolled seizures. A class D drug indicates positive evidence of risk, only to be used if the benefits will outweigh the potential risk. In this case, the patient has the potential of seizure activity, but it has not yet occurred. Therefore, the drug of choice in this case is magnesium sulfate. Magnesium is also a class D drug. However, it is an anticonvulsant to be used for severe preeclampsia and eclampsia. In this case, the benefits of magnesium sulfate outweigh the potential risk.

MATH EQUATIONS

Basic Addition and Subtraction

Addition

1. 4.0 + 5.75 = __________
2. 3.25 + 3.3 + 4 = __________
3. 29.75 + 33.02 = __________
4. 244.33 + 75 + 65.1 + 2 = __________
5. 0.33 + 0.25 = __________

Subtraction

1. 17.20 – 6.25 = __________
2. 33 – 14.85 = __________
3. 25.04 – 17.35 = __________
4. 113.75 – 33.33 = __________
5. 66.05 – 17 = __________

REFERENCES

About.com. *Black box warning.* Retrieved November 18, 2013 from http://drugs.about.com/od/medicationabcs/a/BlackBoxWarning.htm

Beck, R. K. (2012). Introduction to pharmacology. In *Pharmacology for the EMS provider.* New York, NY: Delmar, Cengage Learning.

Deglin, J. H., Vallerand, A. H., and Sanboski, C. A. (2011). *Davis's drug guide for nurses twelfth edition.* Philadelphia, PA: F.A. Davis Company.

Iowa Public Television, Explore More: Genetic Engineering. (2004). Medicine—DNA. Retrieved November 18, 2013 from www.iptv.org/exploremore/ge/uses/use2_medical.cfm

Miller, K. Off-label drug use: What you need to know. Retrieved November 18, 2013 from www.webmd.com/a-to-z-guides/feature/off-label-drug-use-what-you-need-to-know

U.S. Drug Enforcement Administration. Drug scheduling. Retrieved November 17, 2013 from www.justice.gov/dea/druginfo/ds.shtml

Venes, D., ed. (2013). *Taber's cyclopedic medical dictionary* (22nd ed.). Philadelphia, PA: F. A. Davis Company.

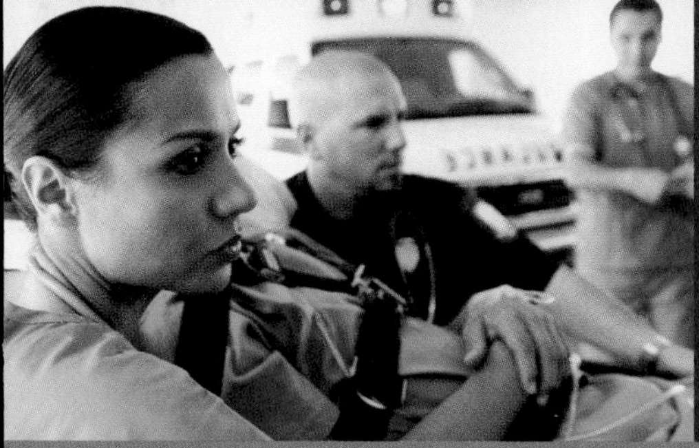

CHAPTER 2

Professionalism

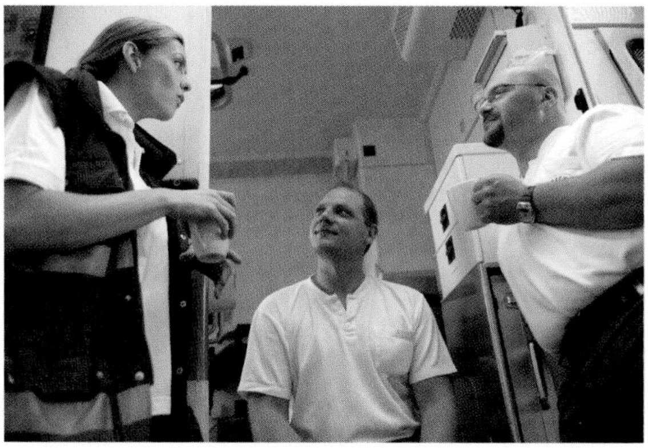

Paramedics discussing an emergency call. *(Photograph © Thinkstock)*

LEARNING OUTCOMES

- Describe the four elements required to prove negligence.
- Describe measures you can take to protect yourself from a claim of negligence.
- Define profession, professionalism, licensure, certification, and credentialing.
- List and briefly discuss the characteristics of the professional paramedic.
- Define ethics.

KEY TERMS

Altruism
Certification
Credentialing
Code of ethics
Courteous
Distance education
Ethics
Health Insurance Portability and Accountability Act of 1996 (HIPAA)
Licensure
Medical ethics
Medical professionalism
Morals
Negligence
Profession
Professional
Professionalism
Registration
Statutes

SCENARIO OPENING

You have been assigned to Rescue 33 as part of your field-internship requirements. Rescue 33 is known to be a rather slow station, so you brought your texts with you to study. As you sit down to study for an OB/GYN exam, a call comes in for a "traffic accident." While you are en route, the dispatcher states that this accident is a head-on crash at an intersection controlled by four stop signs.

When you arrive on the scene, there is an elderly female sitting in the front passenger seat holding her head. When you approach the patient, you notice some blood on her forehead and see that the passenger side of the windshield has been "starred." You introduce yourself, and the patient states that her name is Betty. Betty tells you that you can perform an exam, but "I am not going to any damn hospital. I have a little bit of a headache, but, other than that, I feel fine." Your assessment reveals:

Level of consciousness:	alert, oriented, but agitated
Respirations:	20 breaths/minute
Heart rate:	110 and irregular
Blood pressure:	160/104 mm Hg
Skin:	warm and dry
Allergies:	allergic to codeine
Age:	76 years old

Betty stated that she was not wearing her seat belt, and she is adamant about not going to the hospital.

Introduction

Think of the last time you required the services of the health-care system. You may have had an appointment with your personal physician for an annual physical, or it may have been more serious requiring a trip to the emergency room of your local hospital. Whether your visit was a scheduled appointment or an emergency, how were you treated by the medical staff? How was your family treated?

Now, as an EMT-Paramedic student, how do you treat your patients and their families? As we know, some calls we receive are true emergencies, but the majority of our calls are not considered true emergencies, except to the person calling 911. Thankfully, the majority of our patients are cooperative and truly want our help. But, as we know, some patients can challenge our professionalism.

This chapter will explain the importance of treating all patients with respect and presenting ourselves as professionals at all times.

EMS Licensure, Certification, Registration, and Credentialing

As paramedics, we are granted permission to practice our skills by four processes: **licensure, certification, registration,** and **credentialing.**

- **Licensure:** Granting permission to an individual by an authoritative body to perform professional actions that may not be legally performed by those who do not have such permission
- **Certification:** A document issued by a governing body showing that a person has met requirements to practice specific activities within a profession
- **Registration:** The act or process of entering information about someone into a system of public records
- **Credentialing:** Recognition in a field in which a person has met certain educational, professional, or occupational requirements that permit the person to continue practicing under his or her license or certification

Check the Evidence

Some governmental bodies issue licenses, and some issue certifications to practice paramedicine. Many feel that a license has more authority than a certification. In fact, a certification that grants a right to engage in a profession is a license.

Professionalism in EMS

For many years, EMTs and paramedics were considered not much more than ambulance drivers. Many volunteer rescue services did not require any official training to be a part of their agency and respond to emergency calls. However, over the years, training, education, and performance standards have helped to define EMS personnel as true health-care professionals (Fig. 2-1).

EMS has become its own **profession** within the medical field. A profession is a type of job that requires special

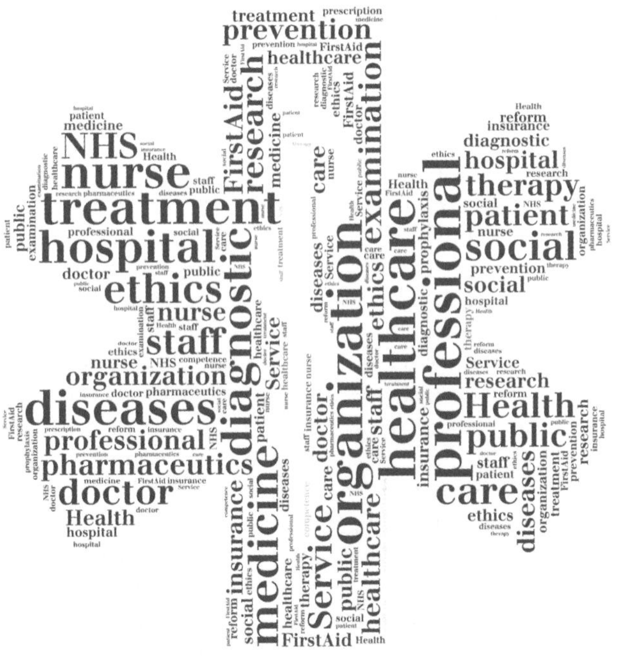

Figure 2-1 Star of life. *(Photograph © Thinkstock)*

education, training, standards, or skills. All four of these requirements have made EMS more of a reputable medical profession. A **professional** is a person who earns a living from his or her profession, while **professionalism** refers to the way that a person follows the standards of a profession. The profession's standards also include a requirement that their personnel adhere to a **code of ethics** approved by the profession.

The professional paramedic must adhere to the following attributes:

- **Altruism:** Feelings and behavior that show both a desire to help other people and a lack of selfishness. An example of altruism is offering to help team members who are busy without expecting anything in return. Each member of an EMS team should know that his or her partner has the attribute of altruism.
- **Integrity:** The quality of being honest and fair. The community in which the EMS team serves assumes that EMS professionals have integrity.
- **Compassion:** The sympathetic consciousness of others' distress together with a desire to alleviate that distress
- **Empathy:** Understanding, being aware of and sensitive to, and experiencing the feelings and thoughts of another, without having the feelings and thoughts fully communicated in an objective manner
- **Appearance and personal hygiene:** Having uniforms that are clean and in good repair as well as reporting to duty with good personal hygiene. If you work at a busy station, there should be a change of clothing ready to wear. Perfumes and cologne should be avoided during shifts, as the odors produced may have a negative effect on patients.

Check the Evidence

Numerous research studies have concluded that people act more professionally when they dress professionally.

- **Communication:** We must be able to communicate effectively both when speaking and in writing. Electronic communication, such as with social media, has made face-to-face communication more difficult for many people. It is important that EMS professionals be able to communicate clearly with patients and their families. EMS professionals must also be able to listen effectively. Patients may not always understand how to provide all of the information requested of them. EMS professionals must be able to convey key information clearly and concisely so no one takes anything for granted.
- **Patient advocate:** Most patients will be glad to see you and will be cooperative. However, there will be times when a patient will be disagreeable or combative or refuse part or all of the treatment necessary. Regardless of the situation, EMS professionals must be patient advocates; they must always place the needs of the patient above their own needs. Patient advocacy is also applicable when it comes to patient confidentiality. EMS professionals must comply with the **Health Insurance Portability and Accountability Act of 1996** (HIPAA). HIPAA protects the privacy of patients' health information, disclosing the minimum amount needed for treatment, billing, and operations. Compliance with HIPAA is mandatory.
- **Respect:** This means understanding that a person is important and deserves to be treated in an appropriate way. We all like to be treated with respect. However, there will be patients who will challenge your professionalism. In such cases, EMS professionals must never use derogatory or demeaning terms when speaking with patients or their family members. Showing disrespect will be a direct reflection on you, your service, and the EMS profession as a whole.
- **Teamwork:** EMS is a part of the entire medical team. Teamwork will break down at the weakest link. The medical team is there for the benefit of the patient. Therefore, EMS professionals must place the team before any personal goals.

Ethics

Most of us have probably faced an occasional ethical dilemma, both in our personal and professional lives. How do we approach and tackle these dilemmas? Once we slip off that slippery slope and tarnish our integrity due to an ethical breach, it is difficult if not impossible to regain that integrity.

Ethics are rules of behavior based on ideas about what is morally good and bad (Fig. 2-2). **Morals** relate to what is right and wrong in human behavior. On the surface, ethics and morals are very similar. However, there is a subtle difference. For example, ethics focus on a social system in which morals are applied. Morals, on the other hand, define personal character.

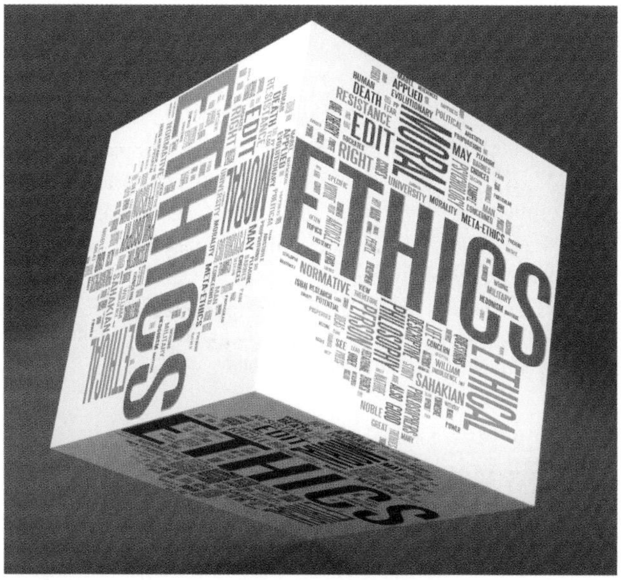

Figure 2-2 Ethics cube. *(Photograph © Thinkstock)*

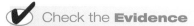

When it comes to morals, good or bad behavior is variable in different groups. Each group will follow its own moral code, which is influenced by its worldview. Some common examples of moral behavior include returning change when the cashier gives you too much, keeping your promises, respecting others, and forgiving others.

Medical ethics refers to moral conduct within the medical professions. These medical ethics are high standards and principles that were developed and are maintained by medical professionals who are willing to adhere to them. Every segment within the medical profession has a code of ethics that its members are expected to follow.

The Code of Ethics for EMS Practitioners was originally written by Charles B. Gillespie, M.D. and was adopted by the National Association of Emergency Medical Technicians in1978. It was revised and adopted by the National Association of Emergency Medical Technicians on June 14, 2013.

effective **Communication**

The Code of Ethics for EMS Practitioners can be found at http://www.naemt.org/about_us/emtoath.aspx.

Ethical Duties

All EMS professionals have an ethical duty to their employer and their community. These duties are defined as **statutes**. EMS statutes are based on the developed standards of medical care. Ethical duties of EMS professionals include the following:

- Respecting the needs of every patient and their families and caregivers
- Maintaining confidentiality
- Maintaining your skill level
- Maintaining all continuing education requirements
- Critiquing one's own performance and making adjustments when necessary
- Complete and honest documentation
- Being a team member
- Adhering to your state and local protocols and following your established standard of care

Check the **Evidence**

EMS laws and the standard of care vary from state to state and in some cases from region to region within a state. Know and understand your ethical duties. Failure to perform your ethical duties can result in criminal or civil liability.

Standard of Care

Paramedics are health-care professionals. As such, paramedics must conform to a **standard of care** set by their training and education level, as well as their EMS regional practice protocols. The EMS standard of care asserts that each paramedic must provide the same knowledge, care, and skill that a similarly trained paramedic would provide under the same circumstance and in the same EMS region. Laws require that only reasonable, ordinary care and skill be provided to each patient.

Paramedics are expected to use all resources available to them when treating patients. This includes taking a thorough appropriate medical history, giving complete patient assessments, and administering appropriate treatment under medical control and their local protocols. Paramedics who violate their standard of care may be liable for negligence.

Negligence

Negligence is the failure of health-care professionals to meet their responsibilities to a patient, with resultant injury. There are four elements of negligence:

1. Duty owed: This refers to the paramedic-patient relationship. Once a paramedic responds to an emergency and initiates patient contact, the relationship has been established.
2. Breach of duty or standard of care: This refers to the paramedic's failure to act as any ordinary and prudent paramedic within the same EMS region would act in a similar circumstance when treating a patient.
3. Proximate cause: This requires the patient to prove that the paramedic's breach of duty was the direct cause of the injury that resulted.
4. Damages or injuries: This refers to any injuries that the patient suffered. The courts may also award compensatory damages to pay for the patient's injuries.

Negligence can also be broken down into three subcategories: ordinary negligence, gross negligence, and contributory negligence. Ordinary negligence is the failure of a paramedic to exercise the care that an ordinary prudent paramedic would exercise under similar circumstances. Gross negligence is any voluntary, intentional, and conscious act or omission committed by a paramedic with reckless disregard for the consequences. Contributory negligence indicates that the patient has contributed to the injury or the deterioration of his or her condition.

EMS professionals must be aware of how their treatment or omission of treatment can pose a threat of litigation for negligence. The following guidelines can help keep EMS professionals protected against negligence:

- Initial education and training
- Regular continuing education and skills retention
- Quality improvement
- Thorough, accurate documentation
- Strong medical direction

Confidentiality

Once a paramedic-patient relationship has been established, a legal contract has been developed. Paramedics, as well as all other health-care professionals who come in contact with patients, have a legal and ethical duty to protect patient privacy. This means refraining from divulging patient information, including the patient's medical history and test results and even the fact that he or she was a patient.

The U.S. Congress passed the **Health Insurance Portability and Accountability Act of 1996 (HIPAA).** HIPAA was enacted to improve the efficiency and effectiveness of the health-care system. All health-care professionals must undergo HIPAA training during their employment orientation. There are three parts to HIPAA: privacy regulations, transaction standards, and security regulations.

HIPAA also extends its rules to computers that are used to house confidential patient information. This means that unauthorized individuals cannot access confidential patient information from a computer. In addition, all e-mails that contain private patient information must include a statement informing the recipient that the information is confidential.

Check the Evidence

If confidential patient information is accidentally transmitted to an unauthorized individual, the sender must notify a supervisor and destroy the information.

Continuing Professional Education

Continuing professional education is the schooling of professionals that extends their learning and teaches concepts that can contribute to the quality of their daily performance (Fig. 2-3). It enables health-care professionals to keep abreast of new knowledge and maintain and enhance their competence. Continuing professional education focuses primarily on an individual's growth and development. It emphasizes the acquiring of knowledge, skills, and performance abilities.

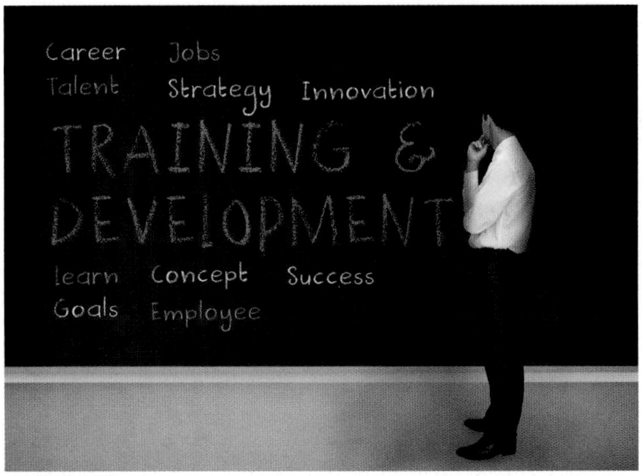

Figure 2-3 Education. *(Photograph © Thinkstock)*

Each EMS region expects its EMS professionals to provide only appropriate medical care, properly executed. To maintain this expected level of care, continuing professional educators attempt to identify the educational activities and programs that will best meet the needs of each EMS region.

Distance Education

Distance education is professional education in which the majority of instruction occurs while the instructor and the participants are at a distance from one another. For example, an instructor can be presenting a continuing class from Chicago to EMS personnel located in Nashville.

Some topics in EMS are better presented in a classroom, but many other topics can be presented as well or even better via distance learning. Not only does distance education have a place in initial EMS education, but many certification agencies are also using it to enable EMS professionals to maintain their credentials. For example, some state legislatures and professional medical bodies such as the American Heart Association have been turning to distance education. Health-care professionals have varied schedules that may make it difficult to complete some required courses. Distance education can make it more convenient for EMS professionals to maintain both their right to practice and their certification within the EMS field.

SCENARIO REVISITED

Do you recall the case of Betty whose head hit and cracked the windshield of an automobile? After you have assessed Betty, you explain to her that, due to the mechanism of injury, her condition could become more serious over time depending on how much damage may have occurred to her brain, blood vessels, and nerves during the accident. When the head hits the windshield, the brain hits the skull and puts an upward tension on the brain stem and spinal cord at the base of the brain. When the head recoils backward, the brain hits the back of the skull. Movement of the brain within the skull also puts pressure on nerves and blood vessels, resulting in possible contusion and intracerebral hemorrhage.

Betty also has to be told that there are two other factors working against her. First, the fact that she is 76 years old increases her chances of developing signs and symptoms due to her accident. People over age 55 are more at risk of serious injury due to trauma. Second, the fact that Betty is agitated is a sign that her brain may not be receiving sufficient blood supply. As a professional, what should the on-scene paramedic do for Betty? She still does not want to go the hospital.

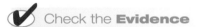

Let's Recap

It is probably safe to say that we all would like to be treated with respect and in a professional manner by the people with whom we come in contact. As EMS professionals, we must treat all of our patients and their families with respect and in a professional manner. Granted, that can be difficult at times, and in some cases it may seem impossible. But we must make every attempt to present ourselves as the professionals that we truly are. Similar to other professions, EMS has a standard of care that we must follow.

Professionalism is not just about how we present ourselves to people. To maintain our professional status within our profession and within the community, we must also maintain our knowledge base and advance our level of care as necessary. This includes maintaining our license/certification status by attending the required continuing professional education classes. Professionalism is a never-ending process. We must always maintain the professional standards as developed for EMS providers.

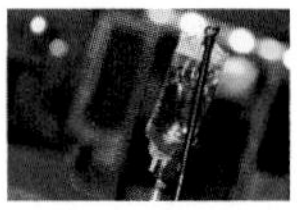

SCENARIO CONCLUSION

Betty must be taken to the hospital. It takes a lot of force to cause damage to the windshield of a vehicle. If someone's head causes damage to a windshield, that person is likely to have a life-threatening injury. Having Betty sign a refusal form is not only unprofessional but also negligent and is considered patient abandonment as well.

After carefully explaining to Betty some of the problems that could develop if she is not seen by a physician, you could call medical control and have the physician talk directly to her. Sometimes, when patients talk directly to a physician, they will agree to be transported. If all else fails, you can have the police arrest Betty and force her to be transported. This scenario presents professional, moral, and ethical issues in patient care.

PRACTICE EXERCISES

1. Granting permission to an individual by an authoritative body to perform professional actions that may not be legally performed by those who do not have such permission is termed:
a. Registration
b. Licensure
c. Certification
d. Credentialing

2. Feelings and behavior that show both a desire to help other people and a lack of selfishness is termed:
a. Integrity
b. Altruism
c. Empathy
d. Compassion

3. ________ are rules of behavior based on ideas about what is morally good and bad.
a. Ethics
b. Morals
c. Teamwork
d. Professionalism

4. Paramedics must conform to a ______________ set by their training and education level, as well as their EMS regional practice protocols.
a. Moral code
b. Code of ethics
c. Standard of care
d. Standard of ethics

5. ________ is the failure of health-care professionals to meet their responsibilities to a patient, with resultant injury.
a. Liability
b. Negligence
c. Breach of duty
d. Malfeasance

6. _______ requires the patient to prove that the paramedic's breach of duty was the direct cause of the injury that resulted.
a. Damage
b. Proximate cause
c. Negligence
d. Malfeasance

7. Once a paramedic-patient relationship has been established, a(n) ______ contract has been developed.
a. Professional
b. Ethical
c. Moral
d. Legal

8. The U.S. Congress passed the Health Insurance Portability and Accountability Act (HIPAA) of ______.
a. 1996
b. 1998
c. 2001
d. 2003

9. If you receive an e-mail containing confidential patient information by mistake, you should:
a. Read it but do not share the contents
b. Tell your supervisor and then delete the e-mail
c. Forward the e-mail to your supervisor
d. Send the e-mail back to the sender

10. _______ is the recognition in a field in which a person has met certain educational, professional, or occupational requirements that permit the person to continue practicing under his or her license or certification.
a. Professionalism
b. The code of ethics
c. Credentialing
d. Licensure

CASE STUDIES

1. You are called to a gentlemen's club for a "fight." While you are en route, the dispatcher tells you that the owner of the club has been hit in the head with a baseball bat. Upon arrival, you find the owner, Big Mike, lying in front of the stage with blood oozing from the back of his head. Mike is conscious but unable to stand. You decide to get Mike into the ambulance before a formal assessment due to the loud music, flashing lights, and patrons of the club getting in your way. There are only two police officers on the scene, and they are unable to control the crowd.

Once in the ambulance, you and your partner do an assessment and find a slight depression on Mike's occipital region. Mike is still conscious and reaches into his front pocket and pulls out $2,000 in cash and gives it to you for safekeeping.

a. Was it appropriate to remove Mike from his club before performing an assessment? Please explain.
b. Should you take the $2,000 that Mike wanted to give you? Please explain.

2. It is that time again. Two years have passed, and it is time to renew your Advanced Cardiovascular Life Support (ACLS) card. After sitting through the lectures and performing the required skills, it is now time to take the written examination. During the exam, you notice that Phil appears to be cheating. It looks like he has the answers to the written exam. You remember that, during the lectures, Phil had a difficult time staying awake. On several occasions, he needed help to get through the skills portion of the class. You always thought Phil was an average paramedic.

a. Do you let this go or should you confront Phil after the class? Please explain.
b. Do you "rat" on a team member to the lead instructor? Please explain.
c. Cheating on an ACLS examination may not seem that big a deal to many paramedics. However, is this also cheating on patient care as well? Please explain.

MATH EQUATIONS

Basic Multiplication and Division

Multiplication

1. $12.5 \times 3.7 =$ __________
2. $25.75 \times 6.04 =$ __________
3. $15.75 \times 10 =$ __________
4. $125.5 \times 20.33 =$ __________
5. $33.02 \times 17 =$ __________

Division

1. $253.680 \div 10.5 =$ __________
2. $50.2990 \div 0.125 =$ __________
3. $6.0 \div 100$ __________
4. $15 \div 10$ __________
5. $687.3422 \div 55.5 =$ __________

REFERENCES

Craig, R. L. (1996). *The ASTD training & development handbook: A guide to human resource development* (4th ed.). New York: McGraw-Hill.
HIPAA Guidelines101.com. HIPAA-HITECH guidelines. Retrieved August 19, 2014 from http://www.hipaaguidelines101.com/
LoveToKnow, Corp. Examples of morals. Retrieved August 19, 2014 from http://examples.yourdictionary.com/examples-of-morals.html
MedicineNet, Inc. Head injury. Retrieved August 15, 2014 from www.medicinenet.com/head_injury/page2.htm
Nowlen, P. M. (1998). *A new approach to continuing education for business and the professions.* New York: American Council on Education and Macmillan.
Sanders, M. J. (2012). *Mosby's paramedic textbook* (4th ed.). St. Louis, MO: Elsevier.
Stern, M. R., and Queeney, D. S. (1992). The scope of continuing professional education: providers, consumers, issues. In: *Hunt, E. S., ed. Professional workers as learners.* Washington, D.C.: Office of Educational Research and Improvement, U.S. Department of Education, 13-34.
Venes, D., ed. (2013). *Taber's cyclopedic medical dictionary* (22nd ed.). Philadelphia, PA: F. A. Davis Company.
Verduin, J. R., Jr., and Clark, T. A. (1991). *Distance education: the foundations of effective practice.* San Francisco, CA: Jossey-Bass.

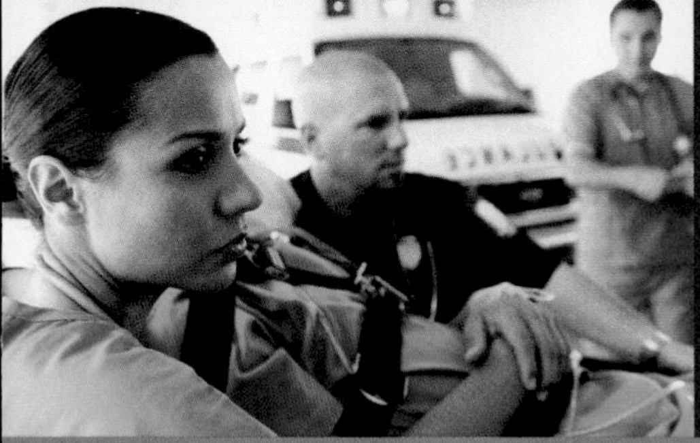

CHAPTER 3

The Basics of Pharmacokinetics and Pharmacodynamics

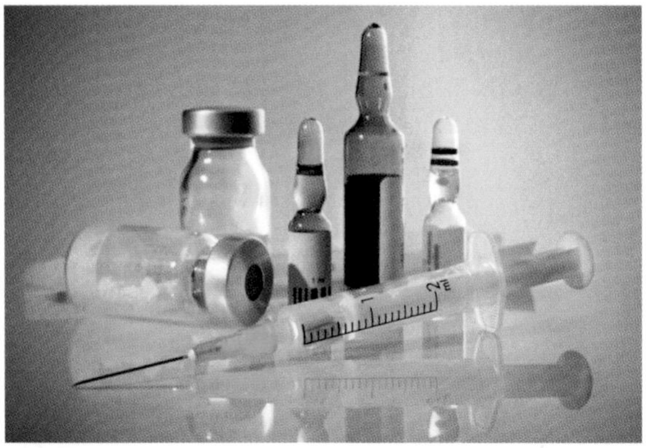

Various drug forms. *(Photograph © Alexander Raths/iStock/Thinkstock)*

LEARNING OUTCOMES

- Define pharmacokinetics and pharmacodynamics.
- Describe the basics of active and passive transport.
- Describe the processes of absorption, distribution, biotransformation, and excretion.
- Explain the phases of drug activity.
- Explain medication therapy for pediatric and geriatric patients.
- Explain medication therapy for patients who are pregnant and patients who are lactating.

KEY TERMS

Absorption
Active transport
Affinity
Agonist
Antagonist
Bioavailability
Biotransformation
Blood-brain barrier
Blood-cerebrospinal fluid barrier
Bound drug
Cumulative drug effects
Diffusion
Distribution
Efficacy
Excretion
Facilitated diffusion
Filtration
Free drug
Half-life
Mechanism of action
Metabolite
Minimum therapeutic concentration
Onset of drug action
Osmosis
Passive transport
pH
Pharmacodynamics
Pharmacokinetics
Prodrug
Receptor
Solubility
Time/action profile
Volatile

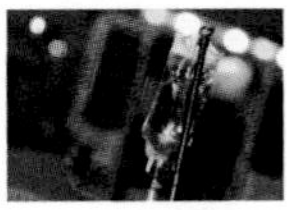

SCENARIO OPENING

You have been assigned to an advanced life support unit as part of your field internship during paramedic school. The unit is called to a pool party for a person who is having trouble breathing. Upon arrival, you find a young female patient named Charlene lying in the grass gasping for air. A friend states that Charlene was stung by "a couple of bees." During a rapid assessment, Charlene has audible strider, has hives on her neck and chest, cannot speak, and is becoming cyanotic. The paramedic team begins oxygen; prepares for an advanced airway, cardiac monitor, and IV; and removes epinephrine and diphenhydramine from the drug box. Charlene's friend states that she does not think Charlene is allergic to anything. Charlene is 22 years old.

Introduction

Drugs must take a complicated journey through the body before they can produce their desired therapeutic effects. Once a drug is given, it is absorbed into the circulatory system, distributed to its site of action, and finally eliminated from the body. **Pharmacokinetics** is the study of drug absorption, distribution, biotransformation (metabolism), and elimination, with emphasis on the time it takes for these processes to take place. In other words, pharmacokinetics studies drug movement.

Once a drug reaches its receptors' sites (sites of action), certain biochemical and physiological actions occur, producing the desired pharmacologic effects. These pharmacologic effects are called the drug's **mechanism of action**. **Pharmacodynamics** is the study of drug actions in the body. Drug pharmacokinetics and pharmacodynamics determine the route, frequency, and dosage of drug administration.

Pharmacokinetics

Basic Transport Physiology

Active Transport

Once a drug enters the body, it must travel or move to its site of action. This movement is dependent on the body's two main physiological mechanisms: active and passive transport (discussed further in chapter 5).

Active transport is the process whereby a cell membrane moves molecules against a concentration or electrochemical gradient (Fig. 3-1). This movement of molecules requires metabolic work, such as adenosine triphosphate. For example, potassium is maintained at high concentrations within cells and low concentrations in extracellular fluid by active transport. Other ions actively transported are sodium, calcium, hydrogen, iron, chloride, iodide, and urate. Several sugars and the amino acids are also actively transported in the small intestine.

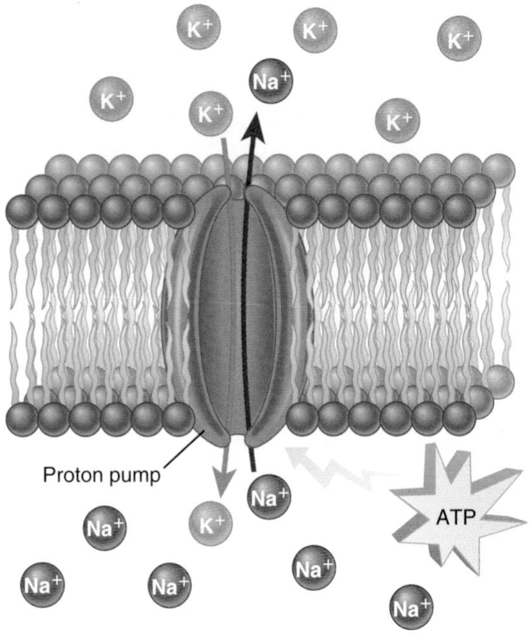

Figure 3-1 Active transport.

Passive Transport

Passive transport is a movement of molecular substances across membranes. Unlike active transport, passive transport does not require chemical energy. The rate of passive transport depends on the permeability of the cell membrane as well as the organization and characteristic of membrane lipids and proteins. Passive transport depends on four mechanisms: (1) filtration, (2) diffusion, (3) facilitated diffusion, and (4) osmosis.

- **Filtration** is the movement of fluid through a membrane, caused by differences in hydrostatic pressure (Fig. 3-2). Hydrostatic pressure is the force exerted by the weight of a solution; it causes the solution to move from an area of higher pressure to an area of lower pressure. In two compartments separated by a permeable or semipermeable membrane, hydrostatic pressure tends

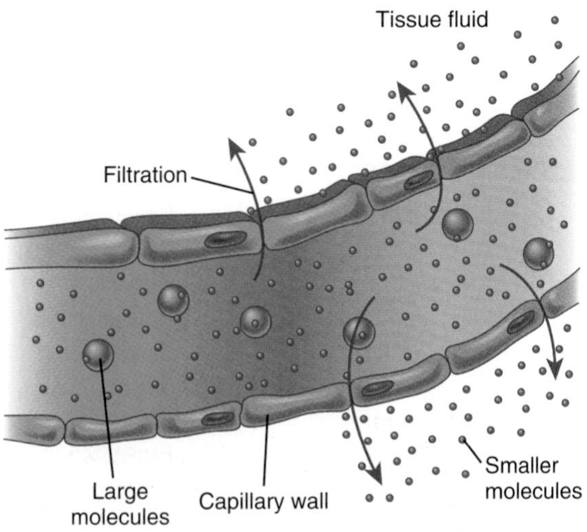

The small molecules exit the capillary since the capillary hydrostatic pressure is greater than the blood osmotic pressure.

Figure 3-2 Filtration caused by hydrostatic pressure.

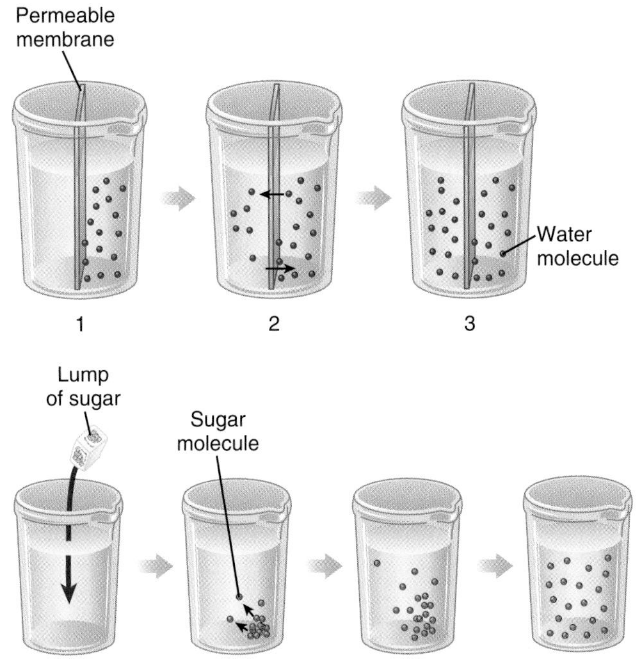

Figure 3-3 Diffusion: (a) through a membrane, (b) in a solution.

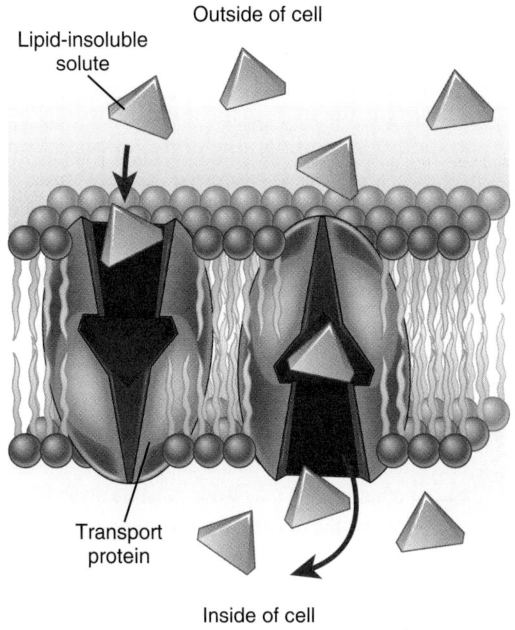

Figure 3-4 Facilitated diffusion.

to cause fluid to move from one compartment to the other until the pressure in both compartments is equal.

- **Diffusion** is the tendency of molecules in solution to distribute equally (Fig. 3-3). In diffusion, molecules, atoms, or ions flow from an area of higher concentration to areas of lower concentration, until the concentration (number of molecules of solute per amount of solution) is the same throughout the solution.
- **Facilitated diffusion**, also called carrier-mediated diffusion, is the movement of molecules across a cell membrane by special transport proteins that are embedded within the cellular membrane (Fig. 3-4). Large molecules, such as glucose, are insoluble in lipids and too large to fit through the membrane pores. Therefore, large molecules will bind with their specific carrier proteins and will then bond to a receptor site and move through the cellular membrane. Solutes move down the concentration gradient without using energy.
- **Osmosis** is the diffusion of solute and/or solvent through a permeable or semipermeable membrane (Fig. 3-5). It is a result of the same force that causes solute molecules or ions within a solution to flow from areas of high concentration to areas of low concentration. With two solutions separated by a semipermeable membrane, a difference in solute concentration creates osmotic pressure, which causes water and (if possible) solute to move across the membrane until the solutions are in equilibrium.

Absorption

Absorption is the passage of a drug from the site of administration (where absorption begins) into the circulatory system. The speed at which a drug is absorbed is very important, because it determines how quickly the drug reaches its target tissue to produce its therapeutic effects. The rate of absorption depends on the following factors:

- **Nature of the absorbing surface:** The absorbing surface area is a determining factor in how quickly a drug is absorbed. The greater the surface area of the absorption site, the faster a drug becomes absorbed, and the quicker it produces its therapeutic effect.
- **Circulatory status:** Poor circulation results in slow drug absorption and, therefore, delayed or inadequate therapeutic response. However, drugs that can be administered via the IV route bypass the absorption process. The IV administration technique permits the drug to go directly into circulation, thereby permitting a faster therapeutic response.

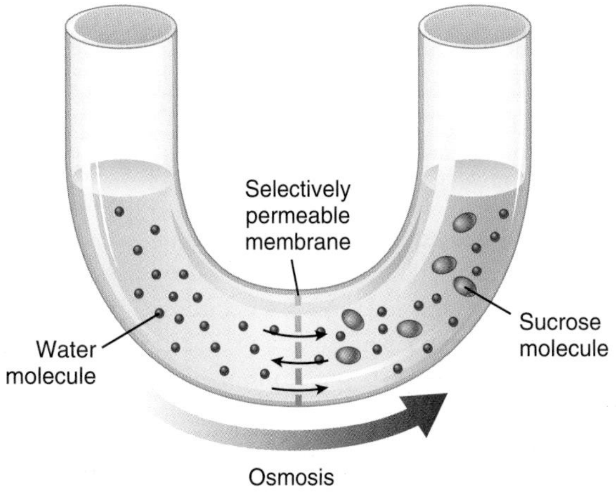

Figure 3-5 Osmosis.

- **Solubility** is the drug's ability to dissolve. The higher a drug's solubility, the faster it enters the circulatory system.
- **Body pH: pH** is the measurement of the hydrogen ion concentration of a solution. The degree of acidity or alkalinity of a substance is expressed as a pH value. A solution that is neither acid nor alkaline has a pH value of 7. Acidosis delays drug absorption in many cases. For example, acidosis can delay the absorption of epinephrine, thus making it inactive. This is why some patients in cardiac arrest do not respond to epinephrine.

effective Communication

Inadequate ventilations and/or chest compressions may leave patients acidotic, limiting the effectiveness of some medications.

Drugs can vary significantly in pH. For example, a drug that is acidic will generally absorb better when introduced into the stomach because of the stomach's acidic environment. Also, an alkaline drug will absorb more quickly when introduced into the alkaline environment of the kidneys. Therefore, both a drug's pH and the pH of the body can affect absorption.

- **Concentration:** Generally, the higher the percentage of drug in the preparation administered, the faster the rate of absorption. Approximately 80 percent of drugs used in medicine are formulated to be taken orally. However, the oral route has two drawbacks. First, it is harder to predict and control the final concentration in the circulatory system of an orally administered drug. This unpredictability results from:
  - Changes in the rate of absorption, depending on the presence or absence of food in the digestive system
  - The destruction of some of the drug by gastric enzymes

Second, the rate of absorption through the digestive system is slower than the rate from subcutaneous injection and intramuscular (IM) injection.

- **Bioavailability:** A sufficient amount of a drug must reach its target site of action in order to produce a therapeutic response. **Bioavailability** is the rate at which a drug enters the general circulation, permitting access to the site of action. This is determined by the measurement of the concentration of the drug in body fluids or by the magnitude of the pharmacologic response.

Table 3-1 lists the routes in which drugs can be given and their rates of absorption.

Table 3-1 Rates of Drug Absorption

Drug Route	Rate of Administration
IV	Immediate
Endotracheal/Transtracheal	Immediate
Intraosseous	Immediate
Inhalation	Rapid
Rectal	Rapid
Intramuscular	Moderate
Topical	Moderate
Intranasal	Moderate
Subcutaneous	Slow
Oral	
Sublingual	Rapid
Intralingual	Rapid
Ingestion	Slow

Distribution

Once a drug is administered and absorbed into the circulatory system, it must travel to its site of action before it can be of any benefit. Once in the bloodstream, the entire dose does not travel to its targeted tissues. Instead, the drug travels throughout the entire body. As Figure 3-6 illustrates, a certain amount of the drug may become bound to blood proteins (such as hemoglobin, albumin, and globulin). When this occurs, the drug is unavailable for further **distribution** until it is released from the blood protein. Drugs can also become stored within the body's fatty tissues. The drug must be released from fatty tissue to be available for distribution. The amount of drug that binds to blood protein, or becomes stored in the body's fatty tissues, is termed **bound drug**. Only the drug not bound, termed **free drug**, can be distributed for metabolism and elimination and is available to targeted tissues.

Because drugs are distributed by way of the circulatory system, they generally concentrate in tissues that are well

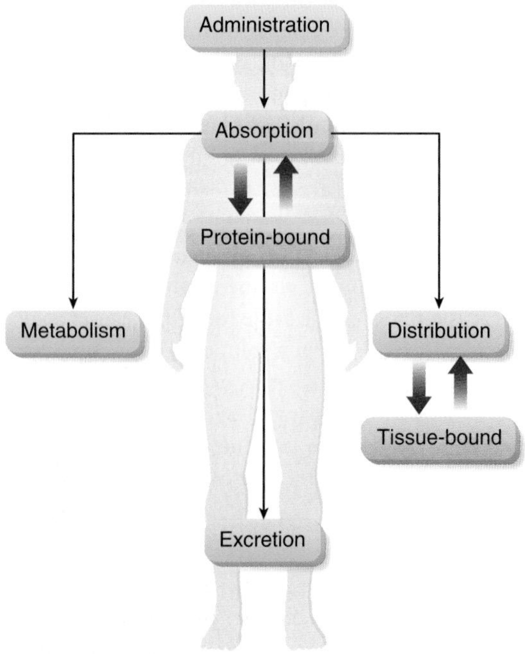

Figure 3-6 The pharmacokinetic phase of drug action.

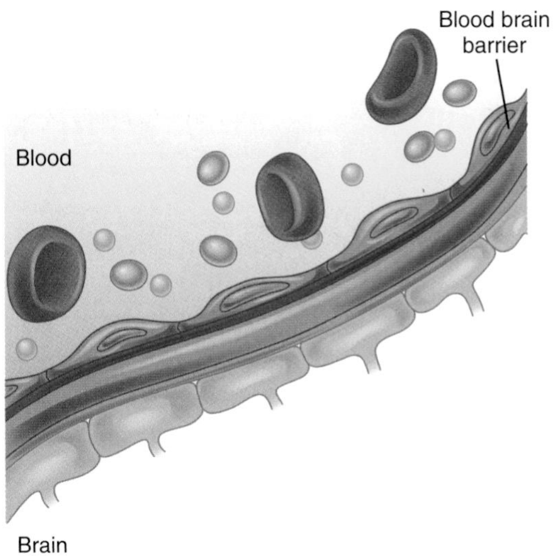

Figure 3-7 The blood-brain barrier.

supplied with blood, such as the heart, liver, kidneys, and brain. The **blood-brain barrier** and the **blood-cerebrospinal fluid barrier**, however, limit delivery of drugs to the brain (Fig. 3-7). These barriers are tightly packed cell membranes that separate the circulating blood from the brain and cerebrospinal fluid. The blood-brain barrier and the blood-cerebrospinal fluid barrier restrict the movement of some damaging drugs and toxins to the brain and cerebrospinal fluid. Only non-protein-bound, highly lipid-soluble drugs can cross these barriers into the central nervous system (CNS). Even these drugs generally enter the brain and spinal fluid at a slower rate than other tissues because of this extra barrier.

Check the **Evidence**

The blood-brain barrier occurs along all capillaries in the brain and consists of tight junctions around the capillaries that do not exist in normal circulation. Endothelial cells restrict the diffusion of microscopic objects and large or hydrophilic molecules into the cerebrospinal fluid, while allowing the diffusion of small hydrophobic molecules.

Biotransformation

There are two ways in which the body eliminates a drug: biotransformation and excretion. **Biotransformation** is the chemical alteration of a drug within the body to an active or inactive water-soluble metabolite. A **metabolite** is any product that results from biotransformation. Changing a drug to a water-soluble metabolite makes excretion from the body easier. Most drugs are inactivated as a result of biotransformation. Some drugs, however, become therapeutically active (**prodrugs**) as a result of biotransformation.

The biotransformation process of a drug to an inactive metabolite begins immediately after drug administration. This actually becomes a race against time. The drug must reach the target site of action at a sufficient therapeutic concentration in the blood before biotransformation converts the drug to an inactive state.

Biotransformation takes place primarily in the liver. It can, however, occur in all body cells and tissues. Biotransformation that takes place in the liver is called *hepatic biotransformation*.

If the rate of drug biotransformation is slowed for any reason, **cumulative drug effects** may occur. Therefore, subsequent doses have more effect. Increasing the rate of biotransformation may produce a state of apparent tolerance, in which the drug effect decreases. Generally, when biotransformation is complete, a drug is no longer able to work therapeutically (unless the drug becomes an active metabolite), and it is excreted.

Excretion

Excretion is the elimination of waste products from the body. Drug excretion takes place through the intestines in the feces, through the kidneys in the urine, through the skin in perspiration, and through the respiratory system in exhaled air.

Volatile (easily evaporated) drugs are excreted from the body through the respiratory system in exhaled air or through the skin in perspiration. Nonvolatile, water-soluble drug metabolites are excreted in the urine. The kidney is the most important site of the excretion of drugs and drug metabolites.

Some drugs are excreted from the body through the alimentary tract. This occurs when the drug passes through the liver, is released into the bile, and is finally eliminated in the feces. Alternatively, the bile enters the small intestine; however, some of the drug travels through the circulatory system until it is finally excreted in the urine. If the reabsorbed drug is in active form, this reabsorption prolongs its actions on the body.

Dosing Considerations

Half-life

Half-life is the time required by the body, tissue, or organ to metabolize or inactivate half the amount of drug that has been administered. Knowing a drug's half-life is an important consideration in determining the proper amount and frequency of drug administration. For example, the half-life for midazolam (Versed) for adults is 2 to 6 hours. For this reason, patients who have been given midazolam cannot drive or perform other activities requiring alertness for up to 24 hours after administration due to the decrease in mental alertness side effect. Most medications will have lost their effectiveness after five half-lives.

effective **Communication**

Patients who have kidney impairment, congestive heart failure, or cirrhosis will have an increased half-life of midazolam. Therefore, these patients may have a longer period of decreased mental alertness.

Time/Action Profile

The **time/action profile** provides the onset of drug action, the drug's peak effect, and the drug's duration of activity. For

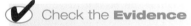

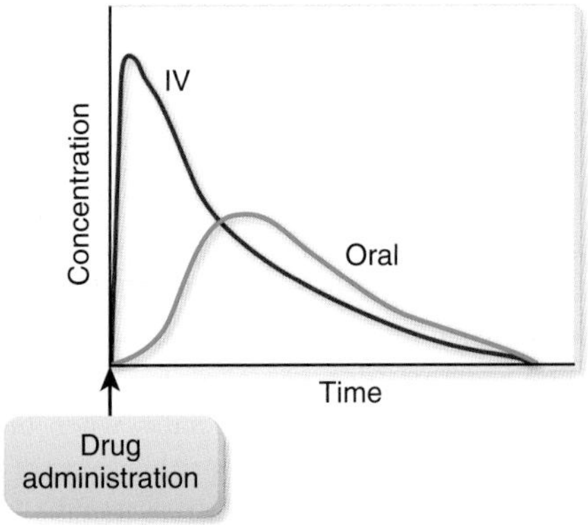

Figure 3-8 Concentration curve of a drug given IV as compared to a drug given orally.

example, midazolam's onset of action for IM injection is approximately 15 minutes, whereas its onset of action for IV injection is only 1.5 to 5 minutes. Therefore, during emergent situations, administering midazolam via IV will be effective more rapidly than the IM route.

Pharmacodynamics

Unless a drug enters the body via the IV, intraosseous, or endotracheal route, some time elapses before the drug reaches its target site of action. The length of time from a drug's first administration until it reaches a concentration necessary to produce a therapeutic response at its target site of action is called the **onset of drug action.** Figure 3-8 compares the onset of action for a drug administered intravenously with the onset of action for the same drug given orally.

Most drugs produce desired effects by inhibiting or increasing the action of targeted **receptors.** A drug receptor is a component of a cell that combines with a drug to initiate a response. In essence, a section of the drug molecule combines with part of the molecular structure on or within a cell to produce a therapeutic effect. Once a drug reaches the site of action, it binds to or unites with the receptor so it can cause the desired therapeutic response. This action at the receptor site is also called the drug's mechanism of action.

Drug receptors (target cells) are often referred to as "locks," and drugs that bind to the receptors are generally referred to as the "keys" that fit the locks. A drug's (key) ability to fit a certain receptor (lock) enables a pharmacologic response to occur (Fig. 3-9). Such a drug is called an **agonist.** In addition, some drugs bind to receptors, but their effect is to inhibit or counteract a response. These drugs are called **antagonists.**

Affinity and efficacy describe the nature of drug–receptor interaction. **Affinity** means attraction; to say that a drug has an affinity for a receptor means that it tends to combine with that receptor. **Efficacy** means the power to produce a desired effect. To say a drug has efficacy means that it has the capacity to produce a pharmacologic response when it interacts with its receptor. Drugs that are agonists have both affinity and efficacy, while antagonist drugs have affinity but not efficacy.

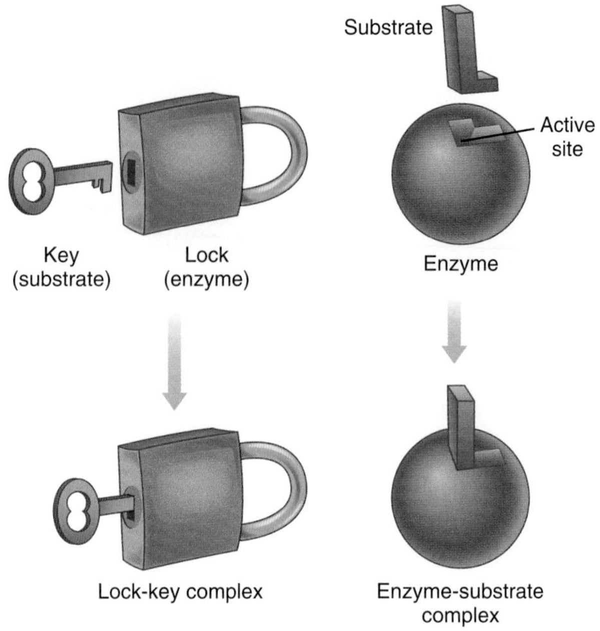

Figure 3-9 Lock-and-key union of drug and receptor.

Phases of Drug Activity

A drug goes through four phases of activity before it produces a desired pharmacologic effect (Table 3-2). The administration phase is the introduction of the drug into the body by the appropriate route. Once administered, the drug enters the pharmaceutical phase. During this phase, the drug dissolves so it can be made available for absorption. Once dissolved, the drug begins the pharmacokinetic phase. Only free drugs capable of reaching their receptors can be said to exist in the pharmacokinetic phase. Once a drug reaches its receptors, the pharmacodynamic phase of drug activity occurs. It is only when the drug binds to its receptor that the pharmacologic effect occurs.

Most drugs have a predetermined standard dosage or one that is determined by body weight. Dosage guidelines are established to achieve **minimum therapeutic concentrations.** Any deviation from established dosage guidelines might be harmful. Remember that the goal for drug therapy is to give the minimum concentration of a drug necessary to obtain the desired therapeutic response.

Special Considerations

Administering drugs can be further complicated by the added factors of patient age, body mass, pregnancy, and lactation. For example, the very young and the elderly are generally more susceptible to the adverse reactions and side effects of drugs. Therefore, drug dosages may have to be modified for these age groups. Some drugs are administered according to body mass. Generally, the larger the patient, the more medication may have to be administered. For example, one of the drugs that can be used for treating adult bradycardia with a pulse is

Table 3-2 The Phases of Drug Activity

Administration Phase	Pharmaceutical Phase	Pharmacokinetic Phase	Pharmacodynamic Phase
IV Intraosseous Transtracheal Intramuscular Subcutaneous Inhalation Oral	Dissolution of the drug Amount of drug available for absorption	Absorption Distribution Biotransformation Excretion Amount of drug available for action	Drug receptor binding Pharmacologic effect

dopamine (Intropin). The adult dosage for dopamine is 2 to 10 mcg/kg/min IV infusion. A patient who weighs 250 pounds will receive more dopamine than a patient who weighs 175 pounds.

Understand the Numbers

If the physician orders dopamine to run at 2 mcg/kg/min for both the 175-pound patient and the 250-pound patient, what is the dosage for each patient?

175 lb ÷ 2.2 kg = 79.5 or 80 kg × 2 mcg/min = 160 mcg/minute

250 lb ÷ 2.2 kg = 113.6 or 114 kg × 2 mcg/min = 228 mcg/minute

Additionally, some drugs can cross the placental barrier and reach the fetus, causing adverse effects. Once the baby is born, certain drugs can also be transferred to the child via the breast milk.

Medications During Pregnancy and Lactation

There are two potential problems that may occur when giving drugs to pregnant patients. First, drugs have the potential to cross the placental barrier and affect the fetus. When giving drugs to pregnant patients, the potential benefits must always be weighed against the risks. The FDA categorizes drugs based on potential risk during pregnancy (Table 3-3).

Second, pregnancy causes several anatomical and physiological changes that must be considered prior to administering drugs. These include:

- An increase in heart rate
- An increase in cardiac output
- An increase of up to 45 percent in blood volume
- A decrease in blood pressure
- A decrease in protein binding
- A decrease in hepatic biotransformation

Another concern may develop after the baby is born. If the mother must begin to take medications for any reason and is also breastfeeding, many drugs can be excreted into the breast milk and ingested by the baby.

Table 3-3 Pregnancy Categories: FDA Assigned

The U.S. Food and Drug Administration's use-in-pregnancy rating system weighs the degree to which available information has ruled out risk to the fetus against the drug's potential benefit to the patient. The ratings, and their interpretation, are as follows:

Category	Interpretation
A	**CONTROLLED STUDIES SHOW NO RISK.** Adequate, well-controlled studies in pregnant women have failed to demonstrate a risk to the fetus in any trimester of pregnancy.
B	**NO EVIDENCE OF RISK IN HUMANS.** Adequate, well-controlled studies in pregnant women have not shown increased risk of fetal abnormalities despite adverse finding in animals, or, in the absence of adequate human studies, animal studies show no fetal risk. The chance of fetal harm is remote but remains a possibility.
C	**RISK CANNOT BE RULED OUT.** Adequate, well-controlled human studies are lacking, and animal studies have shown a risk to the fetus or are lacking as well. There is a chance of fetal harm if the drug is administered during pregnancy, but the potential benefits may outweigh the potential risk.
D	**POSITIVE EVIDENCE OF RISK.** Studies in humans, or investigational or post-marketing data, have demonstrated fetal risk. Nevertheless, potential benefits from the use of the drug may outweigh the potential risk. For example, the drug may be acceptable if needed in a life-threatening situation or serious disease for which safer drugs cannot be used or are ineffective.
X	**CONTRAINDICATED IN PREGNANCY.** Studies in animals or humans, or investigational or post-marketing reports, have demonstrated positive evidence of fetal abnormalities or risk, which clearly outweighs any possible benefit to the patient.
N/A	FDA pregnancy rating not available

Pediatric Patients

Neonates pose a particular concern during drug administration. The major organ for biotransformation is the liver. However, the neonate's liver is not fully developed, impairing biotransformation. Drug excretion through the neonate's kidneys may be impaired as well. Therefore, drug dosages to the neonate have to be modified to account for these factors.

In most cases, drug dosages for the pediatric patient are smaller than those of the adult. Drug dosages for the pediatric patient are generally based on body weight and body surface area. Therefore, EMS providers must determine the body weight of the pediatric patient before administering drugs.

Geriatric Patients

As the baby boomers age, there will be an increased use of the EMS system by this population. As patients become older, they are more likely to develop more than one disease process at a time. When this occurs, generally an increased use of medications must become a part of their daily lives. Body systems will respond to these medications differently than they would in younger years. Common physiological effects of aging include a decrease in:

- Cardiac output
- Brain mass
- Renal function
- Respiratory capacity
- Serum albumin
- Body fat
- Total body water
- Biotransformation
- Excretion

The listed changes that occur with age may also cause a change in pharmacokinetics and pharmacodynamics. Therefore, the dosages of many drugs may have to be reduced when given to the elderly.

Pharmacodynamics Terminology

Pharmacodynamics can be described in a variety of ways. EMS professionals should be familiar with the following descriptive terms:

- **Additive:** An additive effect is the effect that one drug contributes to the action of another. For example, a narcotic analgesic such as morphine may have an additive effect on someone who is taking an antihistamine drug, such as hydroxyzine, because both drugs cause CNS depression.
- **Antagonist:** Antagonism is the mutual opposition in effect between two or more drugs. For example, EMS providers may use naloxone to oppose the effects of a morphine overdose because naloxone and morphine are antagonists.
- **Cumulative:** Cumulative effect is the result of repeated doses of drugs that accumulate in the body to produce symptoms of poisoning.
- **Depressant:** A depressant is a drug that depresses a body function. For example, the drug codeine is a narcotic analgesic that produces generalized CNS depression.
- **Habituation:** Habituation is the act of becoming accustomed. To habituate to a drug is to develop physical tolerance to and dependence on the drug.
- **Hypersensitiveness:** Hypersensitiveness is the excessive susceptibility to the action of a drug.
- **Idiosyncrasy:** Idiosyncrasy is an accelerated, toxic, or uncharacteristic response to the usual therapeutic dose of a drug.
- **Irritation:** An irritation is temporary tissue inflammation caused by drug action.
- **Physiological action:** Physiological action is the effect on a body function produced by a drug.
- **Potentiation:** Potentiation is the enhanced action of two drugs, in which the total effects are greater than the sum of each drug's independent effects.
- **Synergism:** Synergism is the joint action of two drugs producing an effect that neither drug could produce alone.
- **Therapeutics:** Therapeutics is the production of favorable results from application of a remedy, such as a drug, in the management of disease.
- **Tolerance:** Tolerance is the progressive decrease in the effectiveness or response of a drug.
- **Untoward reaction:** An untoward reaction is a harmful side effect of a drug treatment.

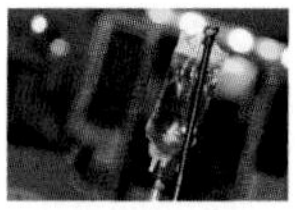

SCENARIO REVISITED

Did you consider the case of Charlene? As you recall, Charlene is experiencing anaphylaxis due to multiple bee stings. She has audible stridor and hives, cannot speak, and is becoming cyanotic, which indicates the development of shock. The EMS team has prioritized this as a life-threatening emergency, has secured an advanced airway, and is monitoring her ECG while administering an IV bolus of 0.3 to 0.5 mg of epinephrine.

Check the Evidence

Epinephrine can be given by SubQ, IM, or IV bolus followed by an IV infusion if necessary. IV epinephrine should be considered immediately if life-threatening signs and symptoms are present.

After the epinephrine bolus, the team will prepare for an IV infusion of epinephrine if necessary. After the epinephrine, Charlene will be given 10 to 50 mg slow IV bolus of diphenhydramine.

Once your team has performed an appropriate assessment, you should proceed using a critical thinking approach to medication administration.

Step 1: Determine signs and symptoms to be treated.
Step 2: Consider both the risks and benefits of treating or not treating your patient.

Step 3: Choose the medication that provides the best possible outcome.

Step 4: Remember the drug's indications, contraindications, and precautions.

Step 5: Decide the best route for administering the medication for the best outcome.

Step 6: Administer the medication(s) according to the 7 Patient Rights.

1. The right patient
2. The right drug
3. The right drug amount
4. The right time
5. The right route
6. The right documentation
7. The right of the patient to accept or refuse the medication(s)

Step 7: Reevaluate the patient for the desired and undesired effects.

Let's Recap

It is not enough for EMS professionals to know how much of a drug to give and when to give it. Understanding basic pharmacokinetics and pharmacodynamics is essential to knowing the desired therapeutic effects and anticipating possible side effects. For each drug administered, you should be aware of such factors as the drug's rate of absorption, minimum therapeutic concentration, toxic levels, and possible and anticipated side effects.

SCENARIO CONCLUSION

After you transport Charlene to the emergency department (ED) (where she does fine), the paramedics explain why both epinephrine and diphenhydramine were given. They explain that epinephrine and diphenhydramine have a potentiation effect. That means the enhanced action of the two drugs produce total effects that are greater than the sum of each drug. For example, Charlene had histamine effects from the bee stings that, for one, caused airway compromise.

The immediate treatment for severe anaphylaxis is oxygen and epinephrine. Epinephrine has both alpha- and beta-adrenergic properties. Stimulation of $beta_1$-adrenergic receptors increases the rate and force of cardiac contractions, resulting in an increase in cardiac output. Stimulation of $beta_2$-adrenergic receptors relaxes the bronchial smooth muscles, thereby increasing vital lung capacity. Epinephrine's stimulation of alpha-receptors causes the arterioles of the bronchioles to constrict, which can help reduce edema. Alpha-adrenergic stimulation also produces peripheral vasoconstriction, which aids in raising arterial blood pressure. Diphenhydramine competes with histamine for H_1 receptor sites. It has significant anticholinergic properties. Diphenhydramine blocks the effects of histamine.

The potentiation of epinephrine (increasing lung capacity, cardiac output, and blood pressure) and that of diphenhydramine (blocking the effects of histamine) can reverse Charlene's anaphylaxis symptoms.

PRACTICE EXERCISES

1. Pharmacodynamics is the study of drug:
   a. Movement
   b. Absorption
   c. Concentration
   d. Mechanism of action
2. Pharmacokinetics is the study of drug:
   a. Movement
   b. Absorption
   c. Concentration
   d. Mechanism of action
3. ____________ effect is the result of repeated doses of drugs that accumulate in the body to produce symptoms of poisoning.
   a. Therapeutic
   b. Potentiation
   c. Depressant
   d. Cumulative
4. Once dissolved, a drug begins the ____________ phase.
   a. Administration
   b. Pharmaceutical
   c. Pharmacokinetic
   d. Pharmacodynamic
5. When a drug tends to combine with its receptor, it is said to have:
   a. Efficacy
   b. Tolerance
   c. Affinity
   d. Cumulative effects
6. The amount of drug that binds to blood proteins or becomes stored in the body's fatty tissues is termed a:
   a. Volatile drug
   b. Metabolite
   c. Bound drug
   d. Free drug
7. A component of a cell that combines with a drug to initiate a response is called a:
   a. Molecule
   b. Synapse
   c. Receptor
   d. "Key"
8. ____________ is the movement of fluid through a membrane caused by differences in hydrostatic pressure.
   a. Facilitated diffusion
   b. Filtration
   c. Diffusion
   d. Osmosis

9. Drugs that bind to receptors to inhibit a response are called:
a. Antagonists
b. Volatile
c. Agonists
d. Prodrugs

10. When a drug's risk to the fetus cannot be ruled out, it is in the FDA's pregnancy category of:
a. A
b. B
c. C
d. D

CASE STUDIES

1. You are assigned to Rescue 8 as a paramedic student, along with two paramedics. Rescue 8 is called out to an overdose patient. Upon arrival, you find an unconscious 45-year-old female who her boyfriend says has taken an unknown amount of heroin. A rapid assessment reveals that she has:
Resp: 8 breaths/minute
Pulse: 64 beats/minute and regular
Skin: Warm and dry
The paramedics immediately begin an IV, oxygen, and ECG monitor and administer naloxone. Once the patient has been transported to the ED, you ask why the paramedics gave naloxone.

The paramedics explain that naloxone is an opioid antagonist used as an opioid antidote. When someone takes heroin, it acts similar to a "key" that fits into the receptors, or the "locks" of the brain, causing CNS depression. When naloxone is given, its key takes over, displaces many of the heroin keys, and blocks many of the heroin effects. In this case, naloxone has affinity (attraction to the receptors) but does not have efficacy (to produce desired effects).

2. You are assigned to Rescue 51 as part of your field internship during paramedic school. Rescue 51 is called to the home of a 60-year-old male who is complaining of weakness and being short of breath. Upon arrival, the patient is sitting in his chair and able to communicate. Patient assessment reveals the following:
Resp: 10 breaths/minute and somewhat labored
Pulse: 48 beats/minutes with an occasional premature ventricular contraction
Blood pressure: 110/60 mm Hg
The patient has no history of cardiac disease. After being thoroughly assessed, the patient is administered atropine to increase his heart rate and transported to the ED for further testing.

After the patient has left for the hospital, you ask the paramedics how the atropine produces its therapeutic effect; it seems to have both affinity and efficacy. However, even though atropine does produce the desired effect of increasing the heart rate, it does so by inhibiting the action of acetylcholine. Atropine is an anticholinergic, or an antagonist. Therefore, atropine has affinity but does not have efficacy.

MATH EQUATIONS

U.S.-to-Metric Conversions and Metric-to-U.S. Conversions

U.S.-to-Metric

1. 125 lb = ______ kg.
2. 54 lb = ______kg.
3. 235 lb = ______kg.
4. 8 lb = ______ kg.
5. 185 lb = ______ kg.

Metric-to-U.S.

1. 84 kg = ______ lb.
2. 100 kg = ______ lb.
3. 15 kg = ______ lb.
4. 54 kg = ______ lb.
5. 107 kg = ______ lb.

REFERENCES

Beck, R. K. (2012). The basics of pharmacokinetics and pharmacodynamics. In *Pharmacology for the EMS provider.* New York, NY: Delmar, Cengage Learning.

Brent, J., ed. (2005). *Atropine in critical care toxicology: Diagnosis and management of the critically poisoned patient.* Philadelphia, PA: Elsevier/Mosby.

Deglin, J. H., Vallerand, A. H., and Sanboski, C. A. (2011). *Davis's drug guide for nurses, twelfth edition.* Philadelphia, PA: F.A. Davis Company.

Elsevier, Inc. Anaphylaxis: summary. (2012). Retrieved October 18, 2013 from www.clinicalkey.com/topics/immunology/anaphylaxis.html

Kruszeinicki, K. S., for ABC Science, Dr. Karl's Great Moments in Science. (2013). How does the blood-brain barrier work? Retrieved October 18, 2013 from http://www.abc.net.au/science/articles/2013/07/23/3808471.htm

U.S. Food and Drug Administration Office of Women's Health R&D. Consistency of pregnancy labeling across different therapeutic classes. (2012). Retrieved October 18, 2013 from http://www.fda.gov/downloads/scienceresearch/specialtopics/womenshealthsearch/ucm308982.pdf

Venes, D., ed. (2013). *Taber's cyclopedic medical dictionary* (22nd ed.). Philadelphia, PA: F. A. Davis Company.

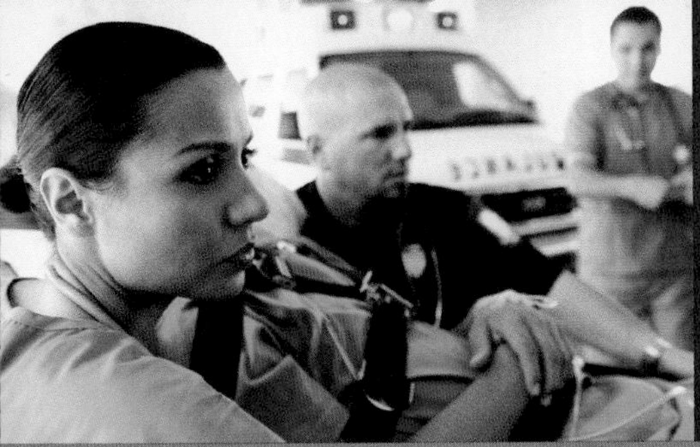

CHAPTER 4

Autonomic Pharmacology

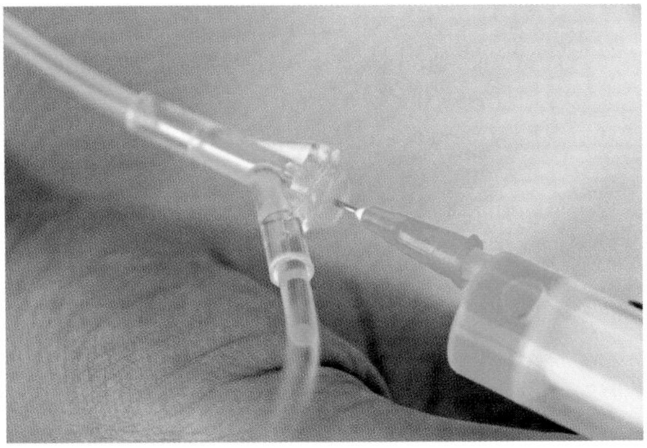

IV bolus drug administration. *(Photograph © GDragan/iStock/Thinkstock)*

LEARNING OUTCOMES

- Describe the organization of the nervous system.
- Explain the process of neurochemical transmission.
- Compare the functions of the parasympathetic and the sympathetic nervous systems.
- Compare the functions of the adrenergic and cholinergic nervous systems.
- List the adrenergic receptors and explain each of their effects on the body.

KEY TERMS

Acetylcholine
Adrenergic
Alpha$_1$-adrenergic receptor
Alpha$_2$-adrenergic receptor
Beta$_1$-adrenergic receptor
Beta$_2$-adrenergic receptor
Central nervous system
Cholinergic
Chronotropic
Effector organ
Epinephrine
Ganglia
Innervate
Inotropic
Motoneurons
Neurotransmitter
Norepinephrine
Parasympathetic nervous system
Parasympatholytic
Parasympathomimetic
Peripheral nervous system
Reflex arc
Sympathetic nervous system
Sympatholytic
Sympathomimetic
Synapse
Vagus nerve

SCENARIO OPENING

You have been assigned to Rescue 22 with two paramedics as your field-internship preceptors. While cleaning the unit, a call comes in for a "man having chest pains." Your 5-minute response time takes you to a local automobile dealership. The sales manager, Dwayne, is sitting in his office holding the center of his chest. One of the salesmen states that Dwayne's pain started about 2 hours ago, but he did not want any help. However, Dwayne has become confused and cannot respond to verbal commands. Dwayne is 54 years old and is approximately 100 pounds overweight. Rapid assessment reveals the following:

Level of Consciousness:	conscious, confused, and disoriented
Respirations:	10 breaths/minute, with clear lung sounds
Pulse:	38 beats/minute and weak a 12-lead ECG shows a sinus bradycardia with a regular rate (Fig. 4-1)
Blood pressure:	74/60
Skin:	pale, cool, and damp
Oxygen saturation (SpO_2):	88 percent
History:	no known illnesses

effective Communication

You should be thinking of some common causes of bradycardia such as tissue damage due to aging or previous myocardial infarction (MI), increased blood pressure, medications (beta-blockers, calcium channel blockers, anti-psychotics), or a recent viral or bacterial illness.

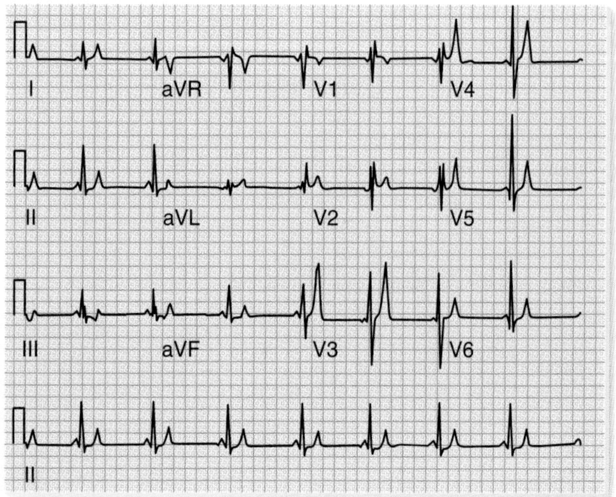

Figure 4-1 Sinus bradycardia.

Introduction

Many of the drugs used by EMS professionals affect tissues that receive their nerve impulses from the **autonomic nervous system.** Most of these drugs produce effects by imitating or opposing neurotransmitters that are released by fibers that innervate (stimulate) smooth muscle, cardiac muscle, and certain glands. A **neurotransmitter** is a chemical substance located on a presynaptic neuron (Fig. 4-2). When the neuron is stimulated, the neurotransmitter travels across the synapse to act on the target cell to either excite or inhibit it. The specific tissues stimulated by the autonomic nervous system are called **effector organs.** The term effector simply means that when a tissue is stimulated, a specific effect should occur.

This chapter presents the general anatomy and physiology of the autonomic nervous system. Included is a discussion of how specific neurotransmitters transmit nerve impulses and how certain drugs can affect the functions of these neurotransmitters. By understanding the basic functions of the autonomic nervous system, one can better predict the various effects drugs may produce on the effector organs stimulated by the autonomic nervous system, as these interactions are the basis of much of the treatment in the out-of-hospital setting.

Physiology of the Nervous System

The nervous system is divided into two major subdivisions: the **central nervous system** (CNS) and the **peripheral nervous system** (PNS). The CNS consists of the brain and spinal cord, and the PNS consists of the cranial nerves and spinal nerves that include the nerves of the autonomic nervous system and its ganglia. Figure 4-3 illustrates the divisions and subdivisions of the nervous system.

The autonomic nervous system is that portion of the PNS that controls the body's automatic or involuntary functions. It helps to control arterial blood pressure, cardiac function, gastrointestinal functions, body temperature, bladder emptying, and many other activities. The autonomic nervous system acts on the various tissue effector organs to reduce or slow their activity or to initiate their function.

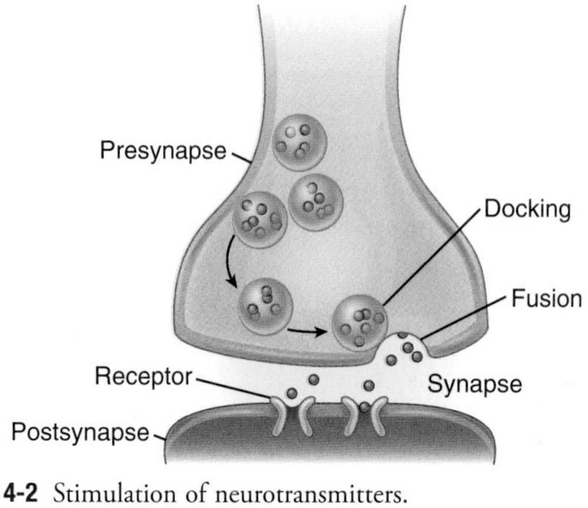

Figure 4-2 Stimulation of neurotransmitters.

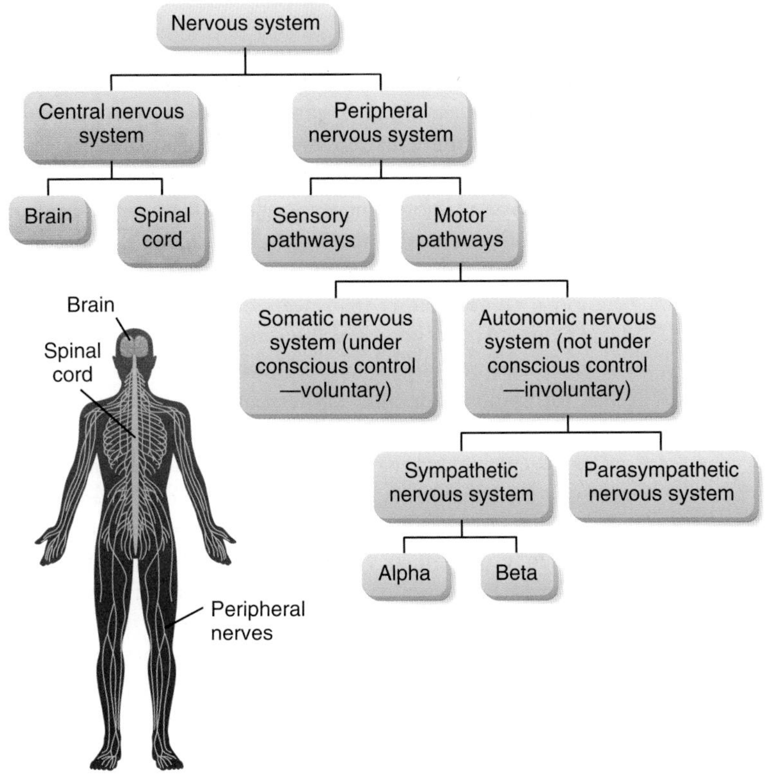

Figure 4-3 Divisions and subdivisions of the nervous system.

The autonomic nervous system is capable of causing rapid changes in the body's automatic functions. For example, it can double the heart rate in 3 to 5 seconds or double the arterial blood pressure within 10 to 15 seconds. Conversely, the autonomic nervous system can lower arterial blood pressure to the point of fainting within 4 to 5 seconds. In short, the autonomic nervous system maintains rapid and effective control of most internal functions of the body.

The autonomic nervous system contains automatic **motoneurons.** Motoneurons are motor neurons that convey impulses to effector tissues from the CNS. In other words, they stimulate effector tissues. Automatic effector tissues include cardiac, smooth muscle, gland, and epithelial tissues.

Neurochemical Transmission

The autonomic nervous system is activated mainly by centers located in the brain and spinal cord. When activated, the autonomic nervous system functions on what is termed the **reflex arc** principle (Fig. 4-4). A reflex arc is the complete circuit of nerves involved in an involuntary movement, from the stimulus to the response: the sensory neuron ending in the spinal cord, the motoneuron from the spinal cord to the effecter organ, and the connecting neurons within the spinal column. There is not an actual connection between two nerve cells or between a nerve cell and the effector organ it **innervates.** The basic units of the system are its neurons and neuronal synapses (Fig. 4-5). A **synapse** is the space between two neurons, or the space between a neuron and an effector organ. An electrical signal travels along the neuron and causes the release of a neurotransmitter (a body-produced chemical) from the *pre*synaptic neuron. The neurotransmitter moves across the synaptic space and combines with receptors on the *post*synaptic neuron. These actions cause an electrical charge in the neuron's membrane ion permeability, which then starts an action impulse potential in the postsynaptic neuron of the effector

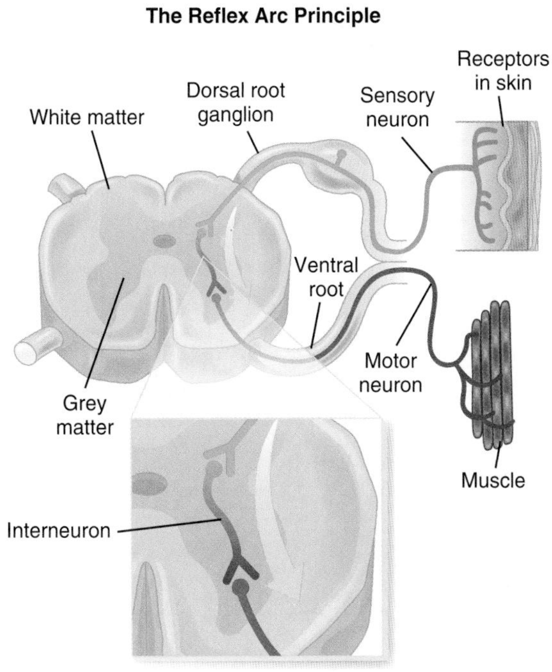

Figure 4-4 Reflex arc.

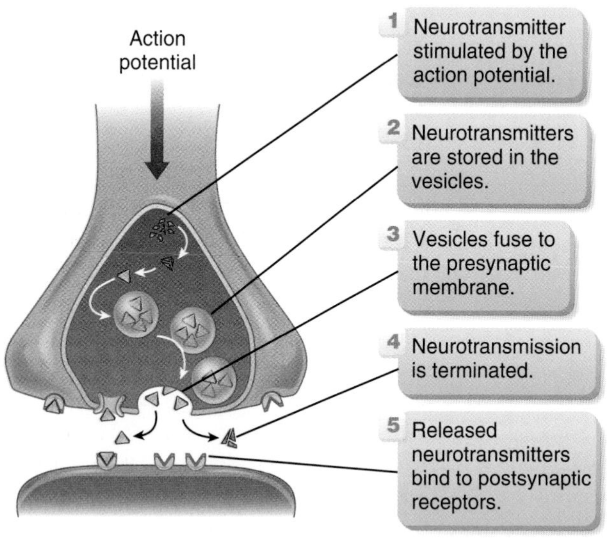

Figure 4-5 Nerve impulse transmission.

organ. The result is continuation of electrical flow causing contraction of a muscle, the secretion of a gland, the contraction of a pupil, or an alteration of the heart.

The Parasympathetic and Sympathetic Nervous Systems

The autonomic nervous system is composed of two anatomically and physiologically separate divisions: the **parasympathetic** and **sympathetic nervous systems.** The parasympathetic nervous system is connected with the CNS through certain cranial nerves and through the middle three sacral segments of the spinal cord. An alternate name that reminds us of its location is *craniosacral.* The **ganglia** (nervous tissue) of the parasympathetic nervous system are located near the effector organs stimulated. The sympathetic nervous system is connected with the CNS through the thoracic and upper lumbar segments of the spinal cord. An alternate name that reminds us of its location is *thoracolumbar.* Its ganglia are located near the spinal column rather than near the effector organs stimulated (Fig. 4-6).

Many effector organs are simultaneously stimulated by both the sympathetic and parasympathetic nervous systems. Physiologically, stimulation by the sympathetic nervous system excites a response, whereas stimulation by the parasympathetic nervous system inhibits a response. The opposition of these two systems works to produce normal automatic body functions. The neural pathways for each system frequently travel together, especially in the thorax, abdomen, and pelvis.

Parasympathetic Nervous System

The major nerves of the parasympathetic nervous system are the two **vagus nerves.** Approximately 75 percent of all parasympathetic nerve fibers are located in the vagus nerves, which travel through the entire thoracic and abdominal region of the body (Fig. 4-7).

The parasympathetic nervous system is the main regulator of many automatic effector organs, including the heart, digestive tract smooth muscle, glands that secrete digestive juices, and endocrine gland cells that secrete insulin. The

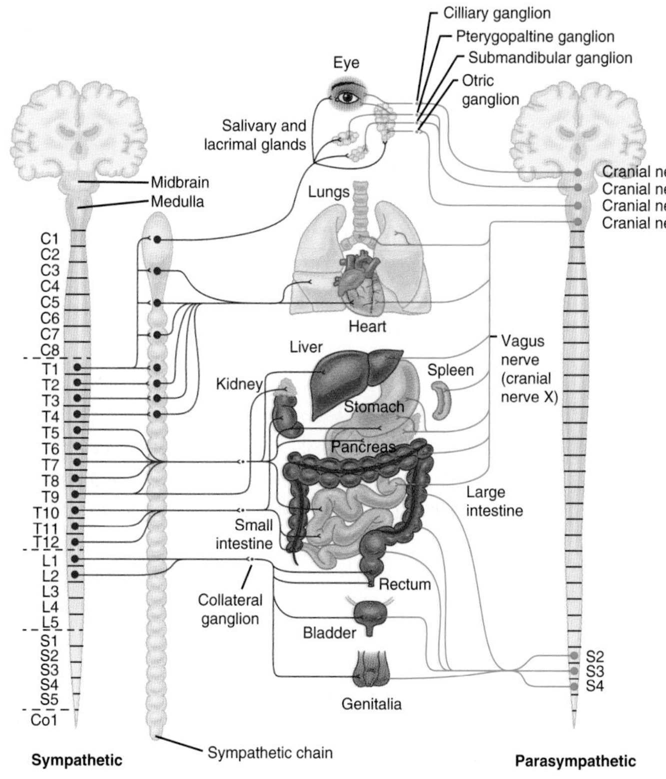

Figure 4-6 Comparison of the parasympathetic and sympathetic nervous systems.

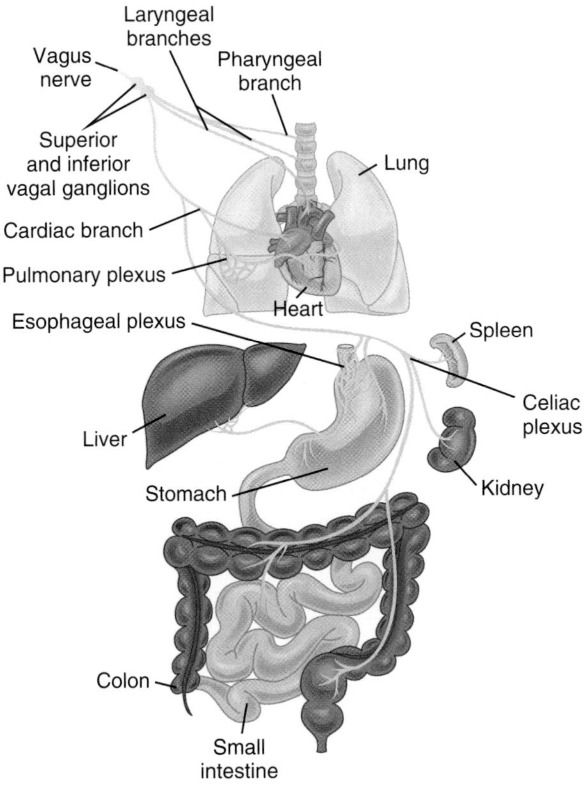

Figure 4-7 The vagus nerve.

parasympathetic division of the autonomic nervous system dominates during nonstressful situations, with the following effect on the body:

- Heart rate slows to a normal rate (negative **chronotropic** effect)
  - Atrioventricular (AV) node conduction velocity decreases
  - Sinoatrial (SA) node rate decreases
  - Atrial muscle contractility decreases
  - Ventricular muscle contractility decreases
- Bronchioles of the lung constrict to a normal size
- Salivary glands increase secretions
- Stomach motility increases
- Digestive juices increase
- Pupil size constricts to normal size
- Glucose storage increases

Vagus nerve fibers do not reach the ventricles of the heart. Therefore, vagal stimulation causes decreased heart rate by its effects on atrial muscle, particularly affecting conduction through the AV node.

Acetylcholine is the neurotransmitter of the parasympathetic nervous system. Most of the effects produced by the parasympathetic nervous system are caused by acetylcholine interacting with cholinergic receptors on the effector cells. There are two main classes of cholinergic receptors: muscarinic and nicotinic. Autonomic effector cells typically have muscarinic receptors.

Check the **Evidence**

Muscarinic receptors are of slow onset but long duration and may be excitatory or inhibitory. These receptors are associated with the neurotransmitter junction.

An example of a drug that affects the parasympathetic nervous system is atropine. Atropine is a parasympathetic blocker. It competes with acetylcholine for receptor sites, blocking its action, thus causing an increase in heart rate. One of the uses for atropine in EMS is in cases of symptomatic bradycardia. Drugs such as atropine are referred to as **parasympatholytics** (anticholinergics). A parasympatholytic drug is one that has the ability to block parasympathetic nerve fibers. Drugs that stimulate the parasympathetic nervous system are called **parasympathomimetics.** A parasympathomimetic drug is one that has the ability to produce effects similar to those resulting from stimulation of the parasympathetic nervous system.

Sympathetic Nervous System

Sympathetic nerves originate in the lateral columns of the thoracic and first three to four lumbar segments of the spinal cord. Stimulation of the sympathetic nervous system prepares the body for emergencies. One of the first steps in the body's reaction to stress is a sudden increase in sympathetic activity, which makes the body ready to use maximum energy and to engage in maximum physical activity. This activity has been historically called the "fight or flight" response. Table 4-1 compares the fight or flight response of the body to sympathetic nervous system stimulation with the body's response to the parasympathetic nervous system.

The sympathetic division of the autonomic nervous system dominates during stressful situations with the following effects on the body:

- Heart rate increases (positive chronotropic effect)
- AV node conduction velocity increases
- SA node rate increases
- Atrial muscle contractility increases (positive **inotropic** effect)
- Ventricular muscle contractility increases (positive inotropic effect)
- Increased stroke volume

effective **Communication**

Drugs with a positive chronotropic effect will increase heart rate, whereas drugs with a positive inotropic effect will increase heart contractility.

- Bronchioles of the lung dilate
- Pupil dilation
- Vasodilation of the skeletal muscles
- Vasoconstriction of the skin, kidneys, and digestive organs
- Increased availability of glucose

Table 4-1 Comparison of the Body's Response to Stimulation of the Sympathetic Nervous System vs. the Parasympathetic Nervous System

Sympathetic Stimulation (Fight or Flight)	Parasympathetic Stimulation
Heart	Heart
AV node conduction velocity—increase	AV node conduction velocity—decrease
SA node rate—increase	SA node rate—decrease
Atrial muscle contractility—increase	Atrial muscle contractility—decrease
Ventricular muscle contractility—increase	Ventricular muscle contractility—decrease
Lungs—Bronchodilation	**Lungs**—Bronchoconstriction
Skin	Skin—N/A
Pilomotor muscle—contraction Secretion (sweat)—increase	
Pupils—dilation	**Pupils**—constriction
Salivary glands—decreased secretion	**Salivary glands**—increased secretion
Kidneys—decreased output	**Kidneys**—N/A
Blood pressure—increases	**Blood pressure**—N/A
Glucose—increased availability	**Glucose**—increased storage

Table 4-2 Physiological Actions of the Adrenergic and Cholinergic Systems

Effector Organ	Adrenergic Response (Sympathetic)	Cholinergic Response (Parasympathetic)
Heart		
Rate of contractions	Increased	Decreased
Force of contractions	Increased	Decreased
Blood pressure	Increased	Decreased
Blood vessels		
Skin/mucous membranes	Constriction	Dilation
Skeletal muscle	Dilation	Dilation
Coronary	Dilation, Constriction	
Renal	Constriction	
Pupils	Dilation	Contraction
Bronchi	Relaxation	Contraction
Adrenal medulla	Secretion of epinephrine and norepinephrine	
Glands		
Sweat	Generalized secretion	Localized secretion
Salivary	Slight secretion	Profuse secretions
Gastrointestinal		Increased secretions
Pancreas (islets)	Inhibit insulin secretion	
Metabolic rate	Increased	

The effects on the cardiovascular system, caused by stimulation of the sympathetic nervous system, increase cardiac output. The sympathetic nervous system stimulates all blood vessels except the capillaries. **Epinephrine** and **norepinephrine** are the main neurotransmitters of the sympathetic nervous system.

The Adrenergic and Cholinergic Nervous Systems

The autonomic nervous system can be further described in terms of **adrenergic** (sympathetic) and **cholinergic** (parasympathetic) components. Neurons and effector organs that are activated by epinephrine are called adrenergic. Neurons and effector organs activated by acetylcholine are defined as cholinergic. Adrenergic drugs are ones that imitate the action of epinephrine, and cholinergic drugs are ones that imitate acetylcholine. Table 4-2 compares the physiological actions of the adrenergic and cholinergic systems.

Drugs that oppose the action of epinephrine are called *anti*adrenergic drugs, and drugs that oppose the action of acetylcholine are called *anti*cholinergic drugs. For example, isoproterenol is classified as a beta-adrenergic agonist related to epinephrine, which is also a beta-adrenergic agonist. The drug atropine is classified as an anticholinergic agent that competes at receptor sites with acetylcholine.

Adrenergic receptors are classified as either alpha-adrenergic receptors or beta-adrenergic receptors. Sympathetic stimulation of alpha-adrenergic receptors produces constriction of blood vessels, dilation of the pupils, relaxation of the smooth muscles of the bronchioles in the lungs and gastrointestinal tract, and vasodilation of blood vessels in the skeletal muscles.

Alpha-adrenergic receptors are identified according to the location of their receptors. **Alpha$_1$-adrenergic-receptor** sites are located on the postsynaptic effector cells, and **alpha$_2$-adrenergic-receptor** sites are located on the presynaptic nerve terminals. Stimulating alpha$_2$-receptors inhibits the release of additional norepinephrine. When alpha$_1$-receptors are stimulated, peripheral and coronary vasoconstriction occurs in part because of the excitatory response when adrenergic agents such as norepinephrine and epinephrine are released.

Beta-adrenergic receptors are also divided into two categories: beta$_1$ and beta$_2$. Most **beta$_1$-adrenergic receptors** are

Table 4-3 Alpha-Adrenergic and Beta-Adrenergic Receptor Sites and Functions

Effector Organ	Alpha	Beta
Heart		
SA node		Increased rate ($beta_1$)
AV node		Increased automaticity and conduction velocity ($beta_1$)
Ventricles		Increased force of contraction and conduction velocity ($beta_1$)
Arterioles	Vasoconstriction ($alpha_1$)	Vasodilation ($beta_2$)
Veins	Vasoconstriction ($alpha_1$)	Vasodilation ($beta_2$)
Lungs		Bronchodilation ($beta_2$)
Pupils	Contraction	
Pancreas (Islets)	Decreased secretions	

located in the heart. Stimulation of $beta_1$-adrenergic receptors causes increased heart rate, increased contractility, and an increase in AV conduction. **$Beta_2$-adrenergic receptors** are located mainly in bronchial and vascular smooth muscle. Stimulation of these receptors causes vasodilation, bronchodilation, and uterine relaxation. Blockage of these receptors opposes the effect of the neurotransmitter. Beta-blocking drugs are either selective for $beta_1$-adrenergic receptors, or they are nonselective. Nonselective blocking drugs block both $beta_1$- and $beta_2$-receptors. Table 4-3 lists the alpha-receptor and beta-receptor sites and their functions.

Drugs that influence the sympathetic nervous system are classified according to the alpha and beta effects they produce. For example, norepinephrine activates all alpha-receptors and some beta-receptors, whereas epinephrine activates all alpha-receptors and all beta-receptors. Isoproterenol is a drug that only activates beta-receptors.

Some drugs block the effects of parasympathetic or sympathetic stimulation. These drugs occupy receptor sites, which prevents parasympathetic or sympathetic neurotransmitters from occupying the sites. For example, atropine blocks the effects of acetylcholine by attaching to the acetylcholine receptor site. Excessive parasympathetic stimulation decreases cardiac output. Atropine increases the heart rate and cardiac output by blocking the parasympathetic effects of acetylcholine on the heart. Drugs that stimulate the sympathetic nervous system are called **sympathomimetics**. Drugs that inhibit the sympathetic nervous system are called **sympatholytics**.

SCENARIO REVISITED

Did you consider the case of Dwayne? As you recall, Dwayne is 54 years old and approximately 100 pounds overweight, and EMS was called because of chest pain that began about 2 hours ago. Patient assessment indicates that Dwayne is going into shock, most likely due to his sinus bradycardia of only 38 beats/minute. It is important the Dwayne be given 100 percent humidified oxygen via a nonrebreather mask and have an IV line established. In the case of symptomatic sinus bradycardia, the first drug of choice is atropine. Atropine is classified as a parasympathetic blocker. Acetylcholine is the neurotransmitter of the parasympathetic nervous system. It binds to the atrial muscle receptor sites to enable vagal nerve stimulation. This stimulation can cause the heart rate to slow, causing bradycardia. Atropine competes with acetylcholine for the same receptor sites, blocking its action, thus causing an increase in heart rate. The initial dosage of atropine is 0.5 mg via IV bolus. Repeat doses may be necessary every 3 to 5 minutes to a maximum of 3 mg.

Understand the Numbers

Your atropine comes packaged 1 mg in a 10 mL prefilled syringe. What is the concentration (C) of the atropine? How much volume (V) will you give for 0.5 mg?

C = Amount of drug (mg) ÷ Volume of solution (mL); C = 1 mg ÷ 10 mL = 0.1 mg/mL.

V = Required drug amount (mg) ÷ Concentration (mg/mL); V = 0.5 mg ÷ 0.1 mg/mL = 5 mL.

Other drugs that may be given to Dwayne include a dopamine infusion or an epinephrine infusion to support blood pressure, if needed. However, before any drug is administered, you must first perform an appropriate assessment using the critical thinking approach to medication administration.

Step 1: Determine signs and symptoms to be treated.
Step 2: Consider both the risks and benefits of treating or not treating your patient.
Step 3: Choose the medication that provides the best possible outcome.
Step 4: Remember the drug's indications, contraindications, and precautions.
Step 5: Decide the best route for administering the medication for the best outcome.
Step 6: Administer the medication(s) according to the 7 Patient Rights.

1. The right patient
2. The right drug
3. The right drug amount
4. The right time
5. The right route
6. The right documentation
7. The right of the patient to accept or refuse the medication(s)

Step 7: Reevaluate the patient for the desired and undesired effects.

Let's Recap

The autonomic nervous system regulates automatic effectors that maintain or quickly restore the state of equilibrium of the body's automatic functions. Doubly stimulated organs receive both sympathetic and parasympathetic impulses, which influence their function in opposing ways. For example, sympathetic impulses make the heart beat faster, and parasympathetic impulses slow the heart down. The relationship between the effects of the two opposing systems determines actual heart rate.

The parasympathetic or cholinergic division of the autonomic nervous system regulates the body's involuntary functions. This is mediated through the vagus nerves by the release of acetylcholine. Vagal stimulation slows the heart rate, but this action can be opposed by parasympathetic blocking drugs (anticholinergics).

The sympathetic or adrenergic division enables the body to respond to emergencies or stress. This system is regulated mainly by the release of norepinephrine or epinephrine. The sympathetic division is further subdivided into alpha-adrenergic and beta-adrenergic receptors. Stimulation of alpha-adrenergic receptors causes vasoconstriction of blood vessels, a decrease in gastrointestinal secretion, and dilation of the pupils. Stimulation of beta-adrenergic receptors causes an increase in the rate and force of contraction of the heart, dilation of the arterioles of skeletal muscles, and dilation of the bronchiolar muscles of the lungs.

SCENARIO CONCLUSION

The initial dose of atropine for symptomatic bradycardia is 0.5 mg IV bolus. Additional doses may be given every 3 to 5 minutes up to a total of 3 mg, if necessary. If blood pressure support is needed, a dopamine infusion or an epinephrine infusion may be ordered. The dosage for dopamine is 2 to 10 mcg/kg/minute. Generally, cardiac stimulation ($beta_1$-adrenergic effects) of dopamine occurs in the dosage range of 5 to 15 mcg/kg/minute. If an epinephrine infusion is used, the dosage is 2 to 10 mcg/minute. Epinephrine affects both $beta_1$- (cardiac) adrenergic receptors and $beta_2$- (pulmonary) adrenergic receptor sites. Epinephrine also has alpha-adrenergic agonist properties, resulting in vasoconstriction.

Understand the Numbers

The physician orders an IV infusion of dopamine at 5 mcg/kg/minute. The dopamine comes premixed at 1,600 mcg/mL in a 250 mL bag. How many gtt/min will be infused using a minidrip set (60 gtt/mL)? Dwayne weighs 325 pounds.

325 lb ÷ 2.2 kg = 147.7 or 148 kg. 5 mcg × 148 kg = 740 mcg to be administered/minute.

There are 1,600 mcg/mL (60 gtt) of dopamine in the IV bag. Therefore, the volume to be infused is: 740 mcg ÷ 1,600 mcg/mL = 0.46 mL/minute. Using a 60 gtt set, the infusion rate is: 0.46 mL × 60 gtt set ÷ 1 min = 27.6 or 28 gtt/minute to deliver 5 mcg/kg/minute to Dwayne.

PRACTICE EXERCISES

1. Stimulation of $alpha_1$-receptor sites causes:
a. Bronchodilation
b. An increase in heart rate
c. Peripheral and coronary vasoconstriction
d. Inhibition of the release of norepinephrine

2. A neurotransmitter is:
a. A body-produced chemical
b. An electrical impulse
c. A postsynaptic neuron
d. A presynaptic neuron

3. Neurons and effector organs that are activated by epinephrine are called:
a. Adrenergic
b. Cholinergic
c. Antiadrenergic
d. Anticholinergic

4. The _____ convey(s) impulses to effector tissues from the CNS.
a. Synapse
b. Reflex arc
c. Motoneurons
d. Neurotransmitter

5. The space between two neurons, or the space between a neuron and an effector organ, is called:
a. Synapse
b. Reflex arc
c. Presynaptic space
d. Postsynaptic space

6. The major nerves of the parasympathetic nervous system are the two:
a. Preganglionic fibers
b. Lumbar nerves
c. Sacral nerves
d. Vagus nerves

7. The neurotransmitter of the parasympathetic nervous system is:
a. Atropine
b. Epinephrine
c. Acetylcholine
d. Norepinephrine

8. The main neurotransmitters of the sympathetic nervous system are:
   a. Epinephrine and atropine
   b. Epinephrine and norepinephrine
   c. Norepinephrine and acetylcholine
   d. Epinephrine and acetylcholine

9. $Alpha_1$-receptor sites are located in the:
   a. Heart
   b. Postsynaptic effector cells
   c. Presynaptic nerve terminals
   d. Bronchial and vascular smooth muscle

10. When $beta_1$-receptors are stimulated, _____ occurs:
   a. Bronchodilation
   b. Increased heart rate
   c. Coronary vasoconstriction
   d. Release of norepinephrine

CASE STUDY

You are called to a possible suicide. Upon arrival, you are directed to Deb's kitchen where she is lying on the floor unconscious. Her husband, Doug, had just come home from work and found her there on the floor. A suicide note is lying on the counter, next to an empty bottle of atenolol. Doug admits that Deb has been going to a counselor for about 3 months due to depression. Deb is 50 years old.

Your assessment reveals Deb's vitals as:

Level of Consciousness: Unconscious—responds to deep pain

Resp: 10 breaths/minute and shallow, with clear lungs

Heart: Rate = 48 beats/minute. ECG indicates bradycardia with a first-degree heart block (Fig. 4-8).

Blood pressure: 70/50 mm Hg

Atenolol (Tenormin) is a beta-blocker used in the management of hypertension and angina pectoris and also in the prevention of MI. Its action blocks stimulation of $beta_1$ (myocardial)—adrenergic receptors. Therapeutic effects of atenolol include decreased blood pressure and heart rate. Emergency treatment for Deb may include:

- Atropine: parasympathetic (anticholinergic) blocker
- Epinephrine: adrenergic, bronchodilator
- Dopamine: adrenergic, inotropic
- Glucagon: hormone that stimulates hepatic production of glucose

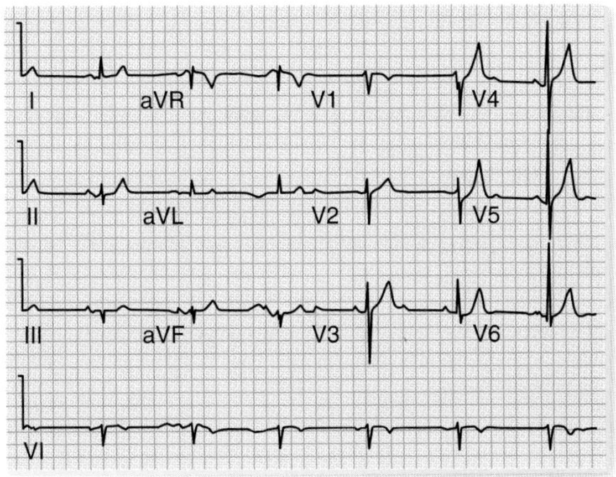

Figure 4-8 Sinus bradycardia with first-degree block.

Check the Evidence

Glucagon increases heart rate and myocardial contractility and improves AV conduction. These effects are unchanged by the presence of beta-receptor blocking drugs. This suggests that glucagon's mechanism of action may bypass the beta-adrenergic receptor site. Because it may bypass the beta-receptor site, glucagon can be considered as an alternative therapy for profound beta-blocker intoxication.

1. A drug with a positive inotropic effect:
   a. Increases the heart rate
   b. Increases the firing rate of the SA node
   c. Increases the strength of cardiac contractions
   d. Maintains the normal strength of cardiac contractions

2. Another term used for anticholinergic is:
   a. Parasympathomimetic
   b. Parasympatholytic
   c. Chronotropic
   d. Inotropic

3. Neurons and effector organs that are activated by epinephrine are called:
   a. Chronotropic
   b. Cholinergic
   c. Adrenergic
   d. Inotropic

MATH EQUATIONS

Metric-to-Metric Conversions

1. 5.25 g = ________ mg
2. 5 L = ________ mL
3. 500 mg = ________ mcg
4. 200 mcg = ________ mg
5. 2,000 mg = ________ g
6. 3.75 g = ________ mcg
7. 250 mL = ________ L
8. 1.5 L = ________ mL
9. 250,000 mg = ________ g
10. 3,250 mcg = ________ mg

REFERENCES

Beck, R. K. (2012). Autonomic pharmacology. In *Pharmacology for the EMS provider.* New York: Delmar, Cengage Learning.

Deglin, J. H., Vallerand, A. H., and Sanboski, C. A. (2011). *Davis's drug guide for nurses.* (12th ed.). Philadelphia, PA: F.A. Davis Company.

Mayo Clinic. Bradycardia: causes. (2011). Retrieved November 11, 2013 from www.mayoclinic.com/health/bradycardia/DS00947/DSECTION=causes

O'Grady, J., Anderson, S., and Pringle, D. (2011). Successful treatment of severe atenolol overdose with calcium chloride. Retrieved November 6, 2013 from www.cjem-online.ca/v3/n3/p224

Peterson, C. D., Leeder, J. S., and Sterner, S. (1984). Glucagon therapy for beta-blocker overdose. Retrieved November 5, 2013 from www.ncbi.nlm.nih.gov/pubmed/6144498

Shamara, A., Tarabar, A. (2013). Beta-blocker toxicity treatment and management. Retrieved November 6, 2013 from www.emedicine.medscape.com/article/813342-treatment

Venes, D., ed. (2013). *Taber's cyclopedic medical dictionary* (22nd ed.). Philadelphia, PA: F. A. Davis Company.

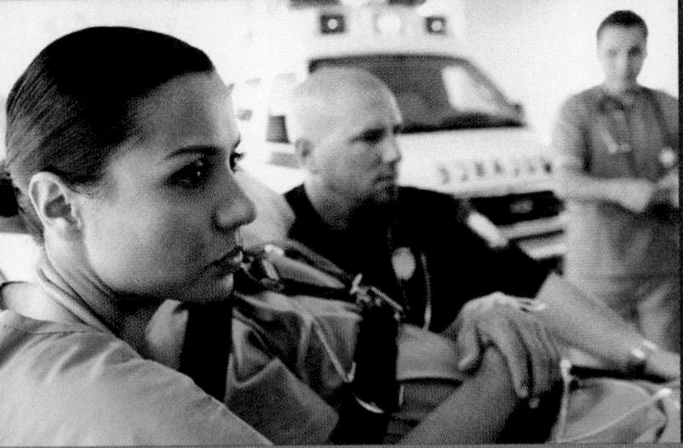

CHAPTER 5

Fluids, Electrolytes, and Intravenous Therapy

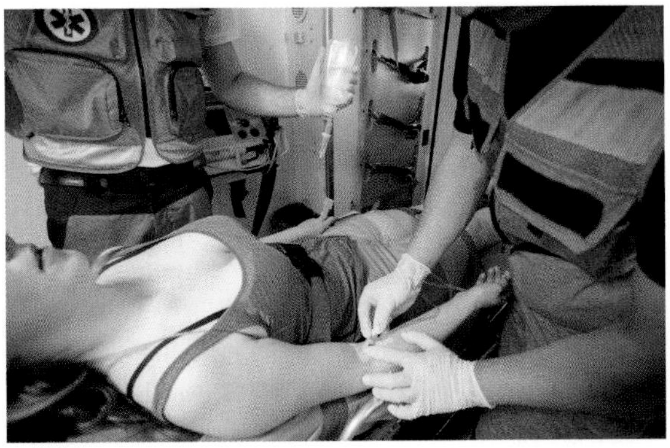

Paramedics starting an IV line. *(Photograph © Thinkstock)*

LEARNING OUTCOMES

- Identify and explain the body water proportions of the major fluid compartments of the body.
- List and describe the roles of the major electrolytes of the body.
- Define and explain the roles of filtration, diffusion, facilitated diffusion, osmosis, and active and passive transport.
- Define and explain the roles of hypotonic, hypertonic, and isotonic solutions.
- List and describe the four clinical situations that result when acid-base balance is disrupted.
- List the various IV fluids and describe the major indications for each.
- Explain the procedure for starting an IV line.

KEY TERMS

Acidosis
Active transport
Alkalosis
Anion
Cation
Colloid
Crystalloid
Diffusion
Electrolyte
Facilitated diffusion
Fluid, body
Fluid, extracellular
Fluid, interstitial
Fluid, intracellular
Fluid, intravascular
Homeostasis
Hydrostatic pressure
Hypertonic
Hypotonic
Ion
Isotonic
Nonelectrolytes
Osmosis
pH
Plasma
Semipermeable membrane

SCENARIO OPENING

You are assigned to two paramedics on Unit #826 at Fire Station #3 during your second field-internship experience. While you are studying notes from last night's class, a call comes in for a "sick woman." Upon arrival, you find a woman (Ellen) who has been experiencing "several episodes" of severe vomiting and diarrhea for the last three hours. When questioned, Ellen's husband states that they attended a pool party where a buffet-style dinner was served. Ellen states that she ate "a lot" of the shrimp and crab dip. She is now resting in bed feeling weak and with some abdominal discomfort.

Physical assessment of Ellen reveals the following:

Level of consciousness:	alert, oriented, weak
Respirations:	22 breaths/minute, clear lung sounds
Blood pressure:	90/66 mm Hg
Heart rate:	130 beats/minute, with no ectopy
Skin:	warm and dry, with poor turgor; dry mucus membranes

Further examination reveals that Ellen's abdomen is soft with deep palpation, but she complains of tenderness. Ellen is not on any medications and is not being treated for any other medical conditions. She is 32 years old.

Questions you should consider include:

1. What do you think Ellen's diagnosis will be?
2. What are the goals of your treatment?
3. What steps will you take to help Ellen?
4. What is your rationale for choosing your treatment options for Ellen?
5. How will you know if the treatment choices are working?

These questions are a few suggestions. You may have other relevant questions as well.

Introduction

Maintaining a proper balance of fluids and electrolytes within the body is necessary for life. Therefore, it is important to be familiar with the basics of body fluids and electrolytes. If, for instance, a patient who is depleted of fluids and electrolytes (such as a patient with severe burns or a patient who is severely dehydrated), it is important to act quickly to help restore the body's internal balance to increase the patient's chances for survival.

This chapter reviews the basics of fluids, electrolytes, and acid-base balance. The chapter also describes some commonly used IV fluids and their roles in the treatment of fluid and electrolyte compromise.

Physiology of Fluids and Electrolytes

Body Fluids

Total **body fluid** varies from individual to individual depending on both sex and age (Table 5-1). However, the average adult has a total body fluid content of approximately 60 percent of body weight. This total body fluid is divided into **intracellular** and **extracellular fluid** compartments (Fig. 5-1). Intracellular fluid (ICF) is the fluid contained inside the body's cells. It accounts for approximately 45 percent of total body weight. Extracellular fluid (ECF) is body fluid outside the cells. It accounts for approximately 15 percent of body weight. Extracellular fluid is further divided into two separate fluid types: **interstitial fluid** and **intravascular fluid** or **plasma**. Interstitial fluid is extracellular fluid located in the spaces between the body's cells. It accounts for approximately 10.5 percent of body weight. Intravascular fluid is the noncellular, fluid portion of blood. It accounts for approximately 4.5 percent of body weight.

To illustrate, a person who weighs 176 pounds (80 kg) has approximately 48 liters (1 L weighs approximately 1 kg) of body fluid. This amount is broken down as follows:

Table 5-1 Approximate Body Water Content as a Percentage of Body Fluids

Age	Total Body Water (TBW)	Extracellular Fluid (ECF)	Intracellular Fluid (ICF)
Infant	74%	40%	34%
Adult Male	60%	28%	32%
Adult Female	50%	25%	25%

Understand the Numbers

80 kg (body weight) × 0.60 (percent of total body water) = 48 L

- Intracellular fluid: 36 L (80 × 0.45 = 36)
- Extracellular fluid: 12 L (80 × 0.15 = 12)
- Interstitial fluid: 8.4 L (80 × 0.105 = 8.4)
- Intravascular fluid: 3.6 L (80 × 0.045 = 3.6)

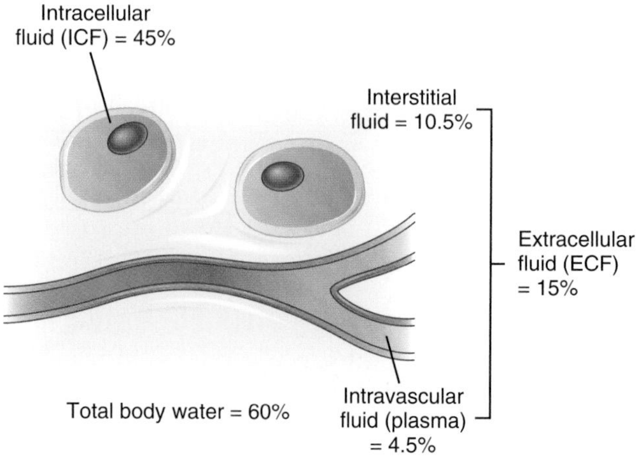

Figure 5-1 Distribution of body fluids.

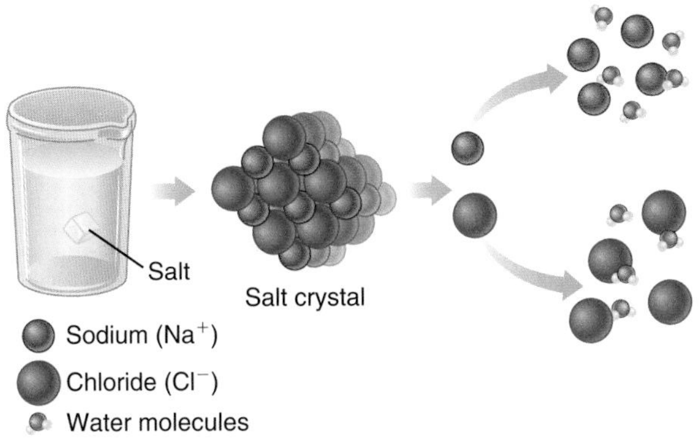

Figure 5-2 Dissociation of electrolytes.

The extracellular fluid aids in controlling the body's internal environment by bathing the cells. The internal environment of the body must be kept within a dynamic state of equilibrium. This state of equilibrium is called **homeostasis.** The body's regulation mechanisms to maintain homeostasis control body temperature, osmotic pressure of blood and its hydrogen ion concentration (pH), and nutrients supplied to the cells. These mechanisms also remove waste products before they accumulate and reach toxic levels.

Electrolytes

An **electrolyte** is a substance that, when placed in water, separates into electrically charged particles called **ions.** A **cation** is a positively charged ion, and an **anion** is a negatively charged ion (Fig. 5-2). The major cations of the body include:

- **Calcium (Ca^{2+}):** Calcium is the most abundant cation in the body. It is required for bone growth, metabolism, blood clotting, normal cardiac function, and the initiation of neuromuscular contractions. Excellent sources of calcium include milk and milk products (except cottage cheese) and calcium-fortified orange juice. Good sources of calcium also include canned sardines and salmon, broccoli, tofu, rhubarb, almonds, figs, and turnip greens.
- **Magnesium (Mg^{2+}):** Magnesium is required for DNA repair, body temperature regulation, protein and carbohydrate metabolism, and neuromuscular contraction. It is a component of enzymes required for the synthesis of adenosine triphosphate (ATP) and the release of energy from ATP.

Check the Evidence

Magnesium deficiency is rare because magnesium is common in foods such as fish, whole grains, fruits, and green vegetables.

- **Potassium (K^+):** Potassium is the major intracellular cation, as well as an important electrolyte in extracellular fluid. It is responsible for acid-base regulation, cell membrane homeostasis, muscle excitability, and nerve impulse conduction. Potassium is found in most foods, such as cereals, dried peas and beans, fresh vegetables, fresh fruits, fruit juices, sunflower seeds, nuts, molasses, cocoa, and fresh fish and meats.
- **Sodium (Na^+):** Sodium is the major extracellular cation. It is the main contributor to osmotic pressure and hydration. Sodium participates in many pumps and receptors on cell membranes and plays a fundamental part in the electrical activities of the body. It is a naturally occurring white crystalline compound—table salt.

The major anions of the body include:

- **Bicarbonate (NCO_3^-):** Bicarbonate is the major buffer of the body. Its main function is to maintain acid-base balance.
- **Chloride (Cl^-):** Chloride is the major extracellular anion. Its main function is to maintain fluid balance.
- **Phosphate (HPO_4^{2-}):** Phosphate is the major intracellular anion. It helps maintain acid-base balance.

Electrolytes are measured in milliequivalents (mEq). A milliequivalent is the concentration of electrolytes in a certain volume of solution, based on the number of available ionic charges. One milliequivalent of a cation will completely react to 1 millequivalent of an anion, forming a new compound. For example:

Na^+ (1 mEq of sodium) and
Cl^- (1 mEq of chloride) combine to form NaCl

Understand the Numbers

2 mEq of calcium (Ca^{2+}) and 1 mEq of chloride (Cl^-) +
1 mEq of chloride (Cl^-) combine to form $CaCl_2$.

Note from Understand the Numbers that Ca^{2+} has two positive charges, or 2 milliequivalents. Therefore, it must have 2 milliequivalents of a singly charged anion (Cl^- + Cl^-) to combine to form calcium chloride. In practice, electrolytes are given as milliequivalents per liter (mEq/L), as in IV solution.

Body fluid also contains compounds with no electrical charges. These substances are called **nonelectrolytes.** Nonelectrolytes are normally measured in milligrams (mg). Nonelectrolytes include:

- **Glucose:** Glucose is a carbohydrate or sugar formed during digestion. It is the most important carbohydrate in metabolism.
- **Urea:** Urea is the major nitrogen end product of protein metabolism. It is formed in the liver.

Fluid Transport

Pharmacologists think of intracellular and extracellular fluid as occupying two separate compartments—the intracellular compartment and the extracellular compartment. For normal metabolism to occur, water, electrolytes, and other substances must pass between these two compartments. To do this, they must cross a **semipermeable membrane** that allows only some molecules to pass through. There are two ways in which

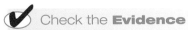

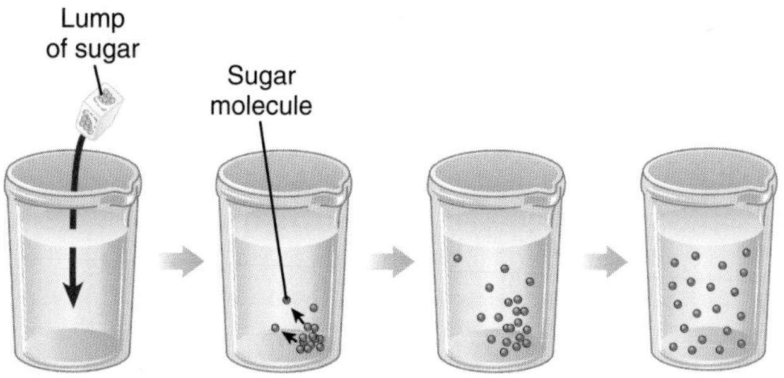

Figure 5-3 The process of diffusion.

this movement occurs: (1) passive transport and (2) active transport.

Passive Transport

Passive transport depends on four mechanisms: (1) filtration, (2) diffusion, (3) facilitated diffusion, and (4) osmosis.

- **Filtration** is the movement of fluid through a membrane caused by differences in hydrostatic pressure. **Hydrostatic pressure** is the force exerted by the weight of a solution; it causes the solution to move from an area of higher pressure to an area of lower pressure. In two compartments separated by a permeable or semipermeable membrane, hydrostatic pressure causes fluid to move from one compartment to the other until the pressure in both compartments is equal.
- **Diffusion** is the tendency of molecules in solution to distribute equally. See diffusion at work by adding a drop of colored dye to a container of water (Fig. 5-3). Soon, without stirring, the dye (solute) spreads itself evenly throughout the water. In diffusion, molecules, atoms, or ions flow from an area of higher concentration to areas of lower concentration, until the concentration (the number of molecules of solute per amount of solution) is the same everywhere in the solution. Diffusion is generally considered a passive process. However, there are instances when the movement of a substance through a cell membrane must happen along a concentration gradient with the help of membrane proteins acting as carrier molecules. This is called **facilitated diffusion.** In the body, oxygen and carbon dioxide move by diffusion.
- **Osmosis** is the diffusion of solute or solvent or both through a permeable or semipermeable membrane. It is a result of the same force that causes solute molecules or ions within a solution to flow from areas of high concentration to areas of low concentration. With two solutions separated by a semipermeable membrane, a difference in solute concentration creates osmotic pressure, which causes water and (if possible) solute to move across the membrane until the solutions are in equilibrium (Fig. 5-4).

Whether both solute and water cross the membrane, or just water, depends on the nature of the solution. There are two

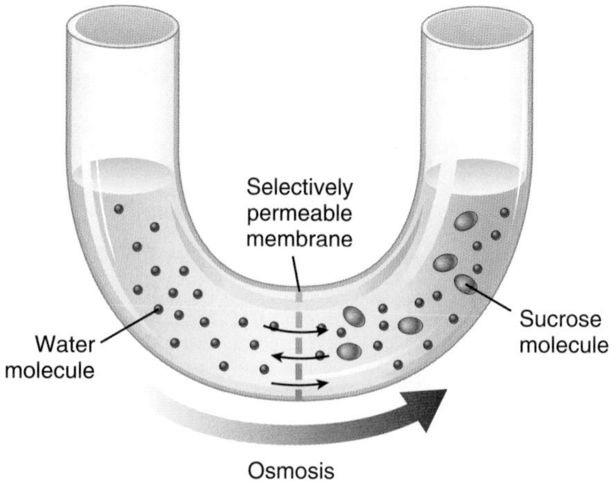

Figure 5-4 Osmosis.

kinds of solutions, with opposite reactions to osmotic pressure: **crystalloid** and **colloid** solutions.

A crystalloid is a substance that truly dissolves—that is, its molecules or atoms separate and disperse completely and equally throughout the solvent. Such a solution is called a *true solution* or a *crystalloid solution.* In a crystalloid solution, the small, individual molecules or atoms of solute easily pass through (diffuse across) a semipermeable membrane. When two crystalloid solutions of unequal concentration are separated by a semipermeable membrane, the osmotic pressure will cause the dissolved molecules or ions to cross the membrane, from the concentrated solution to the solution with lower concentration, until the solute concentration is equal on both sides of the membrane.

Colloids are the physical opposite of crystalloids. When mixed with water, colloids do not truly dissolve. Instead, they form a suspension (sometimes called a *colloid solution*), in which groups of colloid molecules are dispersed throughout the liquid. Unlike crystalloids, colloids do not pass through semipermeable membranes. Therefore, when two colloid solutions of unequal concentration are separated by a semipermeable membrane, osmotic pressure causes the flow of *water* across the membrane, from lower concentration to higher, until the concentration of solute is equal on both sides of the membrane.

effective Communication

In emergency situations, colloids can be used as a plasma expander in place of blood.

In pharmacology, the difference in behavior of the two kinds of solutions allows for different applications. When a crystalloid solution (such as lactated ringers, normal saline, or dextrose 5 percent in water) is injected into the bloodstream, both solute and water can travel across the cell membrane. Crystalloid solutions, therefore, are effective ways of getting water *and* the dissolved substance into the cells. On the other hand, when a colloid solution (such as Dextran or Plasmanate) is injected into the bloodstream, the colloid cannot enter the

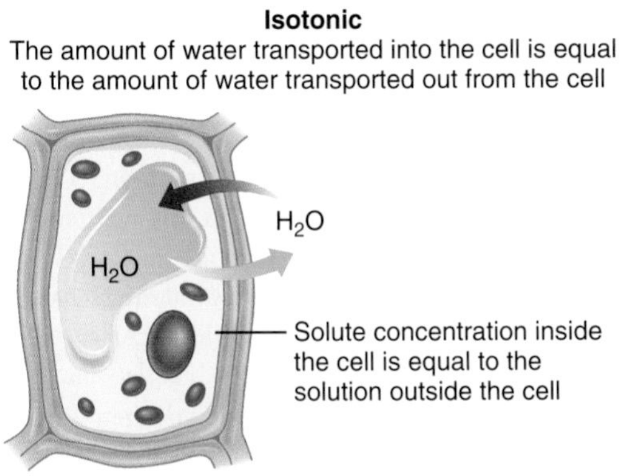
Isotonic
The amount of water transported into the cell is equal to the amount of water transported out from the cell
H_2O
H_2O
Solute concentration inside the cell is equal to the solution outside the cell

Figure 5-5 Passive transport of a cell in an isotonic solution.

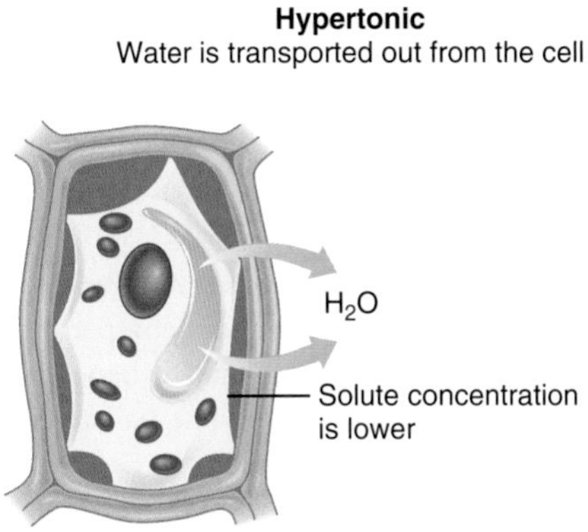
Hypertonic
Water is transported out from the cell
H_2O
Solute concentration is lower

Figure 5-7 Passive transport of a cell in a hypertonic solution.

cells, so osmotic pressure causes water to flow from the cellular compartment into the bloodstream. The flow of water from cell to bloodstream helps maintain vascular volume.

Two solutions may contain different substances but have the same milliequivalence, or ionic potential. Separated by a semipermeable membrane, each has the same osmotic pressure. Such solutions are said to be **isotonic.** For instance, normal saline solution, a common IV solution, is isotonic. Because osmotic pressures on both sides of cell membranes are equal, normal saline solution tends to stay in the extracellular space (primarily the bloodstream) longer than **hypotonic** or **hypertonic** solutions, thus maintaining and increasing vascular volume. Figure 5-5 illustrates the situation in which intracellular and extracellular solutions are isotonic.

A hypertonic solution has a lower ionic potential than the solution with which it is compared. A solution of one-half normal saline, for instance, is hypotonic to normal body fluid. For a normal body cell surrounded by hypotonic fluid, the osmotic pressure on the inside of the cell is greater than on the outside. Water will tend to flow from outside the cell to inside the cell to lower the solute concentration (and therefore the ionic potential). Figure 5-6 illustrates the situation in which extracellular solution is hypotonic to intracellular solution.

A hypertonic solution has a higher solute concentration and ionic potential than the solution with which it is compared. For instance, a solution of dextrose 50 percent in water is hypertonic to normal body fluid. For a cell in a hypertonic solution, the osmotic pressure inside the cell is lower than outside. The higher osmotic pressure outside the cell pulls water out of the cell to lower the solute concentration in the extracellular fluid (Fig. 5-7).

Active Transport

As we have seen, passive transport allows some solutes to travel across cell membranes but only from the concentrated solutions to the less concentrated solutions. Cell metabolism, however, requires substances to travel "upstream," that is, from the less concentrated solution to the more concentrated one (Fig. 5-8). Cell health also requires that the concentration of some substances be higher inside the cell than outside, and vice versa. For instance, under normal conditions, the cellular fluid has more potassium ions than does the extracellular fluid. The process of moving substances across the cell wall from the less concentrated to the more concentrated solution, and keeping the concentration of solutes higher on one side of the cell wall than on the other, is called **active transport**. Active transport

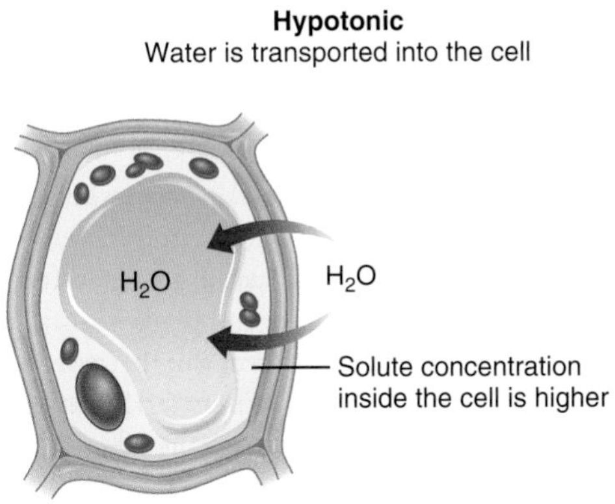
Hypotonic
Water is transported into the cell
H_2O
H_2O
Solute concentration inside the cell is higher

Figure 5-6 Passive transport of a cell in a hypotonic solution.

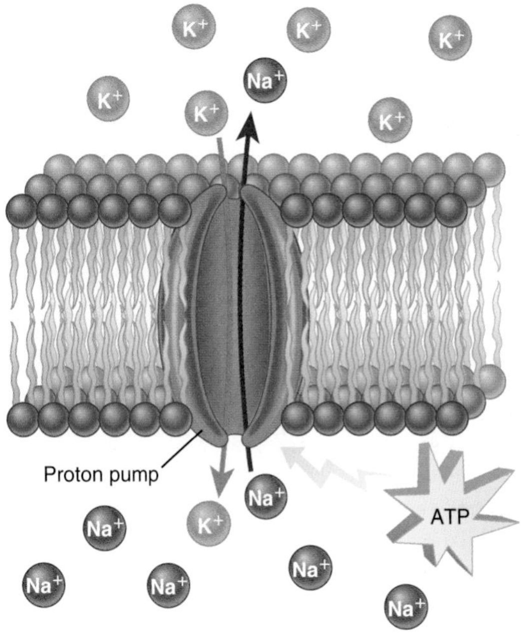
K^+
Na^+
Proton pump
ATP

Figure 5-8 Active transport.

requires metabolic energy. Substances that require active transport across cell membranes include potassium sodium, calcium, hydrogen, chloride, and several sugars and amino acids.

Acid-Base Balance

We have discussed how body chemistry and metabolism work to maintain equilibrium between fluid compartments. A state of equilibrium must also be maintained between the acidity and alkalinity of body fluid. Acid-base balance is the body's way of maintaining this equilibrium.

Body fluid *potential of hydrogen* **(pH)** is the most frequently used measurement of acid-base balance. The pH measurement is inversely related to the body's hydrogen ion concentration. The higher the hydrogen ion centration in a fluid, the lower the pH. Conversely, the lower the hydrogen ion concentration in a fluid, the higher the pH. The pH scale ranges from 1 to 14. A pH reading of 1 means that a substance consists only of hydrogen ions. A pH reading of 14 means that there are no hydrogen ions present. A pH of 7 is neutral.

Arterial blood gases are measured to determine acid-base imbalance using three values: (1) pH, (2) P_aCO_2, and (3) HCO_3. The normal pH of the body ranges from 7.35 to 7.45. When body fluid's pH is greater than 7.45, the body is in a state of **alkalosis.** Body fluid pH of less than 7.35 indicates a state of **acidosis.** Increases or decreases in body pH can be potentially harmful. For example, a significant decrease in the body's pH can cause diminished heart contractions, reduce the body's response to catecholamine release, and inhibit the therapeutic action of drugs. An increase in the body's pH can inhibit the release of oxygen from the red blood cells. Slight changes in H^+ ion concentration can markedly affect rates of chemical reactions in cells. Therefore, regulating H^+ ion concentration is one of the most important facets of homeostasis and is critical to maintaining life.

effective Communication

A body fluid pH higher than 7.8 or lower than 7.0 indicates a very serious, usually fatal condition.

The buffer system is the body's primary mechanism for adjusting and maintaining acid-base balance. The buffer system can act within a fraction of a second to prevent excessive changes in hydrogen ion concentration. This system's effect on acid-base balance is almost instantaneous. Two components of the buffer system include bicarbonate ion (HCO_3^-) and carbonic acid (H_2CO_3), which maintain an equilibrium with the hydrogen ion (H^+):

		20	:	1
H^+	+	HCO_3	$\leftrightarrow$	H_2CO_3
Hydrogen ion		Bicarbonate ion		Carbonic acid

This reaction requires 20 molecules of bicarbonate ion for every molecule of carbonic acid. For the buffer system to maintain body fluid pH, any change in this 20:1 ratio must be immediately corrected.

The respiratory system is the second mechanism for acid-base regulation. If the P_aCO_2 is greater than 45 mm Hg, respiratory acidosis occurs; if P_aCO_2 is less than 35 mm Hg, respiratory alkalosis is present. It takes approximately 1 to 3 minutes for the respiratory system to be effective. The respiratory system works to regulate acid-base balance by altering the carbon dioxide (CO_2) level in the bloodstream. When the respiration rate increases, the lungs excrete more carbon dioxide, which causes a decrease in hydrogen ions and an increase in pH. Conversely, when respirations are decreased, more carbon dioxide remains in the blood, causing hydrogen ions to increase and pH to decrease.

The renal system is the third and slowest mechanism for acid-base regulation. If the P_aCO_2 is less than 24 mEq/L, metabolic acidosis occurs; if it is greater than 28 mEq/L, metabolic alkalosis is present. It takes from several hours to days for this system to correct acid-base imbalance. The kidneys regulate acid-base balance by eliminating excess hydrogen or bicarbonate ions from the bloodstream. For example, if the hydrogen ion concentration of the body increases, the body's pH falls, and the kidneys eliminate more hydrogen ions to restore equilibrium. On the other hand, if the hydrogen ion concentration falls, body pH increases, and the kidneys eliminate bicarbonate ions to restore equilibrium.

There are four clinical situations that result when acid-base balance is disrupted: (1) respiratory acidosis, (2) respiratory alkalosis, (3) metabolic acidosis, and (4) metabolic alkalosis.

- **Respiratory acidosis** *(pH less than 7.35 and P_aCO_2 greater than 45 mm Hg):* This condition results from inadequate ventilation, resulting in the retention of carbon dioxide and an increased level of carbonic acid in the blood. The pH of a person in respiratory acidosis falls as the carbon dioxide level increases. To reverse respiratory acidosis, improve ventilation, using 100 percent oxygen. This removes carbon dioxide from the circulation via the lungs.
- **Respiratory alkalosis** *(pH greater than 7.45 and P_aCO_2 less than 35 mm Hg):* This condition occurs when excessive amounts of carbon dioxide have been eliminated from the patient. In emergency situations, respiratory alkalosis often occurs when a patient hyperventilates, blowing off more carbon dioxide than normal, or if caregivers give excessive mechanical ventilations. When more carbon dioxide than normal is blown off, body pH increases. Treatment of respiratory alkalosis should include having the patient take deep breaths and breathing slowly. EMS professionals can demonstrate a slow, relaxed breathing pattern for the patient. Medications may have to be given to relax the patient and restore a normal breathing pattern.
- **Metabolic acidosis** *(pH greater than 7.35 and HCO_3 less than 24 mEq/L):* This condition occurs when the body produces an excessive amount of metabolic acid. This increase in acid consumes some of the bicarbonate

buffer, causing a further acid buildup and a decrease in base. Metabolic acidosis causes a decrease in pH and bicarbonate, but carbon dioxide levels remain within normal limits. In emergency situations, treat metabolic acidosis by attempting to improve ventilation by using 100 percent oxygen. This removes carbon dioxide and, subsequently, hydrogen ions. When the diagnosis of metabolic acidosis is documented, treatment may also include giving the patient sodium bicarbonate.

Understand the Numbers
A 215-pound patient requires sodium bicarbonate for documented metabolic acidosis. Dosage = 1 mEq/kg IV. 215 pounds ÷ 2.2 kg = 97.7, or 98 kg. 1 mEq × 98 kg = 98 mEq.

- **Metabolic alkalosis** *(pH greater than 7.45 and HCO_3 less than 28 mEq/L):* During metabolic alkalosis, excitability of the CNS occurs. Symptoms may include irritability, mental confusion, and hyperactive reflexes. Hypoventilation may occur as a compensatory mechanism for metabolic alkalosis to conserve the hydrogen ions and carbonic acid. During metabolic alkalosis, the buffer, renal, and respiratory systems try to reestablish balance. In the buffer system, the excess bicarbonate reacts with buffer acid salts to decrease the concentration of carbonic acid. The renal system conserves the hydrogen ions and excretes the sodium, potassium, and bicarbonate ions. The respiratory system maintains balance through hypoventilation. This retains carbon dioxide and increases the concentration of carbonic acid. To treat metabolic alkalosis, EMS professionals need to determine and treat the underlying cause.

Intravenous Therapy

There are two basic reasons for starting an IV line in the out-of-hospital setting: (1) as a route for fluid replacement such as for hemorrhage, severe diarrhea, vomiting, heat exposure, or burns, and (2) as a route for drug administration. Five basic classifications of IV infusions include: crystalloids, colloids, hydrating solutions, hypertonic solutions, and blood or blood components (see Chapter 6). Table 5-2 lists the common indications and contraindications for commonly used IV solutions.

Crystalloids

Crystalloids are solutes that, when placed in a solvent, mix with and dissolve into a solution and cannot be distinguished from the resultant solution. Crystalloids are considered to be true solutions. They are able to diffuse through cell membranes. Crystalloids may be isotonic, hypotonic, or hypertonic solutions.

Colloids

Colloids are substances whose particles do not form a true solution because their molecules, when dispersed in a solvent, do not

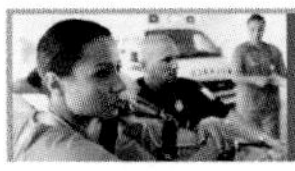

Table 5-2 Indications and Contraindications for Commonly Used Intravenous Solutions

Solution	Indications	Contraindications
Colloids		
Plasma Protein Fraction	Hypovolemic shock, especially from burns	Known hypersensitivity CHF
Dextran	Hypovolemic shock	Known hypersensitivity Patients with CHF or renal failure or those receiving anticoagulants
Hetastarch	Hypovolemic shock, especially from burns Septic shock	Known hypersensitivity Patients with CHF, renal failure, or bleeding disorders
Crystalloids		
Lactated Ringer's	Hypovolemic shock and a keep-open IV route	Patients with CHF or renal failure
Dextrose 5% in water (D_5W)	IV drug route Dilution of concentrated drugs for IV infusion	Patients with a head injury or stroke Volume replacement
Dextrose 10% in water ($D_{10}W$)	Hypoglycemia Neonatal resuscitation	Patients with a head injury or stroke Volume replacement
Normal saline (NS; 0.9% sodium chloride)	IV keep-open line Heat-related emergencies Freshwater drowning Diabetic ketoacidosis (DKA)	Patients with CHF
1/2 Normal saline (1/2NS; 0.45% sodium chloride)	Compromised cardiac or renal function	Emergency rehydration
Dextrose 5% in 1/2 normal saline ($D_5$1/2NS)	Heat emergencies, diabetic emergencies	Emergency rehydration Patients with a head injury or stroke
Dextrose 5% in normal saline (D_5NS)	Heat emergencies, volume replacement, freshwater drowning	Patients with compromised cardiac or renal function, head injury, or stroke
Dextrose 5% in lactated Ringer's (D_5LR)	Volume replacement	Patients with compromised cardiac or renal function, head injury, or stroke

dissolve. Instead, the molecules remain uniformly suspended and distributed throughout the fluid. The particles of colloid solutions are too large to pass through cell membranes; thus, they stay in the bloodstream. Colloid infusions raise colloid osmotic pressure; thus, they are often called plasma or volume expanders. Common colloid infusions are albumin, dextran, plasmanate, and the artificial blood substitute, hetastarch.

Hydrating Solutions

Various IV solutions are given by EMS personnel to patients to supplement caloric intake, supply nutrients, provide water for maintenance or rehydration, or promote effective renal output. Their rate of administration is adjusted so the equilibrium of body fluids is not disturbed. In most cases, glucose solutions are used. When glucose and other nutrients are given in water, they are rapidly metabolized, leaving an excess of water. This is why glucose solutions are often called hydrating solutions. Any water that is not needed by the body is excreted by the kidneys.

Isotonic Solutions

Isotonic solutions have the same tonicity as body fluids. Once infused, isotonic solutions remain within the intravascular space because osmotic pressure is equal between the intracellular and extracellular compartments. For this reason, isotonic solutions are used to treat hypotension resulting from hypovolemia.

Hypotonic Solutions

Hypotonic solutions cause fluid to shift out of the blood and into the cells and interstitial spaces. The rate of administration must be carefully controlled to prevent water from rupturing the red blood cells. As hypotonic solutions hydrate the intracellular compartment, care must be taken to prevent circulatory depletion as fluid moves from the bloodstream into the intracellular compartment. These solutions should not be given to hypotensive patients, as this can further lower blood pressure. Table 5-2 lists the indications for use and precautions for hypotonic solutions. An example of a hypotonic dextrose-containing solution is 5 percent dextrose in water (D_5W).

Hypertonic Solutions

Hypertonic solutions pull fluids from the intracellular and interstitial compartments into the blood vessels. They act to expand the intravascular compartment and are given when there is a serious saline depletion. Caution must be taken when giving hypertonic solutions, as they can cause circulatory overload. They also can cause irritation to the intima of the veins. An example of a hypertonic dextrose-containing solution is 10 percent dextrose in water ($D_{10}W$).

Intravenous Fluid Monographs

Colloids

Plasma Protein Fraction (Albumin, human)
Classifications: Colloid, volume expander
Pregnancy Class: C
Mechanism of Action: Provides colloidal oncotic pressure, which mobilizes fluid from the extravascular tissues back into the intravascular space
Indications: Expansion of plasma volume and maintenance of cardiac output in situations associated with fluid volume deficit, including shock, hemorrhage, and burns

> *effective* **Communication**
>
> While plasma protein fraction is being administered, it is also required for the concurrent administration of an appropriate crystalloid solution.

Contraindications: Known hypersensitivity; should not be given to patients with congestive heart failure (CHF).
Precautions: Use with caution in patients with dehydration or severe liver or kidney disease and in those who require sodium restriction.
Route and Dosage
IV (Adult): 25 g (500 mL); may be repeated within 30 minutes
IV (Pediatric): 0.5–1 g/kg/dose (10–20 mL/kg/dose)
How Supplied
Injection: 5 percent (50 mg/mL), 25 percent (250 mg/mL)
Adverse Reactions and Side Effects
CV: Pulmonary edema, fluid overload, hyper- or hypotension, tachycardia
CNS: Headache
GI: Increased salivation, nausea, vomiting
Derm: Rash
Misc: Chills, fever, flushing
Drug Interactions: None significant
EMS Considerations: Administer 5 percent albumin undiluted. Normal albumin at 25 percent may be administered undiluted or diluted in 0.9 percent NS or D_5W.

Dextran
Classification: Colloid
Pregnancy Class: C
Mechanism of Action: Increases intravascular volume by attracting water from other fluid compartments
Indications: Hypovolemic shock
Contraindications: Known hypersensitivity; should not be given to patients with CHF or renal failure or to those who are receiving anticoagulants
Precautions: Accurate blood-typing may be hindered due to the dextran coating the red blood cells. Therefore, blood samples should be taken before administration.
Route and Dosage
IV: Titrated to patient physiological response
How Supplied
Bottles: 250 mL and 500 mL bottles
Adverse Reactions and Side Effects
Resp: Dyspnea
CV: Chest tightness, hypotension
Derm: Rash, itching
Drug Interactions: Dextran retards blood clotting. Therefore, it should not be given to patients receiving anticoagulants.

EMS Considerations: It is recommended that a crystalloid solution be administered rather than dextran in the management of severe hypovolemic shock.

Hetastarch (Hespan)

Classifications: Colloid, volume expander

Pregnancy Class: C

Mechanism of Action: Hetastarch is a starch-containing colloid that causes water to move from interstitial spaces, increasing the osmotic pressure within the intravascular space.

Indications: Used for patients in hypovolemic shock, especially when caused by burns; also used for patients in septic shock

Contraindications: Known hypersensitivity; should not be used in patients with CHF or renal failure or in those with bleeding disorders

Precautions: Use with caution in patients taking anticoagulants.

Route and Dosage

Note: Dosage should be titrated according to the severity of shock and the patient's hemodynamic response.

IV (Adult): 500–1,000 mL

IV (Pediatric): 10 mL/kg/dose

How Supplied

Bottles: 6 percent hetastarch in 0.9 percent NS in 500 mL bottles

Adverse Reactions and Side Effects

Resp: Pulmonary edema

CV: Arrhythmias, hypotension

GI: Nausea, vomiting

Drug Interactions: Do not administer hetastarch to patients concurrently on anticoagulants.

EMS Considerations: Administration formulas have been established for colloid administration to patients in shock due to burns.

Check the Evidence

EMS professionals must monitor vital signs frequently especially in patients with burn shock. Hypotension in patients with burn shock may develop later than with hemorrhagic causes.

Crystalloid Solutions

Lactated Ringer's

Classification: Isotonic solution

Pregnancy Class: C

Mechanism of Action: Replaces water and the following electrolytes:

Sodium (Na^+)

Potassium (K^+)

Calcium (Ca^{2+})

Chloride (Cl^-)

Indications: Used for patients in hypovolemic shock and for a keep-open IV route

Contraindications: Should not be administered to patients with CHF or to those with renal failure

Precautions: Use with extreme caution in patients with edema or sodium retention.

Route and Dosage

IV: Dosage is dependent on the clinical situation. In severe hypovolemic shock, lactated ringers should be administered through a 14- or 16-gauge IV cannula as rapidly as possible, according to local EMS protocol.

Check the Evidence

Studies have suggested that there is harm associated with prehospital IV placement for victims of trauma—that there may be no survival advantage. These studies have indicated that the routine use of IV fluid administration for all trauma patients should be discouraged.

How Supplied

Bags/bottles: 250 mL, 500 mL, and 1,000 mL

Adverse Reactions and Side Effects

None when used in therapeutic dosages

Drug Interactions: Caution should be used if administered to patients concurrently taking corticosteroids.

EMS Considerations: Lactated ringers should be administered rapidly until a systolic blood pressure of 90 mm Hg to 100 mm Hg is achieved. When the blood pressure reaches this level, the infusion should be reduced to approximately 100 mL/hr.

Dextrose 5 Percent in Water (D_5W)

Classification: Hypotonic dextrose-containing solution

Pregnancy Class: C

Mechanism of Action: Provides nutrients in the form of dextrose and free water

Indications: Used as a keep-open route for the administration of medications; also used for the dilution of concentrated medications for IV infusion

Contraindications: Should not be used for replacement of fluids in hypovolemic patients. Do not administer to patients with head injury or stroke.

Precautions: May produce venous irritation

effective **Communication**

When treating a hypoglycemic patient, it is important to draw a tube of blood before the administration of D_5W or $D_{50}W$.

Route and Dosage

IV: Administered at a "keep-open rate" using a minidrip [60 drops (gtts)/mL] set

How Supplied

Bags/bottles: 50 mL, 100 mL, 150 mL, 250 mL, 500 mL, and 1,000 mL

Adverse Reactions and Side Effects

Rare, when used in therapeutic dosages

Drug Interactions: Should not be used with phenytoin (Dilantin) or inamrinone (Inocor)

EMS Considerations: Closely monitor patients for fluid overload and tissue necrosis.

Dextrose 10 Percent in Water ($D_{10}W$)

Classification: Hypotonic dextrose-containing solution

Pregnancy Class: C

Mechanism of Action: Provides nutrients in the form of dextrose and free water
Indications: Used for patients who are hypoglycemic and during neonatal resuscitation
Contraindications: Should not be used for volume replacement or in patients with head injury or stroke
Precautions: May produce venous irritation
Route and Dosage
IV: The dosage is dependent on the clinical condition of the patient. Local EMS protocols should be followed.
How Supplied
Bags/bottles: 50 mL, 100 mL, 10 mL, 250 mL, 500 mL, and 1,000 mL
Adverse Reactions and Side Effects
Rare, when used in therapeutic dosages
Drug Interactions: Should not be used with phenytoin (Dilantin) or inamrinone (Inocor)
EMS Considerations: Closely monitor patients for fluid overload and tissue necrosis.

Normal Saline (NS, 0.9 percent sodium chloride)
Classification: Isotonic solution
Pregnancy Class: C
Mechanism of Action: Replaces both water and electrolytes
Indications: Commonly used as a keep-open IV line; also used for treatment of heat-related emergencies, hypovolemia, fresh-water drowning, and diabetic ketoacidosis (DKA)
Contraindications: Should not be administered to patients with CHF.
Precautions: Use with caution if large amounts of fluid are needed, because it is possible that electrolytes (other than sodium and chloride) may be depleted.
Route and Dosage
IV: The rate and amount of normal saline to be given is dependent upon the clinical situation being treated. Local EMS protocols should be referenced.
How Supplied
Bags/bottles: 250 mL, 500 mL, and 1,000 mL

effective **Communication**

Sterile normal saline for irrigation should not be confused with the normal saline designated for IV administration.

Adverse Reactions and Side Effects
Rare when used in therapeutic dosages
Drug Interactions: None significant in emergency situations
EMS Considerations: Frequently monitor patients for fluid overload

½ Normal Saline (1/2NS, 0.45 percent sodium chloride)
Classification: Hypotonic solution
Pregnancy Class: C
Mechanism of Action: Replaces electrolytes and water
Indications: Used for patients with compromised cardiac or renal function
Contraindications: Should not be used for rapid rehydration
Precautions: Use with caution if large amounts of fluid are needed, because it is possible that electrolytes (other than sodium and chloride) may be depleted.
Route and Dosage
IV: The rate and amount of 1/2 normal saline to be given is dependent upon the clinical situation being treated. Local EMS protocols should be referenced.
How Supplied
Bags/bottles: 250 mL, 500 mL, and 1,000 mL
Adverse Reactions and Side Effects
Rare, when used in therapeutic dosages
Drug Interactions: None significant in emergency situations
EMS Considerations: Frequently monitor patients for fluid overload.

Dextrose 5 Percent in 1/2 Normal Saline ($D_5$1/2NS)
Classification: Hypertonic dextrose-containing solution
Pregnancy Class: C
Mechanism of Action: Replaces electrolytes and water and provides nutrients in the form of dextrose
Indications: Is used as a keep-open IV line for patients with impaired cardiovascular or renal function; also used for patients with diabetic disorders and in patients with heat exhaustion
Contraindications: Should not be used in patients with head injury or stroke; not to be used when rapid fluid resuscitation is indicated
Precautions: May cause venous irritation or tissue necrosis
Route and Dosage
IV: The rate and amount of dextrose 5 percent 1/2 normal saline to be given is dependent upon the clinical situation being treated. Local EMS protocols should be referenced.
How Supplied
Bags/bottles: 250 mL, 500 mL, and 1,000 mL
Adverse Reactions and Side Effects
Rare, when used in therapeutic dosages
Drug Interactions: Should not be used with phenytoin (Dilantin) or inamrinone (Inocor)
EMS Considerations: Frequently monitor patients for fluid overload. If treating a patient for hypoglycemia, it is important to draw a blood tube before administration of $D_5$1/2NS.

Dextrose 5 Percent in Normal Saline (D_5NS)
Classification: Hypertonic dextrose-containing solution
Pregnancy Class: C
Mechanism of Action: Replaces electrolytes and water and provides nutrients in the form of dextrose
Indications: Used to treat patients with heat-related disorders or hypoglycemia or in victims of fresh-water drowning
Contraindications: Should not be given to patients with impaired cardiac or renal function or to patients with head injury or stroke
Precautions: May cause venous irritation or tissue necrosis
Route and Dosage
IV: The rate and amount of dextrose 5 percent normal saline to be given is dependent upon the clinical situation being treated. Local EMS protocols should be referenced.
How Supplied
Bags/bottles: 250 mL, 500 mL, and 1,000 mL
Adverse Reactions and Side Effects
Rare, when used in therapeutic dosages
Drug Interactions: Should not be used with phenytoin (Dilantin) or inamrinone (Inocor)

EMS Considerations: Frequently monitor patients for fluid overload. If treating a patient for hypoglycemia, it is important to draw a blood tube before administration of D_5NS.

Dextrose 5 Percent in Lactated Ringer's Solution (D_5LR)

Classification: Hypertonic dextrose-containing solution

Pregnancy Class: C

Mechanism of Action: Replaces electrolytes and water and provides nutrients in the form of dextrose

Indications: Used for patients in need of volume replacement due to shock

Contraindications: Should not give to patients with impaired cardiac or renal function or to patients with head injury or stroke

Precautions: May cause venous irritation or tissue necrosis

Route and Dosage

IV: The rate and amount of dextrose 5 percent lactated ringers to be given is dependent upon the clinical situation being treated. Local EMS protocols should be referenced.

How Supplied

Bags/bottles: 250 mL, 500 mL, and 1,000 mL

Adverse Reactions and Side Effects

Rare, when used in therapeutic dosages

Drug Interactions: Should not be used with phenytoin (Dilantin) or inamrinone (Inocor)

EMS Considerations: Frequently monitor patients for fluid overload. If treating a patient for hypoglycemia, it is important to draw a blood tube before administration of D_5LR.

Venous Access

It is common practice in the management of most injured or ill patients for the EMS professional to establish an IV line. The IV line provides a route for fluid replacement in the injured patient and a route for medications for the patient with a medical disorder. The type of medical emergency will determine the size of the catheter to be used when establishing the IV line. For example, the patient involved in trauma may require a large-bore 14- or 16-gauge catheter. On the other hand, the medical patient may only require a smaller 18- or 20-gauge catheter. It is important for EMS personnel to try to plan for the future. For example, if a patient may require the infusion of whole blood, a larger catheter must be initially inserted.

Not only is the IV catheter size important, but so is the type of IV administration set to be used. There are two types of IV administration sets: macro- and minidrip sets. The macrodrip set is generally used for the injured patient, while the minidrip set is generally used for medical patients. Macrodrip IV sets can deliver anywhere from 10 to 20 gtt/mL, while the minidrip set delivers 50 to 60 gtt/mL, depending on the manufacturer.

The IV should be started in a large vein, generally above the wrist (Fig. 5-9). Avoid starting an IV in the hand, as it can be more painful than one in the arm. If, for some reason, an IV cannot be started in the arm, other sites include the leg (Fig. 5-10) and the external jugular in the neck (Fig. 5-11), which are both considered peripheral veins. However, the best vein for IV insertion in the traumatic or cardiac arrest patient is the antecubital vein.

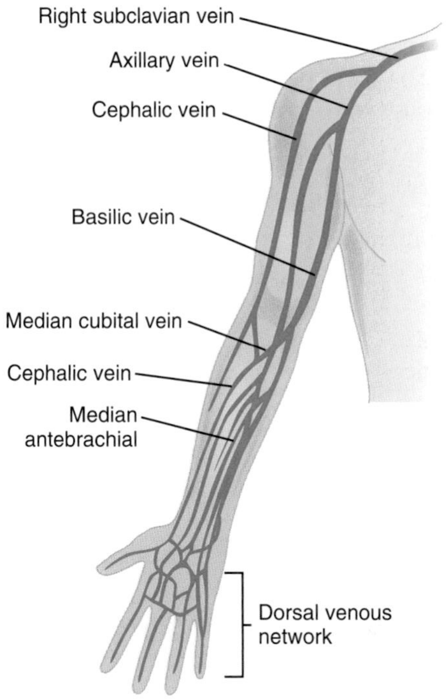

Figure 5-9 Veins of the arm and hand.

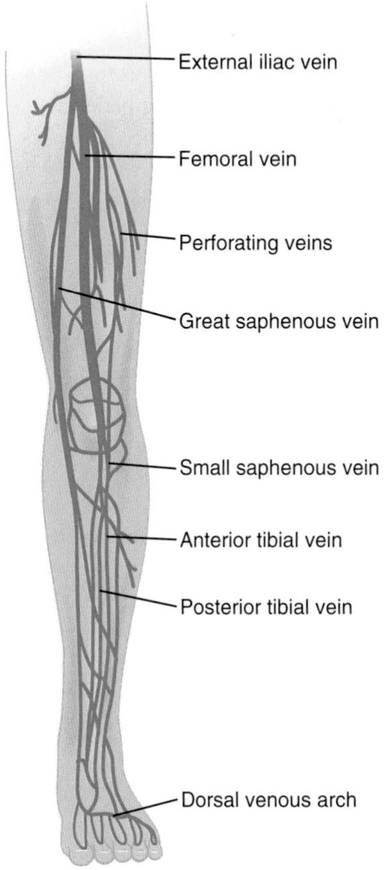

Figure 5-10 Veins of the leg and foot.

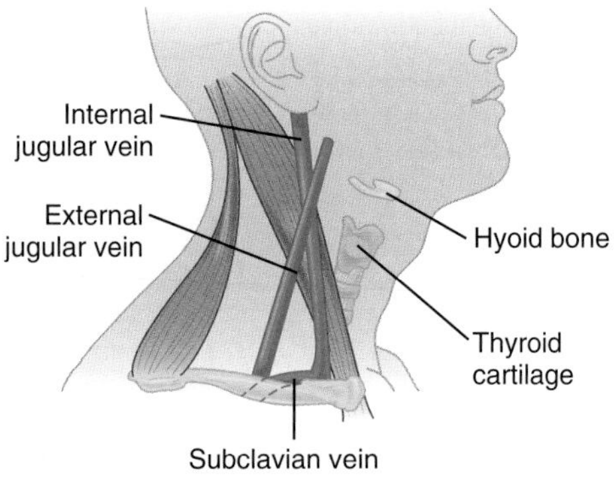

Figure 5-11 External jugular vein.

Procedure for Starting an Intravenous Line

effective **Communication**

While the IV equipment is being prepared, explain the procedure (if the patient is alert and able to understand) and give the reason why the IV will be administered.

1. Observe Standard Precautions.
2. Receive, confirm, and write down the order.
3. Prepare the equipment:
   - IV fluid
   - Administration set (macro- or minidrip)
   - Appropriate indwelling catheter
   - IV extension tubing (some protocols do not use extension tubing for trauma patients)
   - Tourniquet
   - Antibiotic swab
   - 2x2 or 4x4 sterile gauze pads or adhesive bandage
   - 1/2-inch or 1-inch tape
   - Antibiotic ointment
   - Short arm board, if appropriate
4. Remove IV fluid from package. Inspect the fluid for clarity and particulate matter. Do not use if discolored or if particles are present.
5. Open and inspect the IV tubing.
6. Attach extension tubing, if appropriate.
7. Remove the sterile cover from the IV bag and the administration set. Insert the administration set into the IV fluid port.
8. Squeeze the IV tubing drip chamber to fill with fluid and then bleed the air out of the IV tubing.
9. Close the clamp on the IV tubing.
10. Hang the IV bag or have it held at the appropriate height.
11. If appropriate, attach the tourniquet, occluding the patient's venous blood flow.
12. Select an appropriate vein.
13. Clean the selected site using an antibiotic swab.
14. Make the puncture, observe flashback, and advance the catheter while removing the needle.
15. Connect the IV tubing and remove the tourniquet.
16. Open the IV tubing, confirming fluid is flowing with no evidence of infiltration.
17. Apply antibiotic ointment over the puncture site and cover with sterile gauze or adhesive bandage.
18. Tape the IV catheter and tubing in place.
19. Adjust flow rate.
20. If appropriate, attach short arm board.
21. Label the IV bag with patient name, date, time the IV was started, gauge of the catheter, and your initials.
22. Call medical control to confirm successful completion of the IV.
23. Monitor the patient and report any changes.

Intravenous Access via the External Jugular Vein

The external jugular vein in the neck connects into the central circulation via the subclavian vein. Fluids and drugs reach the central circulation of the body rapidly when administered via the external vein. Intravenous access via the external vein should only be done on the unresponsive patient.

1. Observe Standard Precautions.
2. Receive, write down, and confirm the order.
3. Prepare the appropriate equipment:
   - Appropriate IV fluid and administration set
   - Appropriate indwelling catheter
   - Antibacterial swab and ointment and alcohol preps
   - Sterile gauze pads
   - 1/2-inch to 1-inch tape
   - Sharps container
4. Position the patient supine, with the head turned away from the side to be cannulated.
5. After locating the vein, prepare the site.
6. Apply gentle traction on the vein just below the clavicle.
7. Approach the site midway between the angle of the jaw and the clavicle, aiming toward the shoulder, and puncture at a 30-degree angle.
8. Upon entry into the vein, note a flashback of blood and advance the needle and catheter approximately 2 mm to stabilize the needle in the vein.
9. Remove the needle and properly dispose in the sharps container.
10. Connect the IV tubing and slowly open to allow fluid to flow. Confirm that the fluid is flowing freely without evidence of infiltration.
11. Apply antibacterial ointment and cover with a sterile gauze pad or adhesive bandage.
12. Use tape to secure the IV tubing and catheter in place.
13. Adjust flow rate.
14. Confirm and document the successful completion of the infusion.
15. Monitor the patient and report any changes.

Some protocols may require EMS personnel to collect a blood sample when starting the IV. Blood is taken before the IV line is attached to the IV catheter by using a 10-mL syringe.

Once the blood has been taken, the syringe is removed and the IV line attached. Blood collection should be done, if at all possible, before the administration of any medications.

Once the blood has been withdrawn, it is placed into an evacuated blood collection tube. Most of these tubes contain chemicals to prevent the blood from clotting. Each tube has a specific colored rubber top, which determines the use of the contents. After the evacuated blood tube is filled, it should be inverted several times in order to mix thoroughly with the chemical. The patient's name, date, time sampled, and the EMS personnel name should be noted on the tube. If necessary, the tubes may be taped to the IV bag for transport.

Saline Locks

A saline lock is an IV portal, usually placed and left in a vein in one of the patient's arms. There are four major purposes to use saline locks:

1. To maintain venous access in patients without continuous infusion of fluids
2. To minimize the risk of fluid overload and electrolyte imbalance
3. To increase patient comfort and mobility
4. To administer fluid and medications and for the collection of blood samples without repeated venipunctures

Complications of Intravenous Administration

Intravenous administration can be a life-saving procedure for both medical and traumatic emergencies. However, there are possible complications that may include both local and systemic complications.

Local Complications

- **Hematoma:** A hematoma results when blood leaks into tissues surrounding the IV insertion site. Hematomas due to IV cannula insertion are usually small enough that they generally resolve spontaneously. Treatment includes removing the cannula and applying pressure with a sterile dressing.
- **Thrombophlebitis:** Thrombophlebitis is the presence of a blood clot in the vein. It occurs when the vein has been injured. A blood clot in a vein can become a thromboembolism and enter the circulatory system. Treatment includes discontinuing the IV infusion and applying a cold pack to decrease blood flow and increase platelet aggregation, followed by a warm pack, elevating the extremity, and restarting the IV in the opposite extremity.
- **Phlebitis:** Phlebitis is the inflammation of a vein. It may occur due to a catheter that is too large for the vein or because the IV cannula has been left in for an extended period of time. Phlebitis causes localized redness and warmth at the IV insertion site. Treatment includes discontinuing the IV and restarting it in another site. A warm, moist compress should be placed on the affected site.
- **Tissue necrosis:** Tissue death can occur from infiltration of some IV medications, such as $D_{50}W$, sodium bicarbonate, or promethazine. When drugs that may cause necrosis may be administered, the IV should be started in a stable vein of adequate size. Once the IV infusion has been established, the site should be monitored for position and patency before, during, and after drug administration.

Systemic Complications

- **Fluid overload:** It is very important not to infuse too much fluid into a patient. Overloading the circulatory system with excessive IV fluids can cause fluid buildup in the lungs as well as systemically. It is extremely important to frequently monitor vital signs. Signs and symptoms of fluid overload include increased blood pressure; moist crackles of the lungs; edema; dyspnea; and rapid, shallow respirations. Treatment for fluid overload includes decreasing the IV rate and monitoring vital signs frequently.
- **Air embolism:** Fortunately, the risk of air embolism is rare. The greatest risk for an air embolism occurs with cannulation of central veins. Signs and symptoms of an air embolism include dyspnea and cyanosis; hypotension; weak and rapid pulse; loss of consciousness; and chest, shoulder, and low back pain. Treatment includes the immediate clamping of the cannula, placing the patient on the left side, and assessing vital signs frequently. To reduce the possibility of an air embolism, make sure that all IV lines are completely filled with fluid when cannula insertion is performed. An air detection alarm can be installed on IV pumps as well. Complications of air embolism may include shock and death.
- **Septicemia:** Septicemia is a bacterial infection in the bloodstream. It can occur because of contaminated equipment, poor aseptic technique, or prolonged IV therapy. Signs and symptoms of septicemia include sudden temperature increase shortly after the infusion has been started, backache, headache, increased pulse and respiratory rates, nausea and vomiting, diarrhea, chills, and shaking. Treatment is symptomatic and includes culturing of the IV cannula, tubing, or the IV solution.
- **Catheter fragment embolism:** A catheter fragment embolism can result if part of the IV catheter is sheared off and travels in the bloodstream. This can occur in several ways:
  - Poorly secured cannula
  - Cannula inserted in areas of flexion
  - Reinsertion of a needle into a catheter
  - Repeated motion at the cannula's hub

Signs and symptoms of a catheter fragment embolism include sharp pain at the insertion site, chest pain, and tachycardia. If a catheter fragment embolism is suspected, the IV infusion should be stopped, the vein should be palpated for the catheter fragment, and a venous tourniquet should be applied above the fragment to prevent further movement.

effective Communication

An IV needle should never be reinserted through a catheter. As the needle and catheter are inserted, the needle should be removed. Needles only are withdrawn from a catheter, never inserted.

SCENARIO REVISITED

Did you consider Ellen's case?

As you recall, your patient is 32 years old and has been experiencing vomiting and diarrhea for the last three hours. Your paramedic team along with medical control decides that Ellen is suffering from food poisoning due to poor preparation of shrimp or crab or both.

Once a thorough assessment has been completed and a treatment protocol has been decided, you should proceed using a critical thinking approach to IV administration.

Step 1: Determine signs and symptoms to be treated.
Step 2: Consider both the risks and benefits of treating or not treating your patient.
Step 3: Choose the IV fluid that provides the best possible outcome.
Step 4: Remember the solution's indications, contraindications, and precautions.
Step 5: Decide the best rate for administering the IV solution for the best outcome.
Step 6: Administer the IV solution according to the Seven Patient Rights.

1. The right patient
2. The right drug (IV solution)
3. The right amount
4. The right time
5. The right route and rate
6. The right documentation
7. The right of the patient to accept or refuse the IV solution

Step 7: Reevaluate the patient for the desired and undesired effects.

Let's Recap

EMS professionals must be able to recognize and rapidly treat fluid, electrolyte, and acid-base abnormalities. The major key to treatment is rapid fluid-aggressive therapy. To replenish fluids and electrolytes, the proper IV fluids must be chosen and given at the appropriate rate. To maintain appropriate acid-base limits or correct acid-base abnormalities, a patent airway must be maintained and ventilation improved using 100 percent oxygen as needed. The most important drug in correcting acid-base abnormalities is oxygen. Appropriate airway support, coupled with correct cardiopulmonary resuscitation, if needed, can maintain pH levels within or very close to normal limits within the lungs, heart, and brain.

SCENARIO CONCLUSION

After a thorough assessment, Ellen is hypovolemic due to excessive vomiting and diarrhea for more than three hours. It has been determined that, to help restore Ellen's fluid volume, an IV infusion should be started. In this case, an IV fluid bolus of 1,000 mL lactated ringers should be run over a one-hour period.

Understand the Numbers

To infuse 1,000 mL of lactated ringers in 1 hour, the infusion rate is 250 gtt/minute.

1,000 mL $\times$ IV set (15 gtt/mL) $\div$ 60 minutes = 250 gtt/min.

Check the **Evidence**

Lactated ringers is an isotonic crystalloid solution, which is frequently used to manage hypovolemic states. It has the same tonicity as body fluids. Lactated ringers also contains the electrolytes sodium, potassium, calcium, and chloride. In addition, it contains lactic acid, which acts as a buffer.

Upon arrival at the emergency department, Ellen has made a slight improvement after receiving approximately 400 mL of the lactated ringers. Her respirations are now at 16 breaths/minute, heart rate is 116 beats/minute, and her blood pressure is now 116/78 mm Hg.

PRACTICE EXERCISES

1. Fluid located in the spaces between the body's cells, accounting for approximately 10.5 percent of body weight, is called:
a. Interstitial fluid
b. Intracellular fluid
c. Extracellular fluid
d. Intravascular fluid

2. Two major cations of the body are:
a. Calcium and chloride
b. Sodium and bicarbonate
c. Potassium and phosphate
d. Magnesium and potassium

3. A solution equal in milliequivalents to normal body fluid is called a(n):
a. Isotonic solution
b. Colloid solution
c. Hypotonic solution
d. Hypertonic solution

4. The body's primary mechanism for adjusting and maintaining acid-base balance is the:
a. Renal system
b. Buffer system
c. Circulatory system
d. Respiratory system

5. The process of moving substances across the cell wall from the less concentrated to the more concentrated solution, and keeping the concentration of solutes higher on one side of the cell wall than the other, is called:
a. Filtration
b. Diffusion
c. Active transport
d. Passive transport

6. The normal pH of the body ranges from 7.35 to 7.45. When the body fluid's pH is greater than 7.45, the body is in a state of:
a. Alkalosis
b. Acidosis
c. Equilibrium
d. Metabolisis

7. When the body's pH is less than 7.35, the body is in a state of:
a. Alkalosis
b. Acidosis
c. Equilibrium
d. Metabolisis

8. Two components of the buffer system include bicarbonate ion (HCO_3-) and carbonic acid (H_2CO_3), which maintain an equilibrium with the hydrogen ion (H+). This reaction requires _____ molecule(s) of bicarbonate ion for every _____ molecule(s) of carbonic acid.
a. 1:10
b. 10:1
c. 1:20
d. 20:1

9. Substances whose particles do not form a true solution because their molecules, when dispersed in a solvent, do not dissolve, are called:
a. Colloids
b. Crystalloids
c. Hypotonic solutions
d. Hypertonic solutions

10. Solutions that pull fluids from the intracellular and interstitial compartments into the blood vessels are called:
a. Hypertonic solutions
b. Hypotonic solutions
c. Hydrating solutions
d. Isotonic solutions

CASE STUDY

You are called to the home of a "man feeling weak." When you arrive, John is lying in bed stating that he is feeling weak and nauseated. John is 74 years old and states that he has diarrhea and has vomited twice. When asked about any other medical conditions, John states that he is a dialysis patient (dialysis fistula in left arm) and has not had a treatment for two days because he has not felt well. Assessment of John reveals the following:

Respirations: 18 breaths/minute, with clear lung sounds
Pulse rate: 70 beats/minutes. ECG shows "peaked T waves" (Fig. 5-12).
Blood pressure: 150/90 mm Hg
Oxygen saturation: 93 percent

Hyperkalemia (elevated potassium levels) may occur in patients with renal failure. It may present with gastrointestinal symptoms, weakness, and ECG abnormalities such as an elevated T wave or a widened QRS complex. EMS treatment may include an IV of normal saline and drugs such as calcium, sodium bicarbonate, insulin, and $D_{50}W$.

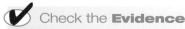

Check the **Evidence**

Sodium bicarbonate shifts potassium into the cells. It works by pushing potassium into the cell in exchange for a hydrogen ion.

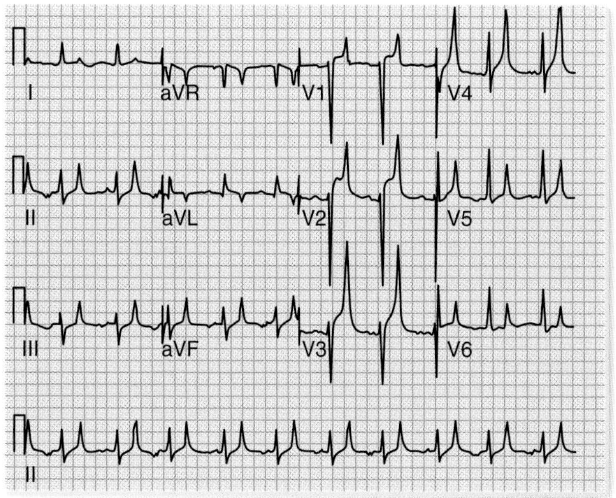

Figure 5-12 ECG showing elevated T waves.

MATH EQUATIONS

Drug Concentration

1. Your drug comes packaged as 40 mg in 4 mL. What is the drug concentration (mg/mL)?
2. You add 1 mg of a drug to 250 mL of solution. What is the resulting concentration (mg/mL)?
3. You add 2 mg of a drug to 500 mL of solution. What is the resulting concentration (mcg/mL)?
4. Your drug comes packaged as a 2 percent concentration in 5 mL of solution. What is the drug concentration (mg/mL)?
5. You add 2 g of a drug to 1,000 mL of solution. What is the resulting concentration (mg/mL)?
6. You add 20 percent concentration of a drug in 500 mL of solution. What is the concentration of the solution (g/mL)?
7. Your drug comes packaged as 100 mg in 20 mL of solution. What is the concentration of the drug (mg/mL)?
8. Your drug comes packaged as 0.1 mg/mL in a 10 mL syringe. How many mg are in the syringe?
9. You add 0.5 mg of a drug to 5 mL of solution. What is the concentration (mcg/mL)?
10. You add 4 mg of a drug in 500 mL of solution. What is the resulting concentration (mg/mL)?

REFERENCES

Beck, R. K. (2012). Fluids, electrolytes, and intravenous therapy. In *Pharmacology for the EMS provider.* New York: Delmar, Cengage Learning.

Deglin, J. H., Vallerand, A. H., and Sanboski, C. A. (2011). *Davis's drug guide for nurses* (12th ed.). Philadelphia, PA: F.A. Davis Company.

Garth, D. Hyperkalemia in emergency medicine. Retrieved November 1, 2013 from emedicine.medscape.com/article/766479-overview

Khanna, A., White, W. B. (2009). The management of hyperkalemia in patients with cardiovascular disease. *The American Journal of Medicine. 122*(3):215-221.

Rx List Inc. Lactated Ringer's: warnings. Retrieved October 25, 2013 from www.rxlist.com/lactated-ringers-drug/warnings/precautions/html

University of Babylon. Managing systemic complications. Retrieved October 28, 2013 from www.uobabylon.edu.iq/eprints/publication_12_4471_233.pdf

Venes, D., ed. (2013). *Taber's cyclopedic medical dictionary* (22nd ed.). Philadelphia, PA: F. A. Davis Company.

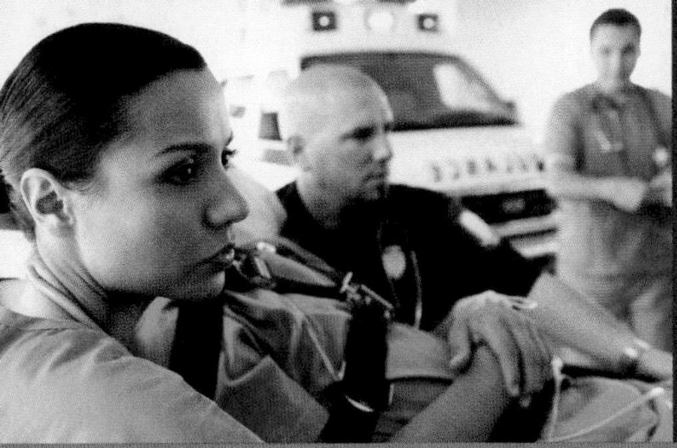

CHAPTER 6

Blood and Blood Product Administration

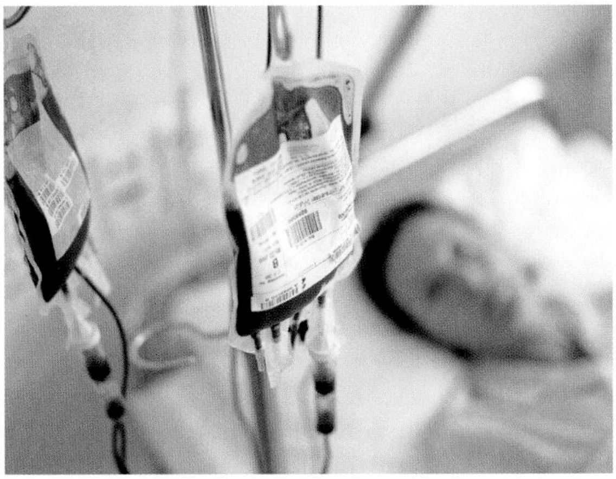

Patient with blood infusion. *(Photograph © Jochen Sands/ Digital Vision/Thinkstock)*

LEARNING OUTCOMES

- Describe the basic components of the blood, including whole blood, packed red blood cells (RBCs), white blood cells (WBCs), platelets, and plasma.
- Describe the basic concepts of immunology to include antigens, antibodies, and immune response.
- Describe the basic concepts of blood grouping.
- Explain the concepts of blood typing and crossmatching.
- List the signs and symptoms of blood transfusion reactions.
- Describe the antihyperlipidemic drugs, including their indications for use, contraindications, and their adverse reactions and side effects.

KEY TERMS

Agglutination
Agglutinins
Agglutinogens
Antibody
Antigen
Blood typing
Crossmatching
Epitope
Genotype
Immune response
Immunity
Isoantigen
Universal donor
Universal recipient

SCENARIO OPENING

You have been assigned to do a field-internship shift on a critical care transport unit #826. You and the critical care team are en route to a small rural hospital to transfer a patient to the local trauma center. The patient is a 24-year-old female who was a passenger in a motor vehicle accident (MVA). Upon arrival, the patient (Emma) responds to verbal commands, and her vital signs are:

LOC:	responds to verbal commands
Respirations:	16 breaths/minute
Blood pressure:	116/70 mm Hg
Heart rate:	104 beats/minute and regular

Prior to your arrival, Emma was given 1 L of normal saline (NS) by the responding paramedics, and another liter is currently infusing. Transport time to the trauma facility is approximately 30 minutes. The weather is not conducive for using rotor-wing transport.

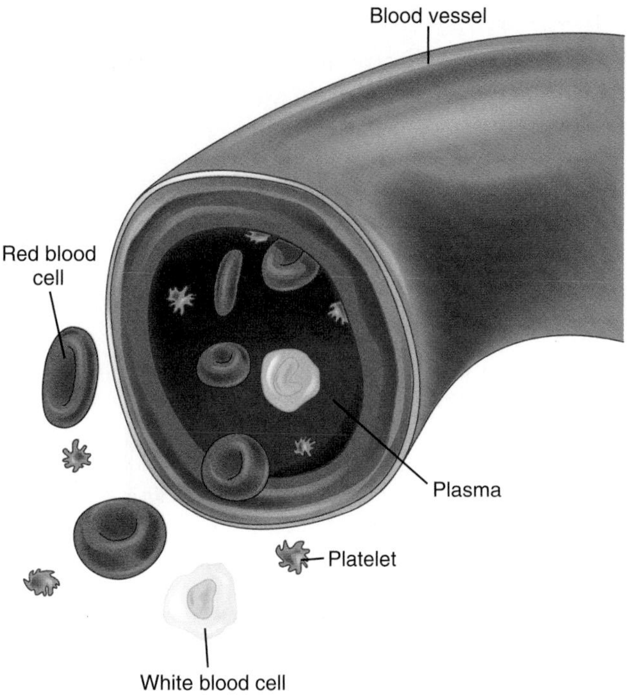

Figure 6-1 Composition of the blood.

Introduction

It is becoming more and more common for EMS professionals to administer blood or blood products or transport patients who are being administered blood or blood products. Therefore, it is important to understand the blood forms that can be administered, the therapeutic results expected, and the side effects administering these products can create. For example, RBCs carry oxygen; WBCs aid in the immune response to infection; platelets are important in blood clotting; and plasma transports nutrients, waste products, hormones, carbon dioxide, and other substances and helps regulate electrolyte balance and body temperature. Adverse reactions and side effects of the cardiovascular system that can occur while administering blood products include chest pain, hypotension, and dysrhythmias.

Physiology of the Blood

The EMS professional may find it necessary to administer or transport a patient receiving whole blood or blood components in an emergency situation. A thorough understanding of blood products will assist in treating these types of patients.

Whole Blood

There may be times when the EMS professional will be called upon to administer whole blood or transport a patient who is receiving whole blood. Whole blood consists of red and white blood cells, platelets, electrolytes, plasma, and stable clotting factors (Fig. 6-1). One unit of blood equals 500 mL. In emergencies, whole blood is indicated for massive blood loss equal to or exceeding 25 percent of a patient's total blood volume.

Human blood is about 52 to 62 percent plasma and 38 to 48 percent cells. The plasma is mostly water, ions, proteins, hormones, and lipids. The cellular components of the blood are the RBCs (erythrocytes), WBCs (leukocytes), and platelets (thrombocytes). A person weighing 154 pounds (70 kg) has a blood volume of approximately 5 L or 70 mL/kg of body weight. Blood constitutes approximately 7 to 8 percent of body weight. The pH of the blood ranges from 7.35 to 7.45.

Understand the Numbers

A patient weighing 85 kg has lost 25 percent of his blood volume. Therefore, how many pounds of his body weight has he lost?

85 kg × 0.25 = 21.25 kg. 21.25 kg × 2.2 lbs. = 46.25 lbs.

Many times, it is difficult and impractical to administer whole blood during an emergency. Therefore, protocols have largely been replaced with the use of blood components. This has allowed one unit of blood to be separated into RBCs, plasma, and platelets, which in turn may be used to treat several different patients. Another advantage of separating whole blood into components is that the ABO blood type incompatibility between blood groups is eliminated. Also, colloidal and crystalloid infusions can often be used when up to one-third of an adult's blood volume is lost.

Whole blood should be administered as rapidly as the patient can tolerate. The loss of potassium from the RBCs into the plasma increases proportionately to the length of time the blood is stored. Therefore, administration of whole blood to cardiac patients may be contraindicated.

effective **Communication**

The only thing that can be mixed with whole blood is 0.9 percent NS.

Packed Red Blood Cells

Packed RBCs have 80 percent of the plasma removed but provide the same amount of RBCs as whole blood. Packed RBCs are indicated for patients who are anemic and do not need fluid volume expansion but who do need to increase their blood's oxygen-carrying ability.

The major advantage of packed RBCs versus whole blood is the reduction of anti-A or anti-B **agglutinins** with the removal of the plasma. During an emergency, when typing and crossmatching are not feasible, packed type O RBCs can be given.

Platelets

Platelets are colorless round or oval-shaped disks that are present in our blood. Their sticky surface lets them, along with other substances, form clots to help stop bleeding. When bleeding from a wound occurs, the platelets gather at the wound and attempt to block the blood flow. Calcium, vitamin K, and a protein called fibrinogen help the platelets form a clot. The platelets, calcium, vitamin K, and fibrinogen begin forming fibrin, which resembles tiny threads. The fibrin threads then begin to form a web-like mesh that traps the blood cells. Blood clotting may be beneficial, as in preventing blood loss from wounds, or harmful if it occurs within arteries as in stroke or myocardial infarction.

Plasma

Plasma is the liquid portion of the blood and lymph. It carries nutrients to body tissues and transports wastes for excretion. Rh crossmatching is not necessary before administering plasma, as plasma contains no RBCs. However, ABO compatibility must be determined. In emergency situations, AB plasma can be given to all ABO patients. This is because plasma does not have anti-A or anti-B agglutinins. During an emergency, if only volume expansion is needed, the patient should be given a crystalloid solution to avoid disease transmission or adverse side effects and reactions.

Basic Immunology

The human immune system protects the body from harm by invading organisms. It accomplishes this through all the body cells, tissues, organs, and physiological processes. **Immunity** is the condition in which a person is protected from disease. The **immune response** is the ability of the immune system to recognize and respond to foreign invaders. Once an invader has been recognized, the immune system neutralizes or eliminates it, so the invader cannot cause damage to the body. An **antigen** is an agent that combines with an antibody to elicit an immune response. An **antibody** is an immunoglobulin (Ig) molecule. The antibody develops in response to an antigen that enters the body and combines with just a portion of the antigen called an **epitope.**

Basic Immunohematology

Within each of us, there is a special combination of genes called a **genotype.** The genotype determines our characteristics for certain traits. Our genetic differences occur because of the variations in cell surface composition. These variations in cell surface composition form the basis for blood compatibility.

Red Blood Cells

RBCs, also called erythrocytes, have an important protein called hemoglobin. Hemoglobin is responsible for the transportation of oxygen and carbon dioxide. Approximately 45 percent of our blood is composed of RBCs (Fig. 6-2).

An **isoantigen** is a substance that can stimulate the production of antibodies when introduced into the body. Blood groups are based on the isoantigens that are present on the surface of RBCs. There have been hundreds of isoantigen groups identified. However, the two most significant isoantigen groups are the ABO system and the Rh system. These two groups are likely to cause blood transfusion reactions because of their cell surface composition.

Blood Groups

A significant segment of the population has two related antigens on the surface of their RBCs, A and B. However, more than 40 percent of the population has neither A nor B antigens on the RBC surface. These people are said to have blood type "O." Every person has two genotypes that decide blood type. These pairs are what determine one of the four blood types: A, B, AB, or O. This pairing of genotypes may be AA, AO, BB, BO, AB, or OO. AA and AO genotypes produce blood type A. BB and BO produce blood type B. AB

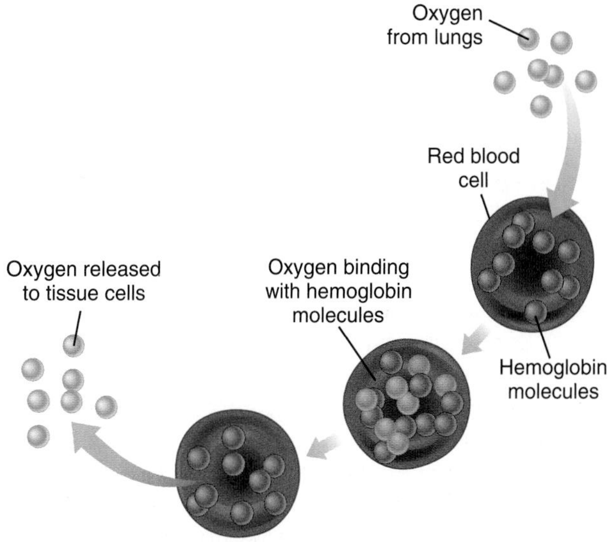

Figure 6-2 Red blood cell illustrating O_2 and CO_2 exchange.

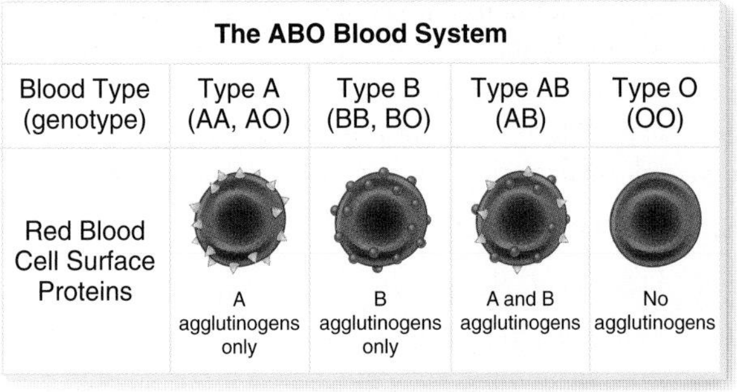

The ABO Blood System
Blood Type (genotype)
Type A (AA, AO)
Type B (BB, BO)
Type AB (AB)
Type O (OO)
Red Blood Cell Surface Proteins
A agglutinogens only
B agglutinogens only
A and B agglutinogens
No agglutinogens

Figure 6-3 The ABO blood typing system.

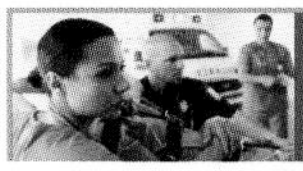

Table 6-1 Blood Compatibilities

Blood Type	Red Blood Cell Antigen	Plasma Antibody	Recipient Status	Donor Status
A	A	B	A or B	A or AB
B	B	A	B or O	B or AB
AB	A & B	None	A, B, AB, O	AB
O	None	A & B	O	A, B, AB, O

produces blood type AB, and genotype OO produces blood type O (Fig. 6-3).

Rh Factor (Type D)

The Rh (D) antigen is a component of the Rh blood groups. When people have an Rh factor on the surface of their RBCs, they are Rh positive (Rh^+). When the Rh factor is not on the surface of the RBCs, they are Rh negative (Rh^-). Approximately 95 percent of all African Americans are Rh^+, approximately 85 percent of Caucasians are Rh^+, and virtually all Native Americans are Rh^+. Antibodies are not present in the plasma in either Rh^+ (in patients not previously exposed to an Rh^+ patient) or Rh^- blood. A patient who is Rh^+ may receive either Rh^+ or Rh^- blood. However, a patient who is Rh^- can only receive Rh^- blood to avoid the formation of antibodies to Rh^+ blood. The first time an Rh^- patient receives Rh^+ blood, a reaction will generally not occur. However, antibodies will slowly develop during a 2-week to 4-month period. If the patient receives another transfusion of Rh^+ blood, the Rh antibodies will clump with the Rh antigens (**agglutinogens**) of the blood being transfused.

Blood Typing

Before blood can be administered to a patient, there must be compatibility between the blood types of the donor and the recipient. The process to determine this compatibility is called blood typing and crossmatching. **Blood typing** is the test run to determine the patient's blood type. **Crossmatching** is the process that determines the compatibility between the blood donor and the patient (recipient). If the blood donor and the recipient are incompatible, **agglutination** occurs, obstructing circulatory flow and ultimately causing death.

Patients who have blood type A should only receive blood type A, and those patients who have blood type B should only receive blood type B. However, in emergency situations, blood type O can be administered to any of the four blood types, because it does not contain either A or B antigens. A person who has blood type O is considered the **universal donor.** In emergency situations, persons who have type AB blood are able to receive all four types of blood, because they have no A or B antibodies. A person who has type AB blood is considered a **universal recipient.** However, unless there is an emergency, blood typing and crossmatching should be done to avoid any type of transfusion reaction. Table 6-1 illustrates blood types and their compatibilities with other blood types.

Blood Transfusion Reactions

The administration of blood or any of its components can cause a transfusion reaction, which may be fatal if not recognized and treated appropriately. EMS professionals must be able to recognize the signs and symptoms associated with a transfusion reaction and carry out interventions necessary to reverse its effects. The best way to recognize the signs and symptoms of a transfusion reaction is to assess the patient by body system. Table 6-2 illustrates the signs and symptoms of a transfusion reaction.

It is important to understand that reactions from blood or blood product transfusions can occur within 5 minutes of the start of the transfusion or as late as 48 hours after the transfusion is discontinued. Some patients have been known to experience a transfusion reaction up to 6 months after the transfusion.

Lipid-Lowering Agents

The National Cholesterol Education Program Exert Panel on Detection, Evaluation, and Treatment of High Cholesterol in Adults has developed guidelines for the treatment of high cholesterol and low-density lipoprotein (LDL) in adults. The adult recommendations for both LDL and high-density lipoprotein (HDL) levels of cholesterol are as follows.

Status of Total Cholesterol

- Desirable: (less than 200 mg/dL)
- Borderline high: (200 to 239 mg/dL)
- High: (greater than 240 mg/dL)

Status of LDL Cholesterol

- Optimal: (less than 100 mg/dL)
- Near optimal: (100 to 129 mg/dL)
- High-risk: (160 to 189 mg/dL)
- Very high-risk: (190 mg/dL or higher)

Status of HDL Cholesterol

- High-risk: (less than 40 mg/dL)
- Average: (40 to 50 mg/dL)
- Low-risk: (greater than 60 mg/dL)

Table 6-2 Signs and Symptoms of a Transfusion Reaction

Respiratory	Apnea Cough Dyspnea Rales Tachypnea Wheezing
Cardiovascular	Shock Chest pain Hyper- or hypotension Bradycardia or tachycardia Weak pulse
Nervous	Apprehension Fever Headache Numbness Tingling Sense of impending doom
Renal	Flank pain Concentrated, dark urine Renal failure
Musculoskeletal	Back pain
Gastrointestinal	Abdominal cramping or pain Diarrhea (may be bloody) Nausea/vomiting
Integumentary	Diaphoresis Urticarial (hives) Itching/rash Edema Cyanosis Facial flushing Cool/clammy or dry/flushed/hot
General	Chest pain Back pain Chills Headache Muscle aches Heat at infusion site

An antihyperlipidemic drug prevents or counteracts the accumulation of fatty substances in the blood. These drugs are used as an adjunct to diet to decrease elevated total LDL cholesterol in patients when the response to diet and other nondrug approaches has been unsuccessful.

Pharmacokinetics

Lipid-lowering drugs are used to help decrease blood lipids in an effort to reduce the morbidity and mortality of atherosclerotic cardiovascular disease and related diseases. HMG-CoA reductase inhibitors inhibit an enzyme involved in cholesterol synthesis. Statins block the production of cholesterol in the liver itself.

Bile acid sequestrants bind cholesterol in the GI tract. These drugs work inside the intestine, where they bind to bile from the liver and prevent it from being reabsorbed into the circulatory system. Bile is made largely from cholesterol, so these drugs work by depleting the body's supply of cholesterol.

Individual Drugs

HMG-CoA Reductase Inhibitors (Statins)

Atorvastatin (a-TORE-va-stat-in)

Lipitor

Classifications: Lipid-lowering drug (HMG-CoA reductase inhibitor)

Pregnancy Class: X

Mechanism of Action: Inhibits the enzyme HMG-CoA reductase, which is responsible for catalyzing an early step in the synthesis of cholesterol

Pharmacokinetics:

Absorption: Rapidly absorbed but undergoes extensive GI and liver metabolism, resulting in 14 percent bioavailability

Onset: Unknown

Duration: 20 to 30 hours

Indications: Primary prevention of cardiovascular disease in patients with multiple risk factors for coronary heart disease; secondary prevention of cardiovascular disease in patients with clinically evident coronary heart disease

Contraindications: Known hypersensitivity. Should not be used in patients with active liver disease. ❗ Potential for fetal anomalies during pregnancy and may disrupt infant lipid metabolism during lactation. ❗ Safety has not been established in children under 8 years of age.

Precautions: Use with caution in patients with a history of liver disease and in patients with a history of alcoholism.

Route and Dosage

PO (Adult): Initially, 10 to 20 mg once daily. Dosage may start with 40 mg daily if LDL should be lowered by more than 45 percent. Dosage may be increased every 2 to 4 weeks up to 80 mg/day.

PO (Pediatric, 10 to 17 years old): 10 mg/day initially. May be increased every 4 weeks up to 20 mg/day.

How Supplied

Tablets: 10 mg, 20 mg, 40 mg, 80 mg

Adverse Reactions and Side Effects

Resp: Bronchitis

CV: Chest pain, peripheral edema

CNS: Dizziness, headache, insomnia, weakness

EENT: Rhinitis

GI: Abdominal cramps, constipation, diarrhea, flatus, heartburn, altered taste, drug-induced hepatitis, dyspepsia, elevated liver enzymes, nausea, pancreatitis

GU: Erectile dysfunction

Derm: Rashes, pruritus

MS: RHABDOMYOLYSIS—An acute, sometimes fatal disease in which the by-products of skeletal muscle destruction accumulate

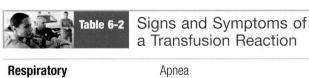

in the renal tubules and produce acute renal failure; arthritis, myalgia, myositis.
Drug Interactions: The effectiveness may be decreased by cholestyramine and colestipol. The risk of myopathy is increased if used with amiodarone, diltiazem, verapamil, and erythromycin. The risk of bleeding may increase with warfarin.
EMS Considerations: None

Fluvastatin (FLOO-va-sta-tin)

Lescol, Lescol XL
Classifications: Lipid-lowering drug (HMG-CoA reductase inhibitor)
Pregnancy Class: X
Mechanism of Action: Inhibits the enzyme HMG-CoA reductase, which is responsible for catalyzing an early step in the synthesis of cholesterol
Pharmacokinetics:
Absorption: 98 percent absorbed after oral administration but undergoes extensive first-pass metabolism resulting in 24 percent bioavailability
Onset: 1 to 2 weeks
Duration: Unknown
Indications: Used in the slow progression of coronary atherosclerosis in patients with coronary heart disease
Contraindications: Known hypersensitivity. Do not use in patients with active liver disease. (!) Potential for fetal anomalies during pregnancy and may disrupt infant lipid metabolism during lactation. (!) Safety has not been established in children under 8 years of age.
Precautions: Use with caution in patients with a history of liver disease and in patients with a history of alcoholism.
Route and Dosage
PO (Adult): 20 mg capsule once daily at bedtime. May start with 40 mg once daily at bedtime if LDL needs to be lowered by 25 percent. May be increased to 80 mg once daily (extended-release tablet) or 40 mg twice daily (capsule).
How Supplied
Capsules: 20 mg, 40 mg
Extended-release tablet: 80 mg
Adverse Reactions and Side Effects
Resp: Bronchitis
CV: Chest pain, peripheral edema
CNS: Dizziness, headache, insomnia, weakness
EENT: Rhinitis
GI: <u>Abdominal cramps</u>, <u>constipation</u>, <u>diarrhea</u>, <u>flatus</u>, <u>heartburn</u>, altered taste, drug-induced hepatitis, dyspepsia, elevated liver enzymes, nausea, pancreatitis
GU: Erectile dysfunction
Derm: <u>Rashes</u>, pruritus
MS: RHABDOMYOLYSIS—An acute, sometimes fatal disease in which the by-products of skeletal muscle destruction accumulate in the renal tubules and produce acute renal failure; arthritis, myalgia, myositis.
Drug Interactions: The effectiveness may be decreased by cholestyramine and colestipol. The risk of myopathy is increased if used with amiodarone, diltiazem, verapamil, and erythromycin. The risk of bleeding may increase with warfarin.
Drug Interactions: May increase digoxin levels. May increase the risk of bleeding if used with warfarin. Fluvastatin levels may increase if used with alcohol, cimetidine, ranitidine, and omeprazole.
EMS Considerations: None

Lovastatin (LOE-va-sta-tin)

Altoprev, Mevacor
Classifications: Lipid-lowering drug (HMG-CoA reductase inhibitor)
Pregnancy Class: X
Mechanism of Action: Inhibits the enzyme HMG-CoA reductase, which is responsible for catalyzing an early step in the synthesis of cholesterol
Pharmacokinetics:
Absorption: Poorly and variably absorbed after oral administration
Onset: 2 weeks
Duration: 6 weeks
Indications: Used in the slow progression of coronary atherosclerosis in patients with coronary heart disease
Contraindications: Known hypersensitivity. Do not use in patients with active liver disease. (!) Potential for fetal anomalies during pregnancy and may disrupt infant lipid metabolism during lactation. (!) Safety has not been established in children under 8 years of age.
Precautions: Use with caution in patients with a history of liver disease and in patients with a history of alcoholism.
Route and Dosage
PO (Adult): 20 mg once daily with evening meal. May be increased at 4-week intervals to a maximum of 80 mg/day (immediate-release) or 60 mg/day (extended-release).
How Supplied
Immediate-release tablets: 10 mg, 20 mg, 40 mg
Extended-release tablets: 10 mg, 20 mg, 40 mg, 60 mg
Adverse Reactions and Side Effects
Resp: Bronchitis
CV: Chest pain, peripheral edema
CNS: Dizziness, headache, insomnia, weakness
EENT: Rhinitis, blurred vision
GI: <u>Abdominal cramps</u>, <u>constipation</u>, <u>diarrhea</u>, <u>flatus</u>, <u>heartburn</u>, altered taste, drug-induced hepatitis, dyspepsia, elevated liver enzymes, nausea, pancreatitis
GU: Erectile dysfunction
Derm: <u>Rashes</u>, pruritus
MS: RHABDOMYOLYSIS—An acute, sometimes fatal disease in which the by-products of skeletal muscle destruction accumulate in the renal tubules and produce acute renal failure; arthritis, myalgia, myositis
Drug Interactions: The effectiveness may be decreased by cholestyramine and colestipol. The risk of myopathy is increased if used with amiodarone, diltiazem, verapamil, and erythromycin. The risk of bleeding may increase with warfarin.
Drug Interactions: Lovastatin levels may be increased if used with amiodarone, cyclosporine, diltiazem, and verapamil. Risk of bleeding increases if used with warfarin.
EMS Considerations: None

Pitavastatin (pi-TAVA-sta-tin)

Livalo

Classifications: Lipid-lowering drug (HMG-CoA reductase inhibitor)
Pregnancy Class: X
Mechanism of Action: Inhibits the enzyme HMG-CoA reductase, which is responsible for catalyzing an early step in the synthesis of cholesterol
Pharmacokinetics:
Absorption: Well absorbed after oral administration
Onset: Within 4 weeks
Duration: Unknown
Indications: Secondary prevention of cardiovascular disease in patients with clinically evident coronary heart disease.
Contraindications: Known hypersensitivity. Should not be given to patients with active liver disease. Do not give to patients with concurrent use of cyclosporine or lopinavir/ritonavir or to those with severe renal impairment.
Precautions: Use with caution in patients with a history of liver disease. Use with caution in patients with hypothyroidism. ❗ Increases the risk of myopathy in patients over the age of 65. ❗ Safety has not been established in children under 8 years of age.

Route and Dosage

PO (Adult): 2 mg once daily initially. May be increased up to 4 mg depending on response. NOTE: Concurrent erythromycin therapy—daily dose should not exceed 1 mg. Concurrent rifampin therapy—daily dose should not exceed 2 mg.

How Supplied

Tablets: 1 mg, 2 mg, 4 mg

Adverse Reactions and Side Effects

Resp: Bronchitis
CV: Chest pain, peripheral edema
CNS: Dizziness, headache, insomnia, weakness
EENT: Rhinitis
GI: <u>Abdominal cramps</u>, <u>constipation</u>, <u>diarrhea</u>, <u>flatus</u>, <u>heartburn</u>, altered taste, drug-induced hepatitis, dyspepsia, elevated liver enzymes, nausea, pancreatitis
GU: Erectile dysfunction
Derm: <u>Rashes</u>, pruritus
MS: RHABDOMYOLYSIS—An acute, sometimes fatal disease in which the by-products of skeletal muscle destruction accumulate in the renal tubules and produce acute renal failure; arthritis, myalgia, myositis
Drug Interactions: The effectiveness may be decreased by cholestyramine and colestipol. The risk of myopathy is increased if used with amiodarone, diltiazem, verapamil, and erythromycin. The risk of bleeding may increase with warfarin.
Drug Interactions: Cyclosporine increases the levels of pitavastatin and the risk of toxicity. Erythromycin and rifampin may increase blood levels of pitavastatin.
EMS Considerations: None

Pravastatin (PRA-va-sta-tin)

Pravachol

Classifications: Lipid-lowering drug (HMG-CoA reductase inhibitor)
Pregnancy Class: X
Mechanism of Action: Inhibits the enzyme HMG-CoA reductase, which is responsible for catalyzing an early step in the synthesis of cholesterol
Pharmacokinetics:
Absorption: Poorly and variably absorbed after oral administration
Onset: Several days
Duration: Unknown
Indications: Primary prevention of coronary heart disease in patients without clinically evident coronary heart disease; secondary prevention of cardiovascular disease in patients with clinically evident coronary heart disease
Contraindications: Known hypersensitivity. Should not be given to patients with active liver disease. ❗ Potential for fetal anomalies during pregnancy and may disrupt infant lipid metabolism during lactation. ❗ Safety has not been established in children under 8 years of age.
Precautions: Use with caution in patients with liver disease and in patients with alcoholism.

Route and Dosage

PO (Adult): 40 mg once daily at bedtime. Dosage may be increased at 4-week intervals up to 80 mg/day. Note: Concurrent cyclosporine therapy—initial dose is 10 mg/day and should not exceed 20 mg/day.
PO (Pediatric, 8 to 13 years): 20 mg once daily
PO (Pediatric, 14 to 18 years): 40 mg once daily

How Supplied

Tablets: 10 mg, 20 mg, 40 mg, 80 mg

Adverse Reactions and Side Effects

Resp: Bronchitis
CV: Chest pain, peripheral edema
CNS: Dizziness, headache, insomnia, weakness
EENT: Rhinitis
GI: <u>Abdominal cramps</u>, <u>constipation</u>, <u>diarrhea</u>, <u>flatus</u>, <u>heartburn</u>, altered taste, drug-induced hepatitis, dyspepsia, elevated liver enzymes, nausea, pancreatitis
GU: Erectile dysfunction
Derm: <u>Rashes</u>, pruritus
MS: RHABDOMYOLYSIS—An acute, sometimes fatal disease in which the by-products of skeletal muscle destruction accumulate in the renal tubules and produce acute renal failure; arthritis, myalgia, myositis
Drug Interactions: None significant
EMS Considerations: None

Rosuvastatin (roe-SOO-va-sta-tin)

Crestor

Classifications: Lipid-lowering drug (HMG-CoA reductase inhibitor)
Pregnancy Class: X
Mechanism of Action: Inhibits the enzyme HMG-CoA reductase, which is responsible for catalyzing an early step in the synthesis of cholesterol
Pharmacokinetics:
Absorption: 20 percent absorbed after oral administration
Onset: Unknown
Duration: Unknown

Indications: Slow progression of coronary atherosclerosis in patients with coronary heart disease
Contraindications: Known hypersensitivity. Should not be given to patients with active liver disease. (!) Potential for fetal anomalies during pregnancy and may disrupt infant lipid metabolism during lactation. (!) Safety has not been established in children under 8 years of age.
Precautions: (!) Use with caution in patients with Asian ancestry because they may develop increased rosuvastatin blood levels and an increased risk of rhabdomyolysis.
Route and Dosage
PO (Adult): 10 mg once daily. Dose may be adjusted at 2- to 4-week intervals up to 40 mg/day. (!) Patients with Asian ancestry should not be given an initial dose of more than 5 mg/day. NOTE: Concurrent cyclosporine therapy—dose should not exceed 5 mg/day.
How Supplied
Tablets: 5 mg, 10 mg, 20 mg, 40 mg
Adverse Reactions and Side Effects
Resp: Bronchitis
CV: Chest pain, peripheral edema
CNS: Dizziness, headache, insomnia, weakness
EENT: Rhinitis
GI: Abdominal cramps, constipation, diarrhea, flatus, heartburn, altered taste, drug-induced hepatitis, dyspepsia, elevated liver enzymes, nausea, pancreatitis
GU: Erectile dysfunction
Derm: Rashes, pruritus
MS: RHABDOMYOLYSIS—An acute, sometimes fatal disease in which the by-products of skeletal muscle destruction accumulate in the renal tubules and produce acute renal failure; arthritis, myalgia, myositis
Drug Interactions: May cause an increase in bleeding if used with warfarin. Antacids decrease the absorption of rosuvastatin. Therefore, antacids should be taken 2 hours after rosuvastatin. Cyclosporine increases the levels and risk of toxicity of rosuvastatin.
EMS Considerations: None

Simvastatin (SIM-va-sta-tin)

Zocor
Classifications: Lipid-lowering drug (HMG-CoA reductase inhibitor)
Pregnancy Class: X
Mechanism of Action: Inhibits the enzyme HMG-CoA reductase, which is responsible for catalyzing an early step in the synthesis of cholesterol
Pharmacokinetics:
Absorption: 85 percent absorbed but rapidly metabolized
Onset: Several days
Duration: Unknown
Indications: Secondary prevention of cardiovascular events in patients with clinically evident coronary heart disease or those at high risk for coronary heart disease
Contraindications: Known hypersensitivity. Should not be given to patients with active liver disease. (!) Potential for fetal anomalies during pregnancy and may disrupt infant lipid metabolism during lactation. (!) Safety has not been established in children under 8 years of age.
Precautions: Use with caution in patients with a history liver disease and in patients with alcoholism.
Route and Dosage
PO (Adult): 5 to 80 mg once daily in the evening. NOTE: Concurrent cyclosporine or danazol therapy—dose should not exceed 10 mg/day. Concurrent amiodarone or verapamil therapy—dose should not exceed 20 mg/day.
PO (Pediatric, 10 to 17 years): 10 mg once daily; may increase dose at 4-week intervals up to 40 mg/day
How Supplied
Tablets: 5 mg, 10 mg, 20 mg, 40 mg, 80 mg
Adverse Reactions and Side Effects
Resp: Bronchitis
CV: Chest pain, peripheral edema
CNS: Dizziness, headache, insomnia, weakness
EENT: Rhinitis
GI: Abdominal cramps, constipation, diarrhea, flatus, heartburn, altered taste, drug-induced hepatitis, dyspepsia, elevated liver enzymes, nausea, pancreatitis
GU: Erectile dysfunction
Derm: Rashes, pruritus
MS: RHABDOMYOLYSIS—An acute, sometimes fatal disease in which the by-products of skeletal muscle destruction accumulate in the renal tubules and produce acute renal failure; arthritis, myalgia, myositis
Drug Interactions: The risk of myopathy is increased with amiodarone, cyclosporine, diltiazem, verapamil, and erythromycin. Risk of bleeding increases with warfarin. Antacids decrease the absorption of simvastatin. Therefore, antacids should be taken 2 hours after simvastatin.
EMS Considerations: None

Bile Acid Sequestrants

Cholestyramine (koe-less-TEAR-a-meen)

LoCHOLEST, LoCHOLEST Light, Prevalite, Questran, Questran Light
Classifications: Lipid-lowering drug/bile acid sequestrant
Pregnancy Class: C
Mechanism of Action: Binds bile acids in the GI tract, resulting in increased clearance of cholesterol
Pharmacokinetics:
Absorption: Action takes place in the GI tract—no absorption occurs.
Onset: 24 to 48 hours
Duration: 2 to 4 weeks
Indications: Used in the management of primary hypercholesterolemia
Contraindications: Known hypersensitivity. Should not be used in patients with biliary obstruction. Some products contain aspartame and should be avoided in patients with phenylketonuria (PKU), a congenital autosomal recessive disease.

Precautions: Use with caution in patients with a history of constipation. (!) Extreme caution must be used in pediatric patients because this drug may cause intestinal obstruction; deaths have been reported.

Route and Dosage

PO (Adult): 4 g 1 to 2 times daily; may be increased as needed/tolerated up to 24 g/day in six divided doses

PO (Pediatric): 240 mg/kg/day in 2 to 3 divided doses. Patients should not receive more than 8 g/day.

> ***Understand the Numbers***
>
> Your 66-pound patient is given a prescription for cholestyramine at 240 mg/kg/day. How many mg will she take in each of three divided doses?
>
> 66 lbs. × 2.2 = 30 kg. 30 kg × 240 mg = 7,200 mg ÷ 3 = 2,400 mg or 2.4 g/dose.

How Supplied

Powder for suspension with aspartame (LoCHOLEST, Prevalite, Questran Light): 4 g packet or scoop

Powder for suspension (LoCHOLEST, Questran, generic): 4 g packet or scoop

Adverse Reactions and Side Effects

EENT: Irritation of the tongue

GI: Abdominal discomfort, constipation, nausea, fecal impaction, flatulence, hemorrhoids, perianal irritation, vomiting

Derm: Irritation, rashes

Metab: Vitamin A, D, and K deficiency

Drug Interactions: May decrease absorption/effects of orally administered acetaminophen, amiodarone, digoxin, diuretics, corticosteroids, phenytoin, propranolol, tetracyclines, and fat-soluble vitamins (A, D, E, and K), as well as many other medications

EMS Considerations: None

Colesevelam (koe-le-SEV-e-lam)

Welchol

Classifications: Lipid-lowering drug/bile acid sequestrant

Pregnancy Class: B

Mechanism of Action: Binds bile acids in the GI tract, resulting in increased clearance of cholesterol

Pharmacokinetics:

Absorption: Action takes place in the GI tract—no absorption occurs.

Onset: 24 to 48 hours

Duration: Unknown

Indications: Adjunctive therapy to diet and exercise for the reduction of LDL cholesterol in patients with primary hypercholesterolemia

Contraindications: Known hypersensitivity. Should not be used in patients with bowel obstruction, in patients with triglycerides greater than 500 mg/dL, and in patients with a history of pancreatitis due to hypertriglyceridemia.

Precautions: Use with caution in patients with triglycerides greater than 300 mg/dL; in patients with dysphagia, swallowing disorders, or severe GI motility disorders; or in patients with major GI tract surgery. (!) Safety has not been established in pregnant or lactating patients or in children.

Route and Dosage

PO (Adult): Three tablets twice daily or six tablets once daily

How Supplied

Tablets: 625 mg

Adverse Reactions and Side Effects

GI: Constipation, dyspepsia

Drug Interactions: May decrease absorption of glyburide, levothyroxine, phenytoin, and estrogen-containing oral contraceptives

EMS Considerations: None

Colestipol (koe-LES-ti-pole)

Colestid

Classifications: Lipid-lowering drug/bile acid sequestrant

Pregnancy Class: Unknown

Mechanism of Action: Binds bile acids in the GI tract, resulting in increased clearance of cholesterol

Pharmacokinetics:

Absorption: Action takes place in the GI tract—no absorption occurs.

Onset: 24 to 48 hours

Duration: 1 month

Indications: Used in the management of primary hypercholesterolemia

Contraindications: Known hypersensitivity. Should not be used in patients with biliary obstruction. Some products contain aspartame and should be avoided in patients with PKU, a congenital autosomal recessive disease.

Precautions: Use with caution in patients with a history of constipation. (!) Extreme caution must be used in pediatric patients because this drug may cause intestinal obstruction; deaths have been reported.

Route and Dosage

PO (Adult):

Granules—5 g 1 to 2 times daily; may be increased every 1 to 2 months up to 30 g/day in 1 to 2 doses

Tablets—2 g 1 to 2 times daily; may be increased every 1 to 2 months up to 16 g/day in 1 to 2 doses

How Supplied

Granules for suspension: 5 g/packet or scoop

Tablets: 1 g

Adverse Reactions and Side Effects

EENT: Irritation of the tongue

GI: Abdominal discomfort, constipation, nausea, fecal impaction, flatulence, hemorrhoids, perianal irritation, vomiting

Derm: Irritation, rashes

Metab: Vitamin A, D, and K deficiency

Drug Interactions: May decrease absorption/effects of orally administered acetaminophen, amiodarone, digoxin, diuretics, corticosteroids, phenytoin, propranolol, tetracyclines, and fat-soluble vitamins (A, D, E, and K), as well as many other medications

EMS Considerations: None

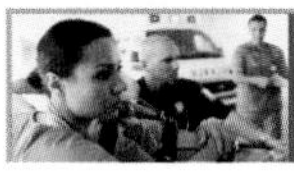

Table 6-3 Common Statin-combination Drugs

Genetic Name	Trade Name	Mechanism of Action
niacin with lovastatin	Advicor	Lowers LDL cholesterol and raises HDL cholesterol
atorvastatin with amlodipine	Caduet	Lowers how much cholesterol the body makes and also lowers blood pressure
gemfibrozil	Lopid	Lowers triglycerides and raises HDL cholesterol; may slightly increase LDL cholesterol
ezetimibe with simvastatin	Vytorin	Lowers how much cholesterol the body makes; also affects how the body absorbs cholesterol
ezetimibe	Zetia	Lowers how much cholesterol the body can absorb

Table 6-3 lists some common statin-combination drugs that are also used to help control high cholesterol levels.

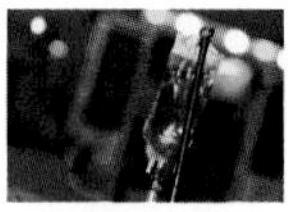

SCENARIO REVISITED

Have you considered the case of Emma?

As you recall, Emma, 24 years old, was a passenger in an MVA and was originally transported to a local rural hospital. Due to her injuries, Emma needs treatment at the local trauma facility. About 10 minutes into the transport, Emma becomes unresponsive, and her vital signs begin to deteriorate. Her heart rate has increased to 112 beats/minute with an occasional PVC, respirations are 18 breaths/minute, and her blood pressure has dropped to 90/60 mm Hg. Medical control has advised your team to infuse 1 U of packed RBCs. All current signs indicate that Emma is probably bleeding internally.

Once you have performed an appropriate assessment, you should proceed using a critical thinking approach to the administration of the packed RBCs.

Step 1: Determine signs and symptoms to be treated.
Step 2: Consider both the risks and benefits of treating or not treating your patient.
Step 3: Choose the medication that provides the best possible outcome. In this case, the hospital sent your team with 1 U of type O Rh^- packed RBCs. This is the optimal type of packed RBCs for out-of-hospital administration.
Step 4: Remember indications, contraindications, and precautions for administering packed RBCs.
Step 5: Decide the best route for administering the medication for the best outcome.
Step 6: Administer the medication(s) according to the 7 Patient Rights.

1. The right patient
2. The right drug (type of packed RBCs)
3. The right drug amount (1 U of packed RBCs is approximately 350 mL)
4. The right time
5. The right route
6. The right documentation
7. The right of the patient to accept or refuse the medication(s)

Check the Evidence

In blood transfusion administration, the greatest risk to the patient is ABO-incompatibility. However, in this case ABO incompatibility is not a concern, because only blood type O is used in the out-of-hospital setting.

Step 7: Reevaluate the patient for the desired and undesired effects.

To prepare for the administration of the packed RBCs, you will need the 1 U of packed RBCs, blood tubing (filtered), NS, and the proper personal protective equipment (PPE).

effective Communication

Only NS is compatible with whole blood and blood products.

After performing the patient assessment, including the Seven Patient Rights, the procedure for administering packed RBCs is as follows:

1. Observe standard precautions.
2. If possible, explain the procedure to the patient and why the procedure is necessary.
3. Assess and document that the proper packed RBC temperature has been maintained.
4. Examine the unit expiration date and the pack numbers on both the transfusion record and on the label of the packed RBCs.
5. Confirm that the RBCs are type O and Rh^-.

Check the Evidence

Rh^+ blood should be avoided in women of childbearing age. If a woman with Rh^- blood receives a transfusion of Rh^+ blood, she may develop antibodies against the Rh factor. This could be harmful to the fetus if pregnancy occurs.

6. Examine the packed RBCs for any leakage, abnormal color, or clumps.
7. Confirm that the packed RBCs will be infused through an IV line flushed with NS.
8. Record all vital signs before the transfusion and every 15 minutes during the transfusion.
9. Attach the unit of packed RBCs to the blood tubing and begin the transfusion.

10. Closely monitor the transfusion during the first 10 to 15 minutes, observing for an acute hemolytic reaction. If any sign of a reaction occurs, discontinue the transfusion immediately. Save the remaining unit for analysis.
11. Document all identifying numbers of the infused unit, infusion times, and all patient vital signs.

Let's Recap

Administering blood and blood products can be lifesaving; however, if done improperly, it can also become deadly. It is imperative that, once blood or a blood product is given, the EMS professional knows the signs and symptoms of an adverse reaction or a transfusion and reports and treats the patient accordingly.

There are many individuals taking medications to help in lowering their cholesterol levels. EMS professionals should become familiar with each of these drugs so they can better understand the disease process of coronary artery disease and hypercholesterolemia. Antihyperlipidemic drugs have helped greatly to combat these disease processes.

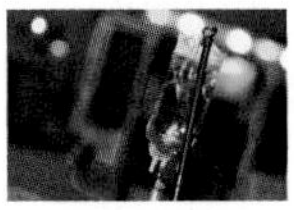

SCENARIO CONCLUSION

During transport to the trauma center, you must constantly monitor Emma for any signs of transfusion reactions. Transfusion reactions can occur rapidly or may occur several hours after the transfusion has completed, or some patients may develop reactions several months later.

The major concern while transporting Emma is the probable internal bleeding from the MVA. This can only be controlled successfully at the receiving facility. The best way to assess Emma during the packed RBC infusion is by body system: respiratory status, cardiovascular status, nervous system status, etc. The most common reactions to the infusion of the packed RBCs for Emma are anaphylaxis, chest pain, back pain, chills, headache, muscle aches, and heat at the infusion site. If any transfusion reactions occur, immediately discontinue the infusion, keep the IV line open using NS, and treat emergency situations using your local protocol.

PRACTICE EXERCISES

1. Within each human being, there is a unique combination of genes called a(n):
a. Antigen
b. Epitope
c. Antibody
d. Genotype

2. A substance that can stimulate the production of antibodies when introduced into the body is called a(n):
a. Isoantigen
b. Genotype
c. Antigen
d. Epitope

3. The process that determines the compatibility between the blood donor and the patient (recipient) is called:
a. Blood typing
b. Crossmatching
c. Agglutinogen
d. Agglutination

4. A person who is called the universal donor has a blood type of:
a. A
b. B
c. O
d. AB

5. A person who is called the universal recipient has a blood type of:
a. A
b. B
c. O
d. AB

6. You are working a clinical rotation in the office of a pediatrician. She orders a patient to begin taking cholestyramine at 240 mg/kg/day in three divided doses. The patient weighs 85 pounds. How much of the drug should be given at each of the three doses? Remember, the maximum daily dose for cholestyramine is 8 g/day for the pediatric patient.
a. 1.50 g (1,500 mg)
b. 1.67 g (1,670 mg)
c. 2.50 g (2,500 mg)
d. 2.67 g (2,670 mg)

7. You are transporting a patient with a blood type of AB. If he requires additional blood to be infused, he must receive blood type(s):
a. O
b. A or O
c. B or O
d. A, B, AB, or O

8. Packed RBCs have _____ of the plasma removed but provide the same amount of RBCs as whole blood.
a. 50 percent
b. 60 percent
c. 70 percent
d. 80 percent

9. It is important to understand that reactions from blood or blood product transfusions can occur within 5 minutes of the start of the transfusion or as late as 48 hours after the transfusion is discontinued. However, some patients have been known to experience a transfusion reaction up to ____ months after the transfusion.
a. 2
b. 4
c. 6
d. 8

10. People are considered at high risk for HDL cholesterol when their mg/dL levels become:
a. less than 200 mg/dL
b. less than 100 mg/dL
c. greater than 40 mg/dL
d. less than 40 mg/dL

CASE STUDY

You are at a clinical rotation in the intensive care unit. Dr. Weiss has ordered a blood transfusion on his patient, Dr. Hill, a retired dentist. Dr. Hill has a blood type of AB, the universal recipient. Your preceptor, Miss Scherer, wants you to observe while Dr. Hill receives the transfusion. Before administering the blood, Dr. Weiss ordered 325 mg of acetaminophen to help prevent a mild fever and 50 mg of diphenhydramine to help mild hypersensitivity reactions.

Approximately 15 minutes into the blood transfusion, Dr. Hill went into severe anaphylaxis. After Dr. Hill was stabilized, Miss Scherer reviewed how paramedics could treat this reaction in the out-of-hospital setting:

- Stop the infusion and replace with NS. It is important to maintain volume levels.
- Secure the patient's airway and administer 100 percent humidified oxygen.
- You may give the following medications, depending on protocols:
  - Furosemide may be given to increase renal flow.
  - Low-dose dopamine may be given to increase renal flow.
  - Diphenhydramine may be given to relieve allergic reactions.
  - Epinephrine may be given for relief of severe allergic reactions and for the management of reversible airway constriction.
  - Various bronchodilators may be given to help combat airway constriction.

It is important to monitor patients receiving blood or blood products in case they experience transfusion adverse reactions.

MATH EQUATIONS

Volume

1. You are ordered to give 200 mg of a drug to your patient. The drug comes as a 10 mL syringe containing 500 mg of the drug. How much of the drug do you give?
2. You are ordered to give 0.3 mg of a drug to your patient. The drug comes as 1 mg in 10 mL. How much of the drug do you give?
3. You are ordered to give 75 mg of a drug to your patient. The drug comes as 150 mg in 100 mL. How much of the drug do you give?
4. You are ordered to give 300 mg of a drug to your patient. The drug comes as 360 mg in 200 mL. How much of the drug do you give?
5. You are ordered to give 40,000 mcg of a drug to your patient. The drug comes as 2,500 mg in 250 mL. How much of the drug do you give?
6. You are ordered to give 40 mg of a drug to your patient. The drug comes as 250 mg in 5 mL. How much of the drug do you give?
7. You are ordered to give 200 mg of a drug to your patient. The drug comes as 800 mg in 10 mL. How much of the drug do you give?
8. You are ordered to give 0.6 mg of a drug to your patient. The drug comes as 1.2 mg in 4 mL. How much of the drug do you give?
9. You are ordered to give 2 mg of a drug to your patient. The drug comes as 10 mg in 5 mL. How much of the drug do you give?
10. You are ordered to give 135 mg of a drug to your patient. The drug comes as 100 mg in 10 mL. How much of the drug do you give?

REFERENCES

American Pregnancy Association. Rh factor. Retrieved December 19, 2013 from www.americanpregnancy.org/pregnancycomplications/rhfactor-2.html

American Red Cross. Learn about blood. Retrieved December 10, 2013 from www.redcrossblood.org/learn-about-blood

Beck, R. K. (2012). Blood and blood product administration. In *Pharmacology for the EMS provider.* New York: Delmar, Cengage Learning.

Deglin, J. H., Vallerand, A. H., and Sanboski, C. A. (2011). *Davis's drug guide for nurses* (12th ed.). Philadelphia, PA: F. A. Davis Company.

Drugs.com. Blood transfusion reactions. Retrieved December 19, 2013 from www.drugs.com/cg/blood-transfusion-reactions.html

The Franklin Institute. The human heart. Retrieved December 10, 2013 from www.fi.edu/learn/heart/blood/platelet.html

Kardon, E. M., and Brenner, B. E. (2012). Transfusion reactions in emergency medicine treatment and management. Retrieved December 19, 2013 from www.emedicine.medscape.com/article/780074-overview

National Heart, Lung, and Blood Institute. (2009). *What you need to know about high cholesterol.* Washington, DC: U.S. Department of Health and Human Services. Retrieved December 13, 2013 from www.nhlbi.nih.gov/health/public/heart/chol/cholesterol_atglance.pdf

Venes, D., ed. (2013). *Taber's cyclopedic medical dictionary* (22nd ed.). Philadelphia, PA: F. A. Davis Company.

WebMD, LLC. High cholesterol: Cholesterol-lowering medication. Retrieved December 10, 2013 from www.webmd.com/cholesterol-management/guide/cholesterol-lowering-medication

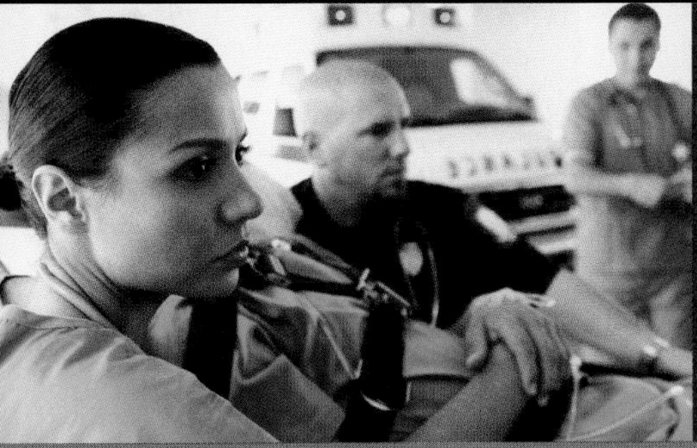

CHAPTER 7

Drug-Dosage Calculations

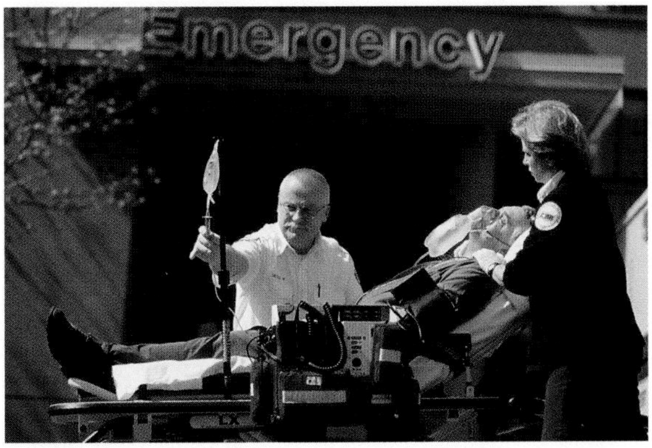

Paramedics calculating an IV infusion rate. *(Photograph © Keith Brofsky/Photodisc/Thinkstock)*

LEARNING OUTCOMES

- Define and briefly discuss the metric system and the apothecaries' system.
- Interpret a medication order accurately.
- Solve the mathematical principles using decimals by adding, subtracting, multiplying, dividing, rounding, and using ratio and proportion.
- Convert quantities from the U.S. system of measurement to the metric system.
- Convert quantities within the metric system.
- Calculate drug dosages for adults and children.
- Calculate drug solutions, including rates of infusion.
- Convert temperature measurements from Fahrenheit to Celsius.

KEY TERMS

Apothecaries' system
Celsius
Concentration
Fahrenheit
Gram
International System of Units (metric system)
Length
Liter
Mass
Meter
Proportion
Ratio
Unit
U.S. system of measurement
U.S.P. unit
Volume

SCENARIO OPENING

You are assigned to Rescue 22 at one of the busiest stations in the city. It is a warm, sunny, summer day. About 20 minutes after you arrive, a call comes in as "a little girl having trouble breathing." Upon arrival, you are directed to the patient's bedroom where you find 5-year-old Gail, who is having trouble breathing. Her mom states that Gail was playing in the screened-in porch when she was bitten by "several" fire ants. Your initial rapid assessment reveals:

Level of consciousness:	alert but very anxious
Respirations:	rapid, with stridor
Pulse:	rapid and regular
Skin:	cool and damp
Eyes:	equal and reactive

You also notice that Gail wants to rub her left ankle, which is red and swollen. Gail's mom states that Gail does not have any known allergies. Gail weighs approximately 45 pounds.

Your assessment determines that Gail is having an anaphylactic reaction to the fire ant bites. Since Gail's breathing is becoming more compromised, the decision is made to treat her with oxygen and IM epinephrine immediately at the scene. While the epinephrine is being prepared, Gail is placed on oxygen and an ECG monitor. The initial dosage for the epinephrine is 0.01 mg/kg of a 1:1000 solution.

Understand the Numbers

The 1:1000 ratio for epinephrine means that there is 1 mg in 1 mL of solution. Epinephrine also comes as a 1:10,000 solution. This means that there is 1 mg in 10 mL of solution.

Introduction

Administering drugs would be much easier if they all came in the same forms and the same concentrations and were packaged in the same way. However, drugs come in a variety of forms, packages, and concentrations (Fig. 7-1). Everyone with the responsibility for administering drugs must (1) be familiar with their various forms and concentrations, (2) know how to prepare the drug for administration, and (3) be able to calculate the dosage and rate of administration. The following list is an example of the bewildering variety of forms in which drugs often used in EMS are packaged:

- **Lidocaine:** 2 grams (2 g) in solution in a 10-milliliter (10-mL) syringe. In this case, the drug concentration is 200 milligrams per milliliter (200 mg/mL). The EMS professional dilutes this in an appropriate intravenous fluid before administration. Lidocaine is also commonly available, for direct intravenous bolus injection, as 100 milligrams of a 20-milligrams-per-milliliter solution in a prefilled 5-milliliter syringe.

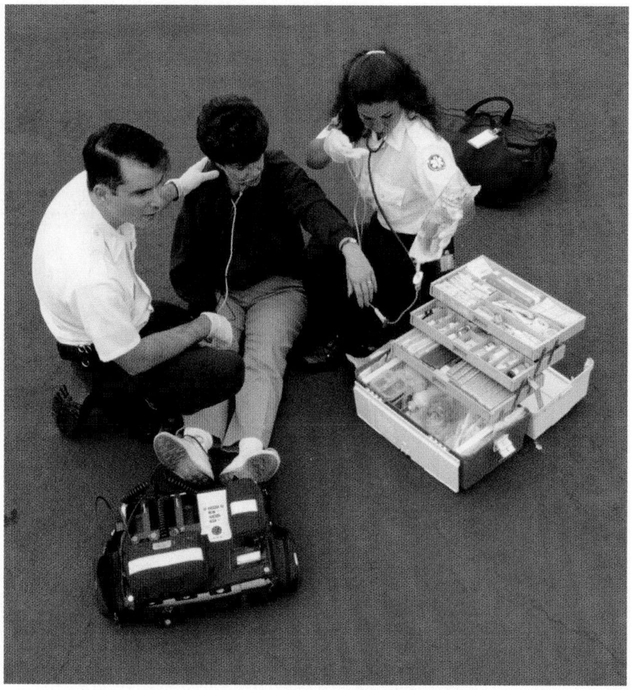

Figure 7-1 Various forms and concentrations of drugs used in EMS. *(Photograph © Keith Brofsky/Photodisc/Thinkstock)*

- **$D_{50}W$ (50 percent dextrose in water):** This widely used EMS drug is commonly available in a 50-milliliter prefilled syringe, which contains 25 grams of dextrose.
- **Furosemide:** 20 milligrams in a 2-milliliter prefilled syringe. Furosemide is also packaged in ampules of different sizes (for example, 20 milligrams in a 2-milliliter ampule, 100 milligrams in a 10-milliliter ampule).
- **Nitroglycerin:** Tablets—Commonly available in 1/150 grain (1/150 gr), which equals 0.4 milligram, or 1/200 grain, which equals 0.3 milligram. (One grain, in apothecaries' measure, equals about 60 milligrams.) Metered spray—0.4 mg/spray. Parenteral: 5 mg/mL; 10 mg/100 mL, 20 mg/100 mL, and 40 mg/100 mL
- **Oxytocin:** Commonly packaged as 10 U.S.P. units in a 1-milliliter ampule. A **unit** is defined as one of anything. It is a specific amount adopted as a standard of measurement. A **U.S.P. unit** is any unit specified in the *United States Pharmacopeia.*
- **Dopamine:** One of the forms in which this drug is packaged is as 200 milligrams in solution in a 5-milliliter prefilled syringe.
- **Sodium bicarbonate:** Sodium bicarbonate is usually packaged in prefilled 50-milliliter syringes, containing either 44.4 or 50 milliequivalents (mEq). A **milliequivalent** is the concentration of electrolytes (see Chapter 5) in a certain volume of solution, usually expressed as milliequivalent per liter (mEq/L).

As the preceding list shows, drugs come in a bewildering variety of forms, concentrations, and packages. EMS professionals who administer drugs must be able to use mathematical calculations to determine the correct dosages. This chapter reviews the necessary calculations involved in the safe administration of drugs to the patient.

effective Communication

Do not administer a drug that is given in the form of volume ("give 2 mL of morphine sulfate"). Drugs can come in varying concentrations. For example, IV injection morphine can come packaged anywhere from 1 mg/mL to 50 mg/mL. Therefore, only accept orders given in specific concentrated dosages, such as "give 4 mg of morphine sulfate."

Weights and Measures

Throughout history, humans have developed various systems of weights and measures—ways of describing the size or amount of physical objects or substances. Each system has units of measure for three physical characteristics:

- **Length:** The distance between two points
- **Mass:** How much matter is in an object or a substance; this is commonly expressed as its weight.
- **Volume:** The amount of space occupied by an object or a substance

Some systems use different measures for dry and liquid volume. For instance, in the system used in the United States (called the **U.S. system of measurement** or household system), the units of dry measure are pint, quart, peck, and bushel, and the units of liquid measure include fluid ounce, pint, quart, and gallon.

Because of the historic roots of pharmacology, drug dosages in the United States are expressed in any one of three systems:

1. The **International System of Units (metric system):** discussed in the next section
2. The **U.S. system of measurement:** The U.S. system is based on the traditional English system.
3. The **apothecaries' system:** Apothecary is the old name for pharmacist. The apothecaries' system has units of measure for weight (mass) and liquid weight (capacity).

Table 7-1 lists the various units of measure in each system. Table 7-2 shows the equivalents between various units in the English and metric systems.

To administer drugs safely, EMS professionals must be able to convert various units of measure:

- You will need to convert an amount expressed in one unit of measure into its equivalent in another unit of measure in the same system. For example, if a physician tells you to administer 1,500 milligrams of a drug and the drug is packaged in tablets, each containing 0.5 grams of the drug, you must convert 0.5 grams to its equivalent in milligrams in order to calculate how many

Table 7-1 Systems of Weights and Measures

U.S. (English)	Metric	Apothecaries'
	Mass (Weight)	
Pound (lb)	Kilogram (kg)	Pound* (lb ap)
Ounce (oz)	Hectogram (hg)	Ounce (oz ap)
Dram (dr)	Dekagram (dag)	Dram (dr ap)
Grain (gr)	Gram (g) Decigram (dg) Centigram (cg) Milligram (mg) Microgram (mcg)	Scruple (s) Grain*
	Volume (Liquid Measure)	
Gallon (gal)	Kiloliter (kL)	Gallon (gal)
Quart (qt)	Hectoliter (hL)	Quart (qt)
Pint (pt)	Dekaliter (daL)	Pint (pt)
Gill (gi)	Liter (L)	Gill (gi)
Fluid ounce (fl oz)	Deciliter (dL)	Fluid ounce (fl oz)
Fluidram (fl dr)	Centiliter (cL)	Fluidram (fl dr)
Minim (min)	Milliliter (mL) Microliter (μL)	Minim (min)
	Length	
Mile (mi)	Kilometer (km)	
Yard (yd)	Hectometer (hm)	
Foot (ft or ')	Dekameter (dam)	
Inch (in or ")	Meter (m) Decimeter (dm) Centimeter (cm) Millimeter (mm) Micrometer (μm)	

*Although the English pound and apothecaries' pound are not equivalent, the English grain and apothecaries' grain are—each is equal to approximately 60 milligrams.

Table 7-2 Commonly Used Equivalents

Metric to English	English to Metric
1 kilogram (k) = 2.2 pounds (lb)	1 pound (lb) = 0.454 kilograms (k)
1 gram (g) = 0.035 ounces (oz)	1 ounce (oz) = 28.35 grams (g)
1 milligram (mg) = 0.015 grains (gr)	1 grain (gr) = 0.0645 grains (gr) or 64.5 milligrams (mg)
1 liter (L) = 1.057 quarts (qt)	1 fluid ounce (fl oz) = 29.57 milligrams (mg)
1 deciliter (dL) = 3.38 fluid ounces (fl oz)	
1 milliliter (mL) = 0.27 fluidram (fl dr)	

Table 7-3 Metric Prefixes

Prefix	Multiple of Base
Mega-	1,000,000
Kilo-	1,000
Hecto-	100
Deka-	10
Base	0
Deci-	1/10
Centi-	1/100
Milli-	1/1,000
Micro-	1/1,000,000

	Thousands			Ones				Decimals			
Millions	Hundred Thousands	Ten Thousands	Thousands	Hundreds	Tens	Ones	Decimal Point	Tenths	Hundredths	Thousandths	Ten Thousandths
5	3	8	2	1	6	1	.	7	9	0	3

Figure 7-2 Decimal placement: In the decimal system, the position of a number in relation to the decimal place determines the name and value of the number.

tablets are required. (You will learn how to do this in the "Decimals" section under "Review of Mathematical Principles.")

- You must also know how to convert an amount expressed in one unit of measure into its equivalent in another system. For example, many drug orders are based on body weight. If the order tells you to administer 0.5 milligrams per kilogram of body weight, and your patient weighs 165 pounds, you must convert pounds to kilograms. (The "U.S.-to-Metric Conversions" section shows you how.)

International System of Units (Metric System)

The International System of Units (SI) or metric system is used in many countries of the world and in all scientific disciplines, including medicine and pharmacology. It is a decimal system, meaning it is based on the number 10. Every unit of length is 10 times larger than the next smaller unit and 10 times smaller than the next larger unit. The basic unit of length is the **meter;** the basic unit of mass (weight) is the **gram;** and the basic unit of volume is the **liter.** The names of all the other units of measure in the metric system are formed by adding prefixes to the names of the basic units. The prefix indicates how many times larger or smaller than the basic unit the new unit will be. For example, a kilometer equals 1,000 meters; a millimeter equals one thousandth of a meter. Table 7-3 illustrates the progression of prefixes used in the metric system.

Review of Mathematical Principles

Decimals

Converting dosages within the metric system is easy because it is a decimal system. A review of decimal arithmetic will show how simple calculating metric dosages can be.

Each amount in the metric system consists of a whole number (in many cases, the whole number is 0) and a decimal fraction separated by the decimal point (for example, 1.5). The whole number is on the left of the decimal point, and the decimal fraction is expressed by the numbers on the right of the decimal point. The position of a number in relation to the decimal point gives that number its name and its value (Fig. 7-2). For example, the first place to the left of the decimal point is the unit place, the second is the 10 place, and so on. A 2 in the second place to the left of the decimal point (for example, 20.00) indicates that there are two 10s in the 10s place. A 0 in the first place to the left of the decimal point indicates that there is nothing in the units place, which means, so far, that the number is 20. A 2 in the second place to the right of the decimal point (for example, 0.02) indicates two one-hundredths. The number 20.02, then, means "20 and two-hundredths."

For amounts less than 1, it is a good idea to place a 0 in the unit place (the first place to the left of the decimal point). For example, the best way to express the fraction 1/2 in decimals is 0.5.

Adding and Subtracting Decimals

When adding decimal numbers, place the second number below the first number, the third below the second, and so on, just as with whole numbers—but remember to line the numbers up on the decimal point.

Example:

Add: 3.3 + 29.75 + 4

Solution:

```
   3.30
 +29.75   [Add 0s to the right of the
 + 4.00    decimal point as needed]
  37.05
```

Subtracting one decimal number from another number also requires lining the two numbers up, one below the other, on the decimal point.

Example:

Subtract: 17.20 − 6.25

Solution:

```
  17.20
−  6.25
  10.95
```

Example:

Subtract: 33.02 − 17

Solution:

```
  33.02
− 17.00
  16.02
```

Understand the Numbers
Add 0s to the right of the decimal point as needed.

Rounding Decimals

For many decimal calculations, it is necessary or convenient to "round" the answer up or down. Round down to the nearest whole number if the decimal fraction is below 0.5 (for example, change 6.4 to 6). If the decimal fraction is 0.5 or higher, round up to the next larger whole number (change 6.5 to 7). It is also possible to round down or up to the next decimal place (change 6.43 to 6.4; change 6.68 to 6.7).

There are other systems for rounding numbers that may be used and that will work efficiently.

Multiplying Decimals

First, multiply decimal numbers together as if they were whole numbers, without regard for the decimal point. Then add the number of decimal places (places to the right of the decimal point) in both of the multipliers. That total is the number of decimal places in the product of the two numbers; the decimal point goes that number of places to the left of the last number in the product.

Example:

Multiply: 12.5 × 3.7

Solution:

```
  12.5   [1 decimal place]
×        [+1 decimal place]

+ 37.5
  46.25  [2 decimal places in the product]
```

Example:

Multiply: 25.75 × 6.04

Solution:

```
   25.75    [2 decimal places]
×   6.04    [+2 decimal places]
  1.0300
+   0000
+154.50
 155.5300   [four decimal places in the product]
```

[After determining where the decimal point goes, drop any final 0s at the right of the decimal point.]

When multiplying by any multiple of 10, a shorter method is to move the decimal point to the right by the number of 0s in the multiple. For example, when multiplying by 10, move the decimal point one place to the right:

15.75 × 10 = 157.50

When multiplying by 100, move the decimal point two places to the right:

15.75 × 100 = 1575.0

When multiplying by 1000, move the decimal point three places to the right:

15.75 × 1000 = 15,750.0

Dividing Decimals

When dividing by a decimal number, place a caret (↑) as many places to the right of the decimal point in both the divisor and the dividend as there are places in the divisor. Then place the decimal point in the quotient above the caret in the dividend.

Example:

Divide: 253.680 ÷ 10.5

Solution:

```
        24.16
10.5)253.1680
     210
      436
      420
        168
        105
         630
         630
```

Example:

Divide: 50.2990 ÷ 0.125

Solution:

```
         402.4
0.125)50.2990
      500
        299
        250
         490
         490
```

There is a shorter method for dividing a decimal number by any multiple of 10. Move the decimal point in the dividend to the left by the number of 0s in the divisor.

Example:

When dividing by 10, move the dividend's decimal point one place to the left:

$15.0 \div 10 = 1.5$

Example:

When dividing a decimal number by a multiple of 100, move the decimal point two places to the left:

$6.0 \div 100 = 0.06$

Ratio and Proportion

Nearly every medication problem can be broken down to simple ratio and proportion. Developing skill in setting up ratios and proportions will be an invaluable aid to every EMS professional in solving drug-dosage problems quickly and accurately.

Ratio

A **ratio** is the relationship of two quantities. It may be expressed in the form 1:10 or 1:3300, or it may be expressed as a fraction—1/10 or 1/3300. The ratio expression 1:10 or 1/10 can be read as one in 10, or one-tenth, or one part in 10 parts.

Example:

For every 15 students, there is one instructor.
The ratio of instructors to students is 1 in 15 or 1:15 or 1/15.

> ***Understand the Numbers***
> The drug epinephrine is an example of how ratios are used with medications. A 1:1000 solution of epinephrine indicates that there is 1 mg in 1 mL of solution. A 1:10,000 solution indicates there is 1 mg in 10 mL of solution.

Proportion

A **proportion** is formed by using two ratios that are equal. For example, 1/2 = 5/10.

When two ratios or fractions are equal, their cross product is also equal. The cross product is obtained by multiplying the denominator of one ratio by the numerator of the other.

Example:

$1/2 = 5/10 = 2 \times 5 = 10 \times 1$

The cross products are equal: 10 = 10.
Therefore, the ratio 1/2 is equal to the ratio 5/10.
Does 1/4 = 3/12?
The cross products are equal: 12 = 12.
Therefore, 1/4 is equal to 3/12.

Practice Problem:

The physician orders you to give 20 mg of a drug to your patient. The drug comes packaged in a 10-mL vial containing 50 mg of the drug. How many milliliters will be needed to give the dose of 20 mg?

Solution:

There are three knowns:

1. 10-mL vial of the drug on hand
2. 50 mg of the drug in the 10-mL vial
3. 20 mg is the ordered dose

A ratio can be stated for the drug on hand:

$$\frac{10\text{ mL}}{50\text{ mg}} \text{ reduced to lowest terms} = \frac{1\text{ mL}}{5\text{ mg}}$$

A ratio can also be stated for the required dosage:

$$\frac{X\text{ mL}}{20\text{ mg}}$$

Thus, the proportion is:

$$\frac{1\text{ mL}}{5\text{ mg}} = \frac{X\text{ mL}}{20\text{ mg}}$$

Note in the proportion that the units are labeled, and like units are located in the same position in each fraction or ratio (1 mL is opposite X mL, and 5 mg is opposite 20 mg). It is important to label the parts of the proportion correctly. Note that the answer label is always the label with "X."

Three conditions must be met when using ratio and proportion:

1. The numerators must have the same units.
2. The denominators must have the same units.
3. Three of the four parts must be known.

To solve the last example, simply find the cross product and solve for the unknown (X).

$$\frac{1\text{ mL}}{5\text{ mg}} = \frac{X\text{ mL}}{20\text{ mg}}$$

$$5 \times X = 1 \times 20$$

$$5X = 20$$

$$X = 4\text{ mL } (20 \div 5)$$

Therefore, 4 mL of the solution contains 20 mg of the drug.

Metric-to-Metric Conversions

Because the metric system is a decimal system, it is easy to convert from one metric unit to another. For example, to convert grams to milligrams, all you have to do is multiply by 1000. As a shortcut, move the decimal point three places to the right.

Example:

Convert 3 grams to milligrams.

Solution:

3.0 g × 1000 = 3000 mg [Multiply by 1000]
or simply move the decimal point three places to the right.
3.0 g = 3,000 mg [Add 0s as needed to move the decimal point]

Example:

Convert 5.25 grams to milligrams

Solution:

5.25 g × 1000 = 5250 mg

or

5.25 g = 5250 mg

To convert milligrams to grams, divide by 1000—move the decimal point three places to the left.

Example:

Convert 4000 milligrams to grams.

Solution:

4 g
4000 mg ÷ 1000

or

4000 mg = 4.000 g

Practice Problem:

You are a paramedic student in the emergency department. A physician orders you to administer 1,500 milligrams of a drug. The drug comes in 0.5-gram tablets. You must convert within the metric system to find out how many milligrams are in each tablet. Then, you must calculate to find out how many tablets are required.

Solution:

To find the number of milligrams in each tablet, move the decimal point three places to the right.

1. Step 1 (Convert): Convert grams to milligrams.
   0.5 g = 500.0 mg [Move the decimal point three places to the right]
   Answer = each tablet contains 500 mg.
2. Step 2 (Calculate): Divide the required dosage by the amount of drug per tablet.
   1500 ÷ 500 = 3
   Three tablets are required for the prescribed dose.

When converting liters to milliliters (larger unit to smaller unit), you must multiply by 1,000 (or just move the decimal point three places to the right). For example:

6 L = 56000 mL (6 × 1000 or 6000)
4.5 L = 54500 mL (4.5 × 1000 or 4500)

To convert milliliters to liters (smaller unit to larger unit), you must divide by 1,000 (or just move the decimal point three places to the left). For example:

5000 mL = 5 L (5000 ÷ 1000 or 5.000)
2500 mL = 2.5 L (2500 ÷ 1000 or 2.500)

The cubic centimeter (cc) is a once-common unit of measure whose use is decreasing. Both a milliliter and cubic centimeter are equal to one-thousandth of a liter. Even though milliliter and cubic centimeter are equivalent expressions, milliliter is the preferred term.

U.S.-to-Metric Conversions

For many drugs administered in EMS, the drug order is expressed as a volume of drug based on body weight. For example, an order for lidocaine might call for administering 1 milligram per kilogram of body weight (1 mg/kg). Most patients do not know their body weight in kilograms, so you must be able to convert pounds (U.S.) to kilograms (metric).

If 2.2 pounds equals 1 kilogram (Table 7-2), 1 pound equals 0.454 kilograms (kg). To convert pounds to kilograms, simply divide the number of pounds by 2.2.

Example:

100 lb = 100 ÷ 2.2 = 45 kg
150 lb = 150 ÷ 2.2 = 68 kg [68.18 is rounded down to 68]
235 lb = 235 ÷ 2.2 = 107 kg [106.82 is rounded up to 107]

The Apothecaries' System

The apothecaries' system of measurement is rarely used by physicians when ordering drugs in EMS. However, some drugs are available only in (apothecary) grains. For this reason, EMS professionals should be able to use the apothecaries' system. The apothecaries' system measures solids in units of grains, drams, ounces, and pounds. It measures liquids in minims, fluidrams, fluid ounces, pints, and gallons.

Apothecary System of Weights

The apothecary system of weights is based on the grain (gr), which is the smallest unit in the system. You will seldom see apothecary units in EMS with the exception of the grain, which is commonly used in ordering drugs such as nitroglycerin (1/150 gr, 1/200 gr), codeine sulfate (1/8 gr, 1/4 gr, 1/2 gr, 1 gr), and morphine sulfate (1/6 gr, 1/8 gr, 1/2 gr). To convert grains to metric units, the following approximate equivalent is used:

Example:

Convert 4 grains to grams.

Solution:

$$\frac{15\text{ gr}}{1\text{ g}} = \frac{4\text{ gr}}{X\text{ g}}$$

$$X = 0.27\text{ g}$$

Calculating Drug Solutions

Many drugs are given in solution—that is, a pure drug in powder or liquid form is dissolved in a liquid. To administer a prescribed amount of a drug in solution, it is important to know the drug concentration of the solution. Drug **concentration** is the amount of drug per unit of volume; it is usually expressed in milligrams per milliliter (mg/mL). The formula for determining concentration is:

$$\text{Concentration} = \frac{\text{Amount of Drug}}{\text{Volume of Solution}}$$

For example, a common preparation of furosemide is a prefilled 4-milliliter (4-mL) syringe containing 40 milligrams (40 mg) of furosemide. In this case, the drug concentration is 10 milligrams per milliliter (10 mg/mL).

$$\text{Concentration} = \frac{40\ \text{mg}}{4\ \text{mL}} = 10\ \text{mg/mL}$$

When you know the drug concentration, you know how much drug is in 1 milliliter of solution. From that, you can determine how much solution is required to deliver the amount of drug ordered. Divide the amount of drug ordered by the drug concentration:

$$\text{Required Volume of Solution} = \frac{\text{Required Drug Amount}}{\text{Drug Concentration}}$$

Practice Problem:

The physician orders a patient to receive 200 milligrams (200 mg) of a drug. The preparation on hand is a 10-milliliter (10-mL) syringe containing 500 milligrams (500 mg) of the drug. How much of the preparation do you administer?

Solution:

First, find the drug concentration (amount of drug per milliliter of solution) in the syringe by dividing the amount of drug in the syringe by the total volume of the solution:

$$\frac{500\ \text{mg}}{10\ \text{mL}} = 50\ \text{mg/mL}$$

Next, find the volume of solution required (mL) to deliver the required drug amount (mg) by dividing the required drug amount by the drug concentration (mg/mL).

$$\frac{200\ \text{mg}}{50\ \text{mg/mL}} = 4\ \text{mL [The answer will be in mL.]}$$

Give the patient 4 milliliters (4 mL) of the solution in the 10-milliliter (10-mL) syringe.

Sometimes, drug concentration is expressed as a percentage. For example, a common preparation of lidocaine is a 2 percent concentration in a 5-milliliter syringe. To find out how much lidocaine is in the syringe, multiply the percentage of drug (expressed as a decimal fraction) in solution by the total volume of the syringe.

$$0.02\ \text{[Concentration]} \times 5\ \text{mL [Volume]} = 0.1\ \text{g}$$

What is the concentration in milligrams per milliliter? Convert grams to milligrams and divide by the number of milliliters in the preparation.

$$0.1\ \text{g} \times 1000 = 100\ \text{mg}$$

$$\frac{100\ \text{mg}}{5\ \text{mL}} = 20\ \text{mg/mL}$$

Sometimes, as with epinephrine, the drug concentration is expressed as a ratio. For example, two often-used preparations are epinephrine in a 1:1000 solution and epinephrine in a 1:10,000 solution. The ratio of 1:1000 indicates that 1 milliliter of solution contains 1 milligram of the drug. The 1:10,000 ratio indicates that there is 1 milligram of drug in 10 milliliters of solution.

Remember, in the metric system, the cubic centimeter, milliliter, and gram are equivalent. One cubic centimeter holds one milliliter of water, and 1 milliliter of water (or most other liquids) weighs 1 gram.

Calculating Rates of Infusion

Intravenous tubing is packaged in macrodrop or microdrop sets. Macrodrop intravenous tubing is available in both 10- and 15-drop sets. With a 10-drop intravenous set, 10 drops equals 1.0 milliliter. With a 15-drop set, 15 drops equals 1.0 milliliter. A microdrop intravenous set takes 60 drops to deliver 1.0 milliliter.

To calculate the drip rate for an intravenous infusion, health-care professionals need to know three values: (1) the volume of fluid required, (2) the intravenous set size, and (3) the total time of the infusion in minutes. For example: How many drops per minute will it take to infuse 500 milliliters of fluid using a 15-drop-per-minute (gtt/min) intravenous set for 45 minutes?

$$\text{Infusion Rate} = \frac{\text{Volume of Solution Required} \times \text{Set Size}}{\text{Infusion Time}}$$

$$= \frac{500\ \text{mL} \times 15\ \text{gtts/min}}{45\ \text{minutes}} = 7500\ \text{mL}$$

$$= \frac{7500\ \text{mL}}{45\ \text{min}} = 167\ \text{gtts/min}$$

Example:

How many drops per minute will it take to infuse 250 milliliters of fluid using a microdrop intravenous (60 drops per milliliter) set for 1 hour?

Solution:

$$\frac{250\ \text{mL} \times 60\ \text{gtts/min}}{60\ \text{minutes}} = 250\ \text{gtts/min}$$

Example:

The paramedic is ordered to prepare a lidocaine infusion by adding 2 grams of lidocaine to 500 milliliters of dextrose 5 percent in water. Once the infusion is prepared, it is to run at 3 milligrams per minute, using a microdrip IV set. What is the concentration (milligrams per milliliter) of the lidocaine infusion, and at what rate (drops per minute) should the infusion run to deliver 3 milligrams of lidocaine per minute?

Solution:

Step 1: Determine the lidocaine concentration.

$$\text{Concentration} = \frac{\text{Amount of Drug}}{\text{Volume of Solution}}$$

$$\frac{2\text{ g}}{500\text{ mL}} = [\text{Convert g to mg}]$$

$$\frac{2000\text{ mg}}{500\text{ mL}} = 4\text{ mg/mL}$$

Step 2: Determine the volume of solution needed to deliver 3 milligrams of lidocaine.

$$\text{Required Volume of Solution} = \frac{\text{Required Drug Amount}}{\text{Drug Concentration}}$$

$$= \frac{3\text{ mg}}{4\text{ mg/mL}} = 0.75\text{ mL}$$

Step 3: Determine the infusion rate required.

$$\text{Infusion Rate} = \frac{\text{Required Volume of Solution} \times \text{Set Size (gtts/min)}}{\text{Infusion Time (minutes)}}$$

$$= \frac{0.75\text{ mL} \times 60\text{ gtts/min}}{1\text{ minute}} = 45\text{ gtt/min}$$

Converting Temperature Measurements

In addition to the metric system of weights and measures, EMS professionals must understand the **Celsius** system of temperature measurement. They need to be able to convert temperatures expressed in Celsius to **Fahrenheit** and vice versa.

Figure 7-3 compares the Fahrenheit and Celsius systems of temperature measurement. The freezing point for Celsius is 0 degrees, and the freezing point for Fahrenheit is 32 degrees. On the Celsius scale, the boiling point of water is 100 degrees; it is 212 degrees on the Fahrenheit scale. Normal body temperature on the Celsius scale is 37 degrees, and normal body temperature on the Fahrenheit scale is 98.6 degrees.

Two formulas will assist conversion between the two systems. To convert Fahrenheit to Celsius, use the following formula:

Degrees Celsius = (Degrees Fahrenheit − 32) × 0.556

Example:

Convert 212 degrees F to Celsius

Solution:

C = (212 − 32) × 0.556 = 100 degrees

To convert Celsius to Fahrenheit, use this formula:

Degrees Fahrenheit = Degrees Celsius × 1.8 + 32

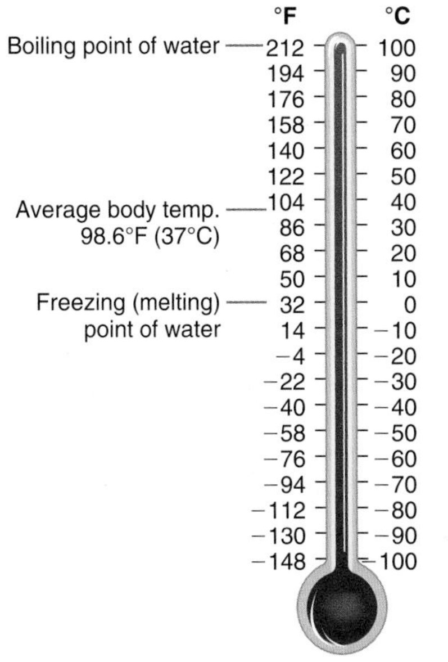

Figure 7-3 The comparison of the Fahrenheit and Celsius scales.

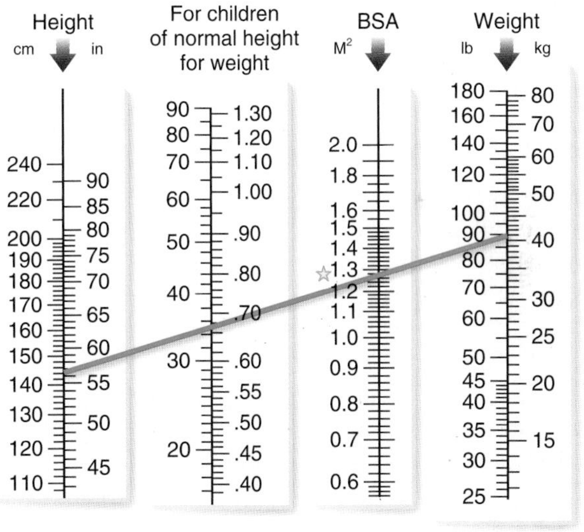

Figure 7-4 Pediatric nomogram.

Example:

Convert 37 degrees C to Fahrenheit.

Solution:

F = 37 × 1.8 = 66.6 + 32 = 98.6 degrees

Pediatric Dosage Calculations

On occasion, a manufacturer's recommended dosage for children is not available. When this occurs, the nomogram is the most accurate method for determining pediatric drug dosages. The nomogram (Fig. 7-4) is a chart that uses the weight and height of a child to estimate body surface area (BSA) in square meters (m^2). This body surface area is then placed in a ratio with the body surface area of an average adult (1.73 m^2). The formula used with the nomogram method is:

$$\text{Pediatric dose} = \text{Pediatric BSA in } m^2 \times \text{adult dose} \div 1.73\ m^2 \text{ (BSA of average adult)}$$

To determine the BSA of a pediatric patient, the weight and height of the child must be known. The nomogram scales contain both metric (kg, cm) and U.S. (lb, in) values for height and weight. Therefore, the BSA can be determined for pounds and inches or kilograms and centimeters without making conversions.

Using the "Pediatric Nomogram," note the three columns labeled height, body surface area, and weight. To determine BSA, a ruler or straightedge is needed. The following steps illustrate the use of the nomogram:

1. Determine the height and weight of the patient. Remember, this information can be metric, U.S., or a combination of both systems.
2. Place a straightedge on the nomogram connecting the two points on the height and weight scales that represent the patient's values. For example, suppose your patient weighs 26.5 pounds and is 33.5 inches tall. Then, 26.5 pounds on the weight scale and 33.5 inches on the height scale are connected with a straightedge.
3. Where the straightedge crosses the center column (BSA), a reading is taken. In this example, BSA = 0.52 m^2.
4. Substitute the BSA value in the formula to calculate the dosage for the patient. For example, the adult dosage of a particular drug is 500 mg. What is the dose for our patient with a calculated BSA of 0.52 m^2?

$$\begin{aligned}\text{Pediatric dose} &= \frac{\text{BSA of Child in } m^2 \times \text{Adult Dose}}{1.73\ m^2 \text{ (BSA of average adult)}}\\ &= \frac{0.52\ m^2 \times 500\ mg}{1.73\ m^2}\\ &= 0.3 \times 500\ mg\\ &= 150\ mg \text{ of the drug}\end{aligned}$$

As with anything else, using the nomogram takes practice. But, once proficient using the nomogram, you will find it a useful tool for calculating pediatric drug dosages.

SCENARIO REVISITED

Do you recall the case of the little girl Gail who is having an anaphylactic reaction to fire ant bites?

Gail needs to be administered 0.01 mg/kg of epinephrine (1:1000) IM immediately. To find out the volume of epinephrine that will give Gail the required dosage, you should do the following:

Step 1: 45 lbs ÷ 2.2 kg = 20.45 kg or 20 kg

Step 2: Dosage of epinephrine: 20 kg × 0.01 mg = 0.2 mg

Step 3: Concentration of the epinephrine: Concentration =

$$\frac{1\ mg}{1\ mL} = 1\ mg/mL$$

Step 4: Volume of epinephrine to equal 0.2 mg:

$$\text{Volume (mL)} = \frac{0.2\ mg}{1\ mg/mL} = 0.2\ mL = 0.2\ mg$$

Let's Recap

When many of us hear the word "math," we immediately have a catecholamine release, sending our stress levels through the roof. The key to feeling comfortable with math is patience and practice. Working with numbers can be similar to putting a puzzle together.

This chapter presents basic information on which to build. As with any skill, math requires frequent practice to maintain acceptable proficiency levels.

Check the **Evidence**

A common learning technique for solving math problems is the STAR method:

<u>S</u>earch the word problem.
<u>T</u>ranslate the words into an equation.
<u>A</u>nswer the problem.
<u>R</u>eview the solution. (Does the answer make sense?)

SCENARIO CONCLUSION

Shortly after receiving the epinephrine, Gail's breathing improves, and she becomes less anxious. At this point, it is recommended to start an IV and monitor Gail's vital signs while en route to the emergency department.

PRACTICE EXERCISES

Conversions

1. 50 kg = ____________ lb

2. 180 lb = ____________ kg

3. 0.2 mg = ____________ mcg

4. 3.0 L = ____________ mL

5. 0.3 g = ____________ mg

6. 10 mL = ____________ cc

7. 3.0 g = ____________ mg

8. 0.06 g = __________ mg
9. 200 lb = __________ kg
10. 4.0 g = __________ mg
11. 0.03 g = __________ mg
12. 8,000 mg = __________ g
13. 200 mL = __________ cc
14. 2.0 mg = __________ mcg
15. 0.1 L = __________ mL

Problem Set A

1. A physician has ordered the administration of 1 mg/kg of a drug to a patient in cardiac arrest. The paramedic estimates that the patient weighs 175 pounds. The drug is packaged as 100 mg in a 5-mL prefilled syringe.
   a. How many milligrams of the drug are required?

   ____

   ____

   b. How many milliliters of solution are needed for the required dose?

   ____

   ____

2. A paramedic is ordered to administer 0.5 mg of a drug by IV bolus. The drug comes packaged as 1 mg in a 10-mL prefilled syringe. How many milliliters will be given?

   ____

   ____

3. A physician orders the administration of a drug infusion. The paramedic is to begin the infusion at 2 mcg/min using a microdrip (60 gtt/min) IV set. The infusion is prepared by adding 1 mg of the drug to 500 mL of normal saline.
   a. What is the concentration of the drug when it is added to the normal saline (mcg/mL)?

   ____

   ____

   b. What infusion rate is needed to administer 2 mcg/min?

   ____

   ____

4. A physician orders the addition of 800 mg of a drug to 500 mL of normal saline solution. What will be the resulting concentration in mcg/mL?

   ____

   ____

5. The paramedic receives an order to administer 20 mg of a drug. The drug comes packaged as 40 mg in a 4-mL prefilled syringe. How many milliliters will be administered?

   ____

   ____

6. A physician orders the administration of 5 mg/kg of a drug. The patient weighs 175 pounds. The drug is packaged as 500 mg in a 10-mL vial.
   a. How many milligrams will be administered?

   ____

   ____

   b. How many milliliters will be administered?

   ____

   ____

Problem Set B

1. The health-care professional has diluted 2 g of a drug in 500 mL of normal saline solution.
   a. What is the resulting concentration (mg/mL)?

   ____

   ____

   b. What infusion rate is needed when using a minidrip (60 gtt/min) IV set to deliver 2 mg/min?

   ____

   ____

2. The paramedic has a 20 percent solution of a drug in 500 mL of IV fluid. The physician orders the administration of 1.5 g/kg of the drug to the patient over 1 hour. The patient weighs 120 pounds. Supplied is a 15 gtt/min IV set.
   a. What is the concentration (g/mL) of the solution?

   ____

   ____

   b. How many gtt/min will be administered to your patient?

   ____

   ____

3. The health-care professional has been ordered to administer 2 L of IV solution over a 3-hour period. How many gtt/min will be administered if the standard IV set yields 10 gtt/min?

   ____

   ____

4. The paramedic has a patient in severe anaphylactic shock. The physician orders 0.5 mg of a 1:10,000 solution of epinephrine by IV bolus. The epinephrine comes packaged as 1 mg in a 10-mL solution. How many milliliters will be administered?

   ____

   ____

5. After the administration of the dose in question 4, the paramedic is requested to start an epinephrine infusion. The physician orders 1 mcg/min. Two milligrams of 1:1000 epinephrine are added to 500 mL of IV solution.
   a. What is the resulting concentration (mcg/mL)?
   ____
   ____
   b. What infusion rate is needed with a microdrip (60 gtt/min) IV set?
   ____
   ____

6. The physician orders an IV infusion at a rate of 2 mcg/min. The paramedic prepares the infusion by adding 4 mg of drug to 500 mL of IV solution.
   a. What is the resulting concentration (mcg/mL)?
   ____
   ____
   b. What infusion rate is needed with a minidrip (60 gtt/min) IV set?
   ____
   ____

CASE STUDIES

1. You respond to a local restaurant where you find a 67-year-old female patient complaining of weakness and feeling faint. She states that she has been feeling this way for about 2 hours, so she decided to go out to eat with a friend hoping a good meal would make her feel better. Initial assessment reveals the following:
   Level of consciousness: Awake but confused and very weak
   Respirations: 10 breaths/minute
   Heart rate: 48 beats/minute and regular
   Skin: Cool and damp
   Patient weight: 135 lbs
   You place the patient on 100 percent humidified oxygen and start an IV of NS at a keep-open rate. The first drug of choice, after oxygen, for adult symptomatic bradycardia is atropine at 0.5 mg IV bolus. This can be repeated every 3 to 5 minutes to a maximum dose of 3 mg. You carry atropine at 1 mg in a 10-mL prefilled syringe.

   What is the volume (mL) of atropine to be given to equal the 0.5 mg initial dose?

   Step 1: Concentration $= \dfrac{1.0 \text{ mg}}{10 \text{ mL}} = 0.1 \text{ mg/mL}$

   Step 2: Volume (mL) $= \dfrac{0.5 \text{ mg}}{\text{mg/mL}} = 5 \text{ mL}$ equals 0.5 mg of atropine

   If the patient does not respond to the atropine, your protocol indicates that dopamine is the next drug of choice for adult symptomatic bradycardia. The dosage for dopamine is 2-10 mcg/kg/min IV infusion. You carry dopamine in a premixed IV bag at 800 mg in 500 mL.

   How many gtts/min will you run the IV with an order of 5 mcg/kg/min of dopamine using a 60 gtt/mL set?

   Step 1: 135 lbs ÷ 2.2 kg = 61 kg

   Step 2: Concentration of IV bag $= \dfrac{800 \text{ mg}}{500 \text{ mL}} =$ 1.6 mg/mL or 1600 mcg/mL

   Step 3: 5 mcg × 61 kg = 305 mcg

   Step 4: Required volume $= \dfrac{305 \text{ mcg}}{1600 \text{ mcg/mL}} = 0.19 \text{ mL}$

   Step 5: Infusion rate $= \dfrac{0.19 \text{ mL} \times 60 \text{ gtt/min}}{1 \text{ minute}} =$ 11 gtts/min

2. You and your team had been working a cardiac arrest for approximately 10 minutes when the patient has return of spontaneous circulation (ROSC). Your patient is a 56-year-old male who weighs approximately 220 pounds. At the point of ROSC, the physician orders an IV infusion of epinephrine with a dosage of 0.4 mcg/kg/min. Your epinephrine comes packaged as 1 mg (1:1000) in a 1-mL ampule. How many drops/min will you run the IV infusion to administer 0.4 mcg/kg/min using a 15 gtt/min set?

   Step 1: 220 lbs ÷ 2.2 kg = 100 kg

   Step 2: IV bag concentration $= \dfrac{1 \text{ mg}}{250 \text{ mL}} = 0.004 \text{ mg/mL}$ or 4 mcg/mL

   Step 3: 0.4 mcg × 100 kg = 40 mcg

   Step 4: Required volume $= \dfrac{40 \text{ mcg}}{4 \text{ mcg/mL}} = 10 \text{ mL}$

   Step 5: Infusion rate $= \dfrac{10 \text{ mL} \times 15 \text{ gtts/min}}{1 \text{ min}} =$ 150 gtts/min

REFERENCES

Beck, R. K. (2012). Drug-dose calculations. In *Pharmacology for the EMS provider.* New York, NY: Delmar, Cengage Learning.

Chernecky, C., Butler, S. W., Graham, P., and Infortuna, M. H. (2002). *Drug calculations and drug administration.* Philadelphia, PA: W. B. Saunders Company.

Deglin, J. H., Vallerand, A. H., and Sanboski, C.A. (2011). *Davis's drug guide for nurses* (12th ed.). Philadelphia, PA: F. A. Davis Company.

Hardy, S. D. (2005). PowerPoint slides. Retrieved March 18, 2014 from http://www.k8accesscenter.org/index.php/category/math/

Venes, D., ed. (2013). *Taber's cyclopedic medical dictionary* (22nd ed.). Philadelphia, PA: F. A. Davis Company.

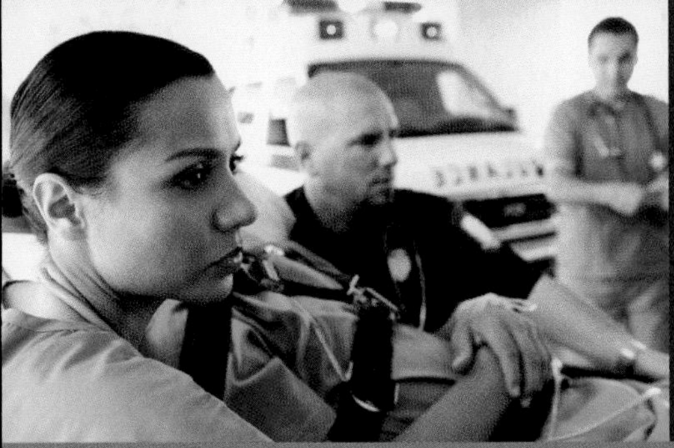

CHAPTER **8**

Drug Administration

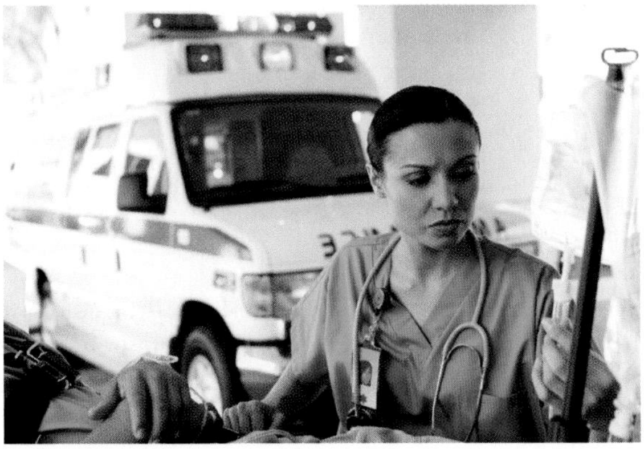

Paramedics preparing an IV infusion. *(Photograph © Fuse/Thinkstock)*

LEARNING OUTCOMES

- Describe the seven rights of drug administration.
- Describe the advantages and disadvantages of alimentary and parenteral drug administration.
- List and describe the alimentary and parenteral drug routes.
- Describe the methods of administering drugs through inhalation.
- Briefly discuss drug administration to the pediatric patient.
- Briefly discuss drug administration to the geriatric patient.
- Briefly discuss contaminated sharps and equipment disposal.

KEY TERMS

Alimentary route
Bolus
Endotracheal (ET)
Inhalation
Inhaler
Intradermal (ID)
Intramuscular (IM)
Intraosseous (IO)
IV
IV infusion
Local
Nasal
Nebulizer
Otic
Parenteral routes
Piggyback
Prophylactic
Rectal
Subcutaneous (SubQ)
Sublingual
Systemic
Transdermal

SCENARIO OPENING

You have been assigned to Medic 14 located between terminals B and C at the airport. Just before lunch, you get a call for a "man down" at one of the airport restaurants in terminal C. When you arrive at the scene, there is a TSA agent preforming CPR on a male patient who appears to be in his early 70s. Your response time was 3 minutes. While your partner begins bag-mask ventilations, you attach defibrillator pads. The screen on the ECG monitor shows course ventricular fibrillation (V-Fib), and you cannot feel a pulse. You immediately defibrillate the patient, and he converts to a sinus rhythm. The patient remains unconscious but begins breathing on his own. While preparing the patient for transport, you place him on humidified oxygen and start an IV of normal saline (NS).

Introduction

Drug administration is one of the most important, demanding, and risky functions the EMS professional will perform. He or she is responsible for interpreting, evaluating the appropriateness of, and administering the drug order. Drug administration requires training, a solid knowledge base, and well-developed decision-making abilities.

To have its intended therapeutic effect, a drug must reach its site of action. To do this, the drug must enter the body, be absorbed into the circulation, and then be transported to the targeted tissues. All these events vary according to the route of administration, which is determined by the amount of drug needed, the rapidity of action desired, and the patient's condition.

There are two ways to introduce drugs into the body: by **alimentary routes** and **parenteral routes.** In EMS, drugs are most often given by parenteral routes, as these are much more rapid and generally more predictable.

The Drug Order

EMS professionals are required to select, prepare, and give many different medications. Before a drug is given, a thorough patient assessment, including the medication assessment, must be performed. Depending on the type of EMS system, drugs are given by written treatment protocols, standing orders, or direct contact with medical control. If the patient assessment is not complete or is inaccurate, the wrong drug could be given.

***effective* Communication**

EMS professionals should be familiar with the written protocols and standing orders of their facility. A copy of these documents should be kept with the professional in case they may be needed for reference.

If an EMS professional receives an order from medical control that is different from the protocols, he or she should contact medical control to have the order clarified. If the physician at medical control insists on the order, give the drug at the dose ordered, documenting carefully. However, if at any time the drug order will harm the patient, do not give the drug. Instead, tell medical control the rationale for not giving the drug and thoroughly document the situation.

Seven Rights of Drug Administration

Before administering drugs, EMS professionals must adhere to the *seven rights of drug administration:*

1. The right drug
2. The right drug amount
3. The right patient
4. The right time
5. The right route
6. The right documentation
7. The rights of the patient

The Right Drug

One of the most common EMS drug administration errors is selecting the incorrect drug. If there are any questions concerning a drug, do not administer it until it has been confirmed. Verify the order with medical control or your partner if there is any doubt about the drug to be given.

EMS professionals must be very careful not to inadvertently pick up the wrong drug. Most EMS drugs come packaged as ampules, vials, or prefilled syringes, and many of these look very much alike. After selecting a drug, read the label and inspect the drug three times, verifying the drug's name, concentration, expiration date, and clarity. Check the drug first when selecting it from its box or cabinet. Then, check the drug again when preparing it. And, finally, check the drug just prior to administration.

The Right Drug Amount

Another common mistake made by health-care professionals is giving the incorrect dosage of a drug. Most of these errors occur because of calculation or preparation errors. It is very important that EMS professionals are familiar with all the drugs that they may be called upon to use. When preparing to give a drug, be certain to calculate and prepare the drug accurately. If appropriate, have a colleague check your accuracy before the drug is given. Remember, in many cases, accuracy may save more lives than speed.

The Right Patient

Most emergency responses will only involve one patient. However, there will be times when multiple patients are at the scene. It is very important that each patient be distinguished by assigning each a label. For example, you can label numerically (for example, patient 1, patient 2, etc.) or alphabetically (for example, patient A, patient B, etc.).

When multiple patients are involved at a scene, it is important not only to correctly identify each patient but also to identify the ambulances as well. Treatment errors will be kept to a minimum by an organized scene management system. Each patient and each ambulance should be identified; this will give medical control a better picture of the scene and the types of patient treatments given before arrival at the emergency department.

The Right Time

Time is a critical factor when giving drugs. Some drugs may only have to be given one time. However, other drugs, such as epinephrine, are given by IV bolus every 3 to 5 minutes during a cardiac arrest. There also are drugs that are given by IV infusion over a specific period. For example, norepinephrine may be ordered at 2 mcg/minute, or aminophylline can be given at 250 mg over 20 minutes. Some drugs should be given by rapid IV bolus, such as adenosine, and some drugs should be given by slow IV bolus, such as morphine. Knowledge of the time factors for each drug to be given will affect the success of the drug therapy. It is a good idea to have a drug reference text available for questions that may arise.

The Right Route

Depending on the emergency, different drugs will be given through different routes. For example, during a cardiac arrest, epinephrine is generally given by IV bolus every 3 to 5 minutes. However, if an IV cannot be started or is delayed, epinephrine can be given down the ET tube. The initial dose of lidocaine is generally given IV bolus and followed with an IV infusion.

There are some drugs that are administered by inhalation, while others are given intramuscularly, subcutaneously, or sublingually. A strong knowledge base of each drug's routes of administration is invaluable for EMS personnel.

The Right Documentation

All health-care professionals who come in contact with patients must know what treatments have already been given, including medications. There is an old saying in EMS: "If it was not written down, it did not happen." All documentation should be completed as soon after treatment as possible. Do not try to rely on your memory when the call is complete. Attempting to provide all documentation after the completion of a call can be detrimental for the patient. The longer the wait to complete documentation, the more likely vital information may be left out or entered incorrectly.

The Rights of the Patient

Do not forget the rights of each patient. Patients have the right to refuse some or all treatment. Also, if a patient elects to accept treatment, he or she has the right to be informed about what a medication is for, how it works, side effects, and so forth. Therefore, when appropriate, explain what drug(s) you are giving, why you are giving the drug(s), and possible side effects the patient may experience.

Venous Access

It is common practice in the management of most injured or ill patients for the EMS professional to establish an IV line. The IV line provides a route for fluid replacement in the injured patient and a route for medications for the patient with a medical disorder. The type of medical emergency will determine the size of the catheter to use when establishing the IV line. For example, the trauma patient may require a large-bore, 14- or 16-gauge catheter. On the other hand, the medical patient will only require a smaller 18- or 20-gauge catheter. It is important for EMS personnel to try to plan for the future. For example, if a patient may require the infusion of whole blood, a larger catheter must be inserted initially.

Not only is the IV catheter size important but so is the type of IV administration set to be used. There are two types of IV administration sets: macrodrip and minidrip. The macrodrip set is generally used for the injured patient, while the minidrip set is generally used for medical patients. Macrodrip IV sets can deliver anywhere from 10 to 20 gtt/mL, while the minidrip set delivers 50 to 60 gtt/mL, depending on the manufacturer.

The IV should be started in a large vein, generally above the wrist. If, for some reason, an IV cannot be started in the arm, other sites include the leg and the external jugular in the neck, which are both considered peripheral veins. However, the best vein for IV insertion in the trauma or cardiac arrest patient is the antecubital vein.

effective **Communication**

Avoid starting an IV in the hand, as it can be more painful than one in the arm. Causing an increase in the patient's pain can produce an increase in the patient's anxiety.

Procedure for Starting an Intravenous Line

1. During the procedure, follow the Centers for Disease Control and Prevention (CDC) Standard Precautions for infection control.
2. Receive, confirm, and write down the order and then confirm the Seven Rights of Drug Administration.
3. Prepare the equipment:
   - IV fluid
   - Administration set (macrodrip or minidrip)
   - Appropriate size indwelling catheter
   - IV extension tubing (some protocols do not use extension tubing for trauma patients)
   - Tourniquet
   - Antibiotic swab
   - 2 × 2 or 4 × 4 sterile gauze pads
   - 1/2-inch or 1-inch tape
   - Antibiotic ointment
   - Short arm board, if appropriate

4. Remove IV fluid from package. Inspect the fluid for clarity and particulate matter. Do not use if discolored or if any particles are present.
5. Open and inspect the IV tubing.
6. Attach extension tubing if appropriate.
7. Remove the sterile cover from the IV bag and the administration set. Insert the administration set into the IV fluid port.
8. Squeeze the IV tubing drip chamber to fill with fluid and then bleed the air out of the IV tubing.
9. Close the clamp on the IV tubing.
10. Hang the IV bag or have it held at the appropriate height.
11. If appropriate, attach the tourniquet, occluding the patient's venous blood flow.
12. Select an appropriate vein.
13. Clean the selected site using an antibiotic swab.
14. Make the puncture, observe flashback, and advance the catheter while removing the needle.
15. Connect the IV tubing and remove the tourniquet.
16. Open the IV tubing, confirming fluid is flowing with no evidence of infiltration.
17. Apply antibiotic ointment on the puncture site and cover with sterile gauze or an adhesive bandage.
18. Tape the IV catheter and tubing in place.
19. Adjust the fluid flow rate.
20. If appropriate, attach a short arm board.
21. Label the IV bag with the patient's name, date, time the IV was started, gauge of the catheter, and your initials.
22. Call medical control to confirm successful completion of the IV.
23. Monitor the patient and report any changes.

Some protocols may require EMS personnel to collect a blood sample when starting the IV. Blood is taken before the IV line is attached to the IV catheter by using a 10-mL syringe. Once the blood has been taken, the syringe is removed and the IV line attached. Blood should be collected, if at all possible, before administering any medicine.

Once the blood has been withdrawn, it is placed into an evacuated blood-collection tube. Most of these tubes contain chemicals to prevent the blood from clotting. Each tube has a specific colored rubber top that determines the use of the contents. After the evacuated blood tube is filled, it should be inverted several times so the blood mixes thoroughly with the chemical. The patient's name, date, time sampled, and EMS personnel name should be noted on the tube. If necessary, the tubes may be taped to the IV bag for transport.

Drug Administration Routes

Nonparenteral Drug Administration

Oral

Oral (PO) administration of drugs provides the most convenient, safe, and economical way to get drugs into the body. Although some orally administered drugs are absorbed from the stomach and colon, most are absorbed from the small intestines. Because they must travel through the mouth, throat, and stomach before entering the bloodstream, the onset of action of oral drugs is slower. The delay in onset sometimes means a decrease in, or a lack of, therapeutic effects. Therefore, when a rapid therapeutic effect is required, such as in life-threatening emergencies, parenteral drug administration is preferred. However, if you are giving an oral medication, the procedure is as follows (during the procedure, follow the CDC's Standard Precautions for infection control):

1. Identify the patient and explain the procedure.
2. Observe the Seven Rights of Drug Administration.
3. Verify the medication order and select the proper drug, checking its name, expiration date, concentration, dosage, and clarity (if a liquid).
4. Assemble any required supplies.
5. Recheck the medication order and drug as in step 3.
6. Prepare the medication for administration.
7. Recheck the medication order and drug as in steps 3 and 5.
8. Administer the medication to the patient. Instruct the patient to swallow the medication completely.
9. Assess the patient for any response to the medication.
10. Document the administration and any patient response.

Oral (Nasogastric/Gastric) Drug Administration

When administering medications by nasogastric or gastric tube, follow these steps (during the procedure, follow the CDC's Standard Precautions for infection control):

1. Identify the patient and explain the procedure.
2. Observe the Seven Rights of Drug Administration.
3. Verify the medication order and select the proper drug, checking its name, expiration date, concentration, dosage, and clarity (if a liquid).
4. Assemble any required supplies.
5. Recheck the medication order and drug as in step 3.
6. Prepare the medication for administration.
7. Recheck the medication order and drug as in steps 3 and 5.
8. Elevate the patient's head.
9. Hold the end of the tube up and remove the clamp, plug, or adapter.
10. Insert the tube, making sure the tube is in the stomach by injecting air into the tube and listening for the sound of air in the stomach. You can also draw back on a syringe attached to the tube to see if any stomach contents flow up into the syringe.
11. Attach the needleless syringe to the port.
12. Flush the tube with NS solution.
13. Administer the medication using the syringe.
14. Flush the tube with NS to make sure all of the medication is in the stomach.
15. Clamp the tube, remove the syringe, and reattach the tube-securing device.

16. Assess the patient for any reactions to the procedure.
17. Document the medication administration and any patient reaction.

Sublingual

To administer a drug **sublingually,** place it under the patient's tongue and give instructions to keep it there until it is dissolved and absorbed into the capillaries.

> **Check the Evidence**
>
> If you are administering a nitroglycerin *tablet* under the patient's tongue, instruct him to remove any remaining tablet once the pain is relieved to avoid possible adverse reactions.

The underside of the tongue is rich in capillaries, which permits rapid absorption and, therefore, rapid drug action. Sublingual drug administration permits the drug to enter the general circulation without passing through the liver or being affected by gastric and intestinal enzymes. This yields a higher concentration of the drug in the circulation than oral administration does.

Obviously, the tongue is in the mouth, which is the beginning of the alimentary tract. However, because the drug is absorbed through the mucosa of the tongue and directly into the circulation without interference from gastric enzymes and other material found in the alimentary tract, the sublingual drug route is considered a parenteral route. An example of an EMS drug administered sublingually is nitroglycerin, which is used to treat anginal attacks and for the long-term **prophylactic** management of angina pectoris. (*Prophylactics* are designed to prevent illness or disease.)

To administer a drug sublingually, follow these steps (during the procedure, follow the CDC's Standard Precautions for infection control):

1. Identify the patient and explain the procedure.
2. Observe the Seven Rights of Drug Administration.
3. Verify the medication order and select the proper drug, checking its name, expiration date, concentration, dosage, and clarity (if a liquid).
4. Assemble any required supplies.
5. Recheck the medication order and drug as in step 3.
6. Prepare the medication for administration.
7. Recheck the medication order and drug as in steps 3 and 5.
8. Administer the medication to the patient. Instruct the patient NOT to swallow the medication.
9. Assess the patient for any response to the medication.
10. Document the administration and any patient response.

Buccal Drug Administration

When giving a drug via the oral buccal route, the drug is placed between the patient's cheek and gum beneath the teeth. The drug moves through the mucous membranes and into the blood capillaries. The drug is quickly absorbed for a rapid onset of action. The most common drug given by the buccal route is glucose for a diabetic patient in need of a rapid increase in blood sugar. The procedure for buccal drug administration is as follows (during the procedure, follow the CDC's Standard Precautions for infection control):

1. Identify the patient and explain the procedure.
2. Observe the Seven Rights of Drug Administration.
3. Verify the medication order and select the proper drug, checking its name, expiration date, concentration, dosage, and clarity (if a liquid).
4. Assemble any required supplies.
5. Recheck the medication order and drug as in step 3.
6. Prepare the medication for administration.
7. Recheck the medication order and drug as in steps 3 and 5.
8. Administer the medication to the patient. Instruct the patient NOT to swallow the medication.
9. Assess the patient for any response to the medication.
10. Document the administration and any patient response.

Administering Drugs by Inhalation

Giving a drug via **inhalation** (directly into the respiratory system by way of the mouth or nasal passage) is a rapid and effective way of getting drugs into the circulatory system. Inhalation medications are commonly given by metered-dose inhalers (MDIs) (Fig. 8-1) or a **nebulizer** (Fig. 8-2).

An MDI is used by a patient for the self-administration of an aerosolized medication. The MDI can deliver accurate doses of medication directly to the respiratory tract. The MDI is a drug canister in an L-shaped mouthpiece, which can be used alone or with a spacer. The spacer is a holding chamber designed to aerosolize the drug so it can more easily reach the lower respiratory tract. The MDI should be sprayed once or twice before initiating use. Drug administration by **inhaler** is performed as follows (during the procedure, follow the CDC's Standard Precautions for infection control):

1. Identify the patient and explain the procedure.
2. Observe the Seven Rights of Drug Administration.

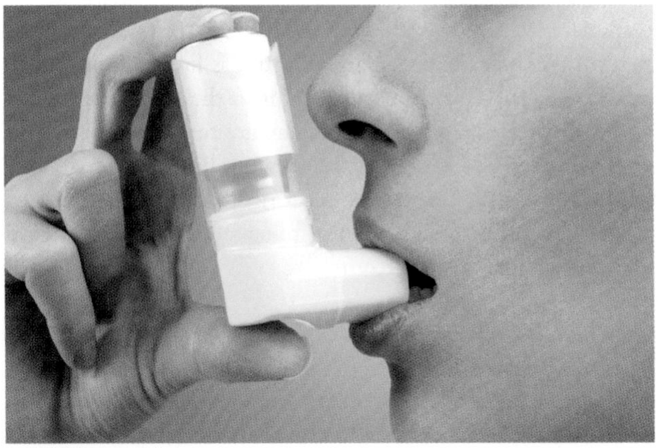

Figure 8-1 Metered-dose inhaler. *(Photograph © Fuse/Thinkstock)*

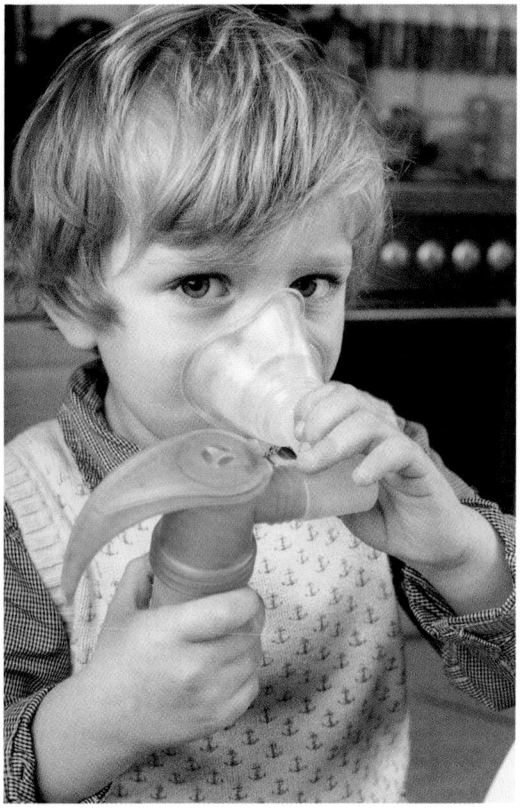

Figure 8-2 Nebulizer treatment. *(Photograph © Remains/iStock/Thinkstock)*

3. Verify the medication order and select the proper drug, checking its name, expiration date, concentration, dosage, and clarity (if a liquid).
4. Assemble any required supplies.
5. Recheck the medication order and drug as in step 3.
6. Prepare the medication for administration.
7. Recheck the medication order and drug as in steps 3 and 5.
8. Ask the patient to exhale.
9. Insert the inhaler into the patient's mouth and depress the container when the patient inhales; repeat for the number of times ordered.
10. Assess the patient for any response to the medication.
11. Document the administration and any patient response.

A nebulizer is used for producing a fine spray or mist that is breathed into the respiratory tract. The nebulizer can be attached to an electric pump. Air is then forced through a liquid medication, or the liquid medication is vibrated at a high frequency so that the particles produced are extremely small. The procedure for nebulizer drug administration is as follows (during the procedure, follow the CDC's Standard Precautions for infection control):

1. Identify the patient and explain the procedure.
2. Observe the Seven Rights of Drug Administration.
3. Verify the medication order and select the proper drug, checking its name, expiration date, concentration, dosage, and clarity (if a liquid).

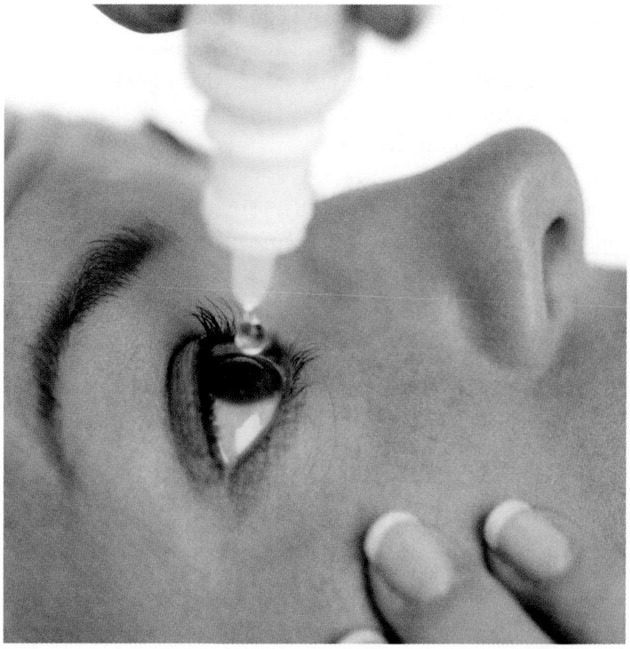

Figure 8-3 Ophthalmic drug administration. *(Photograph © romrodinka/iStock/Thinkstock)*

4. Assemble any required supplies.
5. Recheck the medication order and drug as in step 3.
6. Prepare the medication for administration.
7. Recheck the medication order and drug as in steps 3 and 5.
8. Apply a nasal cannula or mask to the patient.
9. If the nebulizer is electric, turn it on. If it is manual, have the patient breathe deeply.
10. Assess the patient for any response to the medication.
11. Document the administration and any patient response.

Ophthalmic Drug Administration

Ophthalmic drug administration is placing a drug directly on the eye (Fig. 8-3). Ophthalmic drugs come as a liquid or as an ointment. Many patients become very anxious when they realize something must be placed on their eye. Therefore, it is very important to keep the patient informed throughout this procedure.

When placing drops onto the eye, it is important to have the patient slightly tilt his or her head back and look upward. After the drops are given, the patient must close his or her eyes. Closing the eyes helps prevent the medication from entering the nasolacrimal duct, a small tube that runs from the inside corner of the eye to the nose. When giving a drug in the form of an ointment, place the drug into the bottom of the patient's eyelid and not directly onto the eye. The procedure for the administration of ophthalmic medications is outlined here (during the procedure, follow the CDC's Standard Precautions for infection control):

1. Identify the patient and explain the procedure.
2. Observe the Seven Rights of Drug Administration.

3. Verify the medication order and select the proper drug, checking its name, expiration date, concentration, dosage, and clarity (if a liquid).
4. Assemble any required supplies.
5. Recheck the medication order and drug as in step 3.
6. Prepare the medication for administration.
7. Recheck the medication order and drug as in steps 3 and 5.
8. Ask the patient to look upward.
9. Drop the medication onto the affected eye or apply the ointment to the bottom eyelid.
10. For drops, have the patient close his or her eyes for a few seconds. You can also apply gentle pressure on the corner of the eye, which will help prevent the medication from entering the nasolacrimal duct.
11. Assess the patient for any response to the medication.
12. Document the administration and any patient response.

Nasal Drug Administration

Nasal drug administration is giving a medication into the nasal passage. Patients often can self-administer nasal medications, but some patients may require assistance. Nasal medications may be given as drops or as a spray mist. It is important that the patient blow his or her nose before the medication is given. This clears the mucosa for maximum drug absorption. Absorption is also aided by having the patient tilt his or her head back while the drug is being administered. The nasal drug administration procedure is described here (during the procedure, follow the CDC's Standard Precautions for infection control):

1. Identify the patient and explain the procedure.
2. Observe the Seven Rights of Drug Administration.
3. Verify the medication order and select the proper drug, checking its name, expiration date, concentration, dosage, and clarity (if a liquid).
4. Assemble any required supplies.
5. Recheck the medication order and drug as in step 3.
6. Prepare the medication for administration.
7. Recheck the medication order and drug as in steps 3 and 5.
8. Ask the patient to tilt his or her head back.
9. Drop or spray the medication into the affected nostril(s).
10. Assess the patient for any response to the medication.
11. Document the administration and any patient response.

Otic Drug Administration

Otic drug administration is giving a drug into the ear(s) (Fig. 8-4). The patient should lie with the affected ear upward and remain in this position for a few minutes after the drug has been given to allow for maximum absorption. When giving a drug via the otic route, gently pull the pinna (the projected part of the external ear) up and back for the adult patient and pull the outer ear down and backward for the pediatric patient. This technique aids the entrance of the medication into the ear.

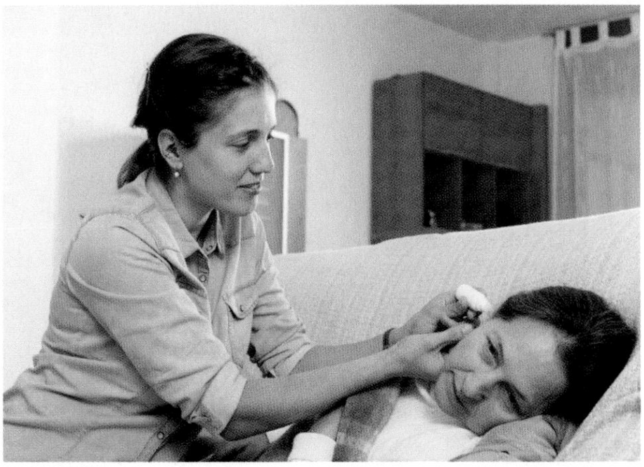

Figure 8-4 Otic drug administration. *(Photograph © Fuse/Thinkstock)*

The otic drug administration procedure is as follows (during the procedure, follow the CDC's Standard Precautions for infection control):

1. Identify the patient and explain the procedure.
2. Observe the Seven Rights of Drug Administration.
3. Verify the medication order and select the proper drug, checking its name, expiration date, concentration, dosage, and clarity (if a liquid).
4. Assemble any required supplies.
5. Recheck the medication order and drug as in step 3.
6. Prepare the medication for administration.
7. Recheck the medication order and drug as in steps 3 and 5.
8. Ask the patient to lie down with the affected ear upward.
9. Drop the medication into the affected ear.
10. Ask the patient to remain still to allow the medication to completely enter the ear. Place a cotton ball to the ear to absorb any medication that may run out.
11. Assess the patient for any response to the medication.
12. Document the administration and any patient response.

Transdermal Drug Administration

Transdermal drug administration is done by placing a medication in a special gel-like matrix that is applied directly to the patient's skin (Fig. 8-5). Each application provides an infusion of medication for anywhere from one to several days at a fixed rate. Transdermal patches consist of three layers: the backing, the medication, and a liner that is peeled off just before application. Once applied, the drug-absorption rate is not affected by the patient's skin texture, thickness, or skin color. However, the patient's skin should be dry and cleaned of lotions, creams, oils, and so on before application. Transdermal patches should not be placed on tattoos or scars.

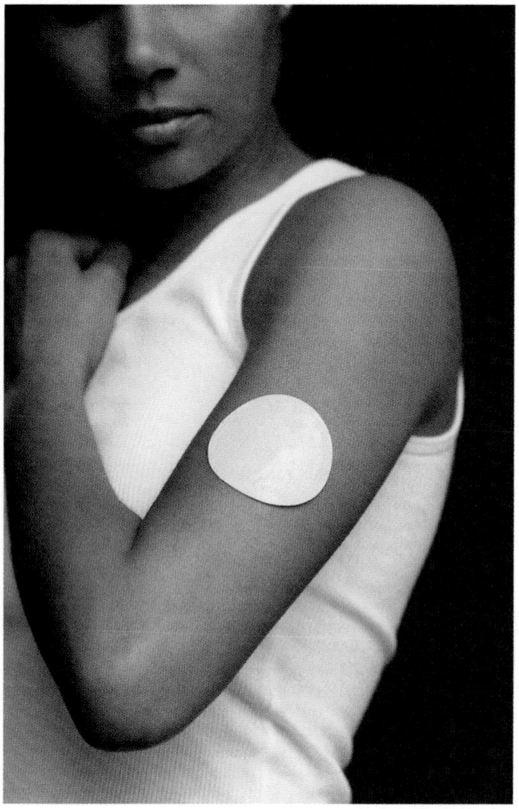

Figure 8-5 Transdermal drug administration. *(Photograph © JackF/iStock/Thinkstock)*

The procedure for applying a transdermal medication patch follows (during the procedure, follow the CDC's Standard Precautions for infection control):

1. Identify the patient and explain the procedure.
2. Observe the Seven Rights of Drug Administration.
3. Verify the medication order and select the proper drug, checking its name, expiration date, concentration, dosage, and clarity (if a liquid).
4. Assemble any required supplies.
5. Recheck the medication order and drug as in step 3.
6. Prepare the medication for administration.
7. Recheck the medication order and drug as in steps 3 and 5.
8. Place the patch on the patient in the area specified on the order.
9. Hold the patch in place with tape if necessary.
10. Assess the patient for any response to the medication.
11. Document the administration and any patient response.

Rectal

Rectal drug administration can have either **local** or systemic effects. **Systemic** drug absorption from rectal administration, however, can be incomplete and unpredictable, especially if the patient is unable to retain the drug. For two reasons, rectal drug administration quickly results in a high concentration of the drug in the circulation. First, the rectum contains a rich network of capillaries. Second, because venous blood from the lower part of the rectum does not pass through the liver, drugs absorbed in the rectum are not biotransformed in the liver before reaching other body sites.

Rectal drug administration may be necessary when oral administration is unsuitable, for example, in unconscious or nauseated patients or small children who are unable to swallow drugs. An example of a drug administered rectally is promethazine (Phenergan), used in the treatment of motion sickness, as a sedative, and as an antiemetic.

effective Communication

It is important to keep rectal medications in a cool environment because, when suppositories become warm, they soften and are more difficult to administer. Therefore, rectal medications should be given immediately after opening.

Rectal drug administration is usually not performed in the out-of-hospital setting. However, if you are ordered to administer a rectal medication, the procedure for administering rectal medications follows (during the procedure, follow the CDC's Standard Precautions for infection control):

1. Identify the patient and explain the procedure.
2. Place the patient on his or her side.
3. Drape the patient for privacy.
4. Place a waterproofing sheet under the patient's buttocks.
5. Observe the Seven Rights of Drug Administration.
6. Verify the medication order and select the proper drug, checking its name, expiration date, concentration, dosage, and so on.
7. Assemble any required supplies.
8. Recheck the medication order and drug as in step 6.
9. Prepare the medication for administration.
10. Recheck the medication order and drug as in steps 6 and 8.
11. Gently separate the patient's buttocks.
12. Insert the suppository with one finger into the patient's rectum.
13. Ask the patient to lie still for a few minutes so the medication can be absorbed.
14. Assess the patient for any response to the medication.
15. Document the administration and any patient response.

Parenteral Drug Routes

Intradermal

Intradermal administration is the injection of a drug into the upper layers of the skin, with the needle almost parallel to the skin surface. These injections are usually done with a fine, short (5/8-inch by 26- to 27-gauge) needle and a small-barrel (1-mL)

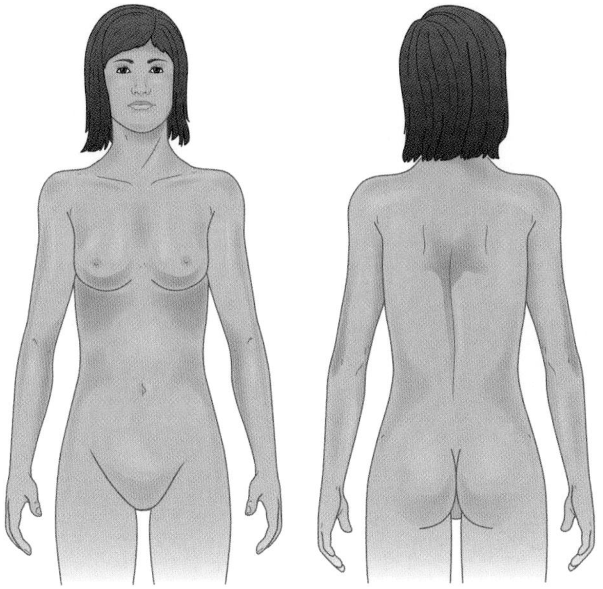

Figure 8-6 Common SubQ injection sites. *(Photograph © moodboard/moodboard/Thinkstock)*

syringe. Intradermal drug administration is used to provide local effects for the treatment of allergies or to perform allergy skin testing. The amount of drug that can be injected intradermally is small; the rate of absorption is slow because absorption is limited to the capillaries of the dermis.

Subcutaneous

A **subcutaneous (SubQ)** injection is performed by inserting a small needle (1/2 to 5/8 inches long, with a gauge of 25 or less) into the fatty tissue above the muscle. Usually, the largest dose that can be injected by this method is 2 mL. SubQ injection causes minimal tissue trauma and avoids damage to large blood vessels and nerves. Figure 8-6 illustrates the common SubQ injection sites.

Drug absorption after a SubQ injection largely depends on the physical condition of the patient. For example, SubQ injection is undesirable for patients with compromised circulatory perfusion, such as those in shock or those with peripheral vascular disease.

An example of an EMS drug administered by SubQ injection is epinephrine (1:1000 solution) used in treating bronchoconstriction associated with anaphylaxis.

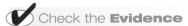

Check the Evidence

Inadvertently injecting a 1:1000 epinephrine solution into an IV line can cause very serious adverse reactions, including death.

The procedure for administering a SubQ injection is as follows (during the procedure, follow the CDC's Standard Precautions for infection control):

1. Perform a thorough patient assessment and history, confirming that the drug is needed and that the patient does not have any allergies that contraindicate the use of the drug.
2. Receive, write down, and confirm the order and observe the Seven Rights of Drug Administration.
3. Calculate the required dosage.
4. Prepare the appropriate equipment:
   - Drug
   - 1- to 2-mL syringe
   - 5/8-inch by 25-gauge needle
   - Antibacterial swab and ointment and alcohol prep
   - 2 × 2 or 4 × 4 gauze pads
   - Adhesive bandage strip
   - Sharps container
5. Explain the procedure to the patient.
6. Examine the drug, reconfirming that:
   - It is the correct medication.
   - It has not expired.
   - It is not discolored.
   - There are no visible particles in the solution.
7. Gently tap the upper part of the ampule or shake the ampule down, forcing the drug to the lower portion of the ampule. Figure 8-7 illustrates the withdrawal of a drug from an ampule.
8. Using a gauze pad or alcohol prep to protect your hand, break off the top of the ampule.
9. Draw the drug into the syringe and expel any excess air from it.

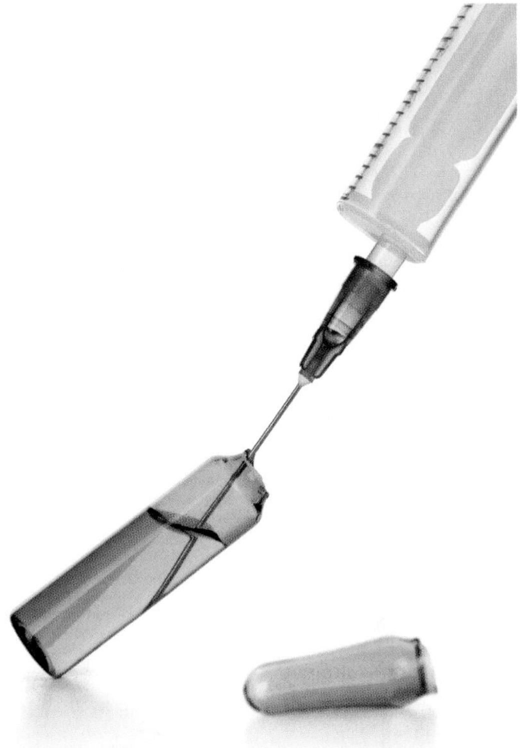

Figure 8-7 Withdrawing a medication from an ampule. *(Photograph © Thinkstock)*

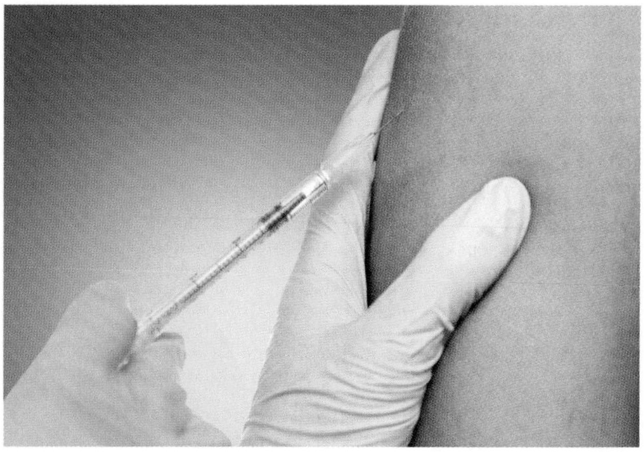

Figure 8-8 Subcutaneous injection. *(Photograph © urfinguss/iStock/Thinkstock)*

10. Choose a suitable administration site. A commonly used site is the SubQ tissue over the triceps brachii muscle on the back of the arm.
11. Cleanse the site with an antibacterial swab.
12. Pinch the skin and insert the needle at a 45-degree angle (Fig. 8-8).
13. Aspirate the syringe (gently pull the plunger back to create suction) to make sure that the needle is not in a blood vessel. If blood enters the syringe, withdraw the needle and prepare another site for another attempt, *using a new needle.*
14. Inject the drug slowly.
15. Remove and properly dispose of the needle.
16. Gently massage the injection site. (This aids in drug absorption, as well as patient comfort.)
17. Cover the site with an adhesive bandage strip.
18. Confirm and document administration of the drug.
19. Closely monitor the patient and report any changes.

*Some drugs come in a vial instead of an ampule. When withdrawing a drug from a vial, first clean the rubber stopper with an antibacterial swab. Insert the needle and inject a volume of air into the vial equal to the volume of drug you need to withdraw. For example, if you need 4 mL of a drug, inject 4 mL of air into the vial. Doing so makes it easier to draw the drug into the syringe.

Intramuscular

Intramuscular (IM) injection is the most common method of administering parenteral drugs. However, it is not common in the out-of-hospital setting. The drug is injected deep into the muscle tissue, where it is absorbed into the capillaries and enters the bloodstream. Drug doses of up to 5 mL can be given via the IM route; this requires needles of 21- to 23-gauge and 1 to 1 1/2 inches in length. If larger amounts of a drug are to be given, it is better to use two injection sites. Figure 8-9 illustrates common sites for intramuscular drug administration.

The rate of absorption of a drug administered by IM injection depends on the physical condition of the patient. For example, IM injection may be contraindicated for patients with decreased peripheral perfusion or inadequate muscle mass. On the other hand, IM drug administration usually yields a predictable absorption rate.

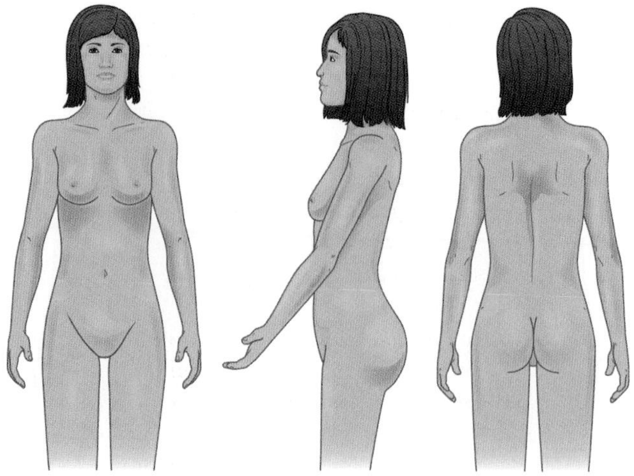

Figure 8-9 Intramuscular injection sites. *(Photograph © Remains/iStock/Thinkstock)*

In emergencies in which an intravenous line cannot be established, IM injection is sometimes the answer. For example, EMS personnel can use IM injection to administer thiamine to patients in a coma of unknown origin or a coma caused by alcohol and to patients suffering delirium tremens. There is also the option of sedating the patient before an IV is started in difficult situations.

effective **Communication**

In most cases, IM injections should be avoided when the patient's chief complaint is chest pain.

An IM injection may cause a rise in the amount of certain muscle enzymes circulating within the bloodstream. The level of these enzymes can help the physician determine if a myocardial infarction (MI) is the cause of the patient's chest pain. An IM injection in the out-of-hospital setting may confuse the picture when measurements of muscle enzymes are evaluated at the hospital. The procedure for IM administration of drugs is as follows (during the procedure, follow the CDC's Standard Precautions for infection control):

1. Perform a thorough patient assessment and history, confirming that the drug is needed and that the patient does not have any allergies that contraindicate the use of the drug.
2. Receive, write down, and confirm the order and perform the Seven Rights of Drug Administration.
3. Calculate the required dosage.
4. Prepare the appropriate equipment:
   - Drug
   - Appropriate size syringe (1- to 3-mL)

- 1- to 1 1/2-inch by 21- to 23-gauge needle
- Antibacterial swab and ointment and alcohol prep
- 2 × 2 or 4 × 4 inch gauze pads
- Adhesive bandage strip
- Sharps container

5. Explain the procedure to the patient.
6. Examine the drug, reconfirming that:
   - It is the correct drug.
   - It has not expired.
   - It is not discolored.
   - There are no visible particles in the solution.
7. Gently tap the upper part of the ampule or shake the ampule down, forcing the drug to the lower part of the ampule.
8. Using a gauze pad or an alcohol prep to protect your hand, break off the top of the ampule.
9. Draw the drug into the syringe and expel any excess air from it.
10. Choose a suitable administration site. A commonly used site is the deltoid muscle of the arm.
11. Cleanse the administration site with an antibacterial swab.
12. Insert the needle into the tissue at a 90-degree angle (Fig. 8-10).
13. Aspirate the syringe to make sure the needle is not in a blood vessel. If blood enters the syringe, withdraw the needle and prepare another site for another attempt, *using a new needle.*
14. Inject the drug slowly.
15. Remove and properly dispose of the needle.
16. Gently massage the injection site. (This aids in drug absorption.)
17. Cover the site with an adhesive bandage strip.
18. Confirm and document administration of the drug.
19. Closely monitor the patient and report any changes.

Intravenous

When the situation calls for a rapid therapeutic effect, **intravenous (IV)** injection allows direct administration of a drug directly into the bloodstream, either as a **bolus** or as an infusion. A bolus is one dose of a drug injected into the vein all at once. Continuous infusion is the controlled introduction (at a specific rate) of a drug into the bloodstream over a period of time. Continuous infusion is a way to keep the amount of drug available to body tissues at a constant level. Most out-of-hospital emergency drugs are administered by IV injection. Drug administration by IV bolus yields quick, predictable therapeutic concentrations, which makes it the route of choice in most emergency situations.

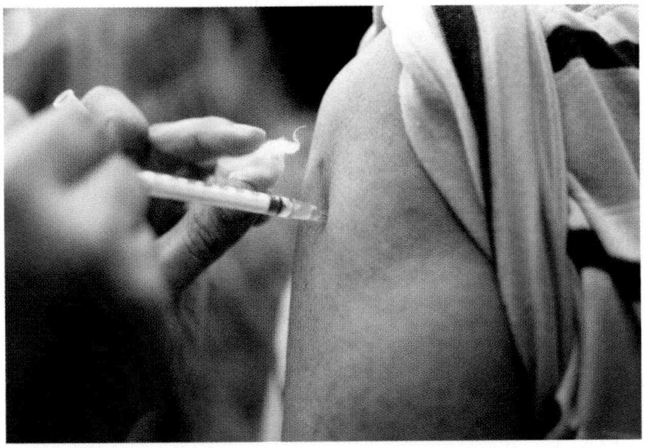

Figure 8-10 IM injection. *(Photograph © Thinkstock)*

effective Communication

The rapidity of absorption of an IV bolus carries the risk of producing immediate adverse reactions and side effects.

The rate of an IV infusion can be set to maintain therapeutic levels of a drug. In some emergency situations, the physician or paramedic first gives an IV bolus to achieve therapeutic levels quickly and then uses an **intravenous infusion** to maintain those established levels. For instance, amiodarone is administered in this way to treat V-Fib. The bolus of amiodarone is used to produce therapeutic levels as quickly as possible. Once circulation has been restored, an infusion maintains the established therapeutic level of amiodarone in the bloodstream.

Intravenous Bolus Injection

Once an IV infusion (IV lifeline) has been established, this enables the administration of a bolus injection through the IV line. This procedure is called an *intravenous bolus injection.* In the following description of the procedure, the bolus is packaged in a single-dose, prefilled syringe. In most emergency situations, this is the case. Sometimes, however, the necessary drug is available only in an ampule or vial, from which you must draw the proper dose.

1. Perform a thorough patient assessment and history, confirming that the drug is needed and that the patient does not have any allergies that contraindicate the use of the drug.
2. Receive, write down, and confirm the order (during the procedure, follow the CDC's Standard Precautions for infection control).
3. Perform the Seven Rights of Drug Administration.
4. Prepare the appropriate equipment:
   - Correct drug (prefilled syringe with needle)
   - Antibacterial swab and alcohol prep
5. Explain the procedure to the patient.
6. Examine the drug, reconfirming that:
   - It is the correct drug.
   - It has not expired.
   - It is not discolored.
   - There are no visible particles in the solution.
7. Calculate the required dosage.
8. Assemble the prefilled syringe and expel any excess air.

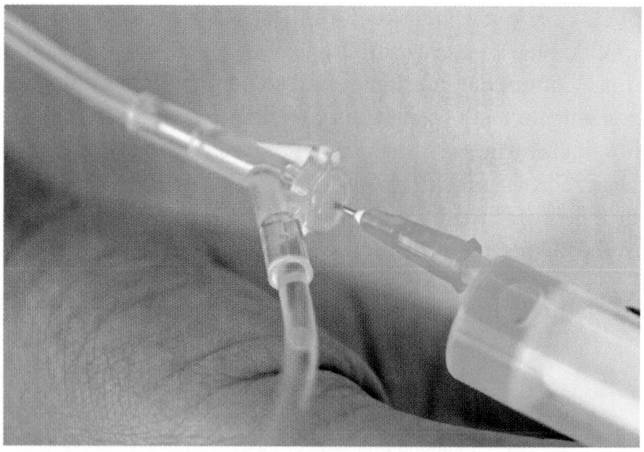

Figure 8-11 IV bolus medication. *(Photograph © kaurmungadd/iStock/Thinkstock)*

9. Verify the patency of the IV line.
10. Clean the medication port on the IV administration set using an antibacterial swab.
11. Recheck the drug.
12. Insert the needle into the medication port (Fig. 8-11).
13. Pinch the tubing off above the medication port.
14. Administer the drug at the appropriate rate. (Rates differ between different types of drugs.)
15. Remove the needle and clean the administration port with an antibacterial swab; properly dispose of the needle and syringe.
16. Release the pinched IV line.
17. Flush the IV line by opening the line wide open for 30 seconds to 1 minute.
18. Confirm and document administration of the drug.
19. Closely monitor the patient and report any changes.

Intravenous Infusion (Piggyback)

1. Perform a thorough patient assessment and history, confirming that the drug is needed and that the patient does not have any allergies that contraindicate the use of the drug.
2. Receive, write down, and confirm the order (during the procedure, follow the CDC's Standard Precautions for infection control).
3. Perform the Seven Rights of Drug Administration.
4. Prepare the appropriate equipment:
   - Correct drug (prefilled syringe with needle)
   - Antibacterial swab and alcohol prep
   - Label for the intravenous bag
5. Explain the procedure to the patient.
6. Examine the drug, reconfirming that:
   - It is the correct drug.
   - It has not expired.
   - It is not discolored.
   - There are no visible particles in the solution.
7. Recheck the drug.
8. Assemble the prefilled syringe.
9. Clean the medication port on the IV bag with an antibacterial swab.

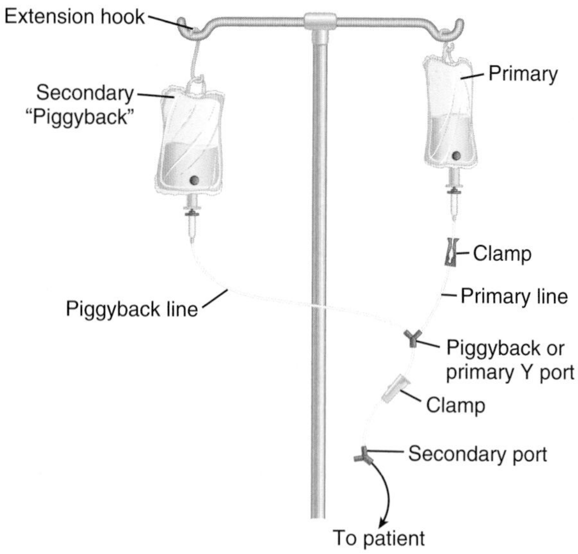

Figure 8-12 IV piggyback. *(Photograph © GDragan/iStock/Thinkstock)*

10. Insert the needle into the medication port of the bag and add the drug.
11. Remove the needle and cleanse the administration port with an antibacterial swab; properly dispose of the syringe and needle.
12. Thoroughly mix the drug in the IV bag.
13. Attach an IV line to the bag, "prime" the line, and attach a 1-inch by 18-gauge needle to the line.
14. Clean the medication port of the already established IV line with an antibacterial swab, insert the needle, and secure with tape (Fig. 8-12).
15. Shut down the previously established IV line and begin flow of the **piggyback** drug line; set the flow to the necessary rate.
16. Label the piggyback IV bag with:
   - The patient's name
   - The date and time that the piggyback infusion was established
   - The name and amount of the drug added to the piggyback IV bag
   - The infusion flow rate
   - The name of the person who established the piggyback infusion
17. Confirm and document the establishment of the piggyback infusion.
18. Monitor the patient and report any changes.

Transtracheal

Some emergency drugs can be administered down an **endotracheal (ET)** tube when an IV line cannot be started or cannot be established quickly enough. Drugs given down the ET tube are absorbed into the capillaries of the lungs. When ET administration is done correctly, the rate of absorption of the drug is just as rapid as when the drug is given by IV injection.

Check the **Evidence**

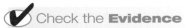

Drugs that can be administered down the ET tube include:

N = naloxone
A = atropine
V = vasopressin
E = epinephrine
L = lidocaine

When giving these drugs down the ET tube, the dosages are 2 to 2.5 times the IV dosages.

Transtracheal Administration

1. Receive, write down, and confirm the order (during the procedure, follow the CDC's Standard Precautions for infection control).
2. Perform the Seven Rights of Drug Administration.
3. Examine the drug, reconfirming that:
   - It is the correct drug.
   - It has not expired.
   - It is not discolored.
   - There are no visible particles in the solution.
4. Assemble the prefilled syringe.
5. Remove the bag-valve-mask device and inject the correct amount of the drug into the ET tube. Properly dispose of the needle and syringe. If the drug order is for a small dose and you must withdraw the drug from an ampule or vial, dilute the drug with 5 to 10 mL of sterile NS solution or sterile water.
6. Replace the bag-valve-mask device and hyperventilate to force the drug down the tube. (Note that some ET tubes have medication ports built into them.)
7. Resume normal ventilations.
8. Confirm and document the administration of the drug.
9. Monitor the patient and report any changes.

Intraosseous

Intraosseous (IO) administration is a safe, rapid, and effective way to introduce fluids and drugs into the bloodstream via the highly vascular bone marrow cavity of both adult and pediatric patients. Giving fluids and drugs via the IO route is just as rapid as via the IV route. The best access for an IO line is the tibia just below the tubercle on the anteromedial surface. Alternate sites include the femur, just above the lateral condyles in the midline for pediatric patients, and the sternum, just below the sternal notch, the tibia, the medial malleolus, and the head of the humerus in adults.

Indications for starting an IO infusion line include cardiopulmonary arrest, critical burns, status seizures, and hemodynamic instability. All drugs and crystalloid solutions that can be administered intravenously can also be given by the IO route. The procedure for establishing an IO line follows:

1. Receive, write down, and confirm the order (during the procedure, follow the CDC's Standard Precautions for infection control).
2. Perform the Seven Rights of Drug Administration.
3. Prepare the appropriate equipment:
   - IV solution, IV tubing, and a stopcock
   - Spinal or bone-marrow needle with a stylet (15- to 18-gauge) or commercial IO access device
   - Syringe filled with NS
   - Antibacterial swab and alcohol preps
4. Examine the solution, reconfirming:
   - It is the correct solution.
   - It has not expired.
   - It is not discolored.
   - There are no visible particles in the solution.
5. Attach a line to the bag, prime the line, and attach the needle.
6. Identify bony landmarks. For example:
   - The proximal tibia: The needle will enter 1 to 3 centimeters below the tibial tuberosity just beneath the knee (Fig. 8-13). The proximal tibia is the preferred site for three reasons: (1) The prominence of the bone makes it easy to find the right injection site. (2) There is little soft tissue over the bone. (3) The flat surface of the bone makes for easier needle insertion.
   - The distal femur: The needle will enter 3 centimeters above the lateral condyle just above the knee (Fig. 8-14).
   - The distal tibia: The needle will enter in the flat surface of the tibia 1 to 3 centimeters above the medial malleolus at the ankle (Fig. 8-15).
   - Humeral head: The proximal aspect or humeral head (Fig. 8-16)
   - Sternum: Just below the sternal notch (Fig. 8-17)
7. Clean the site with an antibacterial swab.
8. Insert the needle with the stylet in place at a 90-degree angle to the bone or at a slight angle *away*

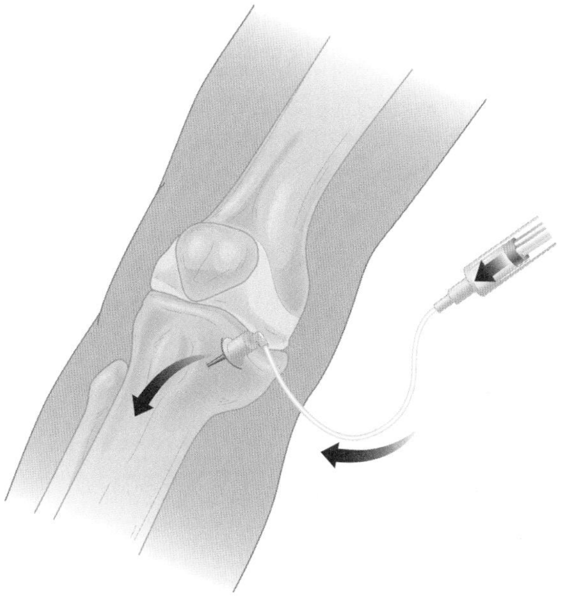

Figure 8-13 IO infusion into the proximal tibia.

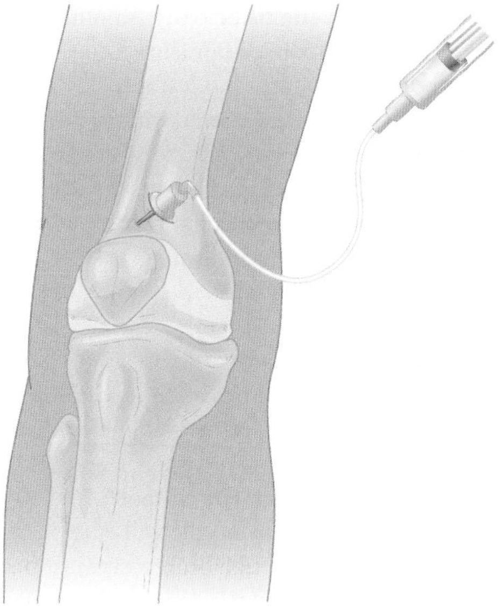

Figure 8-14 IO infusion into the distal femur.

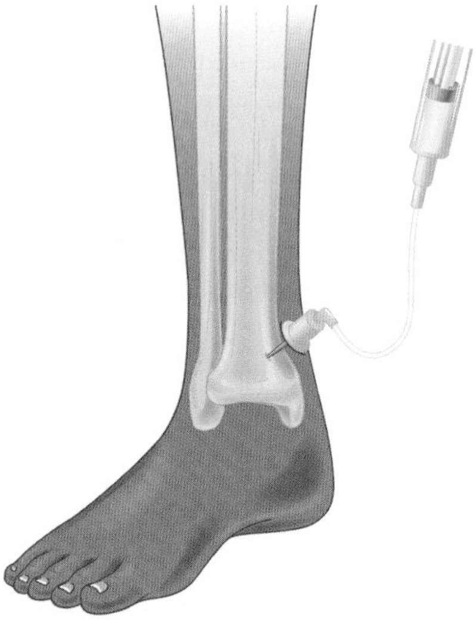

Figure 8-15 IO infusion into the distal tibia.

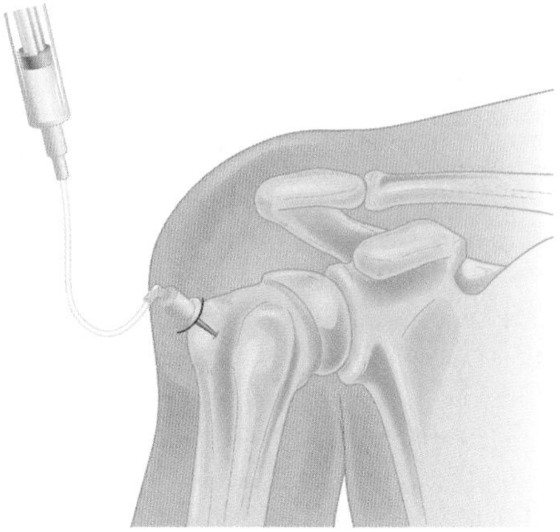

Figure 8-16 IO infusion into the humeral head.

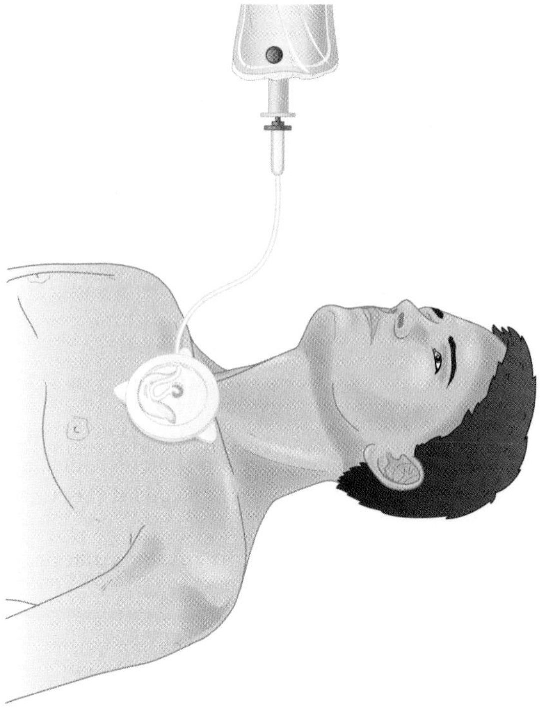

Figure 8-17 IO infusion into the sternum.

from the joint. This is to avoid inserting the needle into the growth plate.

9. Remove the stylet.
10. Attempt to aspirate bone marrow. If no marrow enters the needle, inject a small amount of saline solution into the site. If there is resistance to the injection, or if saline solution infiltrates the soft tissue around the site, the needle is not in the bone marrow.
11. Stabilize the needle (although it should stand unsupported).
12. Connect the tubing and begin the infusion.
13. Confirm and document the establishment of the IO infusion.
14. Monitor the patient and report any changes.

Once the IO infusion has been established, drugs can be administered via IV bolus or piggyback.

Intravenous Access via the External Jugular Vein

The external jugular vein in the neck connects into the central circulation via the subclavian vein. Fluids and drugs reach the central circulation of the body rapidly when administered via the external jugular vein. IV access via the external jugular vein should only be done on an unresponsive patient.

Check the Evidence

The external jugular vein is considered a peripheral IV access line.

The procedure for establishing an external jugular IV includes:

1. Perform a thorough patient assessment and history, confirming that the drug is needed and that the patient does not have any allergies that contraindicate the use of the drug.
2. Receive, write down, and confirm the order (during the procedure, follow the CDC's Standard Precautions for infection control).
3. Perform the Seven Rights of Drug Administration.
4. Prepare the appropriate equipment:
   - Appropriate intravenous fluid and administration set
   - Appropriate indwelling catheter
   - Antibacterial swab and ointment and alcohol preps
   - Sterile gauze pads
   - 1/2- to 1-inch tape
   - Sharps container
5. Position the patient supine, with the head turned away from the side to be cannulated.
6. After locating the vein, prepare the site.
7. Apply gentle traction on the vein just below the clavicle.
8. Approach the site midway between the angle of the jaw and the clavicle, aiming toward the shoulder, and puncture at a 30-degree angle.
9. Upon entry into the vein, note a flashback of blood and advance the needle and catheter approximately 2 mm to stabilize the needle in the vein.
10. Remove the needle and properly dispose of it in the sharps container.
11. Connect the IV tubing and slowly open to allow fluid to flow. Confirm that the fluid is flowing freely without evidence of infiltration.
12. Apply antibacterial ointment and cover with a sterile gauze pad or adhesive bandage.
13. Use tape to secure the IV tubing and catheter in place.
14. Adjust the flow rate.
15. Confirm and document the successful completion of the infusion.
16. Monitor the patient and report any changes.

Patient-Administered Nitrous Oxide–Oxygen Mixture

Inhalation of a 50 percent mixture of nitrous oxide and oxygen produces central nervous system depression, as well as rapid pain relief. The procedure for patient-administered nitrous oxide–oxygen administration is as follows:

1. Perform a thorough patient assessment and history, confirming that the drug is needed and that the patient does not have any allergies or medical conditions that contraindicate the use of the drug.
2. During the procedure, follow the CDC's Standard Precautions for infection control.
3. Perform the Seven Rights of Drug Administration.
4. Prepare the appropriate equipment:
   - Nitrous oxide tank
   - Oxygen tank
   - Demand valve with attached face mask
5. Open the valves on both tanks.
6. Explain the procedure to the patient and advise the patient of the possible side effects that may be experienced.
7. Place the patient in a sitting position and instruct the patient on the use of the device.
8. Explain that, if the patient begins to feel uncomfortable or if the pain is relieved, he or she should remove the mask and breathe normally.
9. Monitor the patient and report any changes.

Epinephrine Autoinjector

Many people who experience allergic reactions carry epinephrine autoinjectors. The adult dose delivered from one of these autoinjectors is 0.3 mg of epinephrine. The pediatric autoinjector dose is 0.15 mg of epinephrine. There may be instances when the EMS professional will be required to use the autoinjector to administer the epinephrine.

1. Perform a thorough patient assessment and history, confirming that the drug is needed and that the patient does not have any allergies that contraindicate the use of the drug.
2. Receive, write down, and confirm the order (during the procedure, follow the CDC's Standard Precautions for infection control).
3. Perform the Seven Rights of Drug Administration.
4. Explain the procedure to the patient.
5. Examine the autoinjector for name, dose, and expiration date.
6. Remove the safety cap from the autoinjector and place it on the patient's outer thigh.
7. Press until you hear the autoinjector function. Hold in place for approximately 5 seconds.
8. Gently massage the injection site for approximately 15 seconds.
9. Monitor the patient and report any changes.

Umbilical Vein Catheterization

In cases when the neonate patient (less than 1 week of age) is in need of an IV line or medications and peripheral access is impossible, the umbilical vein route can be used. The procedure for umbilical vein catheterization is as follows:

1. Perform a thorough patient assessment and history, confirming that the infusion is needed.
2. Receive, write down, and confirm the order (follow the CDC's Standard Precautions for infection control).
3. Perform the Seven Rights of Drug Administration.
4. Prepare the appropriate equipment:
   - IV fluid and administration set
   - Indwelling catheter
   - Antibacterial swab and ointment and alcohol preps

- Sterile gauze pads
- 1/2- to 1-inch tape
- Sharps container

5. Explain to the patient's caregiver(s) the procedure and the possible complications that might result.
6. If necessary, restrain the child.
7. Clean and drape the umbilicus and umbilical area.
8. Loosely tie umbilical tape around the base of the umbilicus.
9. There are two umbilical arteries and one umbilical vein. Locate the umbilical vein. It has a thin wall and larger lumen compared with the thick walls and small lumen of the umbilical arteries. Trim the umbilical vein approximately 1 cm to provide a fresh opening.
10. Insert the tip of a sterile hemostat into the lumen of the umbilical vein and gently open the hemostat to dilate the vein.
11. Advance a heparintized-saline flushed umbilical catheter into the umbilical vein approximately 2 to 4 inches, noting blood return. The catheter is now in the inferior vena cava of the child.
12. Attach a three-way stopcock to the catheter and flush with 1 mL of heparin solution.
13. Secure the catheter with umbilical tape.
14. Attach the IV line to the stopcock to allow for the administration of fluids and drugs.
15. Monitor the child and report any changes.

Drug Administration to the Pediatric Patient

Drug administration to the pediatric population requires special consideration. A standard drug dosage is nearly nonexistent in children. One reason for this is that drug metabolism in the liver of neonates is slow because of immaturity. When children reach the age of 1, most pharmacokinetic patterns are similar to those of the adult, except for those of the liver. At age 1, liver-metabolizing enzymes are increased, causing children to metabolize drugs at a faster rate than adults. Children generally reach adult metabolizing parameters at puberty. Therefore, drugs primarily eliminated by metabolism through the liver (hepatic) may require dosage adjustments or may require an increase in the dosing frequency.

Renal excretion is decreased for children under 1 year of age. Adult parameters for glomerular filtration are reached between 3 and 6 months. Tubular filtration does not mature for children until approximately 1 year of age. The renal excretion rate during childhood may increase and exceed that of the adult. This may cause drug underdosing problems.

Drugs for children are generally ordered according to either their body weight or body surface area (BSA). However, calculations based on the child's body weight are generally inaccurate. Therefore, drugs should be ordered based on BSA.

The BSA nomogram (Chapter 7, Figure 7-4: Pediatric Nomogram) utilizes conversions from weight and height to determine drug dosages for children. Using the weight and height relationship, the BSA nomogram can provide a more precise guide to the maturity of the child's organs and metabolic rate of functioning for pharmacokinetics. Drug dosing should be tailored to the individual child according to the amount of drug per square meter of BSA. The BSA rule for pediatric dosages is:

Approximate pediatric dose = Child's BSA in square meters × Adult dose/1.73

For example, using the BSA nomogram, a child with a weight of 10 kg and a height of 34 inches is considered to have a BSA (m^2) of 0.5. The dosage calculation is:

Child's approximate dose = 0.5 × Adult dose/1.73

Drug Administration to the Geriatric Patient

As people become older, they undergo a variety of physiological changes that may increase their sensitivity to drugs. The loss of body weight, for example, may require initiation of therapy of a lower adult dose. Some older patients are obese, some weigh no more than a large child, some weigh more, and some weigh less. Yet, some of these patients are prescribed the standard adult doses. Other physiological changes that may occur with age include:

- **Blood-brain barrier:** Because the barrier is easily penetrated by fat-soluble drugs, the patient may become confused.
- **Baroreceptor response:** Reduced response exaggerates the hypotensive effects of antihypertensive drugs.
- **Liver:** Smaller liver size can result in toxicity of some drugs.
- **Kidneys:** Decreased blood flow can cause normal dosages to actually become toxic.
- **Poor peripheral venous tone** exaggerates the hypotensive effects of antihypertensive drugs.
- **Stomach:** Slower stomach emptying and an increase in gastric pH can cause stomach irritation with some drugs.

Estimates have suggested that up to 80 percent of adverse drug reactions in the geriatric population are dose related. The physiological changes related to aging may result in a decrease in drug metabolism, poor distribution in the body, and poor renal excretion.

Contaminated Sharps and Equipment Disposal

Body fluids can contain infectious material that endangers not only EMS personnel but also family, friends, and bystanders. Because the patient may be infected with a pathogen without showing any signs or symptoms, EMS professionals must treat every patient as though he or she is infected.

Starting IV fluids and administering drugs involves coming in contact with needles and body fluids. One of the most common problems in health care is inadvertent needle sticks. Needle sticks can easily transmit diseases between the patient and EMS personnel. It is extremely important that needles and other sharps are properly handled before and after each patient use. There are some commonsense precautions that must be taken while using sharps:

- **Slow down:** More lives are saved because of accuracy, not speed. That is also true when it comes to handling sharps and avoiding accidents. When using sharps, take the time to perform the task correctly and safely. You must also be aware of the sudden bumps, turns, and so forth that you encounter in the back of an ambulance or in a helicopter. These environments can create hazards that can contribute to accidents using sharps. Remember, we have a tendency to make more mistakes when in a hurry.
- **Immediately dispose of used sharps:** Never throw used sharps on the floor, on the "buddy" bench, or anywhere other than in an approved sharps container.
- **Avoid recapping needles:** This is especially true in a moving vehicle. If a needle must be recapped, never use two hands. Use only one hand on a stable surface.

SCENARIO REVISITED

Do you recall the converted cardiac arrest patient at the airport? You now place the patient on a pulse oximeter and are ordered to administer amiodarone at 150 mg over 10 minutes, followed by a 1 mg/minute IV infusion to prevent a reoccurrence of V-Fib. Your amiodarone comes packaged as 150 mg in 3 mL of solution (50 mg/mL). In order to administer the amiodarone as ordered, you can set up one piggyback IV for each infusion.

Let's Recap

EMS professionals must be knowledgeable about and competent in every drug administration procedure they need to perform. Again, a strong knowledge base of medical protocols and the routes of each medication is essential. When an emergency arises, time is precious. In an emergency, the EMS professional is required to quickly identify the drug(s) to be given, the necessary dosage, and the most appropriate route. It is important to build a knowledge base that allows comfort with the protocols and drugs administered routinely within the EMS system. Practice and prepare extensively to be able to administer drugs in a safe, rapid, and systematic manner.

SCENARIO CONCLUSION

To set up the 150 mg over 10 minutes, you can add 150 mg of amiodarone in a 100-mL bag of NS and infuse it over 10 minutes.

Understand the Numbers

When you add 3 mL of the amiodarone (150 mg) to your 100-mL bag of NS, how many gtt/minute will be needed to infuse the 150 mg using a 10 gtt/minute set?

103 mL × 10 gtt/minute ÷ 10 minutes = 103 gtt/minute

To set up the 1 mg/minute IV infusion, you can add 150 mg of amiodarone to 250 mL of NS.

Understand the Numbers

How many gtt/minute are required to run your amiodarone at 1 mg/minute using a 10 gtt/minute set?

Add 150 mg to a 500-mL bag of NS. This gives you a concentration of:

C = 150 mg ÷ 500 mL = 0.3 mg/mL

Vol. = 1 mg ÷ 0.3 mg/mL = 3.33 mL

Rate = 3.33 mL × 10 gtt/minute ÷ 1 minute = 33.3 or 33 gtt/minute

PRACTICE EXERCISES

1. The rate of action of a drug is determined by the drug concentration and the route by which the drug is administered. Of the four routes of drug administration listed below, which lists the routes in order from fastest to slowest rate of drug absorption?
a. IM, PO, SubQ, IV
b. IV, ET, PO, IM
c. PO, SubQ, IM, IV
d. IO, IM, SubQ, PO

2. Which of the following steps is not appropriate when administering a drug by IV bolus?
a. Verify the patency of the IV line before administering the drug.
b. Pinch the IV tubing off above the medication injection port.
c. Flush the IV line after drug administration.
d. Recap the needle and save the unused drug.

3. The most convenient, safe, and economical way to get drugs into the body is by:
   a. PO
   b. IO
   c. IV
   d. SubQ

4. The preferred site for IO drug administration in the pediatric patient is in the:
   a. Sternum
   b. Distal tibia
   c. Distal femur
   d. Proximal tibia

5. Pediatrics generally reach adult metabolizing parameters at:
   a. Age 1
   b. Age 5
   c. Age 8
   d. Puberty

6. The adult dose from one epinephrine autoinjector is:
   a. 0.3 mg
   b. 0.5 mg
   c. 1.3 mg
   d. 1.5 mg

7. All of the following drugs can be given down an ET tube except:
   a. Atropine
   b. Naloxone
   c. Vasopressin
   d. Norepinephrine

8. The common method of administering parenteral drugs is by:
   a. SubQ
   b. IM
   c. IV
   d. IO

9. Generally, an IM injection can give drug doses up to:
   a. 2 mL
   b. 3 mL
   c. 4 mL
   d. 5 mL

10. SubQ injections are generally given with needle gauges of:
   a. 20
   b. 22
   c. 23
   d. 25

CASE STUDY

You are called to a high school baseball game for a player who may have broken his left ankle. Upon arrival, you find a player with an obvious deformity of the left ankle. The patient injured himself by sliding into third base. He is complaining of severe pain and does not want you to touch his injured ankle. You contact medical control, and you are ordered to give 2 mg of morphine by slow IV.

The preferred route for administering morphine is by slow IV at 2 to 10 mg. However, morphine can be given IM, at a minimum dose of 5 mg. Morphine is one of the drugs that can be given by more than one route, but dosages are different depending on the route.

Another drug that can be given by more than one route is epinephrine. Epinephrine can be given by SubQ, IM, ET, and IV, depending on the disorder. EMS systems carry epinephrine in 1:1000 and 1:10,000 concentrations. The 1:1000 concentrations are given by the SubQ or IM routes. The 1:10,000 solution is given IV. If a 1:1000 concentration of epinephrine is given IV, serious adverse reactions may occur. Therefore, it is very important that EMS professionals know the route and dosage for each drug they administer.

MATH EQUATIONS

IV Infusions

1. How many drops per minute will it take to infuse 100 mL of fluid using a 60 gtt/mL IV set for 1 hour?
2. You are ordered to prepare an IV infusion by adding 2 grams of a drug to 500 mL of solution. Once prepared, the infusion is to run at 3 mg/minute, using a 60 gtt/mL IV set.
   a. What is the concentration (mg/mL) of the prepared infusion?
   b. How many drops/minute should the infusion run to deliver 3 mg/minute?
3. You are ordered to prepare and run an IV infusion at a rate of 2 mcg/minute. You prepare the infusion by adding 2 mg of the drug to 250 mL of solution.
   a. What is the resulting concentration of the solution (mcg/mL)?
   b. What infusion rate is needed using a 60 gtt/mL IV set?

4. You have a 20 percent solution of a drug in 500 mL of IV fluid. You are ordered to run the IV at a rate of 1.5 g/kg over 1 hour.
   a. What is the concentration of the IV solution (g/mL)?
   b. How many gtt/minute will be given to your patient using a 15 gtt/mL IV set?
5. You are ordered to run 1,000 mL of IV solution over 3 hours using a 15 gtt/mL IV set. How many gtt/minute should you give this IV?
6. You are ordered to run an IV infusion at 2 mcg/minute using a 60 gtt/minute IV set. The infusion is prepared by adding 1 mg of the drug to 500 mL of solution.
   a. What is the concentration of the IV solution after adding the drug (mcg/mL)?
   b. What infusion rate is needed to give 2 mcg/minute?

REFERENCES

Beck, R. K. (2012). Drug administration. In *Pharmacology for the EMS provider.* New York, NY: Delmar, Cengage Learning.

Deglin, J. H., Vallerand, A. H., and Sanoski, C. A. (2011). *Davis's drug guide for nurses* (12th ed.). Philadelphia, PA: F. A. Davis Company.

Venes, D., ed. (2013). *Taber's cyclopedic medical dictionary* (22nd ed.). Philadelphia, PA: F. A. Davis Company.

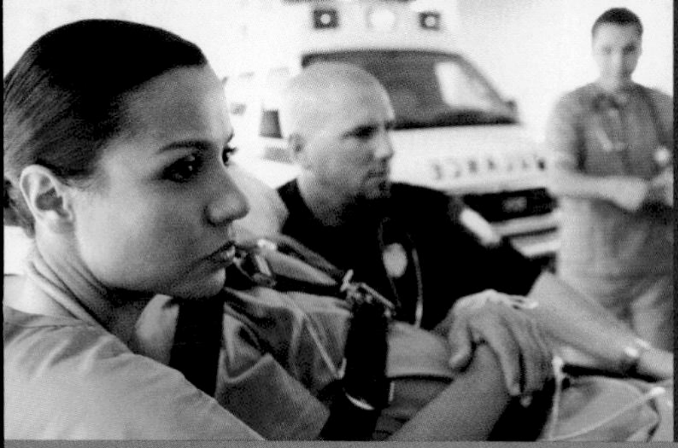

CHAPTER 9

Drug Classifications

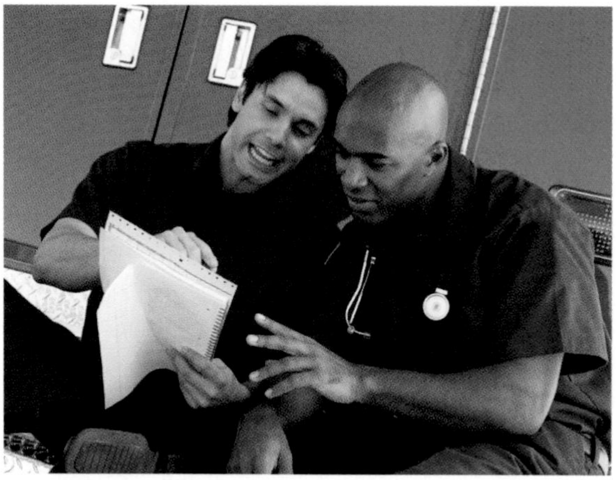

Paramedics discussing a new drug. *(Photograph © Monkey Business Images/Monkey Business/Thinkstock)*

LEARNING OUTCOMES

- Discuss the importance of knowing and understanding drug classifications in EMS.
- Briefly discuss the cardiac membrane action potential.
- Describe the mechanism of action, indications, contraindications, and precautions of each drug classification presented in this chapter.
- Briefly discuss the importance of vitamins.

KEY TERMS

Beta$_1$-adrenergic receptor
Beta$_2$-adrenergic receptor
Cardiac membrane action potential
Generalized anxiety disorder
Hypoglycemic
Loop diuretic
Opiate receptor
Selective serotonin reuptake inhibitors (SSRIs)
Thiazide diuretic
Tricyclic antidepressant

SCENARIO OPENING

Your field internship assignment is with Rescue 11. While getting prepared to do a drug inventory, you are called to a "man having trouble breathing." While you are en route, the dispatcher learns that the patient is a 24-year-old male who was stung by a wasp at a pool party. When you arrive, you find the patient Bob, sitting in the shade audibly wheezing and in obvious respiratory distress. Your initial rapid assessment shows Bob's skin to be warm and flushed, and he has a rapid, irregular heart rate. Bob's girlfriend Kimberly states that Bob is allergic to bees. She also states that she could not find the EpiPen that Bob usually carries. You remember from class that epinephrine is a bronchodilator, which is often used to treat allergic reactions.

Introduction

The classification of a drug is the pharmacologic class to which the drug has been assigned. This information is useful in learning to categorize drugs. For example, the drug albuterol is classified as a sympathomimetic. Sympathomimetics stimulate $beta_2$-receptors of the bronchi, leading to bronchodilation. Therefore, whenever a drug (albuterol, epinephrine, terbutaline) is classified as a sympathomimetic, the reader should know how the drug works, or its mechanism of action. Understanding the drug classification should make it easier to rationalize and understand when to use a drug, its contraindications, and the precautions to take when using it.

The drug classifications contained in this chapter are broad based and cover many subclassifications that are listed under the individual drugs. For example, the drug epinephrine is a sympathomimetic. However, it can also be classified as a direct-acting adrenergic drug, as well as a bronchodilator. These subclassifications are covered when epinephrine is presented (not in this chapter), thereby eliminating unnecessary duplication.

Individual Drug Classifications

Antianginals

Mechanism of Action: Nitrates dilate coronary arteries and cause systemic vasodilation (decreased preload). Calcium channel blockers dilate coronary arteries and can slow heart rate. Beta blockers decrease myocardial oxygen consumption by lowering the heart rate.
Indications: Nitrates are used to treat and prevent acute attacks of angina pectoris. Calcium channel blockers and beta blockers are used prophylactically in the long-term management of angina.
Contraindications: Known hypersensitivity; should not use beta blockers or calcium channel blockers in high-degree heart block, cardiogenic shock, or untreated CHF
Precautions: Use beta blockers with caution in patients with diabetes mellitus, pulmonary disease, or hypothyroidism.
Drug Interactions: Nitrates, calcium channel blockers, and beta blockers may cause hypotension if used with other antihypertensive drugs.
EMS Considerations: Monitor blood pressure and ECG frequently during therapy.

Antianxiety Agents

Mechanism of Action: Most of these drugs cause generalized central nervous system (CNS) depression. They have no analgesic properties.
Indications: Used in the management of various forms of anxiety, including **generalized anxiety disorder**
Contraindications: Known hypersensitivity; should not be given to patients with preexisting CNS depression or to patients with uncontrolled severe pain. Most antianxiety drugs should not be used with MAO inhibitors.
Precautions: Use with caution in patients with liver dysfunction, severe renal impairment, or severe pulmonary disease. Antianxiety drugs should be used with caution in patients who may be suicidal or who may have had previous drug addictions.
Drug Interactions: Additive CNS depression if used with antihistamines, selected antidepressants, opioid analgesics, or phenothiazines
EMS Considerations: Monitor blood pressure, ECG, and respiratory status frequently during therapy.

Antiarrhythmic Drugs

Mechanism of Action: Correct cardiac arrhythmias by a variety of mechanisms, depending on the group used. The choice of antiarrhythmic drug depends on the etiology of the arrhythmia. Antiarrhythmics are classified by their effects on cardiac conduction tissue in the following groups:

- **Group I:** These drugs decrease the rate of entry of sodium during cardiac membrane depolarization and decrease the rate of rise of phase "0" of the **cardiac membrane action potential** (Fig. 9-1). Group I antiarrhythmics are further listed

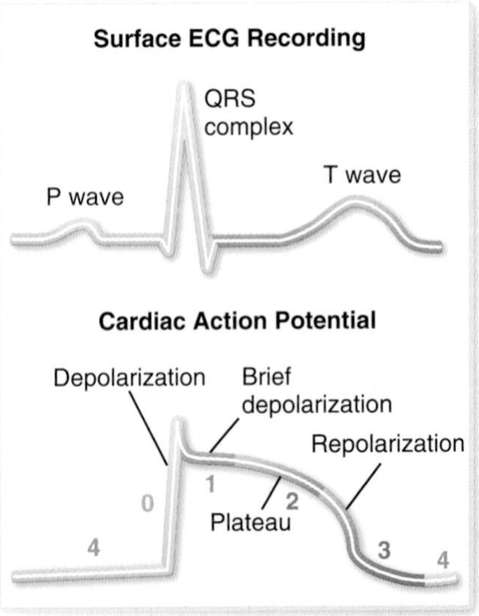

Figure 9-1 Cardiac action potential.

in subgroups according to their effects on action potential duration.

- **Group IA:** Depress phase "0" and prolong the duration of the action potential; for example, procainamide or quinidine
- **Group IB:** Slightly depress phase "0" and shorten the action potential; for example, lidocaine or phenytoin
- **Group IC:** Slight effect on repolarization but marked depression of phase "0" of the action potential; significant slowing of conduction; for example, flecainide or propafenone
- **Group II:** Competitively block beta-adrenergic receptors and depress phase "4" depolarization; for example, acebutolol or propranolol
- **Group III:** Prolong the duration of the relative refractory period without changing the phase of depolarization of the resting membrane potential; for example, amiodarone or sotalol
- **Group IV:** Slow conduction velocity and increase the refractoriness of the AV node; for example, verapamil

Indications: Used for the suppression of cardiac arrhythmias
Contraindications: Known hypersensitivity. Contraindications differ greatly between the various drugs. See individual drugs.
Precautions: Differ greatly between the various drugs; see individual drugs
Drug Interactions: Differ greatly between the various drugs; see individual drugs
EMS Considerations: Monitor ECG and blood pressure continuously during therapy.

Antiasthmatic Drugs

Mechanism of Action: Antiasthmatics treat airway constriction by causing bronchodilation and decreasing airway inflammation.
Indications: Used for the management of acute and chronic episodes of reversible bronchoconstriction
Contraindications: Known hypersensitivity; should not give inhaled corticosteroids or long-acting adrenergic drugs to patients during acute attacks of asthma
Precautions: Use adrenergic bronchodilators and anticholinergics with caution in patients with cardiovascular disease.
Drug Interactions: Adrenergic bronchodilators may have additive CNS and cardiovascular effects if used with other adrenergic drugs. Corticosteroids may decrease the effectiveness of antidiabetics.
EMS Considerations: Assess lung sounds and respiratory function prior to and frequently during therapy. Assess cardiovascular status of patients taking adrenergic bronchodilators or anticholinergics. Monitor patients for ECG changes and chest pain.

Anticholinergics

Mechanism of Action: Anticholinergics competitively inhibit the action of the neurotransmitter acetylcholine.
Indications: Anticholinergics differ in their uses. For example, atropine can be used to treat bradyarrhythmias or excess salivation due to organophosphate poisoning. Ipratropium can be used for bronchospasm or rhinorrhea, and scopolamine can be used to treat nausea and vomiting due to motion sickness and vertigo.
Contraindications: Known hypersensitivity; should not be given to patients with narrow-angle glaucoma, severe hemorrhage, or tachycardia caused by cardiac insufficiency
Precautions: Use with caution in patients with chronic renal, liver, pulmonary, or cardiac disease. Geriatric and pediatric patients are more likely to experience adverse effects.
Drug Interactions: Additive anticholinergic effects if used with other anticholinergic drugs such as antihistamines or antidepressants
EMS Considerations: Assess vital signs, including ECG, frequently during therapy.

Anticoagulants

Mechanism of Action: Act by preventing blood clot extensions and formation. Anticoagulants do not dissolve clots.
Indications: Used in the prevention and treatment of thromboembolic disorders including deep vein thrombosis, pulmonary embolism, and atrial fibrillation with embolization. Anticoagulants are also used in the management of myocardial infarction, alone or in combination with thrombolytics or antiplatelet drugs.
Contraindications: Known hypersensitivity; should not be given to patients with coagulation disorders, ulcer disease, malignancy, recent surgery, or any active bleeding
Precautions: Use with caution in patients with any potential site for bleeding.
Drug Interactions: Drug interactions depend on which drug is displaced. Bleeding may be potentiated by aspirin, NSAIDs, or large doses of penicillin or penicillin-like drugs.
EMS Considerations: Question patients about bleeding from their gums; blood in their urine, stools, or vomit; and bruises. Apply pressure to all venipuncture and injection sites to prevent bleeding and hematoma formation.

Anticonvulsants

Mechanism of Action: Depress the abnormal neuronal discharges in the CNS that may result in seizures. Anticonvulsants may work by preventing the spread of seizure activity, depressing the motor cortex, raising the seizure threshold, or altering the levels of neurotransmitters, depending on the group. See individual drugs.
Indications: Used to decrease the incidence and severity of seizures due to various etiologies
Contraindications: Known hypersensitivity
Precautions: Use with caution in patients with severe liver or renal disease.
Drug Interactions: Barbiturates stimulate the metabolism of other drugs that are metabolized by the liver, decreasing their effectiveness. Many drugs are capable of lowering the seizure threshold and may decrease the effectiveness of anticonvulsants.
EMS Considerations: Assess the patient for orientation to time, place, affect, reflexes, and vital signs. Observe signs and symptoms of impending seizures. With IV administration, monitor for respiratory depression and cardiovascular collapse. Note any evidence of CNS side effects, such as blurred vision, slurred speech, or confusion. Observe the patient for muscle twitching, loss of muscle tone, episodes of bizarre behavior, or subsequent amnesia.

Check the Evidence

The goal of antihypertensives is to lower blood pressure to a normal level (less than 90 mm Hg diastolic) or to the lowest level tolerated.

Indications: Used for the treatment of essential hypertension. Parenteral medications are used in the treatment of hypertensive emergencies.
Contraindications: Known hypersensitivity
Precautions: Some antihypertensives cause sodium and water retention and are generally combined with a diuretic. See individual drugs for more precautions.

effective **Communication**

Abrupt discontinuation of alpha-adrenergic agonists and beta blockers may result in a rapid and excessive rise in blood pressure (rebound phenomenon).

Drug Interactions: Antihistamines, NSAIDs, sympathomimetic bronchodilators, decongestants, antidepressants, and MAO inhibitors can negate the therapeutic effects of antihypertensives.
EMS Considerations: Monitor vital signs frequently, especially blood pressure and ECG.

Antiplatelet Drugs

Mechanism of Action: Inhibit platelet aggregation and prolong bleeding time
Indications: Used to treat and prevent thromboembolic disorders such as stroke and MI
Contraindications: Known hypersensitivity; should not be given to patients with ulcer disease or active bleeding or to those who have had recent surgery
Precautions: Use with caution in patients at risk of bleeding and in those with a history of ulcer disease.
Drug Interactions: May cause a risk of bleeding if used concurrently with NSAIDs, heparin, thrombolytics, or warfarin
EMS Considerations: Monitor patient vital signs frequently during therapy.

Antipsychotics

Mechanism of Action: Block dopamine receptors in the brain and also alter dopamine release
Indications: Used for the treatment of acute and chronic psychoses, especially when accompanied by an increase in psychomotor activity
Contraindications: Known hypersensitivity; should not be given to patients who have CNS depression or to those with angle-closure glaucoma
Precautions: Use with caution in patients with diabetes, respiratory insufficiency, prostatic hypertrophy, or intestinal obstruction.
Drug Interactions: Additive hypotension if used with antihypertensives or nitrates; additive CNS depression if used with other medications that cause CNS depression
EMS Considerations: Monitor orthostatic blood pressure, ECG, and respiratory rate frequently during therapy.

Antipyretics

Mechanism of Action: Lower fever by affecting the thermoregulation center in the CNS and by inhibiting the action of prostaglandins peripherally
Indications: Used to lower fever due to many causes
Contraindications: Known hypersensitivity; should not give aspirin, ibuprofen, or ketoprofen to patients with bleeding disorders. Aspirin should not be given to pediatric patients.
Precautions: Use aspirin, ibuprofen, or ketoprofen with caution in patients with ulcer disease.
Drug Interactions: Additive GI irritation with aspirin, ibuprofen, and other NSAIDs or corticosteroids
EMS Considerations: When assessing a patient's fever, also check for associated symptoms such as diaphoresis, tachycardia, and weakness.

Antiretrovirals

Mechanism of Action: Due to the rapid emergence of resistance and toxicities of individual antiretroviral medications, HIV infection is generally managed by a combination of drugs. The selection of drugs and doses is dependent on individual patients.

Check the Evidence

More than 100 prospective drugs are currently being tested in addition to the current FDA-approved drugs on the market.

Indications: Antiretroviral therapy in the management of HIV infection is to improve cell counts and decrease viral load. Many times this results in slowed progression of the disease and an improved quality of life.
Contraindications: Known hypersensitivity
Precautions: Use with caution in patients with diabetes and in those who are hemophiliacs.
Drug Interactions: Many antiretroviral drugs are affected by medications that alter metabolism.
EMS Considerations: None

Antiviral Drugs

Mechanism of Action: Inhibit viral replication
Indications: Used in the treatment of viral infections
Contraindications: Known hypersensitivity
Precautions: Use with caution in patients with renal impairment; dosage adjustment may be required.
Drug Interactions: Additive CNS and nephrotoxicity with drugs that cause similar adverse reactions
EMS Consideration: None

Beta Blockers

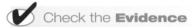

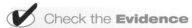

Mechanism of Action: Beta blockers compete with adrenergic neurotransmitters for adrenergic receptor sites. **Beta$_1$-adrenergic receptor** sites are located mainly in the heart where stimulation causes an increased heart rate, increased contractility, and increased AV conduction. **Beta$_2$-adrenergic receptors** are located mainly in the bronchial and vascular smooth muscle and in the uterus. Stimulation of beta$_2$-adrenergic receptors causes vasodilation, bronchodilation, and uterine relaxation.

Blockage of beta-adrenergic receptors antagonizes the effects of the neurotransmitters. Beta blockers may be selective for beta$_1$-adrenergic receptors, or they may be nonselective.
Indications: Beta blockers can be used in the management of hypertension, angina pectoris, tachyarrhythmias, and hypertrophic subaortic stenosis; the prevention of MI; and for treating CHF. Beta blockers can also be given as prophylaxis for migraine headache and to manage the symptoms of hyperthyroidism.
Contraindications: Known hypersensitivity; should not be given to patients with uncompensated CHF, acute bronchospasm, bradyarrhyhthmias, heart block, and certain forms of valvular heart disease
Precautions: Use with caution in patients with any form of lung disease, underlying compensated CHF, diabetes, or severe liver disease.

effective **Communication**

Beta blockers should not be abruptly discontinued in anyone with cardiovascular disease.

Drug Interactions: May cause additive myocardial depression and bradycardia when used with digoxin and some other antiarrhythmics; may alter the requirements for insulin or hypoglycemic drugs when given to diabetic patients
EMS Considerations: Monitor heart rate and blood pressure frequently during therapy. Observe for increasing dyspnea, coughing, any difficulty in breathing, or any symptoms of CHF. With a diabetic patient, monitor for symptoms of hypoglycemia (tachycardia, hypertension).

Bronchodilators

Mechanism of Action: Beta-adrenergic agonists produce bronchodilation by stimulating the production of cyclic adenosine monophosphate (cAMP). Newer drugs are selective for pulmonary (beta$_2$) receptors, and older drugs also produce cardiac stimulation (beta$_1$) in addition to bronchodilation.
Indications: Used in the treatment of reversible airway obstruction due to asthma or COPD

Check the **Evidence**

Revised recommendations for management of asthma suggest that rapid-acting inhaled beta-agonist bronchodilators be reserved for use as acute relievers of bronchospasm.

Contraindications: Known hypersensitivity; should not be given to patients with uncontrolled cardiac arrhythmias
Precautions: Use with caution in patients with diabetes, cardiovascular disease, or hyperthyroidism.
Drug Interactions: Using bronchodilators with beta blockers may antagonize therapeutic effectiveness. Cardiovascular effects may be potentiated by antidepressants or MAO inhibitors.
EMS Considerations: Assess all vital signs, including characters of lung secretions before and frequently throughout therapy. Monitor patients with a history of cardiovascular disease for ECG changes and chest pain.

Calcium Channel Blockers

Mechanism of Action: Block the entry of calcium into the cells of vascular smooth muscle and the myocardium. They also dilate coronary arteries and inhibit coronary artery spasm.
Indications: Depending on the drug, some calcium channel blockers are used in the treatment of hypertension, some are used in the treatment and prophylaxis of angina or coronary artery spasm, and some are used as antiarrhythmics.
Contraindications: Known hypersensitivity; should not be given to patients with bradycardia, second- or third-degree AV heart block, or uncompensated CHF
Precautions: Use with caution in patients with uncontrolled cardiac arrhythmias and in those with liver disease.
Drug Interactions: Additive myocardial depression if used with beta blockers
EMS Considerations: Monitor patient blood pressure and ECG frequently during therapy.

Corticosteroids

Mechanism of Action: Modify the normal immune response and suppress inflammation
Indications: Used for their anti-inflammatory or immunosuppressive functions. Some inhaled corticosteroids can be used in the chronic management of asthma.
Contraindications: Known hypersensitivity; should not be given to patients with serious infections
Precautions: Safety in pregnancy and lactation has not been established.
Drug Interactions: May increase the requirements for insulin or oral hypoglycemic drugs
EMS Considerations: See individual drugs.

Diuretics

Mechanism of Action: Diuretics enhance the excretion of various electrolytes and water by affecting renal mechanisms for tubular secretion and reabsorption.
Indications: **Loop** and **thiazide** diuretics are used alone or in combination in the treatment of hypertension or edema due to CHF.
Contraindications: Known hypersensitivity
Precautions: Use with caution in patients with renal or liver disease.
Drug Interactions: Additive hypotension if used with other antihypertensives or nitrates
EMS Considerations: Monitor vital signs, especially lung sounds, frequently during therapy.

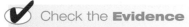

Lipid-Lowering Agents

Mechanism of Action: HMG-CoA reductase inhibitors inhibit an enzyme involved in cholesterol synthesis, and bile acid sequestrants bind cholesterol in the GI tract.
Indications: Used as a part of a total plan including diet and exercise to reduce blood lipids
Contraindications: Known hypersensitivity
Precautions: Safety in pregnancy, lactation, and pediatrics has not been established.
Drug Interactions: Bile acid sequestrants may bind lipid-soluble vitamins and other concurrently administered drugs in the GI tract.
EMS Considerations: None

Minerals/Electrolytes/pH Modifiers

Mechanism of Action: Maintenance of these agents within normal limits is required for many physiological processes such as cardiac, nerve, and muscle function; bone growth and stability; and a number of other activities.
Indications: Used for the maintenance of optimal acid/base balance for homeostasis
Contraindications: Known hypersensitivity

effective **Communication**

Potassium chloride should not be given undiluted.

Precautions: Use with caution in patients with liver or renal disease and in patients with adrenal or pituitary disorders.
Drug Interactions: Depends on individual agents
EMS Considerations: None

Natural and Herbal Products

Mechanism of Action: The FDA has little control over these types of agents. Currently, there is little standardization for natural and herbal products.
Indications: The use of these types of agents is based on historical and anecdotal evidence. These remedies are used for a wide variety of conditions. Prescriptions are not required.
Contraindications: Known hypersensitivity. Many of these agents are plant extracts and may contain a variety of impurities.
Precautions: Patients with serious chronic medical conditions should consult with their health-care professional before using these products.
Drug Interactions: These agents have the ability to interact with prescription drugs. St. John's wort and kava-kava have the greatest risk for interactions.
EMS Considerations: Follow local protocols and contact medical control if necessary.

Nonopioid Analgesics

Mechanism of Action: Inhibit prostaglandin synthesis peripherally for analgesic effects and centrally for antipyretic effects
Indications: Used to control mild to moderate pain or fever
Contraindications: Known hypersensitivity
Precautions: Use with caution in patients with severe liver or renal disease and in those with chronic alcohol use or abuse.
Drug Interactions: Additive risk of CNS depression if used with other CNS depressants. NSAIDs may decrease the effectiveness of diuretics and antihypertensives.
EMS Considerations: Patients who have asthma, allergies, and nasal polyps are at an increased risk of developing hypersensitivity reactions.

NSAIDs

Mechanism of Action: NSAIDs have analgesic, antipyretic, and anti-inflammatory properties. Analgesic and anti-inflammatory effects are due to inhibition of prostaglandin synthesis, and antipyretic action is due to vasodilation and inhibition of prostaglandin synthesis.
Indications: Used to control mild to moderate pain, fever, and various inflammatory conditions
Contraindications: Known hypersensitivity
Precautions: Use with caution in patients with a history of bleeding disorders and severe liver, renal, or cardiovascular disease.
Drug Interactions: NSAIDs prolong bleeding time and potentiate the effect of warfarin, thrombolytic drugs, some cephalosporins, antiplatelet drugs, and valproates.
EMS Considerations: Patients who have asthma, allergies, and nasal polyps are at an increased risk for developing hypersensitivity reactions.

Opioid Analgesics

Mechanism of Action: Bind to **opiate receptors** in the CNS, acting as antagonists, altering the perception of and response to pain
Indications: Management of moderate to severe pain
Contraindications: Known hypersensitivity
Precautions: Use with caution in patients with undiagnosed abdominal pain, head trauma, liver disease, or a history of opioid addiction.
Drug Interactions: Increases the CNS depressant properties of alcohol, antihistamines, antidepressants, sedative/hypnotics, phenothiazines, and MAO inhibitors
EMS Considerations: Assess vital signs prior to and frequently during therapy. If the patient's respiratory rate is less than 10/minute, assess the level of sedation. Dosage may have to be decreased by up to 50 percent.

Sedative/Hypnotics

Mechanism of Action: Cause generalized CNS depression. However, sedative/hypnotics have no analgesic properties.
Indications: Used to provide sedation. Selected drugs are used as anticonvulsants, skeletal muscle relaxants, adjuncts in the management of alcohol withdrawal syndrome, adjuncts to general anesthesia, or amnestics.
Contraindications: Known hypersensitivity; should not be given to patients with preexisting CNS depression or to those in severe pain

Precautions: Use with caution in patients with liver dysfunction, severe renal impairment, or severe underlying pulmonary disease and in those who may be suicidal or who have previous drug addictions.
Drug Interactions: Additive CNS depression when used with other drugs that may cause CNS depression; should not be given to patients who are taking MAO inhibitors
EMS Considerations: Monitor all vital signs frequently during therapy.

Skeletal Muscle Relaxants

Mechanism of Action: Decrease muscle tone and involuntary movement by depressing spinal polysynaptic reflexes
Indications: Used for spasticity associated with spinal cord disease or lesions or as adjunctive therapy in the symptomatic relief of acute painful musculoskeletal conditions
Contraindications: Known hypersensitivity
Precautions: Use with caution in patients with a previous history of liver disease.
Drug Interactions: Additive CNS depression if used with other CNS-depressant drugs
EMS Considerations: Assess patients for pain, muscle stiffness, and range of motion before and frequently during therapy.

Thrombolytics

Mechanism of Action: Converts plasminogen to plasmin, which then degrades fibrin in blood clots
Indications: Used for the acute management of coronary thrombosis and stroke
Contraindications: Known hypersensitivity; should not be given to patients with active internal bleeding, history of a stroke, recent CNS trauma or surgery, or neoplasm
Precautions: Use with caution in patients with recent (within 10 days) surgery, trauma, or GI or GU bleeding and in patients with severe liver or renal disease.
Drug Interactions: Concurrent use with aspirin, NSAIDs, warfarin, or heparins may increase the risk of bleeding.
EMS Considerations: Monitor vital signs, including temperature, frequently during therapy. Assess the patient for signs or symptoms of bleeding every 15 minutes.

effective **Communication**

Do not use the patient's lower extremities to monitor blood pressure.

Vitamins

General Statement: Vitamins are essential, noncaloric substances required for normal metabolism. They are produced by living organisms such as plants and animals and are obtained by diet. Vitamins are necessary for promoting growth, health, and life. They are necessary for the metabolic processes responsible for transforming foods into tissue and energy. However, vitamins do not provide energy because they do not contain calories. Table 9-1 lists the common vitamin requirements for the body, Table 9-2 shows the vitamins and their uses, and Table 9-3 shows the vitamin deficiency states.
Mechanism of Action: Components of enzyme systems that catalyze numerous metabolic reactions. Vitamins are necessary for homeostasis.
Indications: Used in the prevention and treatment of vitamin deficiencies and as supplements in various metabolic disorders
Contraindications: Known hypersensitivity to additives, preservatives, or colorants
Precautions: Doses should be adjusted to avoid toxicity, especially for fat-soluble vitamins.
Drug Interactions: Large amounts of pyridoxine may interfere with the effectiveness of levodopa. Cholestyramine, colestipol, and mineral oil decrease the absorption of fat-soluble vitamins.
EMS Considerations: None

SCENARIO REVISITED

Do you recall the case of Bob who was stung by a wasp while attending a pool party? While talking with Kimberly, you also find out that Bob takes atenolol for his high blood pressure. Atenolol is an antihypertensive that works by blocking the stimulation of beta$_2$-adrenergic (myocardial) receptors.

When Bob was exposed to an allergen due to the wasp sting, cells in his body released histamine, serotonin, and bradykinin. The main chemical released during an allergic reaction is histamine, causing vasodilation, increased capillary permeability, and smooth muscle spasm. According to the ECG, Bob's irregular heart rate is caused by frequent premature ventricular contractions (PVCs) (Fig. 9-2).

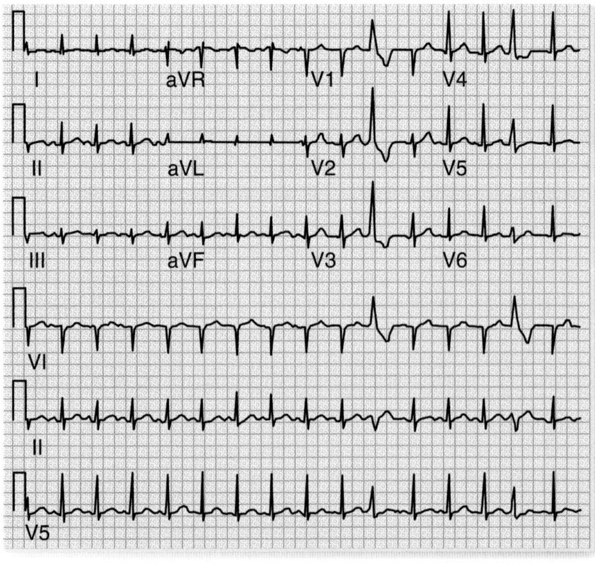

Figure 9-2 Sinus tachycardia with PVCs.

Table 9-1 Common Vitamin Requirements

Vitamin	RDA	Physiological Effects Essential for:
A (retinol, retinaldehyde, retinoic acid)	1,400–6,000 IU	Growth and development, epithelial tissue maintenance, and reproduction; prevents night blindness
B complex:		
B_1 (thiamine)	0.3–1.5 mg	Energy metabolism; normal nerve function
B_2 (riboflavin)	0.4–1.8 mg	Reactions in energy cycle that produce ATP; oxidation of amino acids and hydroxyl acids; oxidation of purines
B_3 (niacin, nicotinic acid, nicotinamide)	5–19 mg	Synthesis of fatty acids and cholesterol; blockage of FFA; conversion of phenylalanine to tyrosine
B_6 (pyridoxine, pyridoxal, pyridoxamine)	0.3–2.5 mg	Amino acid metabolism, glycogenolyis, RBC/Hb synthesis; formation of neurotransmitters, formation of antibodies
Folacin (folic acid, pteroylglutamic acid)	50–800 mcg	DNA synthesis; formation of RBCs in bone marrow with cyanocobalamin
Pantothenic acid (calcium pantothenate, dexpanthenol)	10 mg	Synthesis of sterols, steroid hormones, porphyrins; oxidative metabolism of carbohydrates, gluconeogenesis
B_{12} (cyanocobalamin, hydroxocobalamin, extrinsic factor)	0.3–4.0 mcg	DNA synthesis in bone marrow; RBC production with folacin; nerve tissue maintenance
B_7 (biotin)	No recommendation	Synthesis of fatty acids; generation of tricarboxylic acid cycle; formation of purines; coenzyme in carbohydrate metabolism
C (ascorbic acid, ascorbate)	60 mg	Formation of collagen; conversion of cholesterol to bile acids; protects vitamins A and E and polyunsaturated fats from excessive oxidation; absorption and utilization of iron; converts folacin to folinic acid; some role in clotting, adrenocortical hormones, and reabsorption
D (calcitriol, cholecalciferol, dihydrotachysterol, ergocalciferol, viosterol)	400 IU	Intestinal absorption and metabolism of calcium and phosphorus as well as renal reabsorption; release of calcium from bone and reabsorption
E (tocopherol)	4–15 IU	May oppose destruction of vitamin A and fats by oxygen fragments called free radicals; antioxidant; may affect production of prostaglandins, which regulate a variety of body process
K (menadione, phytonadione)	No recommendations	Formation of prothrombin and other clotting proteins by the liver; blood coagulation

Table 9-2 Vitamins and Uses

Vitamin	Effect	Uses
A (retinoic acid)	Reduces formation of comedones; suppresses keratin production	Treats acne, psoriasis, ichthyosis, Darier disease, xerophthalmia, and intestinal infections; prevents night blindness
Niacin	Reduction of blood cholesterol and triglycerides; blocks FFA release	Hypercholesterolemia, hyperbetalipoproteinemia
D (dihydrotachysterol)	Maintains calcium and phosphorus levels in bone and blood	Hypoparathyroidism; increases intestinal absorption of calcium
C	Reduces urine pH; converts methemoglobin to hemoglobin	Idiopathic methemoglobin; recurrent UTIs in high-risk patients; aids in iron absorption
E	Reduces endogenous peroxidases	Hemolytic anemia in premature infants; protects cell membranes from oxidation
K	Increases liver production of thrombin	Warfarin toxicity; essential for blood coagulation

Table 9-3 Vitamin Deficiency States

Vitamin	Deficiency	Signs and Symptoms
A	Xerophthalmia	Progressive eye changes; night blindness to xerosis of conjunctiva and cornea with scarring
A	Keratomalacia	Degeneration of epithelial cells with hardening and shrinking
B_6	Beriberi	Fatigue, weight loss, weakness, irritability, headaches, insomnia, peripheral neuropathy, CHF, cardiomyopathy
Niacin	Pellagra	Depression, anorexia, beefy red glossitis, cheilosis, dermatitis
B_{12}	Pernicious anemia	Macrocytic anemia, megaloblastic anemia, progressive neuropathy, R/T demyelination
C	Scurvy	Joint pain, growth retardation, anemia, poor wound healing with increased susceptibility to infection, petechial hemorrhages
D	Rickets (child) Osteomalacia (adult)	Demineralization of bones and teeth with bone pain and skeletal muscle deformities
E	Hemolytic anemia in low birth weight infants	Macrocytic anemia, increased hemolysis of RBCs, and increased capillary fragility
K	Hemorrhagic disease in newborns	Increased tendency to hemorrhage

Check the **Evidence**

The most common cause of death from an allergic reaction is obstruction of the patient's airway. The first-line drug to be given, unless contraindicated, is the bronchodilator epinephrine.

Let's Recap

The classification of drugs is the orderly grouping of drugs that have the same or similar mechanisms of action. Attempting to memorize each individual drug as to its mechanism, indications, contraindications, and precautions is a tedious learning method. However, placing drugs in orderly groups based on how they work eliminates much of the repetition in the learning process. Therefore, it is best to place drugs in their groups or classifications to give a more systematic approach to learning.

SCENARIO CONCLUSION

Epinephrine is the first-line drug to be given for an allergic reaction because its beta$_2$-adrenergic stimulation produces bronchodilation, its alpha-receptor stimulation produces vasoconstriction, and it reduces the release of chemical mediators from mast cells.

Other drugs to give Bob include albuterol for its bronchodilation, diphenhydramine to reverse the effects of histamine, and methylprednisolone to reduce inflammation. In this case, Bob may be unresponsive to epinephrine (beta stimulator) because he is taking a beta blocker (atenolol). If Bob does not respond to epinephrine, you may give him the hormone glucagon.

PRACTICE EXERCISES

1. Your patient is a 60-year-old female experiencing an asthma attack. Which class of drug would you expect to administer to her?
a. Alpha$_1$-adrenergic blocking drug
b. Antihistamine (H_1 blocker)
c. Corticosteroid
d. Sympathomimetic

2. While conducting your medication assessment, your 55-year-old male patient states that he is taking a pill for high cholesterol. Drugs that lower cholesterol are classified as:
a. Sulfonamides
b. ACE inhibitors
c. Lipid-lowering agents
d. Anticoagulants

3. A(n) ______________ can be used to treat high blood pressure.
a. Antiarrhythmic
b. Neuromuscular blocker
c. Theophylline derivative
d. Thyroid drug

4. A patient suffering from a urinary tract infection would most likely be taking:
a. Sulfonamides
b. Tetracyclines
c. Anti-inflammatories
d. A general anti-infective

5. A common classification of drugs that are used to treat anxiety is:
a. Neuromuscular blocking drug
b. Tricyclic antidepressant
c. Antipsychotic drug
d. Aminophylline

6. A common contraindication for administering a beta-adrenergic blocking drug is:
a. Sinus bradycardia
b. Sinus tachycardia
c. Hypertension
d. Ventricular arrhythmias

7. An indication for the use of a corticosteroid is:
a. Inflammation
b. Hypertension
c. Hypersensitivity
d. Anxiety

8. Calcium channel blockers are contraindicated in patients with:
a. Liver disease
b. Renal disease
c. Third-degree heart block
d. Angle-closure glaucoma

9. Antihistamines work by blocking the effects of histamines at the:
a. $Alpha_1$ receptors
b. $Beta_1$ receptors
c. H_1 receptors
d. H_2 receptors

10. Anticoagulants work by:
a. Dissolving blood clots
b. Stopping blood clot formation
c. Lowering lipid levels in the blood
d. Causing systemic arterial vasodilation

CASE STUDIES

1. You respond to the home of a known cocaine abuser. On arrival, you find a 21-year-old male lying unresponsive in a closet. He has a pair of panty hose tied around his right upper arm. There are obvious "tracks" on both arms. The patient's neighbor says that Edmond had been high on cocaine and suddenly became unresponsive. Further assessment reveals:
Level of Consciousness: Unconscious; responds to painful stimuli by occasional tonic-clonic movements and incoherent speech
Respirations: 28 breaths/minute, and irregular
Pulse: 124 beats/minute (Fig. 9-3)
Blood pressure: 190/102
Skin: Warm and moist
Pupils: Dilated and slow to react

A. You start an IV of NS at a keep-open rate. The class of drug Edmond needs is:
a. Benzodiazepine (such as diazepam)
b. Opioid antagonist (such as naloxone)
c. Anticholinergic (such as atropine)
d. Anticholinesterase inhibitor (such as pralidoxime)

B. Your patient is a 52-year-old male who says, "My heart feels like it is racing." The ECG shows ventricular tachycardia (Fig. 9-4). Currently, the patient is hemodynamically stable. In this situation, what class of drug should you give him?
a. Antiarrhythmic, class III (such as amiodarone)
b. Antiarrhythmic, class IV (such as verapamil)
c. Antiarrhythmic, class IB (such as lidocaine)
d. Antiarrhythmic, cholinergic blocker (such as atropine)

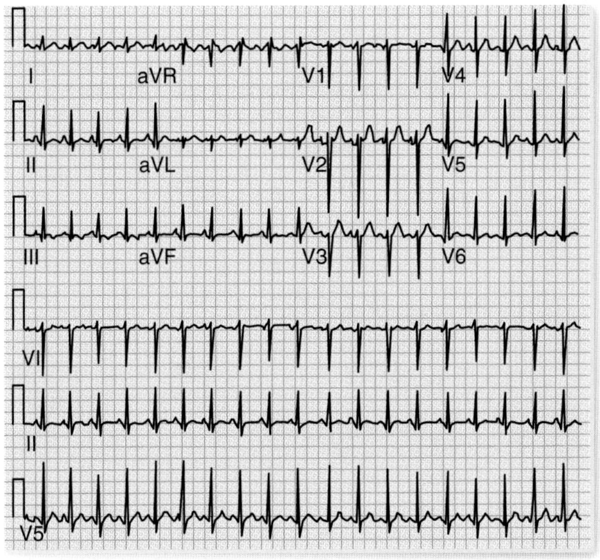

Figure 9-3 Sinus tachycardia.

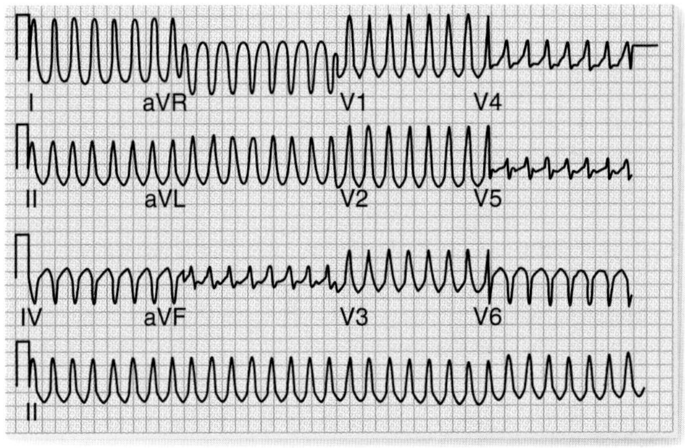

Figure 9-4 Ventricular tachycardia.

MATH EQUATIONS

Mixed Problems

1. Your drug is given as 5 mg/kg IV. Your patient states that she weighs 125 lbs.
   a. How many kg does your patient weigh?
   b. How much drug should you administer to her?
2. 2500 mL = _______ L.
3. How many gtt/minute will it take to infuse 500 mL of IV fluid using a 60 gtt/mL IV set for 2 hours?
4. 2.5 g = _______ mcg.
5. You are ordered to give 200 mg of a drug to your patient. The drug comes packaged as a 10 mL syringe containing 500 mg of the drug. How much of the preparation do you administer (mL)?
6. 215 lb = _______ kg.
7. You are doing a clinical rotation in the emergency department. The physician orders you to give 1500 mg of a drug. The drug comes in 0.5 g tablets.
   a. How many mg are in each tablet?
   b. How many tablets are required to administer to your patient?
8. You are ordered to give 2 mcg/kg/minute IV infusion of a drug. Your patient weighs 190 lbs. The infusion is prepared by adding 8 mg of the drug to 1000 mL of solution.
   a. How many kg does your patient weigh?
   b. What is the concentration of the IV solution (mcg/mL)?
   c. How many gtt/minute, using a 60 gtt/mL IV set, is the infusion run?

REFERENCES

Beck, R. K. (2012). Therapeutic drug classifications. In *Pharmacology for the EMS provider.* New York, NY: Delmar, Cengage Learning.

Deglin, J. H., Vallerand, A. H., and Sanboski, C. A. (2011). *Davis's drug guide for nurses, twelfth edition.* Philadelphia, PA: F. A. Davis Company.

Kalabunde, R. E. (2007). Antiarrhythmic drugs. Retrieved May 19, 2014 from www.cvpharmacology.com/antiarrhy/antiarrhythmic.htm.

U.S. National Library of Medicine. Vitamins. Retrieved May 19, 2014 from www.nlm.nih.gov/medlineplus/vitamins.html.

Venes, D., ed. (2013). *Taber's cyclopedic medical dictionary* (22nd ed.). Philadelphia, PA: F. A. Davis Company.

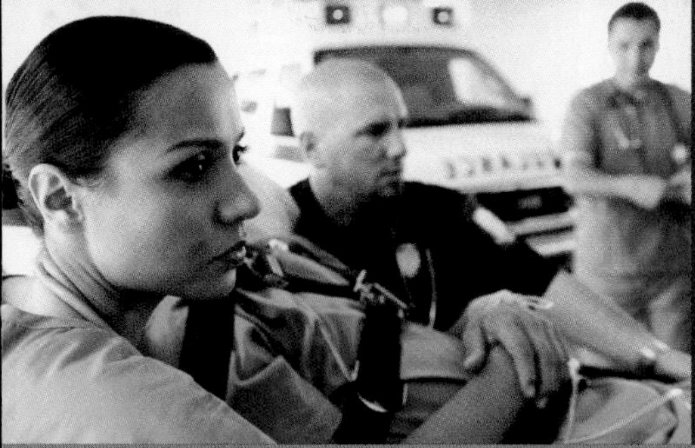

CHAPTER 10

Drugs Used to Treat Respiratory Emergencies

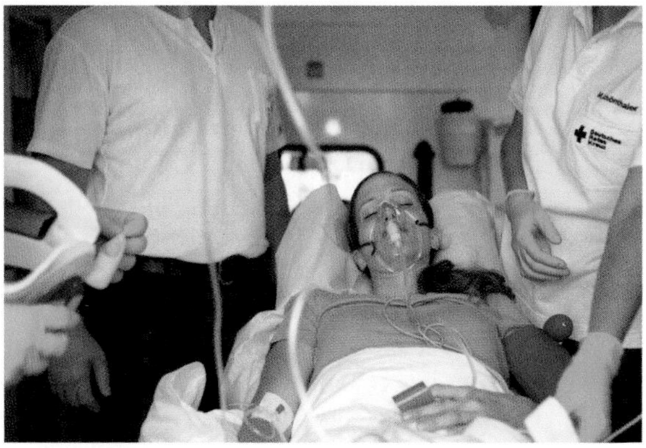

Paramedics administering a respiratory treatment. *(Photograph © Jochen Sand/Digital Vision/Thinkstock)*

LEARNING OUTCOMES

- Briefly describe the out-of-hospital uses for pulse oximetry, peak flow, and capnography.
- Briefly describe the pathophysiology of an allergic reaction, asthma, and chronic obstructive pulmonary disease (COPD).
- List the mechanism of action, uses, contraindications, precautions, route and dosage, and the adverse reactions and side effects of the adrenergic drugs epinephrine, metaproterenol sulfate, and racemic epinephrine.
- List the mechanism of action, uses, contraindications, precautions, route and dosage, and the adverse reactions and side effects of the anticholinergics atropine and ipratropium bromide.
- List the mechanism of action, uses, contraindications, precautions, route and dosage, and the adverse reactions and side effects of the antihistamine diphenhydramine.
- List the mechanism of action, uses, contraindications, precautions, route and dosage, and the adverse reactions and side effects of the bronchodilators albuterol, aminophylline, levalbuterol, and terbutaline sulfate.
- List the mechanism of action, uses, contraindications, precautions, route and dosage, and the adverse reactions and side effects of the corticosteroid hydrocortisone.
- List the mechanism of action, uses, contraindications, precautions, route and dosage, and the adverse reactions and side effects of the electrolyte magnesium sulfate.
- List the mechanism of action, uses, contraindications, precautions, route and dosage, and the adverse reactions and side effects of the glucocorticoids dexamethasone and methylprednisolone.
- List the mechanism of action, uses, contraindications, precautions, route and dosage, and the adverse reactions and side effects of the neuromuscular blocking drugs pancuronium bromide, rocuronium bromide, succinylcholine chloride, and vecuronium bromide.
- List the mechanism of action, uses, contraindications, precautions, route and dosage, and the adverse reactions and side effects of the nondepolarizing skeletal muscle relaxants atracurium and tubocurarine chloride.
- List the mechanism of action, uses, contraindications, precautions, route and dosage, and the adverse reactions and side effects of oxygen.
- Describe the steps in performing rapid-sequence intubation (RSI).

KEY TERMS

Adrenergic
Anticholinergic
Antihistamine
Asthma
Bronchodilator
Capnography
Chronic obstructive pulmonary disease (COPD)
Corticosteroids
End-tidal carbon dioxide detector
Glucocorticoid
Neuromuscular blocking agent
Peak expiratory flow rate (PEFR)
Peak flow meter
Pulse oximetry
Status asthmaticus

SCENARIO OPENING

You are assigned to Rescue 34 as part of your field-internship requirement for paramedic school. So far, it is a quiet shift, so you are studying for a major exam on respiratory emergencies. While reviewing your notes on asthma, a call comes in for a "man fallen." Upon arrival, you and your team find a 58-year-old man (Jackson) who had fallen in the kitchen "hours ago." On initial assessment, you find Jackson is oriented but pale, with signs of peripheral cyanosis, and he has rapid, deep respirations without noticeable distress and a rapid pulse rate.

The information gained from your initial assessment may be misleading and may also give you a false sense of security. Jackson is alert and oriented, yet his vital signs suggest he may quickly become a high-priority patient. For example, his symptoms could be indicators of the following:

Pallor:	associated with poor perfusion
Cyanosis:	hypoxemia—a broad variety of conditions including asthma, pneumonia, COPD, CHF, trauma, etc.
Rapid respirations:	respiratory or cardiac problems
Rapid heart rate:	many conditions including shock, respiratory or cardiac compromise, trauma, etc.

Introduction

Responding to a respiratory emergency is a common occurrence for EMS professionals. A familiar scenario consists of a patient in a sitting position, leaning forward, and fighting to breathe, using accessory muscles. Wheezing is usually present but may become fainter as the patient's condition becomes more severe. The problem is an acute asthma attack.

Fighting for breath can be a terrifying and potentially fatal experience. An EMS professional must be able to act quickly and accurately when treating respiratory emergencies. In many emergencies, a calm EMS professional and 100 percent humidified oxygen are all that is required to provide the patient with relief. However, if needed, several drugs are effective in relieving respiratory distress.

With the exception of oxygen, most of the drugs presented in this chapter work therapeutically as bronchodilators. A **bronchodilator** acts by relaxing the smooth muscles of the bronchial airways and pulmonary blood vessels, making it easier for the patient to breathe.

Most bronchodilators are classified pharmacologically as adrenergic drugs. **Adrenergic** drugs primarily act on $beta_2$-receptors, relaxing bronchial smooth muscles. When $beta_2$-receptors are stimulated, however, $beta_1$-receptors are also stimulated to a lesser extent. $Beta_1$-stimulation causes the heart to increase in both rate and contractile force.

Pulse oximetry has long been the standard of care in out-of-hospital emergency medicine. The pulse oximeter is another tool we can use to help objectively determine the oxygenation status of our patients (Fig. 10-1). It should be immediately applied to the patient to help establish baseline vital signs. The normal oxygen saturation of the blood (SaO_2) should be between 95 and 100 percent. If the SaO_2 reading is below 95 percent but above 90 percent (91 to 94 percent), the patient is experiencing mild hypoxia and should be administered humidified oxygen. The patient is experiencing moderate hypoxia when the SaO_2 reading is below 91 percent but above 85 percent (86 to 90 percent). In this case, continually assess the patient and administer 100 percent humidified oxygen. A SaO_2 reading below 86 percent is an indication that the patient is experiencing severe hypoxia and needs 100 percent humidified oxygen and possibly advanced airway assistance.

Peak flow meters are used in pulmonary function tests (Fig. 10-2). This test measures a patient's **peak expiratory flow rate (PEFR).** PEFR shows how fast the patient can exhale air. It is most often used to help determine the severity of an asthma attack. To measure PEFR, patients must be able to inflate their

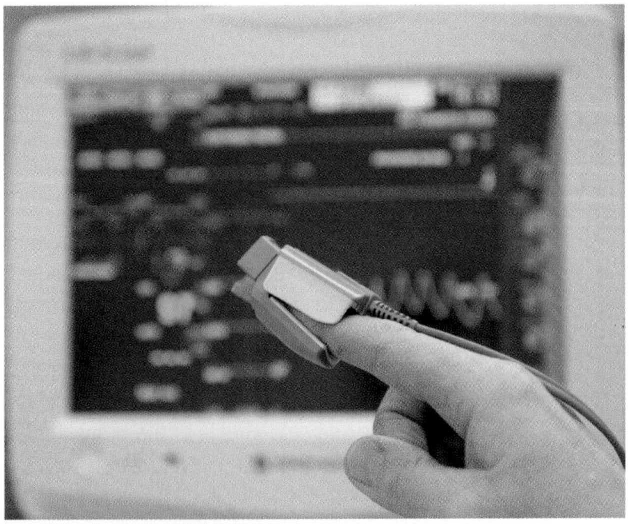

Figure 10-1 Patient with a pulse oximeter. *(Photograph © Jochen Sand/Digital Vision/Thinkstock)*

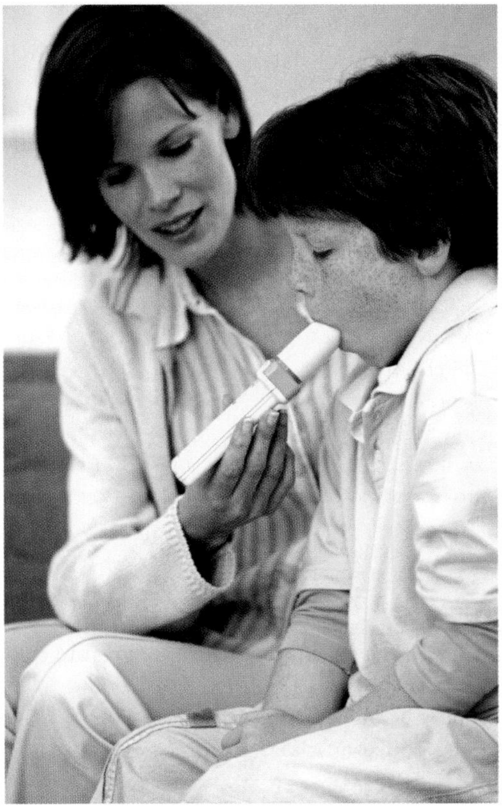

Figure 10-2 Pediatric patient using a peak flow meter. *(Photograph © arnoaltix/iStock/Thinkstock)*

lungs fully and forcefully exhale as quickly as possible into the flow meter. The meter reading is measured in liters per minute. To be effective, the patient should take this test three times before medications are administered, if possible. A PEFR measurement less than 20 percent is considered mild, 20 to 30 percent is moderate, and more than 30 percent is severe. Peak flow readings should be repeated throughout treatment to evaluate the patient's response to therapy.

Capnography, the continuous monitoring of carbon dioxide (CO_2) levels in expired air of patients, has also become the standard of care in out-of-hospital emergency medicine (Fig. 10-3). Capnography measurements are taken from a filter attached to a face mask, nasal cannula, or endotracheal (ET) tube. A graphic representation is displayed as a waveform throughout the respiratory cycle. Each waveform consists of the following four phases (Fig. 10-4).

- **Phase 1 (A-B):** exhaled air from the airways with a low level of CO_2
- **Phase 2 (B-C):** a mixture of air from the anatomical dead space and alveolar gas. CO_2 levels begin to rise.
- **Phase 3 (C-D):** alveolar plateau—alveolar plateau as alveolar gas is exhaled
- **Phase 4 (D-E):** inspiration washout, where D = peak concentration and E = decline in CO_2

It is important not to rely on any one device when assessing a patient.

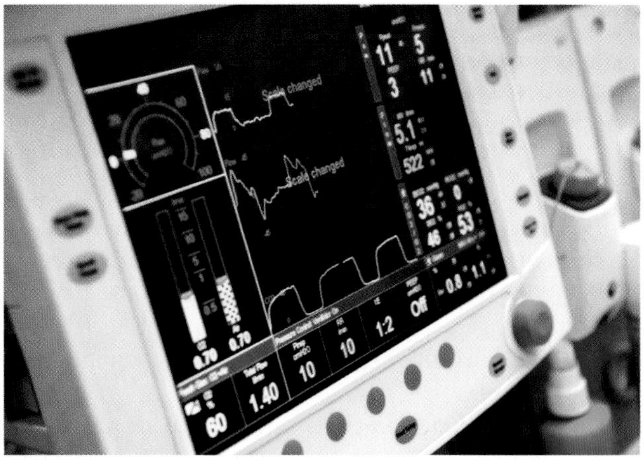

Figure 10-3 Capnography. *(Photograph © Stockbyte/Stockbyte/Thinkstock)*

Check the Evidence

The American Heart Association ACLS Guidelines recommend the use of continuous waveform capnography in all patients who have suffered cardiac arrest to evaluate both the quality of chest compressions and to indicate the return of a patient's spontaneous circulation.

Pathophysiology of Respiratory Disorders

Allergic Reactions

An allergic reaction occurs when the body's immune functions are activated by an agent containing alien antigens. Once the immune system has been sensitized, subsequent exposure results in the binding of specific immunoglobulins or the activation of immunologically active cells. These can release inflammatory chemicals (histamines, kinins, interleukins) that create allergic symptoms. Allergic responses may be initiated by occupational exposure to allergens and by foods, animals, fungal spores, metals, and rubber products.

Allergic symptoms may include nasal inflammation, mucus production, watery eyes, itching, rashes, tissue swelling, bronchospasm, stridor, and shock.

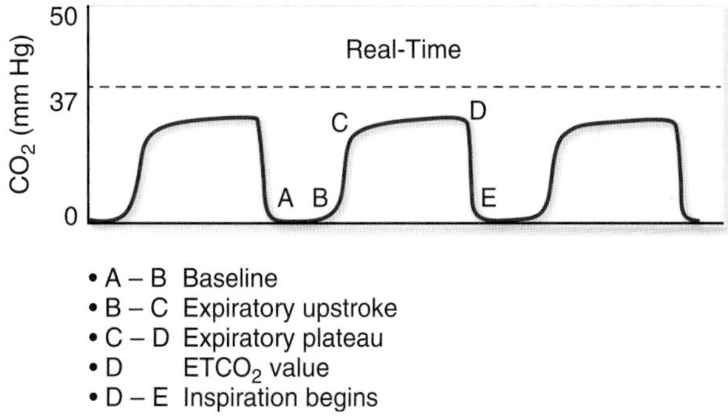

Figure 10-4 Capnography waveform.

Asthma

Asthma is a disease caused by a narrowing and inflammation of the tracheobronchial tree by various stimuli (Fig. 10-5). When this occurs, patients generally present with wheezing, shortness of breath, and coughing. Most patients have mild-to-moderate asthma. However, some patients have continuous asthma attacks called **status asthmaticus,** which may be fatal.

The recurrence and severity of asthma attacks are influenced by *triggers,* or the causes of the asthma attacks. Some examples of asthma triggers include such influences as allergens, dust, various medicines, dyes, odors, exercise, or exposure to occupational hazards.

Generally, asthma occurs most often in children or young adults. However, asthma can occur at any age. Asthma occurs more often in boys than girls before puberty. However, in adults, asthma is equally distributed between the sexes.

Chronic Obstructive Pulmonary Disease (COPD)

Chronic obstructive pulmonary disease (COPD) is a group of debilitating, progressive, and potentially fatal lung diseases that have in common increased resistance to air movement, prolongation of the expiratory phase of respiration, and loss of the normal elasticity of the lung (Fig. 10-6). COPD diseases include emphysema, chronic bronchitis, and asthmatic bronchitis.

- **Emphysema:** A respiratory disease marked by an abnormal increase in the size of air spaces distal to the terminal bronchiole, with destruction of the alveolar walls. This results in patients having difficulty exhaling air.
- **Chronic bronchitis:** Marked by an increased mucus secretion by the tracheobronchial tree. Chronic irritation by inhaled irritants and repeated infections are the primary risk factors.
- **Asthmatic bronchitis:** Bronchitis compounded by wheezing caused by spasm of hyperactive airways.

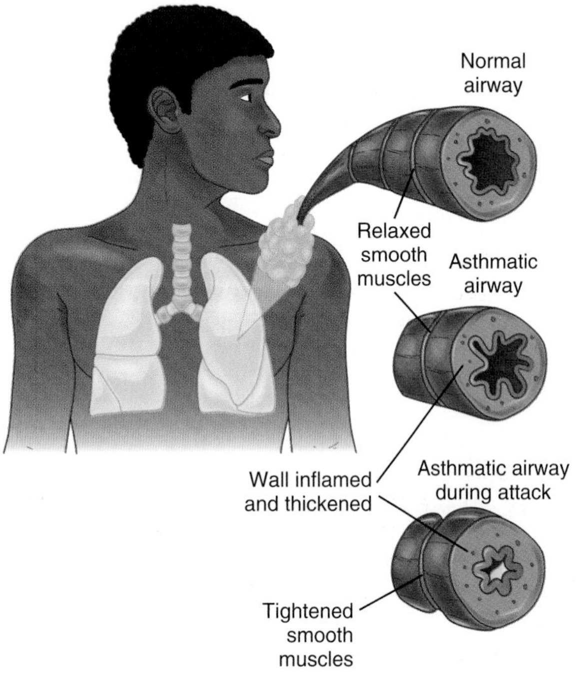

Figure 10-5 Pathophysiology of asthma.

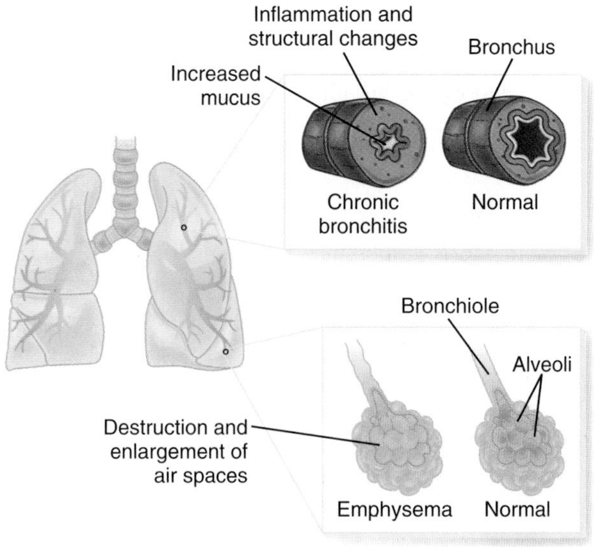

Figure 10-6 Pathophysiology of COPD.

Pharmacokinetics

Adrenergics

Adrenergic drugs are also called sympathomimetic drugs. They are drugs that work by stimulating the sympathetic nervous system (SNS). Adrenergic drugs stimulate nerves by either mimicking the action of the neurotransmitter norepinephrine or stimulating its release.

Anticholinergics

Anticholinergics are a class of drugs that block the action of the neurotransmitter acetylcholine in the brain. They can be used to treat asthma, incontinence, gastrointestinal cramps, and muscular spasms. They also balance the production of dopamine and acetylcholine in the body.

Antihistamines

Antihistamines relieve the symptoms associated with allergies. They block the effects of histamine at the H_1 receptor. They do not block histamine release, antibody production, or antigen-antibody reactions. Most antihistamines have anticholinergic properties.

Bronchodilators

Bronchodilators are used in the treatment of reversible airway obstruction due to asthma or COPD. Beta-adrenergic agonists produce bronchodilation by stimulating the production of cyclic adenosine monophosphate (cAMP). The newer bronchodilators are selective for pulmonary ($beta_2$) receptors. However, older bronchodilators produce cardiac stimulation ($beta_1$-adrenergic effects) in addition to bronchodilation.

Corticosteroids

Corticosteroids are used in replacement doses systemically to treat adrenocortical insufficiency. They produce metabolic effects in addition to modifying the normal immune response and suppressing inflammation.

Electrolytes

An electrolyte is a substance that, in solution, conducts an electric current and is decomposed by its passage. Acids, bases, and salts are common electrolytes. The major electrolytes include sodium, potassium, calcium, magnesium, chloride, bicarbonate, phosphate, and sulfate.

Glucocorticoids

Glucocorticoids are steroids that reduce inflammation throughout the body. They stop inflammation by moving into cells and suppressing the proteins that go on to promote inflammation. Glucocorticoids also affect metabolism by causing cells in the liver to make more sugar. This may lead to too much sugar in the blood and cause steroid-induced diabetes mellitus.

Medicinal Gas

A gas is one of the basic forms of matter. Gas molecules are free and move in all directions. The most often used gas in EMS is oxygen; a colorless, odorless, and tasteless gas. It is carried from the lungs to the body's tissues by hemoglobin in the red blood cells.

Neuromuscular Blockers

Neuromuscular blockers bind to acetylcholine receptors postsynaptically and inhibit the action of acetylcholine. This blocks neuromuscular transmission and causes paralysis of the muscle.

Neuromuscular blockers are used as an adjunct to anesthesia, only when artificial ventilation is available, to produce muscle relaxation in order to prevent movement.

Nondepolarizing Skeletal Muscle Relaxants

Nondepolarizing skeletal muscle relaxants prevent the action of acetylcholine by competing for cholinergic receptors. These drugs are used as a skeletal muscle relaxant during ET intubation.

Individual Drugs

Albuterol (al-BYOO-ter-ole)

AccuNeb, 🍁 Apo-Salvent, 🍁 Gen-Salbutamol, 🍁 Novo-Salmol, ProAir HFA, Proventil HFA, 🍁 Ventodisk, Ventolin HFA, 🍁 Ventolin Nebules, VoSpire ER

Classsifications: Adrenergic, bronchodilator

Pregnancy Class: C

Mechanism of Action: Binds to beta$_2$-adrenergic receptors in airway smooth muscle causing bronchodilation

Pharmacokinetics

Absorption: Well absorbed but rapidly undergoes metabolism

Onset: Inhalation—5 to 15 minutes

Duration: Inhalation—3 to 6 hours

Indications: Used as a bronchodilator to control and prevent reversible airway obstruction caused by asthma or COPD

Contraindications: Known hypersensitivity; should not be given to patients hypersensitive to adrenergic amines

Precautions: Use with caution in patients with cardiac disease, hypertension, hyperthyroidism, diabetes, glaucoma, and seizure disorders. ❗ Safety is not established for pregnant women near term, breastfeeding women, and pediatric patients less than two years old.

Effective **Communication**

Excessive use of inhaler may cause paradoxical bronchospasm.

Route and Dosage

Inhalation (Adults and Pediatrics More Than 4 years old): Via metered-dose inhaler—2 inhalations every 4 to 6 hours. NIH Guidelines for acute asthma exacerbation *(Pediatrics):* 4 to 8 puffs every 20 minutes for 3 doses, then every 1 to 4 hours. *(Adults):* 4 to 8 puffs every 20 minutes for up to 4 hours, then every 1 to 4 hours when needed.

Inhalation (Adults and Pediatrics More Than 12 years old): NIH Guidelines for acute asthma exacerbation via nebulization or IPPB—2.5 to 5 mg every 20 minutes for 3 doses, then 2.5 to 10 mg every 1–4 hours when needed. Continuous nebulization—10 to 15 mg/hr

Inhalation (Pediatric 2 to 12 years): NIH Guidelines for acute asthma exacerbation via nebulization or IPPB—0.15 mg/kg/dose (minimum dose 2.5 mg) every 20 minutes for 3 doses, then 0.15 to 0.3 mg/kg (not to exceed 10 mg) every 1 to 4 hours when needed or 1.25 mg 3 to 4 times daily for pediatrics. 10 to 15 kg or 2.5 mg 3 to 4 times daily for pediatrics more than 15 kg. Continuous nebulization: 0.5 to 3 mg/kg/hr

Understand the Numbers

You have been ordered to give 0.2 mg/kg of albuterol via nebulizer to your 4-year-old patient who weighs 35 pounds. Your initial dose for your patient should be:

35 lbs ÷ 2.2 kg = 15.9 or 16 kg. Then 16 kg × 0.2 mg = 3.2 mg

How Supplied

Metered-Dose Aerosol: 90 mcg/inhalation in 6.7-g, 8.5-g, 17-g, and 18-g dose. 🍁 100 mcg/spray

Inhalation Solution: 0.63 mg/3 mL, 1.25 mg/3 mL, 0.83 mg/mL in vials and 3-mL unit dose, 🍁 1 mg/mL, 🍁 2 mg/mL, 5 mg/mL

Powder for Inhalation (Ventodisk): 🍁 200 mcg, 🍁 400 mcg

Adverse Reactions and Side Effects
Resp: PARADOXICAL BRONCHOSPASM (excessive use of inhalers)
CV: Chest pain, palpitations, angina, arrhythmias, hypertension
CNS: Nervousness, restlessness, tremor, headache, insomnia
GI: Nausea, vomiting
Drug Interactions: Concurrent use with other adrenergic drugs will result in increased adrenergic side effects. Use with MAO inhibitors may lead to hypertensive crisis. Beta blockers may negate therapeutic effect.
EMS Considerations: Assess vital signs before and during therapy. Note amount, color, and character of any sputum. Monitor pulmonary function tests before initiating therapy. Observe for paradoxical bronchospasm (wheezing).

Aminophylline (am-in-OFF-i-lin)

Phyllocontin, Truphylline
Classifications: Bronchodilator, xanthine
Pregnancy Class: C
Mechanism of Action: Produces increased tissue concentrations of cAMP causing bronchodilation and CNS stimulation and producing positive inotropic (increased force of cardiac contractions) and chronotropic (increased heart rate) effects
Pharmacokinetics
Absorption: Well absorbed
Onset: Rapid
Duration: 6 to 8 hours
Aminophylline is converted to theophylline after administration. Theophylline is 90 percent metabolized by the liver to several metabolites, including caffeine, which may accumulate in neonates.
Indications: Used for the long-term control of reversible airway obstruction caused by asthma of COPD
Contraindications: Known hypersensitivity to aminophylline or theophylline
Precautions: Use with caution in patients with CHF, liver disease, or hypothyroidism (reduced dosage); also use cautiously in patients with cardiac arrhythmias or seizure disorders.
Route and Dosage
IV (Adult): Loading dose—6 mg/kg (4.7 mg/kg of theophylline) over 20 to 30 minutes, followed by 0.7 mg/kg/hr (0.56 mg/kg/hr of theophylline) by continuous infusion (non-smokers); an infusion rate of 0.9 mg/kg/hr (0.72 mg/kg/hr of theophylline) for smokers
IV (Geriatrics and Adults With Cor Pulmonale): Loading dose—6 mg/kg (4.7 mg/kg of theophylline) over 20 to 30 minutes, followed by 0.6 mg/kg/hr (0.47 mg/kg/hr of theophylline) IV infusion
IV (Adults With CHF or Liver Failure): Loading dose—6 mg/kg (4.7 mg/kg of theophylline) over 20 to 30 minutes, followed by 0.5 mg/kg/hr (0.39 mg/kg/hr of theophylline) IV infusion
Note: To prepare the IV infusion, add 250 to 500 mg of aminophylline to 50 to 100 mL of IV solution. This yields a concentration of 5 mg/mL (250 mg in 50 mL) to 5 mg/mL (500 mg in 100 mL).

Check the Evidence

Cor pulmonale is hypertrophy or failure of the right ventricle resulting from disorders of the lungs, pulmonary vessels, or the respiratory center of the brain.

Understand the Numbers

You are ordered to give a loading dose of 6 mg/kg of aminophylline over 20 minutes to your 67-year-old, 185-pound patient. However, all you have on board is theophylline. What is the loading dose of the theophylline? 185 lbs ÷ 2.2 kg = 84 kg. Therefore, 4.7 mg × 84 kg = 394.8 or 395 mg over 20 minutes.

IV (Pediatric): Consult your protocol or medical control.
How Supplied
Injection: 25 mg/mL
Adverse Reactions and Side Effects
CV: ARRHYTHMIAS, tachycardia, angina, palpitations
CNS: SEIZURES, anxiety, headache, insomnia, irritability
GI: Nausea, vomiting, anorexia
Derm: Rashes
Drug Interactions: There can be additive CV and CNS side effects when used concurrently use adrenergics. Nicotine, barbiturates, and phenytoin may increase metabolism and may decrease the effectiveness of aminophylline.
EMS Considerations: Rapid administration of aminophylline can cause severe hypotension or ventricular fibrillation. Monitor patients with a history of cardiovascular disorders for chest pain and ECG changes. Resuscitative equipment should be readily available.

Atracurium (ah-trah-KYOUR-ee-um)

Tracrium
Classification: Nondepolarizing skeletal muscle relaxant
Pregnancy Class: C
Mechanism of Action: Prevents the action of acetylcholine by competing for cholinergic receptors
Pharmacokinetics
Absorption: Rapid
Onset: 3 to 5 minutes
Duration: 60 to 70 minutes
Indications: Used as a skeletal muscle relaxant during ET intubation
Contraindications: Known hypersensitivity; should not be given to patients with electrolyte disorders or those with bronchial asthma
Precautions: Use with caution in patients during labor and delivery and in patients who are experiencing histamine release.
Route and Dosage
IV (Adult and Pediatric More Than 2 years old): 0.4 to 0.5 mg/kg IV bolus
How Supplied
Injection: 10 mg/mL
Adverse Reactions and Side Effects
Resp: Dyspnea, laryngospasm
CV: Tachycardia

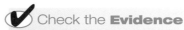

Drug Interactions: None significant
EMS Considerations: Atropine may be used if bradycardia develops. Do not mix atracurium with alkaline solutions, including lactated ringers (LR).

Atropine (AT-ro-peen)

AtroPen
Classifications: Anticholinergic, antimuscarinic
Pregnancy Class: C
Mechanism of Action: Atropine is an **anticholinergic** drug that competes with the neurotransmitter acetylcholine for receptor sites, blocking the stimulation of parasympathetic nerve fibers.
Pharmacokinetics
 Absorption: Well absorbed
 Onset: Rapid via inhalation administration
 Duration: 4 to 6 hours
Indications: Used to reverse exercise-induced bronchospasm
Contraindications: Known hypersensitivity; should not be given to patients with angle-closure glaucoma, acute hemorrhage, or tachycardia secondary to cardiac insufficiency or thyrotoxicosis
Precautions: Use with caution in patients with intra-abdominal infections, prostatic hyperplasia, or chronic renal, liver, pulmonary, or cardiac disease.
Route and Dosage
Nebulizer (Adult): 0.025 to 0.05 mg/kg/dose every 4 to 6 hours as needed; maximum = 2.5 mg/dose
Nebulizer (Pediatric): 0.03 to 0.05 mg/kg/dose, 3 to 4 times/day; maximum = 2.5 mg/dose

Understand the Numbers
You are ordered to administer 0.05 mg/kg of atropine by nebulizer to your 37-year-old, 250-pound patient. What is your initial dose?
250 lb ÷ 2.2 kg = 113.6 or 114 kg. Therefore, 114 kg × 0.5 mg = 5.7 mg. However, the maximum single dose is 2.5 mg.

How Supplied
Injection: 0.05 mg/mL, 0.1 mg/mL, 0.4 mg/mL, 1 mg/mL
Adverse Reactions and Side Effects
Resp: Tachypnea, pulmonary edema
CV: Tachycardia, palpitations, arrhythmias
CNS: Drowsiness, confusion
GI: Dry mouth, constipation, impaired motility of the GI tract
Misc: Flushing, decreased sweating
Drug Interactions: Increased anticholinergic effects with other anticholinergics. Antacids decrease absorption of anticholinergics.
EMS Considerations: The patient's lung sounds should be assessed and peak flow rate measured before and after administration.

Dexamethasone (dex-a-METH-a-sone)

DexPak
Classifications: Antiasthmatic, corticosteroid
Pregnancy Class: C
Mechanism of Action: Suppresses inflammation and the normal immune response
Pharmacokinetics
 Absorption: Well absorbed
 Onset: Rapid
 Duration: 2.75 days
Indications: Used systemically in treating inflammatory and allergic disorders; used in patients for extubation
Contraindications: Known hypersensitivity; should not be given to patients with active untreated infections or to those with known alcohol, bisulfite, or tartrazine hypersensitivity
Precautions: Use with caution in patients with hypothyroidism or cirrhosis.
Route and Dosage
IV, IM (Adult): Anti-inflammatory—0.75 to 9 mg daily in divided doses every 6 to 12 hours Airway edema or extubation—0.5 to 2 mg/kg/day divided every 6 hours. Begin treatment 24 hours prior to extubation and continue for 24 hours postextubation.
IV, IM (Pediatric): Airway edema or extubation—0.5 to 2 mg/kg/day divided every 6 hours. Begin treatment 24 hours prior to extubation and continue for 24 hours postextubation.
How Supplied
Solution for Injection: 4 mg/mL, 10 mg/mL
Adverse Reactions and Side Effects
CV: Hypertension
CNS: Depression, euphoria, headache, increased intracranial pressure (pediatric only), personality changes, psychoses, restlessness
GI: PEPTIC ULCERATION, anorexia, nausea, vomiting
Hemat: THROMBOEMBOLISM, thrombophlebitis
Derm: Acne, decreased wound healing, ecchymoses, petechiae
MS: Muscle wasting, osteoporosis, muscle pain

Effective Communication
Adverse reactions and side effects are much more common with high-dose/long-term therapy.

Drug Interactions: May increase the risk of adverse GI effects with NSAIDs, including aspirin; may increase requirement for insulin or oral hypoglycemic agents
EMS Considerations: Dexamethasone is sensitive to temperature extremes.

DiphenhydrAMINE (dye-fen-HYE-dra-meen)

Allerdryl, Benadryl
Classification: Antihistamine
Pregnancy Class: B
Mechanism of Action: Antagonizes the effects of histamine at the H_1-receptor sites; does not bind to or inactivate histamine; has CNS depressant and anticholinergic properties
Pharmacokinetics
 Absorption: Well absorbed
 Onset: IM—20 to 30 minutes; IV—rapid
 Duration: IM and IV—4 to 8 hours

Indications: Used for the relief of allergic symptoms caused by histamine release
Contraindications: Known hypersensitivity; should not be given to patients with acute attacks of asthma
Precautions: Use with caution in patients with severe liver disease, angle-closure glaucoma, seizure disorders, prostatic hyperplasia, and peptic ulcers. ! Geriatric patients are more susceptible to adverse drug reactions and anticholinergic effects.

Route and Dosage
IM, IV (Adult): 25 to 50 mg every 4 hours
IM, IV (Pediatric): 1.25 mg/kg 4 times daily

How Supplied
Injection: 10 mg/mL, 50 mg/mL

Adverse Reactions and Side Effects
Resp: Chest tightness, thickened bronchial secretions, wheezing
CV: Hypotension, palpitations
CNS: Drowsiness, dizziness, headache, paradoxical excitation (increased in pediatrics)
EENT: Blurred vision, tinnitus
GI: Anorexia, dry mouth, constipation, nausea
Drug Interactions: Increased risk of CNS depression with other antihistamines, opioid analgesics, and sedative or hypnotics. MAO inhibitors intensify and prolong the anticholinergic effects of antihistamines.

Effective **Communication**

Do not confuse Benadryl (diphenhydramine) with Benylin (dextromethorphan).

EMS Considerations: Assess the patient's airway, lung sounds, and respiratory function frequently.

Epinephrine (e-pi-NEF-rin)

Adrenalin, Ana-Guard, Asthmahaler Mist, AsthmaNefrin (racepinephrine), EpiPen, Micronefrin (racepinephrine), S-2 (racepinephrine)
Classifications: Antiasthmatic, bronchodilator, adrenergic, vasopressor
Pregnancy Class: C
Mechanism of Action: Affects both beta$_1$ (cardiac)—adrenergic receptor and beta$_2$ (pulmonary)—adrenergic receptor sites; produces bronchodilation; also has alpha-adrenergic agonist properties resulting in vasoconstriction
Pharmacokinetics
Absorption: Well absorbed following inhalation, SubQ, IM, and IV administration
Onset: Inhalation—1 minute; SubQ—5 to 10 minutes; IM—6 to 12 minutes; IV—Rapid
Duration: Inhalation—1 to 3 hours; SubQ and IM—1 to 4 hours; IV—20 to 30 minutes
Indications: Inhalation, SubQ, IV—used for the management of reversible airway disease due to asthma or COPD; SubQ, IM, IV—used for the management of severe allergic reactions; Inhalation—used for the management of upper-airway obstruction and croup (racemic epinephrine).
Contraindications: Known hypersensitivity; should not be given to patients who are hypersensitive to adrenergic amines, have cardiac arrhythmias, or are hypersensitive to bisulfites
Precautions: Use with caution in patients with cardiac disease and in those with hypertension, hyperthyroidism, diabetes, or cerebral arteriosclerosis.

Route and Dosage
SubQ, IM (Adult): Anaphylactic reactions/asthma—0.1 to 0.5 mg (single dose not to exceed 1 mg). Dose may be repeated every 10 to 15 minutes for anaphylactic shock or every 20 minutes to 4 hours for asthma.
SubQ (Pediatric More Than 1 month old): Anaphylactic reactions/asthma—0.01 mg/kg (not to exceed 0.5 mg/dose) every 15 minutes for 3 doses, then every 4 hours
IV (Adult): Severe anaphylaxis—0.1 to 0.25 mg every 5 to 15 minutes. This may be followed by a 1 to 4 mcg/minute continuous infusion.
IV (Pediatric): Severe anaphylaxis—0.1 mg. This may be followed by 0.1 mcg/kg/minute of a continuous infusion.
Inhalation (Adult): Metered-dose inhaler—1 inhalation (160 to 250 mcg). This may be repeated in 1 to 2 minutes.
Inhalation (Pediatric More Than 1 month old): 0.25 to 0.5 mL of 2.25 percent racemic epinephrine solution diluted in 3 mL of normal saline (NS)

How Supplied
Inhalation Aerosol (OTC): 0.125 percent (300 inhalations/15 mL), 0.5 percent (300 inhalations/15 mL), 300 mcg/spray (300 inhalations/15 mL)
Inhalation Solution (OTC): 1 percent
Injection: 0.1 mg/mL (1:10,000), 1 mg/mL (1:1000)
Autoinjector (EpiPen): 0.15 mg/0.3 mL (1:2,000), 0.3 mg/0.3 mL (1:1000)

Adverse Reactions and Side Effects
Resp: Paradoxical bronchospasm (excessive use of inhalers)
CV: Angina, arrhythmias, hypertension, tachycardia
CNS: Nervousness, restlessness, tremor, headache, insomnia
GI: Nausea, vomiting
Drug Interactions: Concurrent use with other adrenergic drugs will have additive adrenergic side effects. Use with MAO inhibitors may cause hypertensive crisis. Beta blockers may block the therapeutic effects. Tricyclic antidepressants enhance pressor response to epinephrine.
EMS Considerations: Monitor vital signs closely, paying special attention to blood pressure, pulse rate, and ECG status. Assess lung sounds before and after administration.

Effective **Communication**

An IV bolus injection of a 1:1000 solution of epinephrine may cause sudden hypertension or cerebral edema.

Hydrocortisone (hye-droe-KOR-ti-sone)

Cortef, Cortenema, Solu-Cortef
Classifications: Antiasthmatic, corticosteroid
Pregnancy Class: C
Mechanism of Action: Suppresses inflammation and the normal immune response. It also replaces endogenous cortisol in deficiency states.
Pharmacokinetics
Absorption: Rapid
Onset: Rapid
Duration: Unknown
Indications: Allergic reactions, asthma, COPD
Contraindications: Known hypersensitivity; should not be given to patients with active untreated infections or known alcohol, bisulfite, or tartrazine hypersensitivity
Precautions: Use with caution in patients with hypothyroidism or cirrhosis.
Route and Dosage
IM, IV (Adult): Allergic reactions—100 to 500 mg
IM, IV (Pediatric): Allergic reactions—2 to 4 mg/kg/day
IM, IV (Adult): Asthma and COPD—100 to 500 mg
IM, IV (Pediatric): Asthma—1 mg/kg. The dosage may be adjusted by medical control in response to the severity of the asthma.
How Supplied
Powder for Injection: 100 mg, 250 mg, 500 mg, 1 g
Adverse Reactions and Side Effects
CV: Hypertension
CNS: Depression, euphoria, headache, increased intracranial pressure (pediatric only), personality changes, psychoses, restlessness
GI: PEPTIC ULCERATION, anorexia, nausea, vomiting
Hemat: THROMBOEMBOLISM, thrombophlebitis
Derm: Acne, decreased wound healing, ecchymoses, petechiae
MS: Muscle wasting, osteoporosis, muscle pain

Effective Communication

Adverse reactions and side effects are much more common with high-dose/long-term therapy.

Drug Interactions: May increase the risk of adverse GI effects with NSAIDs, including aspirin; may increase the requirement for insulin or oral hypoglycemic agents
EMS Considerations: Assess patient vital signs frequently.

Ipratropium (i-pra-TROE-pee-um)

Atrovent
Classifications: Anticholinergic, bronchodilator
Pregnancy Class: B
Mechanism of Action: Used as maintenance therapy of reversible airway obstruction due to COPD, including chronic bronchitis and emphysema

Check the **Evidence**

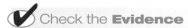

Ipratropium may be used as adjunctive management of bronchospasm caused by asthma (unlabeled use).

Contraindications: Known hypersensitivity; should not be given to patients hypersensitive to atropine or bromide. Do not use in patients during acute bronchospasm.
Precautions: Use with caution in patients with bladder neck obstruction, prostatic hyperplasia, glaucoma, or urinary retention.
Route and Dosage
Inhalation (Adult and Pediatric More Than 12 years old): Metered-dose inhaler (nonacute)—2 inhalations 4 times daily (do not exceed 12 inhalations/24-hour period). Metered-dose inhaler (acute)—4 to 8 puffs using a spacer device as needed. Nebulization (nonacute)—500 mcg 3 to 4 times daily. Nebulization (acute)—500 mcg every 30 minutes for 3 doses, then every 2 to 4 hours as needed.
How Supplied
Inhalation Solution: 🍁 0.0125 percent, 0.02 percent in single-dose vials containing 500 mcg, 🍁 0.025 percent
Adverse Reactions and Side Effects
Resp: Bronchospasm, cough
CV: Hypotension, palpitations
CNS: Dizziness, headache, nervousness
EENT: Blurred vision, sore throat
GI: GI irritability, nausea
Derm: Rash
Drug Interactions: Increased anticholinergic effects if given with other drugs with anticholinergic properties
EMS Considerations: Assess respiratory status before and after administration. ❗ Do not confuse Atrovent with Alupent (metaproterenol).

Check the **Evidence**

Ipratropium may be mixed with albuterol in the nebulizer if used within 1 hour.

Levalbuterol (leev-al-BYOO-ter-ole)

Xopenex
Classifications: Adrenergic, bronchodilator
Pregnancy Class: C
Mechanism of Action: Binds to beta$_2$-adrenergic receptors in airway smooth muscle causing bronchodilation
Pharmacokinetics
Absorption: Some absorption occurs following inhalation.
Onset: 10 to 17 minutes
Duration: 5 to 6 hours
Indications: Used as a short-term control drug to treat bronchodilation due to reversible airway disease
Contraindications: Known hypersensitivity; should not be given to patients with a hypersensitivity to albuterol

Precautions: Use with caution in patients with hypertension, coronary insufficiency, arrhythmias, or a history of seizures, hypokalemia, or diabetes mellitus.

Route and Dosage

Inhalation (Adult and Pediatric More Than 12 years old): 0.63 mg via nebulization 3 times daily

Inhalation (Pediatric Under 12 years old): 0.31 mg via nebulization 3 times daily

How Supplied

Metered-Dose Inhaler: 45 mcg/actuation in 15-g canisters

Inhalation Solution: 0.31 mg/3 mL, 0.63 mg/3 mL, 1.25 mg/3 mL, 1.25 mg/0.5 mL

Adverse Reactions and Side Effects

Resp: PARADOXICAL BRONCHOSPASM (excessive use of inhalers), increased cough, turbinate edema

CV: Tachycardia

CNS: Anxiety, dizziness, headache, nervousness

GI: Vomiting

Endo: Hyperglycemia

Drug Interactions: Concurrent use or use within 2 weeks of tricyclic antidepressants or MAO inhibitors may increase the risk of adverse cardiovascular reactions (use with extreme caution). Beta blockers block the beneficial pulmonary effects of adrenergic bronchodilators.

EMS Considerations: Before giving levalbuterol, be sure to obtain baseline vital signs and monitor the patient closely. Observe for paradoxical bronchospasm (wheezing). If this occurs, contact medical control.

Magnesium sulfate (mag-NEE-zhum SUL-fate)

Classifications: Mineral/electrolyte

Pregnancy Class: D

Mechanism of Action: Essential for the activity of many enzymes; plays an important role in neurotransmission and muscular excitation

Pharmacokinetics

- *Absorption:* IV results in complete bioavailability; well absorbed from IM sites
- *Onset:* IM—60 minutes; IV—Immediate
- *Duration:* IM—3 to 4 hours; IV—30 minutes

Indications: Can be used as adjunctive treatment for bronchodilation in moderate-to-severe cases of acute asthma

Contraindications: Known hypersensitivity; should not be given to patients with hypermagnesemia, hypocalcemia, or heart block

Precautions: Use with caution in patients with renal insufficiency. Geriatric patients may require a decreased dose due to age-related decrease in renal function.

Route and Dosage

IV (Adult): 1.2 to 2 g over 20 minutes

IV (Pediatric): 25 to 50 mg/kg diluted in D_5W and given over 10 to 20 minutes

***Effective* Communication**

Accidental overdose of IV magnesium sulfate has resulted in serious patient harm, including death.

How Supplied

Injection: 500 mg/mL (50 percent)

Premixed infusions: 1 g/100 mL, 2 g/100 mL, 4 g/50 mL, 4 g/100 mL, 20 g/500 mL, 40 g/1,000 mL

Adverse Reactions and Side Effects

Resp: Decreased respiratory rate

CV: Arrhythmias, bradycardia, hypotension

CNS: Drowsiness

GI: Diarrhea

Drug Interactions: May potentiate calcium channel blockers and neuromuscular blocking agents

EMS Considerations: Rapid IV administration may cause respiratory or cardiac arrest. An overdose of magnesium sulfate may cause respiratory depression or heart block. To reverse these effects, you may be ordered to ventilate the patient with 100 percent humidified oxygen and administer an IV bolus of 10 percent calcium gluconate at 5 to 10 mEq (10 to 20 mL).

Metaproterenol (met-ah-proh-TER-ih-nohl)

Alupent

Classifications: Adrenergic, bronchodilator

Pregnancy Class: C

Mechanism of Action: A strong beta$_2$-adrenergic agonist, having a strong effect on pulmonary receptors, relaxing bronchial smooth muscles. This results in an increase in lung capacity and a decrease in airway resistance. Its minimal beta$_1$-adrenergic effects produce CNS and cardiac stimulation.

Pharmacokinetics

- *Absorption:* Rapid
- *Onset:* 1 minute
- *Duration:* 1 to 5 hours

Indications: Used to treat asthma, bronchitis, emphysema, and other conditions associated with reversible bronchospasms

Contraindications: Known hypersensitivity; should not be given to patients with preexisting cardiac arrhythmias associated with tachycardia

Precautions: Use with caution in patients with hypertension, coronary artery disease (CAD), CHF, or diabetes.

Route and Dosage

Metered-Dose Inhaler (Adult): 0.3 mL (range—0.2 to 0.3 mL) of a 5 percent solution diluted to 2.5 mL in normal saline

How Supplied

Metered-Dose Inhaler: 0.63 mg/inhalation

Adverse Reactions and Side Effects

CV: Hypertension, arrhythmias, chest pain

CNS: Nervousness, tremor, headache

GI: Diarrhea, nausea, vomiting

Drug Interactions: Possible potentiation of adrenergic effects if used before or after other sympathomimetic bronchodilators

EMS Considerations: Excessive use of inhalers can result in tolerance and paradoxical bronchospasm. Assess patient's blood pressure, pulse rate, respirations, and lung sounds before and after administration. Measure patient's peak flow rate before and after drug administration.

MethyLPREDNISolone (meth-ill-pred-NISS-oh-lone)

Solu-Medrol

Classifications: Antiasthmatic, corticosteroid

Pregnancy Class: C

Mechanism of Action: Suppresses inflammation and the normal immune response. It also replaces endogenous cortisol in deficiency states.

Pharmacokinetics

Absorption: Well absorbed

Onset: Rapid

Duration: Unknown

Indications: Used for treating patients with severe asthma

Contraindications: Known hypersensitivity; should not be given to patients with active untreated infections or known alcohol, bisulfite, or tartrazine hypersensitivity

Precautions: Use with caution in patients with hypothyroidism or cirrhosis.

Route and Dosage

IV (Adult): 2 mg/kg, then 0.5 to 1 mg/kg every 6 hours for up to 5 days

How Supplied

Powder for Injection: 40 mg, 125 mg, 1 g, 2 g

Adverse Reactions and Side Effects

CV: Hypertension

CNS: Depression, euphoria, headache, increased intracranial pressure (pediatric only), personality changes, psychoses, restlessness

GI: PEPTIC ULCERATION, anorexia, nausea, vomiting

Hemat: THROMBOEMBOLISM, thrombophlebitis

Derm: Acne, decreased wound healing, ecchymoses, petechiae

MS: Muscle wasting, osteoporosis, muscle pain

Effective Communication

Adverse reactions and side effects are much more common with high-dose/long-term therapy.

Drug Interactions: May increase the risk of adverse GI effects with NSAIDs, including aspirin; may increase the requirement for insulin or oral hypoglycemic agents

EMS Considerations: Assess patient vital signs frequently.

Oxygen (OX-ah-gin)

Classification: Medicinal gas

Pregnancy Class: A

Mechanism of Action: Oxygen is required to enable the cells to break down glucose into a usable energy form. Oxygen is a colorless, odorless, tasteless gas, essential to respiration. At sea level, oxygen is made up of approximately 10 to 16 percent venous blood and 17 to 21 percent arterial blood. Oxygen is carried from the lungs to the body's tissue by hemoglobin in the red blood cells. The administration of oxygen increases arterial oxygen tension (PaO_2) and hemoglobin saturation. This improves tissue oxygenation when circulation is adequately maintained.

Pharmacokinetics

Absorption: Oxygen is inhaled into the alveoli and then diffuses into the pulmonary capillary bed. The uptake from the lungs is rapid, and carbon dioxide is simultaneously excreted in the expelled air.

Onset: Immediate

Distribution: The delivery of oxygen to the tissues depends on arterial oxygenation, cardiac output, tissue perfusion, and oxygen delivery systems.

Duration: Approximately 2 minutes

Indications: Oxygen is used: 1) to treat severe chest pain that may be caused by cardiac ischemia, 2) to treat hypoxemia from any cause, and 3) in the treatment of cardiac arrest.

Contraindications: None for out-of-hospital use (see Check the Evidence)

Check the Evidence

Oxygen is contraindicated in patients who are suffering from paraquat poisoning unless they are suffering from severe respiratory distress or respiratory arrest. ! Oxygen can increase the toxicity of the paraquat. Paraquat is a toxic chemical used in agriculture to kill certain weeds.

Precautions: If the patient has a history of COPD, begin oxygen administration at a lower flow rate, increasing the rate as necessary.

Route and Dosage

Inhalation (Adult): Low-dose oxygen—1 to 6 L/minute using a nasal cannula giving oxygen concentrations of 24 to 44 percent. Mid-dose oxygen—8 to 10 L/minutes using a simple face mask giving oxygen concentrations of 40 to 60 percent. High-dose oxygen—10 to 15 L/minute using a face mask with oxygen reservoir (nonrebreather) giving oxygen concentrations of almost 100 percent oxygen.

Inhalation (Pediatric): Same as the adult

How Supplied

Cylinders in various sizes

Adverse Reactions and Side Effects

There are no adverse reactions or side effects in emergency situations. High concentrations of oxygen *may* cause decreased level of consciousness (LOC) and respiratory depression in patients with chronic carbon dioxide retention.

Effective Communication

Never withhold oxygen from any critically ill patient.

Drug Interactions: None

EMS Considerations: Reassure patients who are anxious about face masks but who require high concentrations of oxygen.

Pancuronium (pan-kyou-ROH-nee-um)

Pavulon
Classification: Neuromuscular blocker
Pregnancy Class: C
Mechanism of Action: Pancuronium competes with acetylcholine for the receptor sites in the muscle cells, causing paralysis. Muscle paralysis is sequential in the following order: heaviness of the eyelids, difficulty swallowing and talking, diplopia, progressive weakening of the extremities and neck, relaxation of the trunk and spine. The respiratory system is affected last. Pancuronium does not affect consciousness.
Pharmacokinetics
Absorption: Rapid
Onset: 30 to 45 seconds
Duration: 30 to 60 minutes
Indications: Used to produce muscle relaxation to facilitate ET intubation
Contraindications: Known hypersensitivity; should not be given to patients with a known hypersensitivity to bromides
Precautions: Use with caution in patients with heart or renal disease.
Route and Dosage
IV (Adult and Pediatric): 0.06 to 0.1 mg/kg IV bolus

> ***Understand the Numbers***
> You are ordered to administer 0.06 mg/kg of pancuronium to your 55-pound patient. What is your initial dose?
> 55 lb ÷ 2.2 kg = 25 kg. 0.06 mg × 25 kg = 1.5 mg

How Supplied
Solution for Injection: 1 mg/mL, 2 mg/mL
Adverse Reactions and Side Effects
Resp: Bronchospasm, apnea, respiratory insufficiency
CV: Tachycardia, hypotension
Misc: Salivation, flushing, rash
Drug Interactions: Additive neuromuscular blocking action if used with procainamide, lidocaine, beta blockers, and magnesium sulfate
EMS Considerations: Monitor vital signs and ECG frequently. Pancuronium may cause vagal stimulation producing bradycardia, hypotension, and arrhythmias. Pancuronium does not affect consciousness. Therefore, explain all procedures and provide emotional support for the patient.

Propofol (PROE-poe-fol)

Diprivan
Classification: General anesthetic
Pregnancy Class: B
Mechanism of Action: Short-acting hypnotic. Mechanism of action is unknown. It produces amnesia but has no analgesic properties.
Pharmacokinetics
Absorption: Complete absorption
Onset: IV—40 seconds
Duration: IV—3 to 5 minutes
Indications: Used for sedation of intubated, mechanically ventilated patients
Contraindications: Known hypersensitivity; should not be given to patients hypersensitive to soybean oil, egg lecithin, or glycerol
Precautions: Use with caution in patients with cardiovascular disease, increased intracranial pressure, cerebrovascular disorders, or hypovolemia. Lower induction and maintenance dose reduction are recommended for geriatric patients.
Route and Dosage
IV (Adult More Than 55 Years in Age): Induction—40 mg every 10 seconds until induction achieved. Maintenance—100 to 200 mcg/kg/minute
IV (Geriatric patients, Cardiac patients, Debilitated patients, or Hypovolemic patients): Induction—20 mg every 10 seconds until induction achieved. Maintenance—50 to 100 mcg/kg/minute
How Supplied
Injection: 10 mg/mL
Adverse Reactions and Side Effects
Resp: APNEA, cough
CV: Bradycardia, hypotension, hypertension
CNS: Dizziness, headache
GI: Abdominal cramping, hiccups, nausea, vomiting
Derm: Flushing
Local: Burning, pain, stinging, coldness, numbness, tingling at the IV site
GU: Discoloration of the urine (green)
Misc: PROPOFOL INFUSION SYNDROME, fever

> Check the **Evidence**
> The clinical features of propofol infusion syndrome (PRIS) are acute refractory bradycardia leading to asystole. This is rare but is related to high or long-term use of propofol.

Drug Interactions: Additive CNS and respiratory depression with alcohol, antihistamines, opioid analgesics, and sedatives or hypnotics
EMS Considerations: Assess respiratory status, pulse, and blood pressure continuously during propofol therapy. Propofol can cause apnea lasting more than 60 seconds.

Rocuronium (roh-kyou-ROH-nee-um)

Zemuron
Classification: Neuromuscular blocker
Pregnancy Class: B
Mechanism of Action: Competes with acetylcholine for receptor sites causing muscular paralysis; must be accompanied by adequate sedation; does not affect consciousness or pain threshold
Pharmacokinetics
Absorption: Rapid
Onset: 2 to 8 minutes
Duration: 30 minutes
Indications: Used as an adjunct to facilitate rapid sequence or routine intubation

Contraindications: Known hypersensitivity; should not be given to patients with hypersensitivity to bromide
Precautions: Use with caution in patients with heart disease or liver disease.
Route and Dosage
IV (Adult): 0.6 to 1.2 mg/kg slow IV in premedicated patients
IV (Pediatric): 0.6 mg/kg
How Supplied
Injection: 10 mg/mL
Adverse Reactions and Side Effects
Resp: Symptoms of asthma (bronchospasm, wheezing, rhonchi)
CV: Arrhythmias, tachycardia, transient hypotension and hypertension
GI: Nausea, vomiting
Drug Interactions: Additive paralysis with succinylcholine, lidocaine, quinidine, procainamide, beta-adrenergic blockers, or magnesium sulfate
EMS Considerations: Monitor vital signs frequently during therapy.

Succinylcholine (suck-sin-ill-KOH-leen)

Anectine
Classification: Depolarizing neuromuscular blocker
Pregnancy Class: C
Mechanism of Action: Prevents muscles from contracting by prolonging time during which the receptors at the neuromuscular junction cannot respond to acetylcholine
Pharmacokinetics
Absorption: Rapid
Onset: IM—2 to 3 minutes; IV—30 to 60 seconds
Duration: IM—10 to 30 minutes; IV—2 to 3 minutes
Indication: Used as an adjunct to facilitate ET intubation
Contraindications: Known hypersensitivity; should not be given to patients with acute narrow-angle glaucoma or penetrating eye injuries
Precautions: Use with caution in patients with fractures, because they may receive additional trauma caused by succinylcholine-induced muscle spasms. Pediatric patients may receive fractures when given neuromuscular blockers due to severe muscle spasms that may occur.
Route and Dosage
IM (Adult): 3 to 4 mg/kg; maximum dose = 150 mg
IV (Adult): 0.6 mg/kg

Understand the Numbers
You are ordered to give 4 mg/kg of succinylcholine to your 230-pound adult patient. What is your initial dose?
230 lb ÷ 2.2 kg = 104.5 or 105 kg. 4 mg × 105 kg = 420 mg. However, the maximum dose for IM succinylcholine is 150 mg.

IM (Pediatric): 3 to 4 mg/kg; maximum dose = 150 mg
IV (Pediatric): 1 to 2 mg/kg
How Supplied
Injection: 20 mg/mL, 50 mg/mL, 100 mg/mL
Adverse Reactions and Side Effects
Resp: Apnea, respiratory depression
CV: Bradycardia or tachycardia, hypotension or hypertension; SEVERE BRADYCARDIA OR ASYTOLE, especially after the second dose (pediatric patients)
MS: Muscle spasms, muscle pain
GI: Salivation

Check the Evidence
To reduce the incidence of severe bradycardia or asystole, pediatric patients can be premedicated with atropine.

Drug Interactions: Additive neuromuscular blocking action with lidocaine, procainamide, beta blockers, and magnesium sulfate
EMS Considerations: For IV infusion, use 1- or 2-mg/mL solution of succinylcholine in D_5W or 0.9 percent NS. Succinylcholine is not compatible with alkaline solutions.

Terbutaline (ter-BYOO-ta-leen)

Brethine
Classifications: Adrenergic, bronchodilator
Pregnancy Class: B
Mechanism of Action: Selective of $beta_1$ (pulmonary)-adrenergic receptors sites, with less effect on $beta_1$ (cardiac)-adrenergic receptors. Terbutaline causes bronchodilation.
Pharmacokinetics
Absorption: Well absorbed following SubQ administration
Onset: SubQ—within 15 minutes
Duration: SubQ—1.5 to 4 hours
Indications: Use for the management of reversible airway disease due to asthma or COPD.
Contraindications: Known hypersensitivity; should not be given to patients hypersensitive to adrenergic amines
Precautions: Use with caution in patients with cardiac disease, hypertension, diabetes, glaucoma, and hyperthyroidism. Geriatric patients are more susceptible to adverse reactions and therefore may require decreased doses.
Route and Dosage
SubQ (Adults and Pediatrics More Than 12 years old): 250 mcg. May be repeated in 15 to 30 minutes. Do not exceed 500 mcg/4 hours.
SubQ (Pediatrics Under 12 years old): 0.005 to 0.01 mg/kg; may be repeated in 15 to 20 minutes
How Supplied
Injection: 1 mg/mL
Adverse Reactions and Side Effects
CV: Angina, arrhythmias, hypertension, tachycardia
CNS: Nervousness, restlessness, tremor, headache, insomnia
GI: Nausea, vomiting
Drug Interactions: Concurrent use with other adrenergic drugs will cause additive adrenergic side effects. Use with MAO inhibitors may cause a hypertensive crisis. Beta blockers may negate the therapeutic effect of terbutaline.

EMS Considerations: Auscultate and document lung assessments. Assess patients for evidence of lung tolerance and bronchospasm.

Vecuronium (veh-kyour-OH-nee-um)

Norcuron

Classification: Nondepolarizing neuromuscular blocker

Pregnancy Class: C

Mechanism of Action: Competitive nondepolarizing drug that competes with acetylcholine for receptor sites in the muscle cells, preventing the muscles from contracting

Pharmacokinetics

Absorption: Rapid

Onset: Less than 1 minute

Duration: 30 to 40 minutes

Indications: Used to cause skeletal muscle relaxation to facilitate ET intubation

Contraindications: Known hypersensitivity; should not be given to patients with hypersensitivity to bromides

Precautions: Use with caution in patients with heart disease or liver disease.

Route and Dosage

IV (Adults and Pediatrics More Than 10 years old): 0.08 to 0.1 mg/kg

How Supplied

Powder for Injection: 10 mg, 20 mg

Adverse Reactions and Side Effects

Resp: Bronchospasms, respiratory paralysis

CV: Arrhythmias, bradycardia, hypotension, CARDIAC ARREST

GI: Excessive salivation

Drug Interactions: Additive neuromuscular blocking action with lidocaine, procainamide, beta blockers, and magnesium sulfate

EMS Considerations: Monitor vital signs frequently. Vecuronium can cause vagal stimulation resulting in bradycardia, hypotension, and arrhythmias.

Rapid-Sequence Intubation

Situations may arise when ET intubation is not immediately possible. For example, a patient may resist ventilations because of pain. A semiconscious or combative patient may also resist ventilation. In situations such as these, it may be necessary to administer a series of drugs designed to temporarily paralyze the patient so an ET tube can be inserted.

Rapid-sequence intubation is necessary to facilitate intubation in the conscious or semiconscious patient. A potent sedative is administered simultaneously with a **neuromuscular blocking agent** so the patient can tolerate intubation and then the airway can be effectively controlled.

Indications for rapid-sequence intubation include acute intracranial lesions overdose, status epilepticus, combative patients requiring immediate intubation, possible cervical spine fracture where immobilization is not possible because of delirium, and so forth. Before performing the actual intubation, the patient is given a brief neurological assessment involving level of consciousness, motor response, verbal response, and pupillary response.

Procedure for Rapid-Sequence Intubation

Preparation

- Assemble equipment and ensure everything is operational:
  - Various ET tube sizes/stylets/syringes; test balloon prior to insertion
  - Various types and sizes of laryngoscope handles and blades
  - Two patent IV lines
  - Suction ready
  - Cardiac monitor
  - Pulse oximetry
  - BVM, 100 percent oxygen
  - Appropriate medications with specific dosages
  - End-tidal CO_2 detector; capnography, if available
  - Method to secure ET tube once inserted
  - Adjunct airways available; King airway Combitube, LMA, and surgical cricothyrotomy equipment

Preoxygenation

- Apply a nonrebreather mask at 15 L/minute. If possible, the patient should breathe high-flow oxygen for 5 minutes prior to intubation. This establishes an oxygen reservoir in the lungs by replacing nitrogen, allowing the patient to maintain saturation during paralysis and intubation.

Check the **Evidence**

Administering high-flow oxygen for 5 minutes gives patients several minutes of apnea before desaturation (less than 90 percent) occurs.

Pretreatment

- *Lidocaine, 1 to 1.5 mg/kg IV:* The use of lidocaine in RSI may blunt the intracranial pressure rise associated with RSI.
- *Fentanyl, 2 to 9 mcg/kg, IV:* Fentanyl significantly reduces the hemodynamic response to ET intubation.
- *Atropine (Pediatrics):* 0.02 mg/kg IV (minimum of 0.1 mg). (Adults): 0.5 to 1 mg IV. Atropine is used for pediatrics to prevent bradycardia or asystole due to the side effects of succinylcholine. It can be used in adults to prevent bradycardia due to the side effects of succinylcholine.

Induction With Paralysis

This process involves the administration of an *induction* drug, rapidly followed by a *paralytic* drug, giving this procedure the name "rapid sequence."

Induction Drugs: provide a rapid loss of consciousness that facilitates intubation

- **Etomidate:** 0.3 mg/kg IV
- **Ketamine:** 1 to 2 mg/kg IV
- **Propofol:** 2 mg/kg IV

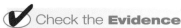

Effective Communication

Many protocols do not advocate the use of midazolam as an induction drug due to the possibility of developing hypotension and the prolonged duration of action.

Paralysis Drugs

Paralysis drugs are administered immediately after the induction drug:

- **Succinylcholine** (depolarizing neuromuscular blocker): 1 to 1.5 mg/kg IV
- **Rocuronium** (nondepolarizing neuromuscular blocker): 1 to 1.2 mg/kg IV
- **Vecuronium** (nondepolarizing neuromuscular blocker): 0.1 to 0.2 mg/kg IV

Check the **Evidence**

Paralysis drugs do not provide sedation, analgesia, or amnesia. Therefore, potent induction is essential.

Positioning

- Ensure that the patient position is ideal to improve visualization during the intubation process.
- In cases of suspected cervical spine injury, intubation must be performed without movement of the patient's head.
- The Sellicks maneuver may be performed to prevent gastric contents regurgitating into the patient's lungs.

Check the **Evidence**

Several studies now show that cricoid pressure (The Sellicks maneuver) does not significantly decrease the risk of aspiration or enhance visualization of the glottis opening.

Verify Endotracheal Tube Placement

- Visualize the ET tube passing through the patient's vocal cord.
- Confirm ET tube placement.
  - Note color change on end-tidal CO_2 detector.
  - Utilize waveform capnography.
  - Listen to the patient's lung fields for the presence of good breath sounds.

Post-Intubation Management

- Note the depth of the ET tube placement and secure the tube in place.
- Initiate mechanical ventilation.
- Administer sedative or analgesia for patient comfort.
- Document all aspects of the procedure.
- Maintain frequent patient monitoring for continued ventilation effectiveness, depth of sedation or paralysis, hemodynamic stability, and continued patient comfort.

Succinylcholine is the most often used short-acting neuromuscular blocking agent for rapid-sequence intubation. After it is given, the patient undergoes fasciculations and muscle cramps, which are followed by flaccid paralysis. The patient will generally experience paralysis within 30 to 60 seconds. Paralysis will last approximately 4 to 6 minutes. Side effects, which may develop, include:

Resp: Respiratory depression, apnea, wheezing
CV: Bradycardia, sinus arrest, hypertension or hypotension
EENT: Intraocular pressure
GI: Nausea, vomiting

Rapid-sequence intubation protocols may also include any of the following drugs:

- **Pancuronium:** Onset of paralysis within approximately 3 minutes, with a therapeutic duration of approximately 40 minutes
- **Propofol:** An induction drug with an onset of approximately 40 seconds and a therapeutic duration of approximately 3 to 5 minutes
- **Atracurium and Vecuronium:** Both drugs are short-acting nondepolarizing muscle relaxants. They have an onset time of approximately 2 to 3 minutes and a therapeutic duration of approximately 20 to 40 minutes.

SCENARIO REVISITED

Do you recall the case of Jackson who fell in the kitchen? Due to your initial findings, Jackson should be considered a high priority. He must be evaluated for potential respiratory and cardiac problems. For example, examine Jackson for chest symmetry, breath sounds, pulses, SpO_2, and ECG evaluation. Jackson should be placed on humidified oxygen to treat his hypoxia and for possible shock.

While placing Jackson on oxygen and an ECG monitor, the following is determined:

- He has a 40-year habit of smoking two packs of cigarettes per day. He states that his doctor told him that he has "mild COPD."
- He has diminished breath sounds with rhonchi bilaterally.
- His vital signs are:
  - Resp: 40 breaths/minute with a productive cough
  - HR: 130 beats/minute and regular (Fig. 10-7)
  - BP: 90/50 mm Hg
  - SpO_2: 78 percent
  - Temp: 102.1° F

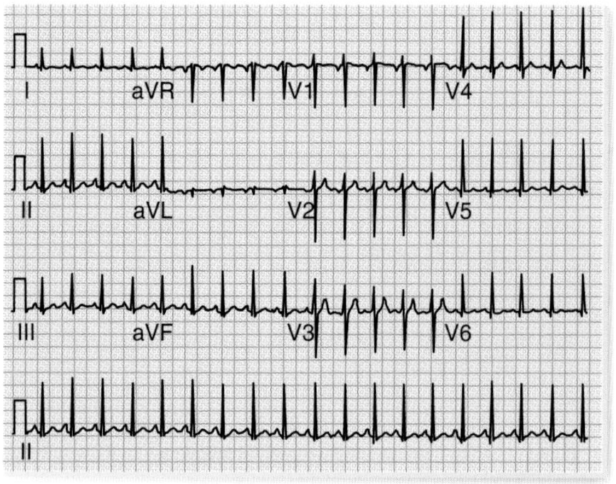

Figure 10-7 Sinus tachycardia (130 beats/minute).

Let's Recap

Having to fight for each breath can be very frightening for patients. Rapid assessment and proper recognition of presenting signs and symptoms by the EMS professional can save lives.

The most important drug used during a respiratory emergency is oxygen. However, conditions such as reversible airway obstruction caused by asthma or COPD may require additional drug options such as bronchodilators, antiasthmatics, or anti-inflammatory drugs. It is important to know each drug classification included in your protocols and how they work so each patient can receive rapid, appropriate treatment.

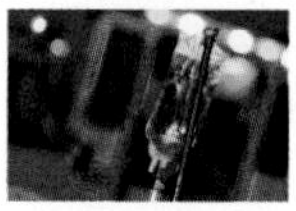

SCENARIO CONCLUSION

You must now try to determine a probable chief complaint to effectively continue treatment and communicate your findings and treatment to the receiving facility.

Jackson's history of smoking and COPD makes him at risk for pneumonia. This is supported by his presentation with fever and productive cough. Therefore, immediate treatment should include transport (as per local protocol), high-flow humidified oxygen to address his hypoxia and developing shock, and an IV to address developing shock. While en route to the receiving facility, reassess Jackson every 3 to 5 minutes and have advanced life support equipment ready to intervene, if needed.

PRACTICE EXERCISES

1. Bronchodilators are used to treat reversible airway obstruction. They work by:
   a. Decreasing edema
   b. Reducing carbon dioxide content
   c. Relaxing the bronchial smooth muscles
   d. Increasing breathing by stimulating the CNS
2. To administer albuterol to a 13-year-old patient, the dosage using a metered-dose inhaler should be:
   a. One-half the adult dose
   b. One inhalation (90 mcg)
   c. Two inhalations (180 mcg)
   d. Three inhalations (270 mcg)
3. Aminophylline is contraindicated in patients:
   a. Who suffer from uncontrolled cardiac arrhythmias
   b. Hypersensitive to theophylline
   c. With CHF
   d. Over 60 years in age
4. The adult dosage for epinephrine to treat bronchial asthma is:
   a. 0.3 to 0.5 mg IV bolus of a 1:10,000 solution
   b. 0.3 to 0.5 mc SubQ of a 1:1000 solution
   c. 3 to 5 mg SubQ of a 1:1000 solution
   d. 0.01 mg/kg SubQ of a 1:1000 solution
5. The most frequent CNS side effect of diphenhydramine is:
   a. Drowsiness
   b. Dizziness
   c. Headache
   d. Anorexia
6. Magnesium sulfate is contraindicated in patients with:
   a. Renal insufficiency
   b. Heart block
   c. Bradycardia
   d. Hypotension
7. Atropine is an anticholinergic drug that competes with the neurotransmitter:
   a. Norepinephrine
   b. Acetylcholine
   c. Epinephrine
   d. Adenosine
8. Diphenhydramine is classified as a(n):
   a. $Beta_1$-adrenergic blocker
   b. $Beta_2$-adrenergic blocker
   c. H_1-receptor agonist
   d. H_2-receptor agonist
9. Lidocaine may be given prior to RSI to prevent or reduce:
   a. Asystole
   b. Bradycardia
   c. Intracranial pressure
   d. Hemodynamic response to intubation
10. Adrenergic drugs primarily act on:
    a. $Beta_1$-receptors
    b. $Beta_2$-receptors
    c. $Alpha_1$-receptors
    d. $Alpha_2$-receptors

CASE STUDIES

1. You are called to a local playground for a child "having trouble breathing." When you arrive, you find a 13-year-old male who is complaining of chest tightness and having trouble breathing. You find out that your patient had been playing "touch football" with his friends. He admits to you that he has asthma and should not have been playing football.

Your initial assessment reveals your patient has wheezing with labored breathing, is pale, and has a rapid heart rate.

A. According to local protocol, your first-line drug for asthma (other than oxygen) is albuterol at an initial dose of:
a. Two inhalations (180 mcg) from a metered-dose inhaler
b. One inhalation (90 mcg) from a metered-dose inhaler
c. 0.01 mcg/kg SubQ
d. 50 mg slow IV

B. A possible life-threatening respiratory side effect of albuterol that you should be assessing for is:
a. Increased wheezing
b. Increased labored breathing
c. Paradoxical bronchospasm
d. Life-threatening tachycardia

2. You are called to the home of a "man having trouble breathing." When you arrive, you find a 44-year-old male on his front porch having difficulty breathing. His wife states that "Charlie got stung by a bee while mowing the lawn. He is allergic to bees." Your initial assessment reveals Charlie has hives, is flushed in appearance, and has audible wheezing.

A. After oxygen, epinephrine is the first-line drug for the treatment of severe anaphylaxis. The initial dosage in this case is 0.1 to 0.5 mg IV, not to exceed:
a. 0.5 mg
b. 1.0 mg
c. 1.5 mg
d. 2.0 mg

B. A second-line drug that may be used after epinephrine while treating anaphylaxis is:
a. Diphenhydramine
b. Albuterol
c. Atropine
d. Terbutaline

MATH EQUATIONS

1. You are ordered to give 1.25 mg/kg of diphenhydramine to your 25 lb pediatric patient. How many mg will you administer to this patient?
2. You are ordered to 4 mcg of epinephrine per minute to your 55-year-old patient. The infusion is prepared by adding 1 mg of a 1:10,000 solution of epinephrine to 500 mL of solution.
   a. What is the resulting concentration of the infusion (mcg/mL)?
   b. How many gtt/minute is infused using a 60 gtt/mL IV set?
3. You are ordered to give 25 mg IV of diphenhydramine to your 50-year-old patient. The diphenhydramine comes packaged as 250 mg in 5 mL.
   a. What is the concentration of the diphenhydramine (mg/mL)?
   b. How much (mL) of the diphenhydramine will you administer?
4. You are ordered to give 0.005 mg/kg of terbutaline to your 30 lb pediatric patient.
   a. How many kg does your patient weigh?
   b. How much volume of terbutaline will you give?
5. You are ordered to give 0.1 mg of epinephrine, followed by a 0.1 mcg/kg/minute continuous infusion of epinephrine. Your pediatric patient weighs 25 lbs. Your epinephrine comes packaged as 1 mg in a 10 mL, 1:10,000 vial.
   a. How many kg does your patient weigh?
   b. What is the concentration of the epinephrine vial (mg/mL)?
   c. How many gtt/minute, using a 60 gtt/mL IV set, are needed to infuse 0.1 mcg/kg/minute.

REFERENCES

Atracurium besylate. Retrieved May 12, 2014 from www.drugs.com/monograph/atracurium-besylate.html

Beck, R. K. (2012). Drugs used to treat pulmonary emergencies. In *Pharmacology for the EMS provider.* New York, NY: Delmar, Cengage Learning.

Cafasso, J. What are adrenergic drugs? Retrieved May 11, 2014 from www.healthline.com/health/adrenergic-drugs#Overview

Cafasso, J. What are anticholinergics? Retrieved May 12, 2014 from www.healthline.com/health/anticholinergics#Overview

Case-Lo, C. What are glucocorticoids? Retrieved May 12, 2014 from www.healthline.com/health/glucocorticoids#Overview

Deglin, J. H., Vallerand, A. H., and Sanboski, C. A. (2011). *Davis's drug guide for nurses* (12th ed.). Philadelphia, PA: F. A. Davis Company.

Kam, P. C. and Cardone, D. (2007). Propofol infusion syndrome. *Anaesthesia, 62,* 690–701.

Neuromuscular blocking agents. Retrieved May 10, 2014 from www.drugs.com/drug-class/neuromuscular-blocking-agents.html

Venes, D., ed. (2013). *Taber's cyclopedic medical dictionary* (22nd ed.). Philadelphia, PA: F. A. Davis Company.

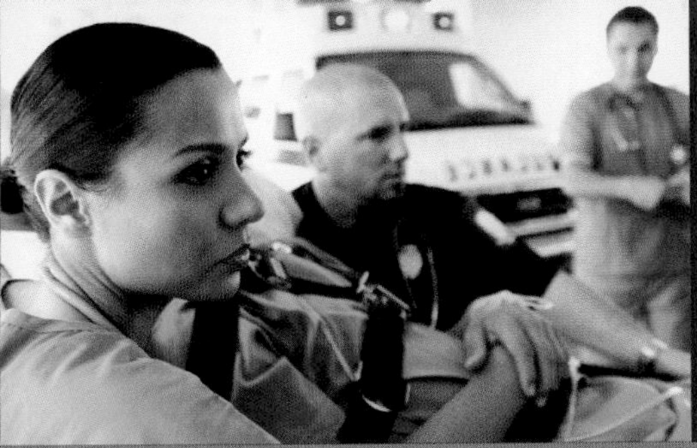

CHAPTER 11

Drugs Used to Treat Cardiovascular Emergencies

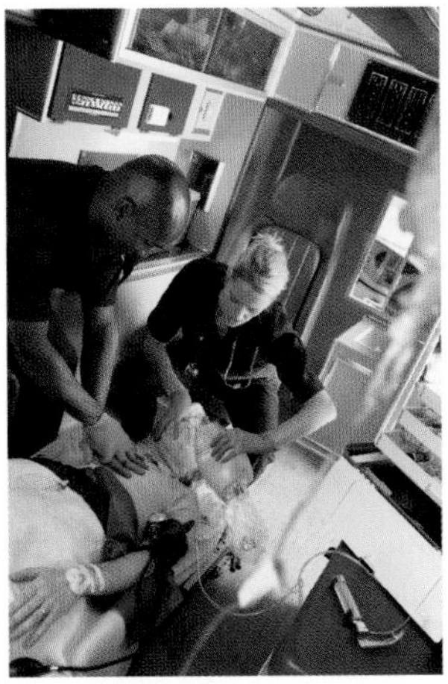

Paramedics working on a cardiac arrest. *(Photograph © Monkey Business Images/Monkey Business/Thinkstock)*

LEARNING OUTCOMES

- Describe the mechanism of action, indications, contraindications, precautions, and adverse reactions and side effects for the following:
  - the antiarrhythmic drugs adenosine, amiodarone, atropine, digoxin, esmolol, lidocaine, phenytoin, procainamide, and sotalol
  - the antianginal drugs atenolol, diltiazem, labetalol, metoprolol, nicardipine, nifedipine, nitroglycerin, propranolol, and verapamil
  - the alkalinizing agent sodium bicarbonate
  - the anticoagulant drugs enoxaparin and heparin
  - the antihypertensive drugs captopril, clevidipine, hydralazine, and lisinopril
  - the antiplatelet drugs abciximab, clopidogrel, enalaprilat, eptifibatide, and tirofiban
  - the diuretic drugs bumetanide and furosemide
  - the medicinal gases nitrous oxide-oxygen mixture and oxygen
  - the mineral/electrolyte/pH modifier magnesium sulfate
  - the nonopioid analgesic aspirin
  - the opioid analgesic morphine
  - the sympathomimetic drugs dobutamine, dopamine, epinephrine, milrinone, norepinephrine, phenylephrine, and vasopressin
  - the thrombolytic drugs alteplase, reteplase, streptokinase, and tenecteplase
- Discuss the roles of cardioversion and defibrillation in cardiovascular emergencies.

KEY TERMS

Antianginal	Cardiogenic shock	Diuretic	Thrombolytic
Antiarrhythmic	Cardioversion	Inotropic agents	Transcutaneous cardiac pacing
Antihypertensive	Congestive heart failure (CHF)	Nonopioid analgesic	Wolff-Parkinson-White syndrome
Antiplatelet	Defibrillation	Opioid analgesic	
Cardiac action potential		Sympathomimetic	

SCENARIO OPENING

You have been assigned to Fire Station 3 for another field-internship clinical rotation. You are just about to eat your first piece of pizza when a call comes in for "chest pain and trouble breathing." When you and the team arrive, a 53-year-old male, Kelvin, is found lying on the living room sofa complaining of substernal chest pain that radiates to his left shoulder and jaw. Kelvin says that he was watching television when the pain began about an hour ago. He passed the pain off as indigestion until it began radiating into his left shoulder and jaw. Kelvin weighs 250 pounds, has no previous cardiac history, and is not taking any medications. The initial examination reveals the following:

Level of consciousness:	alert and oriented, but apprehensive
Respirations:	30 breaths/minute
Breath sounds:	clear bilaterally
Blood pressure:	160/96 mm Hg
Skin condition:	cool and clammy

Introduction

The leading cause of death in the United States and Canada is cardiovascular disease. Often, the initial presentation of cardiovascular disease occurs as an emergency in the out-of-hospital setting. EMS professionals play an integral role in the treatment of cardiovascular emergencies. The treatment for cardiovascular emergencies is the most extensive of any disease state for which EMS professionals are called.

This chapter focuses on the initial treatment including the drugs used in out-of-hospital cardiovascular emergencies. Several categories of drugs are discussed in this chapter. Many of the drugs provide multiple therapeutic actions and are included in several therapeutic categories. Within specific categories, the drugs work via various mechanisms of action, and each is presented in detail within the chapter. For example, **antiarrhythmic** drugs are administered to terminate cardiac arrhythmias. These drugs are classified according to their mechanism of action and their effects on the **cardiac action potential** of cardiac cells. **Inotropic agents** are utilized to increase the force of contractions and improve cardiac output in the setting of **cardiogenic shock. Antihypertensives** act through various mechanisms to reduce blood pressure, while vasopressors cause vasoconstriction to increase blood pressure. Included in this chapter are **antianginal** agents, which are administered to decrease the workload on the heart, reduce the oxygen demands of the heart, and increase coronary blood flow to the heart. **Diuretics** act to reduce pulmonary edema and blood pressure. This chapter also discusses the use of thrombolytic agents to dissolve thrombi and therefore restore blood flow through obstructed vessels.

The appropriate and timely administration of the drugs presented in this chapter has resulted in a significant decrease in morbidity and mortality associated with cardiovascular emergencies. It is vital that EMS professionals be vigilant about maintaining their knowledge of these drugs.

Pathophysiology of Cardiac Disorders

Coronary Artery Disease (CAD)

Coronary artery disease is the narrowing of the coronary arteries in the heart, usually as a result of atherosclerosis (Fig. 11-1). If a blockage within one or more of the coronary arteries occurs, which limits the flow of oxygenated blood to the heart muscle, ischemia or infarction of the heart muscle may occur.

Cardiac Dysrhythmia (Arrhythmia)

A cardiac dysrhythmia is an abnormal rhythm of the heart caused by physiological or pathological disorders in the discharge of electrical impulses from the sinoatrial (SA) node or electrical transmission through the conductive tissue of the heart (Fig. 11-2).

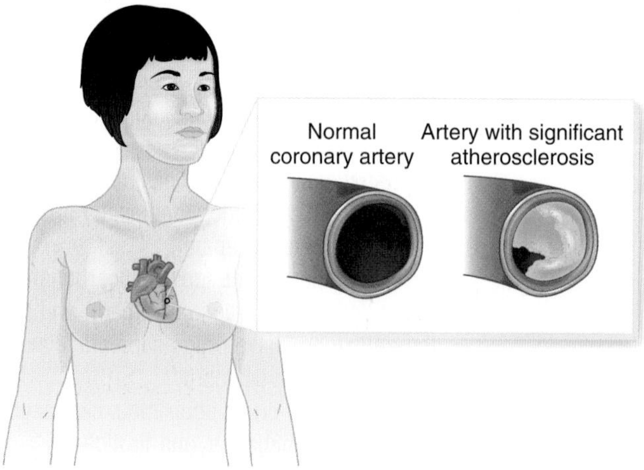

Figure 11-1 A normal coronary artery and an atherosclerotic coronary artery. *(Photograph © Monkey Business Images/Monkey Business/Thinkstock)*

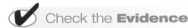

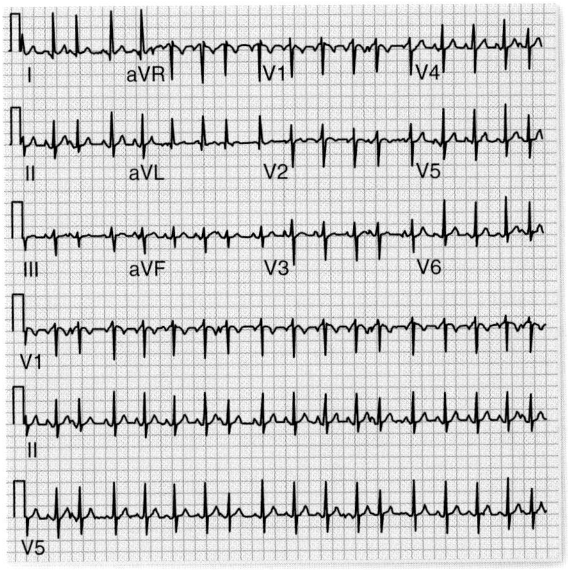

Figure 11-2 Cardiac dysrhythmia—sinus rhythm with PACs.

Congestive Heart Failure (CHF)

Congestive heart failure is the inability of the heart to circulate blood effectively enough to meet the body's needs. It may affect the left ventricle, the right ventricle, or both. CHF can result from either a reduced ability of the heart muscle to contract or from a mechanical problem that limits the ability of the heart's chambers to fill with blood. When weakened, the heart is unable to keep up with the demand. When this happens, blood returns to the heart faster than it can be pumped out so that it gets backed up or congested.

Heart Valve Disorders

- Valve stenosis: Stenosis is when a valve does not open properly. The flaps of a valve thicken, stiffen, or fuse together, resulting in the valve not being able to fully open. If stenosis occurs, the heart has to work harder to pump blood through the valve, and the body may suffer from a reduced supply of oxygen.
- Valve regurgitation: Valve regurgitation is caused by a leaking heart valve, placing a strain on the heart. It can cause the heart to work harder to pump the same amount of blood.
- Mitral valve prolapse (MVP): Mitral valve prolapse is a condition in which the two valve flaps of the mitral valve do not close smoothly or evenly. When the heart contracts, part of one or both mitral flaps collapses backward into the left atrium. In some cases, the prolapsed valve lets a small amount of blood leak backward through the valve, which may cause a heart murmur.

Congenital Heart Defects

A congenital heart defect is a disorder with the structure of the heart. The defects can involve the walls of the heart, the valves of the heart, and the arteries and veins near the heart. The blood flow through the heart can slow down, go in the wrong direction or to the wrong place, or be blocked completely.

> **Check the Evidence**
>
> Congenital heart defects are the most common type of birth defect.

Pacing, Cardioversion, and Defibrillation

The heart is able to beat due to electrical activity beginning in the SA node, progressing through the conduction network of the atria, proceeding to the atrioventricular (AV) node, and finally moving through the conduction network of the ventricles. Since the heart functions due to electricity, there are instances when EMS professionals use electricity to stabilize or restart the heart, alone or in combination with cardiac medications.

Transcutaneous Cardiac Pacing

Transcutaneous cardiac pacing (TCP) emits periodic electrical discharges to help stabilize symptomatic cardiac dysrhythmias such as bradycardia, heart blocks, and the suppression of some ventricular tachydysrhythmias. TCP can function in one of two modes, asynchronous or demand pacing.

Asynchronous pacing delivers electrical impulses at a preselected timed interval regardless of the patient's own cardiac activity. Demand pacing can sense the patient's own QRS complex and produces stimuli only when needed. If the demand mode does not sense any beats, the pacemaker will deliver pacing stimuli at a preselected rate, usually at 70 beats per minute.

Cardioversion

Cardioversion relies on the delivery of synchronized shock of direct electrical current. It is used to terminate dysrhythmias such as atrial fibrillation, atrial flutter, supraventricular tachycardia, and well-tolerated ventricular tachycardia. The electrical stimuli of cardioversion is timed to avoid the T wave of cardiac repolarization to avoid triggering a malignant dysrhythmia.

> **Check the Evidence**
>
> Cardioversion should not be used in patients who have recently eaten (risk of vomiting), in patients with severe electrolyte abnormalities, or in patients with drug overdoses.

Defibrillation

Defibrillation (unsynchronized cardioversion) delivers an electrical stimulus decided by the person operating the defibrillator regardless of where the shock occurs during the cardiac cycle. The defibrillation shock depolarizes the majority of the myocardial cells, placing the heart in brief asystole and giving it a chance for its normal pacemaker to resume discharging. Defibrillation is the single most important intervention EMS can make in patients who have suffered cardiac arrest due to ventricular fibrillation (V-Fib) or pulseless ventricular tachycardia (PVT). Once cardioversion or defibrillation has restored the patient's cardiac function, pharmacologic interventions can be administered to help stabilize the patient's heart.

Pharmacokinetics

Alkalinizing Agents

Alkalinizing drugs are used to buffer acid buildup, raising the body's pH.

Antianginals

Nitrates dilate coronary arteries and cause systemic vasodilation (decreased preload). Calcium channel blockers dilate coronary arteries and can slow heart rate. Beta blockers decrease myocardial oxygen consumption by decreasing the heart rate.

Antiarrhythmic Drugs

Antiarrhythmic drugs correct cardiac arrhythmias through a variety of mechanisms, depending on the group used. The choice of antiarrhythmic drug depends on the etiology of the arrhythmia. Antiarrhythmics are classified by their effects on cardiac conduction tissue in the following groups:

- **Group I:** These drugs decrease the rate of entry of sodium during cardiac membrane depolarization and decrease the rate of rise of phase "O" of the cardiac membrane action potential (see Fig. 9-3). Antiarrhythmics are further listed in subgroups according to their effects on action potential duration:
  - **Group IA:** Depress phase "O" and prolong the duration of the action potential

  For example, procainamide or quinidine.
  - **Group IB:** Slightly depress phase "O" and shorten the action potential

  For example, lidocaine or phenytoin.
  - **Group IC:** Slight effect on repolarization but marked depression of phase "O" of the action potential; significant slowing of conduction

  For example, flecainide or propafenone.
- **Group II:** Competitively block beta-adrenergic receptors and depress phase "4" depolarization
  For example, acebutolol or propranolol.
- **Group III:** Prolong the duration of the relative refractory period without changing the phase of depolarization of the resting membrane potential
  For example, amiodarone or sotalol.
- **Group IV:** Slow conduction velocity and increase the refractoriness of the AV node
  For example, verapamil.

Anticoagulants

Anticoagulants act by preventing blood clot extensions and formation. Anticoagulants do not dissolve clots.

Antihypertensives

Antihypertensives are classified into groups according to their site of action. These include:

- Peripherally acting antiadrenergics
- Centrally acting alpha-adrenergics
- Beta blockers
- Vasodilators
- ACE inhibitors
- Angiotension II antagonists
- Calcium channel blockers
- Diuretics

Check the Evidence

The goal of antihypertensives is to lower blood pressure to a normal level (less than 90 mm Hg diastolic) or to the lowest level tolerated.

Antiplatelet Drugs

Antiplatelet drugs inhibit platelet aggregation and prolong bleeding time.

Diuretics

Diuretics enhance the excretion of various electrolytes and water by affecting renal mechanisms for tubular secretion and reabsorption.

Minerals/Electrolytes/pH Modifiers

Maintenance of these agents within normal limits is required for many physiological processes such as cardiac, nerve, and muscle function; bone growth and stability; and a number of other activities.

Nonopioid Analgesics

Nonopioid analgesics inhibit prostaglandin synthesis peripherally for analgesic effects and centrally for antipyretic effects.

Opioid Analgesics

Opioid analgesics bind to opiate receptors in the CNS, acting as antagonists, altering the perception of and response to pain.

Sympathomimetic Drugs

Sympathomimetic drugs produce effects resembling those from stimulation of the sympathetic nervous system.

Thrombolytics

Thrombolytic drugs convert plasminogen to plasmin, which then degrades fibrin in blood clots.

Individual Drugs

Abciximab (ab-SIX-i-mab)

ReoPro

Classification: Glycoprotein IIb/IIIa inhibitor

Pregnancy Class: C

Mechanism of Action: Inhibits the integrin GP IIb/IIIa receptor, preventing the aggregation of platelets
Pharmacokinetics
Absorption: Well absorbed
Onset: 2 hours
Duration: 24 to 48 hours after infusion is stopped
Indications: Used for UA/NSTEMI patients undergoing planned or emergency percutaneous coronary intervention (PCI)
Contraindications: Known hypersensitivity; should not be given to patients with a bleeding disorder or any active bleeding or to patients with intracranial hemorrhage, neoplasm, AV malformation, aneurysm, or stroke within 2 years; should not be given to patients with major surgery within 6 weeks or to patients with aortic dissection, pericarditis, and severe hypertension
Precautions: Use with caution in patients who may have an increased risk of bleeding.
Route and Dosage
IV (Adult): PCI only—0.25 mg/kg, followed by IV infusion of 10 mcg/minute UA/NSTEMI with planned PCI within 24 hours—0.25 mg/kg 10 to 60 minutes prior to procedure, then 0.125 mcg/kg/minute by IV infusion
How Supplied
Injection: 2 mg/mL
Adverse Reactions and Side Effects
Resp: Anaphylactic shock
CV: Hypotension
CNS: Intracranial hemorrhage, stroke
GI: GI bleeding
GU: Hematuria
Misc: Internal bleeding
Drug Interactions: Incompatibility with dextran
EMS Considerations: Readministration may cause anaphylaxis.

Adenosine (a-DEN-oh-seen)

Adenocard, Adenoscan
Classification: Antiarrhythmic
Pregnancy Class: C
Mechanism of Action: Restores normal sinus rhythm (NSR) by interrupting reentry pathways in the AV node; slows conduction through the AV node and causes coronary artery vasodilation
Pharmacokinetics
Absorption: Complete absorption
Onset: Immediate
Duration: 1 to 2 minutes
Indications: Used for the conversion of paroxysmal supraventricular tachycardia (PSVT), including **Wolff-Parkinson-White syndrome** (Fig. 11-3), to a NSR
Contraindications: Known hypersensitivity; should not be given to patients in second- or third-degree AV block or to patients in **sick sinus syndrome**
Precautions: Use with caution in patients with a history of asthma and in patients with unstable angina.

Check the Evidence
Adenosine may induce bronchospasm in asthma patients.

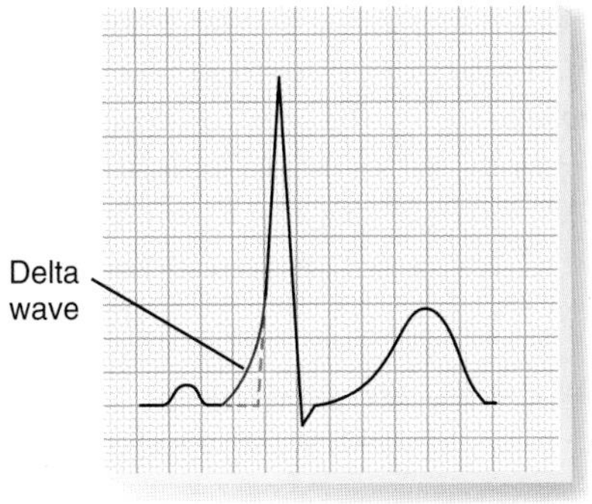

Figure 11-3 Wolff-Parkinson-White Syndrome.

Route and Dosage
IV [Adult and Pediatric greater than 50 kg (110 lbs)]: 6 mg by rapid IV bolus. If unsuccessful, repeat in 1 to 2 minutes at 12 mg bolus. The 12-mg dose may be repeated.
IV [Pediatric less than 50 kg (110 lbs)]: 0.05 to 0.1 mg/kg as a rapid bolus dose. May be repeated in 1 to 2 minutes. If unsuccessful, the dose may be increased by 0.05 to 0.1 mg/kg until sinus rhythm is established or a maximum dose of 0.3 mg/kg is used.
How Supplied
Injection: 6 mg/2-mL vial (Adenocard), 3 mg/1 mL in 30-mL vial (Adenoscan)
Adverse Reactions and Side Effects
Resp: Shortness of breath, chest pressure, hyperventilation
CV: Transient arrhythmias, chest pain, hypotension, palpitations
CNS: Apprehension, dizziness, headache, head pressure, light-headedness
EENT: Blurred vision, throat tightness
GI: Metallic taste, nausea
Derm: Burning sensation, facial flushing
Drug Interactions: Concurrent use with digoxin may increase the risk of ventricular fibrillation.
EMS Considerations: Assess patient vital signs frequently.

Alteplase (AL-te-plase)

Activase, 🍁 Activase t-PA, Cathflo Activase, tissue plasminogen activator, t-PA
Classifications: Thrombolytic, plasminogen activator
Pregnancy Class: C
Mechanism of Action: Converts plasminogen to plasmin, which is then able to degrade fibrin present in blood clots
Pharmacokinetics
Absorption: Complete absorption after IV administration
Onset: 30 minutes
Duration: Unknown
Indications: Used for the treatment of acute MI and acute stroke
Contraindications: Known hypersensitivity; should not be given to patients with a history of stroke, recent intracranial or intraspinal injury or trauma, intracranial neoplasm, or AV malformation or aneurysm
Precautions: Use with caution in patients with recent major surgery, trauma, GI or GU bleeding, severe liver or renal disease,

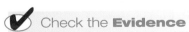

hemorrhagic ophthalmic conditions, or recent streptococcal infection.

Route and Dosage

MI: IV (Adult)—15 mg bolus, then 0.75 mg/kg, up to 50 mg, over 30 minutes, then 0.5 mg/kg, up to 35 mg, over the next 60 minutes

***effective* Communication**

The dosage for myocardial infarction (MI) is usually accompanied by heparin therapy.

Acute Ischemic Stroke: IV (Adult) —0.9 mg/kg, not to exceed 90 mg, IV infusion over 1 hour, with 10 percent of the dose given as a bolus over the first minute

Understand the Numbers

You are ordered to give 0.9 mg/kg of alteplase to your 130-pound patient over 1 hour. What is the bolus dose over the first minute for this patient?

130 lb ÷ 2.2 kg = 59 kg. 0.9 mg × 59 kg = 53 mg. 10% of 53 kg = 5.3 mg IV bolus over 1 minute.

How Supplied

Powder for injection: 2 mg/vial, 50 mg/vial, 100 mg/vial

Adverse Reactions and Side Effects

Resp: Bronchospasm

CV: Hypotension, reperfusion arrhythmias

CNS: INTRACRANIAL HEMORRHAGE

EENT: Epistaxis, gingival bleeding

GI: GI BLEEDING, RETROPERITONEAL BLEEDING, nausea, vomiting

GU: GU TRACT BLEEDING

Local: Phlebitis at IV site

Misc: ANAPHYLAXIS

Drug Interactions: Concurrent use of aspirin and other NSAIDs, warfarin, and heparin may increase the risk of bleeding.

EMS Considerations: (!) Overdosing and underdosing have resulted in patient harm, including death. Monitor vital signs frequently during therapy. Notify medical control if systolic BP higher than 180 mm Hg or diastolic BP higher than 110 mm Hg.

Amiodarone (am-ee-OH-da-rone)

Cordarone, Nexterone, Pacerone

Classification: Class III antiarrhythmic

Pregnancy Class: D

Mechanism of Action: Prolongs the action potential and the refractory period; slows the sinus rate, increasing the PR interval (Fig. 11-4) and the QT interval (Fig. 11-5); and decreases peripheral vascular resistance

Pharmacokinetics

Absorption: Complete bioavailability with IV administration

Onset: IV—2 hours

Duration: IV—unknown

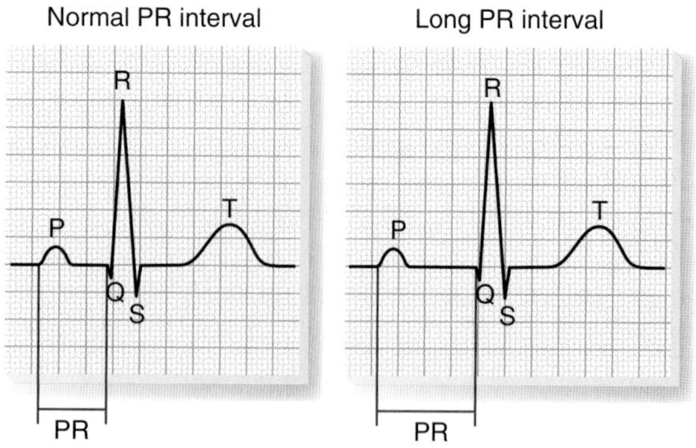

Figure 11-4 Increased PR interval.

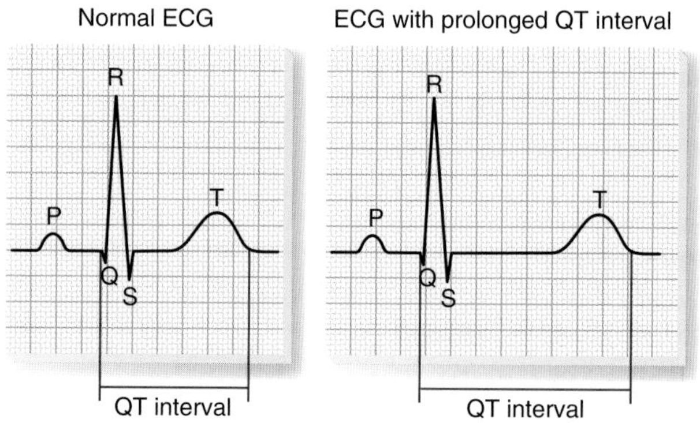

Figure 11-5 Increased QT interval.

Indications: Used as part of the Advanced Cardiac Life Support (ACLS) and Pediatric Advanced Life Support (PALS) guidelines for the management of ventricular fibrillation and PVT after CPR and defibrillation have failed; can be used for other life-threatening tachyarrhythmias as well

Contraindications: Known hypersensitivity; should not be given to patients with cardiogenic shock or to patients with second- and third-degree AV block. (!) Amiodarone enters breast milk and causes harm to the neonate.

Precautions: Use with caution in patients with a history of CHF or thyroid disorders and in those with severe pulmonary or liver disease.

Route and Dosage

IV/IO (Adult): ACLS guidelines for pulseless V-Fib/V-Tach—300 mg bolus; may be repeated in 3 to 5 minutes at 150 mg bolus. Ventricular arrhythmias—150 mg over 10 minutes, followed by 360 mg over the next 6 hours

IV/IO (Pediatric): PALS guidelines for pulseless V-Fib/V-Tach—5 mg/kg bolus. Perfusion tachycardia—5 mg/kg over 20 to 60 minutes

How Supplied

Injection: 50 mg/mL

Adverse Reactions and Side Effects

Resp: ADULT RESPIRATORY DISTRESS SYNDROME (ARDS), PULMONARY FIBROSIS, PULMONARY TOXICITY

CV: CHF, DETERIORATING OF ARRHYTHMIAS, <u>bradycardia</u>, <u>hypotension</u>

CNS: Dizziness, fatigue, malaise, headache, insomnia, confusion, disorientation, hallucinations
GI: Anorexia, constipation, nausea, vomiting, abdominal pain, abnormal sense of taste
Neuro: Ataxia, involuntary movement, paresthesia, peripheral neuropathy, poor coordination, tremor
Derm: TOXIC EPIDERMAL NECROLYSIS (rare)
Drug Interactions: Increased risk of bradyarrhythmias, sinus arrest, or AV heart block with beta blockers or calcium channel blockers
EMS Considerations: During administration, the ECG should be monitored for increased PR and QRS intervals, increased arrhythmias, and bradycardia. Respiratory status and blood pressure should be monitored closely.

Aspirin (AS-pir-in)

🍁 Apo-ASA, 🍁 Arthrinol, 🍁 Arthrisin, 🍁 Artria S.R., ASA, 🍁 Asaphen, Ascriptin, Aspercin, Aspergum, Aspirtab, 🍁 Astrin, Bayer Aspirin, Bufferin, 🍁 Coryphen, Easprin, Ecotrin, 🍁 Entrophen, Genacote, Halfprin, 🍁 Headache Tablets, Healthprin, 🍁 Novasen, 🍁 PMS-ASA, 🍁 Rivasa, St. Joseph Adult Chewable Aspirin, ZORprin

Classifications: Antipyretic, nonopioid analgesic, salicylate
Pregnancy Class: D (first trimester)
Mechanism of Action: Produces analgesia and reduces inflammation and fever by inhibiting the production of prostaglandins; decreases platelet aggregation
Pharmacokinetics
Absorption: Well absorbed from the upper small intestine. Absorption from enteric-coated aspirin is unreliable. Rectal absorption is slow and variable.
Onset: PO—5 to 30 minutes; Rectal—1 to 2 hours
Duration: PO—3 to 6 hours; Rectal—7 hours
Indications: Used as a prophylaxis of MI and transient ischemic attacks
Contraindications: Known hypersensitivity; should not be given to patients with bleeding disorders

effective Communication

Aspirin should not be given to children or adolescents with viral infections due to the risk of developing Reye syndrome.

Precautions: Use with caution in patients with a history of GI bleeding or ulcer disease, in patients with chronic alcohol use or severe renal disease, and in patients with severe liver disease.

Route and Dosage

PO (Adult): 50 to 325 mg once daily

How Supplied (All OTC)

Tablets: 81 mg, 162.5 mg, 325 mg, 500 mg, 650 mg, 🍁 975 mg
Chewable tablets: 🍁 80 mg, 81 mg
Chewing gum: 227 mg
Dispersible tablets: 325 mg, 500 mg
Enteric-coated (delayed-release) tablets: 80 mg, 165 mg, 🍁 600 mg, 650 mg, 975 mg
Extended-release tablets: 🍁 325 mg, 650 mg, 800 mg
Delayed-release capsules: 🍁 325 mg, 🍁 500 mg
Suppositories: 60 mg, 120 mg, 125 mg, 130 mg, 🍁 150 mg, 🍁 160 mg, 195 mg, 200 mg, 300 mg, 🍁 320 mg, 325 mg, 600 mg, 🍁 640 mg, 650 mg, 1.2 g

Adverse Reactions and Side Effects

EENT: Tinnitus
GI: GI BLEEDING, dyspepsia, epigastric distress, nausea, abdominal pain, anorexia, vomiting
Hemat: Anemia, increased bleeding time
Misc: ANAPHYLAXIS, LARYNGEAL EDEMA
Drug Interactions: May increase the risk of bleeding when taken with thrombolytic medications; increased risk of GI irritation when taken with NSAIDs
EMS Considerations: Aspirin should be administered as soon as possible if a TIA, stroke, or MI is suspected.

Check the **Evidence**

Patients who have asthma, allergies, and nasal polyps or who are hypersensitive to tartrazine are at an increased risk for developing hypersensitive reactions.

Atenolol (a-TEN-oh-lole)

🍁 Apo-Atenolol, 🍁 Novo-Atenolol, Tenormin

Classifications: Antianginal, antihypertensive, beta blocker
Pregnancy Class: D
Mechanism of Action: Blocks stimulation of $beta_2$ (myocardial)-adrenergic receptors
Pharmacokinetics
Absorption: 50 to 60 percent after PO administration
Onset: PO—1 hour
Duration: PO—24 hours
Indications: Used for the management of hypertension and angina pectoris and for the prevention of MI
Contraindications: Known hypersensitivity; should not be given to patients with uncompensated CHF, pulmonary edema, cardiogenic shock, bradycardia, or heart block
Precautions: Use with caution in patients with renal impairment, liver impairment, pulmonary disease, or diabetes mellitus and in patients with a history of severe allergic reactions. ❗ Atenolol crosses the placenta and may cause fetal/neonatal bradycardia, hypotension, hypoglycemia, or respiratory depression.

Route and Dosage

PO (Adult): Antianginal—50 mg once daily; may be increased after 1 week to 100 mg/day; Antihypertensive—25 to 50 mg once daily; may be increased after 2 weeks to 50 to 100 mg once daily; MI—50 mg to start, then 50 mg 12 hours later and 100 mg/day as a single dose or in two divided doses until hospital discharge

effective **Communication**

Take apical pulse and compare with ECG monitor before administration. If heart rate is less than 50 beats/minute or if arrhythmia occurs, notify medical control.

How Supplied
Tablets: 25 mg, 50 mg, 100 mg
Adverse Reactions and Side Effects
Resp: Bronchospasm, wheezing
CV: BRADYCARDIA, CHF, PULMONARY EDEMA
CNS: Fatigue, weakness, anxiety, depression, dizziness, drowsiness, insomnia, memory loss, mental status changes, nervousness, nightmares
EENT: Blurred vision, stuffy nose
GI: Constipation, diarrhea, nausea, vomiting
GU: Erectile dysfunction, decreased libido, urinary frequency
Drug Interactions: IV phenytoin and verapamil may cause additive myocardial depression. Additive bradycardia may occur with digoxin, and additive hypotension may occur with other antihypertensives.
EMS Considerations: Do not administer if the patient's heart rate is less than 50 beats/minute or systolic BP is lower than 90 mm Hg. With diabetic patients, watch for symptoms of hypoglycemia (hypotension or tachycardia).

Atropine (AT-ro-peen)

AtroPen
Classifications: Antiarrhythmic, anticholinergic
Pregnancy Class: C
Mechanism of Action: Atropine is an anticholinergic drug that competes with the neurotransmitter acetylcholine for receptor sites, blocking the stimulation of parasympathetic nerve fibers.
Pharmacokinetics
Absorption: Well absorbed
Onset: Rapid via inhalation administration
Duration: 4 to 6 hours
Indications: Used for the treatment of sinus bradycardia and heart block
Contraindications: Known hypersensitivity; should not be given to patients with angle-closure glaucoma, acute hemorrhage, or tachycardia secondary to cardiac insufficiency or thyrotoxicosis
Precautions: Use with caution in patients with intra-abdominal infections or prostatic hyperplasia and in patients with chronic renal, liver, pulmonary, or cardiac disease.
Route and Dosage
IV (Adult): 0.5 to 1 mg over 1 minute. May be repeated every 3 to 5 minutes, but not to exceed a total of 3 mg. Rapid administration (less than 1 minute) may be used during cardiac arrest and followed by a saline flush.
IV (Pediatric): 0.02 mg/kg over 1 minute. May repeat one time; minimum dose = 0.1 mg, and a maximum single dose = 0.5 mg. Rapid administration (less than 1 minute) may be used during cardiac arrest and followed by a saline flush.

Check the Evidence

Slow administration of atropine (longer than 1 minute) may cause paradoxical bradycardia, which usually resolves in approximately 2 minutes.

How Supplied
Injection: 0.05 mg/mL, 0.1 mg/mL, 0.4 mg/mL, 1 mg/mL
Adverse Reactions and Side Effects
Resp: Tachypnea, pulmonary edema
CV: Tachycardia, palpitations, arrhythmias
CNS: Drowsiness, confusion
GI: Dry mouth, constipation, impaired motility of the GI tract
Misc: Flushing, decreased sweating
Drug Interactions: Increased anticholinergic effects with other anticholinergics. Antacids decrease absorption of anticholinergics.
EMS Considerations: Assess vital signs and ECG frequently during therapy. Report any significant changes in HR or BP or signs of increased ventricular ectopy to medical control.

Bumetanide (byoo-MET-a-nide)

Bumex, ✦ Burinex
Classification: Loop diuretic
Pregnancy Class: C
Mechanism of Action: Inhibits the reabsorption of sodium and chloride from Henle's loop and the distal renal tubule
Pharmacokinetics
Absorption: Well absorbed after IM administration
Onset: IM—30 to 60 minutes; IV—2 minutes
Duration: IM—4 to 6 hours; IV—2 to 3 hours
Indications: Used to treat edema due to heart failure
Contraindications: Known hypersensitivity; should not be given to patients with anuria
Precautions: Use with caution in patients with severe liver disease or electrolyte depletion and to patients who are diabetic.
Route and Dosage
IM, IV (Adult): 0.5 to 1 mg/dose; may be repeated every 2 to 3 hours as needed, up to 10 mg/day
How Supplied
Injection: 0.25 mg/mL
Adverse Reactions and Side Effects
CV: Hypotension
CNS: Dizziness, encephalopathy, headache
EENT: Hearing loss, tinnitus
F and E: Dehydration, hypochloremia, hypokalemia, hypomagnesemia, hyponatremia, hypovolemia, metabolic alkalosis
Drug Interactions: Increased hypotension with other antihypertensives or nitrates; an increased risk of hypokalemia if used with other diuretics
EMS Considerations: Frequently monitor vital signs and lung sounds looking for edema or signs of developing dehydration.

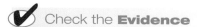

effective Communication

Excessive amounts of bumetanide can ultimately lead to circulatory collapse.

Captopril (KAP-toe-pril)

Capoten

Classifications: Antihypertensive, ACE inhibitor
Pregnancy Class: C (first trimester), D (second and third trimesters)
Mechanism of Action: Blocks the conversion of angiotensin I to the vasoconstrictor angiotensin II, resulting in systemic vasodilation
Pharmacokinetics

Absorption: 60 to 70 percent absorbed after PO administration. Absorption is decreased by the presence of food in the stomach.
Onset: 15 to 60 minutes
Duration: 6 to12 hours

Indications: Used for the management of CHF
Contraindications: Known hypersensitivity; should not be given to patients with a history of angioedema with previous use of ACE inhibitors
Precautions: Use with caution in patients with liver impairment, hypovolemia, or hyponatremia or in those on concurrent diuretic therapy. ❗ Black patients are at an increased risk of angioedema.

Route and Dosage

PO (Adult): Hypertension—12.5 to 25 mg two to three times daily. CHF—25 mg three times daily. Post MI—6.25-mg test dose, followed by 12.5 mg three times daily

✔ Check the Evidence

A severe drop in blood pressure may occur during the first 1 to 3 hours after the first dose of captopril. This may require volume expansion with NS. However, this is not generally considered an indication for stopping therapy.

How Supplied

Tablets: 12.5 mg, 25 mg, 50 mg, 40 mg

Adverse Reactions and Side Effects

Resp: Cough, dyspnea
CV: Hypotension, chest pain, edema, tachycardia
CNS: Dizziness, drowsiness, fatigue, headache, insomnia, vertigo, weakness
GI: Taste disturbances, abdominal pain, anorexia, constipation, diarrhea, nausea, vomiting
Derm: Flushing, rashes
Misc: ANGIOEDEMA, fever
Drug Interactions: Excessive hypotension may occur with concurrent use of diuretics and antihypertensives. Antihypertensive response may be decreased by NSAIDs.
EMS Considerations: If possible, correct volume depletion before the initiation of therapy. Monitor vital signs frequently.

Clevidipine (kle-VI-di-peen)

Cleviprex

Classifications: Antihypertensive, calcium channel blocker
Pregnancy Class: C
Mechanism of Action: Inhibits the calcium transport into vascular smooth muscle; decreases systemic vascular resistance but does not reduce preload
Pharmacokinetics

Absorption: Complete bioavailability
Onset: 2 to 4 minutes
Duration: Until the end of infusion

Indications: Used for the reduction of blood pressure when oral therapy is not feasible
Contraindications: Known hypersensitivity; should not be given to patients with an allergy to soybeans or eggs/egg products, pancreatitis, or severe aortic stenosis
Precautions: Use with caution in patients with decreased liver, renal, or cardiac function. ❗ Geriatric patients should have therapy beginning at the low end of the dose range.

Route and Dosage

IV (Adult): Initial dose is 1 to 2 mg/hour. Titrate dosing according to medical control and local protocol. The usual dose required is 4 to 6 mg/hour.

effective Communication

Patients with severe hypertension may require higher doses with a maximum of 16 mg/hour.

How Supplied

Emulsion for injection 0.5 mg/mL: 50-mL vial, 100-mL vial

Adverse Reactions and Side Effects

CV: CHF, hypotension, rebound hypertension, reflex tachycardia
CNS: Headache
GI: Nausea, vomiting
Drug Interactions: Increased risk of excessive hypotension with other antihypertensives
EMS Considerations: Monitor vital signs frequently during therapy. Hypotension and reflex tachycardia may occur with a rapid upward titration.

Clopidogrel (kloh-PID-oh-grel)

Plavix

Classification: Antiplatelet agent
Pregnancy Class: B
Mechanism of Action: Inhibits platelet aggregation by irreversibly inhibiting the binding of adenosine triphosphate (ATP) to platelet receptors
Pharmacokinetics

Absorption: Well absorbed
Onset: Within 24 hours
Duration: 5 days following discontinuation

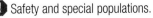

Indications: Used for the reduction of atherosclerotic events in patients at risk, including those with recent MI, acute coronary syndrome, stroke, and vascular death
Contraindications: Known hypersensitivity; should not be given to patients with pathological bleeding disorders such as peptic ulcer or intracranial hemorrhage
Precautions: Use with caution in patients at risk for bleeding and in patients with severe liver impairment or a history of GI bleeding/ulcer disease, etc.
Route and Dosage
PO (Adult): Recent MI, stroke, or peripheral vascular disease—75 mg once daily. Acute coronary syndrome—300 mg initially, then 75 mg once daily. Give aspirin 75 mg to 325 mg once daily concurrently.
How Supplied
Tablets: 75 mg, 300 mg
Adverse Reactions and Side Effects
Resp: Cough, dyspnea
CV: Chest pain, edema, hypertension
CNS: Depression, dizziness, fatigue, headache
EENT: Epistaxis
GI: GI BLEEDING, abdominal pain, diarrhea, gastritis
Hemat: BLEEDING, NEUTROPENIA, THROMBOTIC THROMBOCYTOPENIC PURPURA
Drug Interactions: Concurrent use of aspirin, NSAIDs, heparin, thrombolytic agents, or warfarin may increase the risk of bleeding.
EMS Considerations: None

Digoxin (di-JOX-in)

Lanoxin
Classifications: Antiarrhythmic, inotropic, digitalis glycoside
Pregnancy Class: C
Mechanism of Action: Increases the force of myocardial contractions, prolongs the refractory period of the AV node, and decreases conduction through the SA and AV nodes
Pharmacokinetics
  Absorption: Well absorbed via IV
  Onset: 5 to 30 minutes
  Duration: 2 to 4 days with normal kidney function
Indications: Used for atrial fibrillation and atrial flutter to slow ventricular rate, paroxysmal atrial tachycardia (PAT), and heart failure
Contraindications: Known hypersensitivity; should not be given to patients with uncontrolled ventricular arrhythmias, AV block, idiopathic hypertrophic subaortic stenosis, and constrictive pericarditis
Precautions: Use with caution in patients with hypokalemia, hypercalcemia, hypomagnesemia, renal impairment, and MI.

❗ Geriatric patients are very sensitive to toxic effects—dose adjustments are required.
Route and Dosage
IV (Adult): 0.5 to 1 mg given as 50 percent of the dose initially (0.25 to 0.5 mg)
How Supplied
Injection: 0.25 mg/mL
Adverse Reactions and Side Effects
CV: ARRHYTHMIAS, bradycardia, ECG changes, AV block, SA block
CNS: Fatigue, headache, weakness
EENT: Blurred vision, yellow or green vision
GI: Anorexia, nausea, vomiting, diarrhea
Drug Interactions: Thiazide and loop diuretics and excessive use of laxatives may cause hypokalemia, which may increase the risk of toxicity. Concurrent use of sympathomimetics may increase the risk of arrhythmias.
EMS Considerations: Do not administer digoxin if the patient's ECG is less than 60 beats/minute. Notify medical control if there are any significant ECG changes in rate, rhythm, or quality of the patient's pulse.

Diltiazem (dil-TYE-a-zem)

🍁 Apo-Diltiaz, Cardizem, 🍁 Novo-Diltiazem, 🍁 Syn-Diltiazem
Classifications: Antianginal, class IV antiarrhythmic, antihypertensive, calcium channel blocker
Pregnancy Class: C
Mechanism of Action: Inhibits the transport of calcium into myocardial and vascular smooth muscle cells
Pharmacokinetics
  Absorption: Well absorbed but rapidly metabolized
  Onset: 2 to 5 minutes
  Duration: Unknown
Indications: Used in the management of angina pectoris and vasospastic (Prinzmetal) angina and supraventricular tachycardia (SVT) and in rapid ventricular rates in atrial fibrillation or atrial flutter
Contraindications: Known hypersensitivity; should not be given to patients with sick sinus syndrome, second- or third-degree AV block, recent MI, or pulmonary congestion or to patients with a systolic BP lower than 90 mm Hg
Precautions: Use with caution in patients with severe liver impairment, severe renal impairment, serious ventricular arrhythmias, or CHF.
Route and Dosage
IV (Adult): 0.25 mg/kg; may be repeated within 15 minutes with a dose of 0.35 mg/kg; may follow with an infusion (range 5 to 15 mg/hour) for up to 24 hours

effective Communication

The dosage for obese patients should be based on ideal weight and not actual weight.

Understand the Numbers

Your patient is a 33-year-old 195-pound patient. What is your first and repeat dose of diltiazem?
195 lb ÷ 2.2 kg = 88.6 or 89 kg. 89 kg × 0.25 mg = 22.25 mg (first dose). 89 kg × 0.35 mg = 31.15 mg (second dose).

How Supplied
Injection: 5 mg/mL
Adverse Reactions and Side Effects
Resp: Cough, dyspnea
CV: ARRHYTHMIAS, CHF, peripheral edema, bradycardia, chest pain, hypotension, palpitations, syncope, tachycardia
CNS: Abnormal dreams, anxiety, confusion, dizziness, drowsiness, headache, nervousness, psychiatric disturbances, weakness
EENT: Blurred vision, disturbed equilibrium, epistaxis, tinnitus
GI: Anorexia, constipation, diarrhea, dry mouth, dyspepsia, nausea, vomiting
GU: Nocturia, polyuria, sexual dysfunction, urinary frequency
Derm: Flushing, sweating, photosensitivity, rash
Misc: STEVENS-JOHNSON SYNDROME
Drug Interactions: Increased hypotension may occur when used with other antihypertensives. Concurrent use with beta blockers, digoxin, or phenytoin may result in bradycardia, conduction defects, or CHF.
EMS Considerations: Monitor vital signs and ECG frequently during therapy. Assess for signs of CHF during therapy.

Dobutamine (doe-BYOO-ta-meen)

Dobutrex
Classifications: Inotropic, adrenergic
Pregnancy Class: B
Mechanism of Action: Stimulates $beta_1$- (myocardial) adrenergic receptors with a minor effect on the heart rate or on the peripheral blood vessels
Pharmacokinetics
Absorption: Complete bioavailability
Onset: 1 to 2 minutes
Duration: Minutes
Indications: Used for the short-term management of heart failure caused by depressed contractility
Contraindications: Known hypersensitivity; should not be given to patients hypersensitive to bisulfites or to patients with idiopathic hypertrophic subaortic stenosis
Precautions: Use with caution in patients with a history of hypertension, MI, or atrial fibrillation and in patients with history of ventricular atopic activity.

effective **Communication**

Patients should have hypovolemia corrected before administration of dobutamine.

Route and Dosage
IV (Adult and Pediatric): 2.5 to 15 mcg/kg/minute, titrated to response. Maximum dose is generally up to 40 mcg/kg/minute.

effective **Communication**

Administer dobutamine into a large vein and assess frequently. Extravasation may cause pain and inflammation.

How Supplied
Injection: 12.5 mg/mL in 20-, 40-, 60-, and 100-mL vials
Premixed infusion: 250 mg/250 mL, 500 mg/500 mL, 500 mg/250 mL, 1,000 mg/250 mL
Adverse Reactions and Side Effects
Resp: Shortness of breath
CV: Hypertension, increased heart rate, PVCs, angina pectoris, arrhythmias, hypotension, palpitations
CNS: Headache
GI: Nausea, vomiting
Drug Interactions: Beta blockers may negate the effect of dobutamine. There is increased risk of arrhythmias or hypertension with some MAO inhibitors, oxytocics, or tricyclic antidepressants.
EMS Considerations: Monitor patient vital signs frequently. An increase of systolic BP of 10 to 20 mm Hg and an increase in heart rate of 5 to 15 beats/minute are considered normal.

Dopamine (DOPE-a-meen)

Intropin, ✥ Revimine
Classifications: Inotropic, vasopressor, adrenergic
Pregnancy Class: C
Mechanism of Action: Dopamine stimulates both alpha- and beta-adrenergic receptors and dopaminergic receptors in a dose-dependent fashion. Table 11-1 lists the various dose levels of dopamine, the receptors stimulated, and the actions produced on the body. Dopamine increases blood pressure and cardiac output and improves blood flow through the kidneys.
Pharmacokinetics
Absorption: Complete bioavailability
Onset: 1 to 2 minutes
Duration: Less than 10 minutes
Indications: Used as an adjunct to standard measures of improving BP, cardiac output, and urine output in the treatment of shock unresponsive to fluid replacement
Contraindications: Known hypersensitivity; should not be given to patients with tachyarrhythmias, pheochromocytoma, or hypersensitivity to bisulfites.

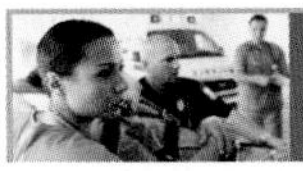

Table 11-1 Dosage-Related Responses to Dopamine

Home	Major Receptors Stimulated	Response
1–5 mcg/kg/minute	Dopaminergic	Vasodilation of renal, mesenteric, and cerebral arteries; no effect on the heart or blood pressure
5–15 mcg/kg/minute	$Beta_1$-adrenergic effects	Cardiac stimulation
>15 mcg/kg/minute	Alpha-adrenergic effects	Increased peripheral vascular resistance

Check the Evidence

Pheochromocytoma is a tumor of the sympathetic nervous system responsible for approximately 0.1 to 2 percent of all cases of hypertension.

Precautions: Use with caution in patients with hypovolemia or MI. (!) Geriatric patients may be more susceptible to adverse effects.

Route and Dosage

IV (Adult): Dopaminergic effects—1 to 5 mcg/kg/minute; Beta-adrenergic effects—5 to 15 mcg/kg/minute; Alpha-adrenergic effects—greater than 15 mcg/kg/minute

Understand the Numbers

You are ordered to give 10 mcg/kg/minute of dopamine to your 44-year-old, 175-pound patient. Your premixed IV bag contains 800 mg of dopamine in 500 mL of NS. What is the drip rate using a 60 gtt/mL infusion set?

175 lb ÷ 2.2 kg = 79.5 or 80 kg. 80 kg × 10 mcg = 800 mcg/minute

Concentration = 800 mg ÷ 500 mL = 1.6 mg/mL or 1,600 mcg/mL

Required volume = 800 mcg ÷ 1,600 mcg/mL = 0.5 mL

Infusion rate = 0.5 mL × 60 gtt/mL = 30 gtts ÷ 1 minute = 30 gtt/minute

How Supplied

Injection for dilution: 40 mg/mL, 80 mg/mL, 160 mg/mL

Premixed injection: 200 mg/250 mL, 400 mg/250 mL, 800 mg/250 mL, 800 mg/500 mL

Adverse Reactions and Side Effects

Resp: Dyspnea

CV: Arrhythmias, hypotension, angina, ECG changes, palpitations, vasoconstriction

CNS: Headache

GI: Nausea, vomiting

Local: Irritation at the IV site

Drug Interactions: Use with MAO inhibitors or some antidepressants may result in severe hypertension. Use with IV phenytoin may cause hypotension and bradycardia. Beta blockers may antagonize cardiac effects.

EMS Considerations: Hypovolemia should be corrected before giving dopamine. Monitor vital signs and ECG continuously.

Enalaprilat (e-NAL-a-pril-at)

Vasotec IV

Classifications: antihypertensive, ACE inhibitor

Pregnancy Class: C (first trimester), D (second and third trimesters)

Mechanism of Action: Blocks the conversion of angiotensin I to the vasoconstrictor angiotensin II, resulting in systemic vasodilation

Pharmacokinetics

Absorption: Complete bioavailability

Onset: 15 minutes

Duration: 4 to 6 hours

Indications: Used for the management of CHF

Contraindications: Known hypersensitivity; should not be given to patients with a history of angioedema with previous use of ACE inhibitors

Precautions: Use with caution in patients with liver impairment, hypovolemia, or hyponatremia and in those on concurrent diuretic therapy. (!) Black patients are at an increased risk of angioedema.

Route and Dosage

IV (Adult): Hypertension—0.625 to 1.25 mg every 6 hours. Dose can be titrated up to 5 mg.

***effective* Communication**

Dosage should be 0.625 mg if the patient is receiving diuretics.

How Supplied

Injection: 1.25 mg/mL

Adverse Reactions and Side Effects

Resp: Cough, dyspnea

CV: Hypotension, chest pain, edema, tachycardia

CNS: Dizziness, drowsiness, fatigue, headache, insomnia, vertigo, weakness

GI: Taste disturbances, abdominal pain, anorexia, constipation, diarrhea, nausea, vomiting

Derm: Flushing, rashes

Misc: ANGIOEDEMA, fever

Drug Interactions: Excessive hypotension may occur with concurrent use of diuretics and antihypertensives. Antihypertensive response may be decreased by NSAIDs.

EMS Considerations: If possible, correct volume depletion before the initiation of therapy. Monitor vital signs frequently.

Enoxaparin (e-nox-a-PA-rin)

Lovenox

Classifications: Anticoagulant, antithrombotic

Pregnancy Class: B

Mechanism of Action: Potentiates the inhibitory effect of antithrombin on factor Xa and thrombin, preventing thrombus formation

Pharmacokinetics

Absorption: 92 percent absorbed after administration

Onset: Unknown

Duration: 12 hours

Indications: Used in the treatment of acute ST-segment elevation MI

Contraindications: Known hypersensitivity; should not be given to patients hypersensitive to port products or to patients with major active bleeding

Precautions: Use with *extreme* caution in patients with severe uncontrolled hypertension, bacterial endocarditis, or bleeding disorders. Use with caution in patients with severe liver or kidney disease.

Route and Dosage
SubQ (Adult): Unstable angina/non-ST segment elevation MI—1 mg/kg every 12 hours for 2 to 8 days, with aspirin
SubQ, IV (Adult Under 75 years old): Acute ST-segment elevation MI—30 mg IV bolus, plus 1 mg/kg SubQ
SubQ (Adult Under 75 years old): Acute ST-segment elevation MI—0.75 mg/kg every 12 hours
How Supplied
Solution for injection (prefilled syringes): 30 mg/0.3 mL, 40 mg/0.4 mL, 60 mg/0.6 mL, 80 mg/0.8 mL, 100 mg/1 mL, 120 mg/0.8 mL, 150 mg/mL
Solution for injection (multidose vials): 300 mg/3 mL
Adverse Reactions and Side Effects
CV: Edema
CNS: Dizziness, headache, insomnia
GI: Constipation, nausea, vomiting
Hemat: BLEEDING, anemia, thrombocytopenia
Drug Interactions: Increased risk of bleeding with the concurrent use of drugs that affect platelet function and coagulation
EMS Considerations: Assess patients for signs of bleeding and hemorrhage during therapy.

Epinephrine (e-pi-NEF-rin)

Adrenalin
Classifications: Antiasthmatic, bronchodilator, adrenergic, vasopressor
Pregnancy Class: C
Mechanism of Action: Affects both beta$_1$- (cardiac) adrenergic receptor and beta$_2$- (pulmonary) adrenergic receptor sites; produces bronchodilation; also has alpha-adrenergic agonist properties resulting in vasoconstriction
Pharmacokinetics
Absorption: Well absorbed after inhalation, SubQ, IM, and IV administration
Onset: Inhalation—1 minute; SubQ—5 to 10 minutes; IM—6 to 12 minutes; IV—rapid
Duration: Inhalation—1 to 3 hours; SubQ and IM—1 to 4 hours; IV—20 to 30 minutes
Indications: Can be used for the treatment of cardiac arrest or symptomatic bradycardia
Contraindications: Known hypersensitivity; should not be given to patients who are hypersensitive to adrenergic amines or to patients with cardiac arrhythmias or those who are hypersensitive to bisulfites
Precautions: Use with caution in patients with cardiac disease and in patients with hypertension, hyperthyroidism, diabetes, or cerebral arteriosclerosis.
Route and Dosage
IV, IO (Adult): Cardiopulmonary resuscitation (ACLS guidelines)—1 mg every 3 to 5 minutes; Bradycardia—2 to 10 mcg/minute
IV, IO, ET (Pediatric): Symptomatic bradycardia/pulseless arrest (PALS guidelines)—0.01 mg/kg (0.1 mL/kg of a 1:10,000 concentration) every 3 to 5 minutes. If no IV/IO access, you may give an ET dose of 0.1 mg/kg (0.1 mL of a 1:1000 concentration) diluted to a volume of 3 to 5 mL with NS followed by several positive pressure ventilations.
How Supplied
Injection: 0.1 mg/mL (1:10,000), 1 mg/mL (1:1000)
Adverse Reactions and Side Effects
Resp: Paradoxical bronchospasm (excessive use of inhalers)
CV: Angina, arrhythmias, hypertension, tachycardia
CNS: Nervousness, restlessness, tremor, headache, insomnia
GI: Nausea, vomiting
Drug Interactions: Concurrent use with other adrenergic drugs will have additive adrenergic side effects. Use with MAO inhibitors may cause hypertensive crisis. Beta blockers may block the therapeutic effects. Tricyclic antidepressants enhance pressor response to epinephrine.
EMS Considerations: Monitor vital signs closely, paying special attention to blood pressure, pulse rate, and ECG status. Assess lung sounds before and after administration.

effective **Communication**

An IV bolus injection of a 1:1000 solution of epinephrine may cause sudden hypertension or cerebral edema.

Eptifibatide (ep-ti-FIB-a-tide)

Integrilin
Classifications: Antiplatelet agent, glycoprotein Iib/IIIa inhibitor
Pregnancy: B
Mechanism of Action: Decreases platelet aggregation by reversibly antagonizing the binding of fibrinogen to the glycoprotein IIb/IIIa binding site on platelet surfaces
Pharmacokinetics
Absorption: Complete bioavailability
Onset: Immediate
Duration: Brief—minutes
Indications: Used in the management of acute coronary syndrome, including patients who will be managed medically and those who will undergo percutaneous coronary intervention (PCI)
Contraindications: Known hypersensitivity; should not be given to patients with active bleeding or a history of bleeding within the last 30 days; should not be given to patients with severe uncontrolled hypertension or those with a history of stroke or hemorrhage
Precautions: (!) Geriatric patients have an increased risk of bleeding.
Route and Dosage
IV (Adult): Acute coronary syndrome (ACS)—180 mcg/kg as an IV bolus, followed by 2 mcg/kg/minute; Percutaneous coronary intervention (PCI)—180 mcg/kg as an IV bolus immediately before PCI, followed by 2 mcg/kg/minute infusion. A second bolus of 180 mcg/kg is given 10 minutes after the first bolus dose.

Check the **Evidence**

Accidental overdose of antiplatelet medications can result in severe patient harm, including death.

How Supplied
Solution for injection: 20 mg/10 mL, 75 mg/100 mL, 200 mg/100 mL
Adverse Reactions and Side Effects
CV: Hypotension
Hemat: BLEEDING, including GI and intracranial bleeding
Drug Interactions: Increased risk of bleeding if used with drugs that affect hemostasis
EMS Considerations: Frequently assess vital signs and monitor patients for signs of bleeding.

Esmolol (ES-moe-lole)

Brevibloc
Classifications: Class II antiarrhythmic, beta blocker
Pregnancy Class: C
Mechanism of Action: Blocks the stimulation of beta$_1$-(myocardial) adrenergic receptors
Pharmacokinetics
Absorption: Complete bioavailability
Onset: Within minutes
Duration: 1 to 20 minutes
Indications: Used in the management of sinus tachycardia and supraventricular arrhythmias
Contraindications: Known hypersensitivity; should not be given to patients with uncompensated CHF, pulmonary edema, cardiogenic shock, bradycardia, or heart block
Precautions: Use with caution in patients with diabetes mellitus, thyrotoxicosis, or a history of severe allergic reactions. (!) Geriatric patients have an increased sensitivity to beta blockers.
Route and Dosage
IV (Adult): 500 mcg/kg loading dose over 1 minute initially, followed by 50 mcg/kg/minute infusion for 4 minutes
IV (Pediatric): 50 mcg/kg/minute; may be increased every 10 minutes up to 300 mcg/kg/minute
How Supplied
Solution for injection (prediluted for use as a loading dose): 10 mg/mL, 20 mg/mL
Premixed infusion: 2,000 mg/100 mL, 2,500 mg/250 mL

Check the Evidence

Patient deaths have occurred when the loading dose vial is confused with concentrated solution for injection, which contains 2,500 mg in 10 mL (250 mg/mL) and must be diluted.

Adverse Reactions and Side Effects
CV: Hypotension, peripheral ischemia
CNS: Fatigue, agitation, confusion, dizziness, drowsiness, weakness
GI: Nausea, vomiting
Derm: Sweating
Local: Injection site reactions

effective Communication

If administration site irritation occurs, stop the infusion and begin at another site.

Drug Interactions: IV phenytoin and verapamil may cause additive myocardial depression. Additive bradycardia may occur with digoxin. Additive hypotension may occur with other antihypertensives.
EMS Considerations: Monitor patient vital signs frequently during therapy.

Furosemide (fur-OH-se-mide)

🍁 Apo-Furosemide, Lasix, 🍁 Lasix Special, 🍁 Novosemide, 🍁 Nu-Furosemide, 🍁 PMS-Furosemide
Classification: Loop diuretic
Pregnancy Class: C
Mechanism of Action: Inhibits the reabsorption of sodium and chloride from Henle's loop and distal renal tubule; increases the renal excretion of water, sodium, chloride, magnesium, potassium, and calcium
Pharmacokinetics
Absorption: Absorbed well from both IM and IV sites
Onset: IM—10 to 30 minutes; IV—5 minutes
Duration: IM—4 to 8 hours; IV—2 hours
Indications: Used to treat edema due to heart failure, liver impairment, or renal disease; also used to treat hypertension
Contraindications: Known hypersensitivity; should not be given to patients with hepatic enciphaloathy or anuria
Precautions: Use with caution in patients with severe liver disease or diabetes mellitus. (!) Geriatric patients may have an increased risk of hypotension and electrolyte imbalance at usual doses.
Route and Dosage
IM, IV (Adult): 20 to 40 mg. Continuous infusion—bolus 0.1 mg/kg followed by 0.1 mg/kg/hour
IM, IV (Pediatric): 1 to 2 mg/kg/dose. Continuous infusion—0.05 mg/kg/hour, titrated to effect
How Supplied
Solution for injection: 10 mg/mL
Adverse Reactions and Side Effects
CV: Hypotension
CNS: Blurred vision, dizziness, headache, vertigo
EENT: Hearing loss, tinnitus
GI: Anorexia, constipation, diarrhea, dry mouth, dyspepsia, nausea, vomiting
F and E: Dehydration, hypochloremia, hypokalemia, hypomagnesemia, hyponatremia, hypovolemia, metabolic alkalosis, hypocalcemia
Drug Interactions: Increased hypotension if used with antihypertensives or nitrates; increased risk of hypokalemia if used with other diuretics
EMS Considerations: Because of furosemide's diuretic effect, monitor the patient's BP closely. Assess lung sounds before

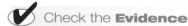

giving furosemide and monitor lung sounds closely after administration.

Heparin (HEP-a-rin)

Calcilean, Calciparine, Hepalean, Heparin Leo, Hep-Lock, Hep-Lock U/P

Classifications: Anticoagulant, antithrombotic
Pregnancy Class: C
Mechanism of Action: Potentiates the inhibitory effect of antithrombin on factor Xa and thrombin
Pharmacokinetics
Absorption: Erratically absorbed after SubQ or IV administration
Onset: SubQ—20 to 60 minutes; IV—Immediate
Duration: SubQ—8 to12 hours; IV—2 to 6 hours
Indications: Used for the prophylaxis and treatment of various thromboembolic disorders
Contraindications: Known hypersensitivity; should not be given to patients with uncontrolled bleeding, severe thrombocytopenia, or open wounds
Precautions: Use with *extreme* caution in patients with severe uncontrolled hypertension, bacterial endocarditis, bleeding disorders, hemorrhage, or stroke and in patients with recent CNS or ophthalmologic surgery. Use with caution in patients with severe liver or kidney disease, retinopathy, untreated hypertension, ulcer disease, spinal cord or brain injury, or malignancy.

Route and Dosage

Therapeutic Anticoagulation
IV (Adult): Intermittent bolus—10,000 units, followed by 5,000 to 10,000 units every 4 to 6 hours; Continuous infusion—5,000 units followed by 20,000 to 40,000 units infused over 24 hours
SubQ (Adult): 5,000 units IV, followed by initial SubQ dose of 10,000 to 20,000 units
Prophylaxis of Thromboembolism
SubQ (Adult): 5,000 units every 8 to 12 hours
Line Flushing
IV (Adult and Pediatric): 10 to 100 units/mL solution to fill heparin lock set to needle hub. Replace after each use.

How Supplied

Solution for injection: 10 units/mL, 100 units/mL, 1,000 units/mL, 5,000 units/mL, 7,500 units/mL, 10,000 units/mL, 20,000 units/mL, 40,000 units/mL
Premixed solution: 1,000 units/500 mL, 2,000 units/1,000 mL, 12,500 units/250 mL, 25,000 units/250 mL, and 25,000 units/500 mL

Adverse Reactions and Side Effects

Derm: Rashes, urticaria
Hemat: BLEEDING, anemia, thrombocytopenia
Local: Pain at injection site
Drug Interactions: Increased risk of bleeding if used concurrently with drugs that affect platelet function. Digoxin, tetracyclines, nicotine, and antihistamines may decrease the anticoagulant effect of heparin.

Check the Evidence

Heparin is frequently used concurrently or sequentially with other drugs affecting coagulation. Serious interaction is greatest with full anticoagulation.

EMS Considerations: Continuously monitor the patient for evidence of bleeding (bleeding gums, nosebleed, hypotension, etc.).

Hydralazine (hye-DRAL-a-zeen)

Apresoline, Novo-Hylazin

Classifications: Antihypertensive, vasodilator
Pregnancy Class: C
Mechanism of Action: Direct-acting peripheral arteriolar vasodilator
Pharmacokinetics
Absorption: Well absorbed
Onset: IM—10 to 30 minutes; IV—5 to 20 minutes
Duration: IM—3 to 8 hours; IV—2 to 6 hours
Indications: Used to treat moderate-to-severe hypertension
Contraindications: Known hypersensitivity; should not be given to patients with an intolerance to tartrazine
Precautions: Use with caution in patients with cardiovascular or cerebrovascular disease and in patients with severe liver or kidney disease.

Route and Dosage

IM, IV (Adult): 5 to 40 mg repeated as needed

How Supplied

Injection: 20 mg/mL

Check the Evidence

Hydralazine may be given concurrently with diuretics or beta blockers to permit lower doses and minimize any side effects.

Adverse Reactions and Side Effects

CV: Tachycardia, angina, arrhythmias, edema, orthostatic hypotension
CNS: Dizziness, drowsiness, headache
GI: Diarrhea, nausea, vomiting
Derm: Rashes
F and E: Sodium retention
Drug Interactions: Increased risk of hypotension if used concurrently with other antihypertensives, MAO inhibitors, or nitrates. NSAIDs may decrease antihypertensive response.
EMS Considerations: Monitor vital signs frequently during therapy.

Labetalol (la-BET-a-lole)

Trandate

Classifications: Antianginal, antihypertensive, beta blocker
Pregnancy Class: C
Mechanism of Action: Blocks the stimulation of $beta_1$- (myocardial), $beta_2$- (pulmonary), and $alpha_1$- (vascular) adrenergic receptor sites

Pharmacokinetics

Absorption: Well absorbed but rapidly undergoes extensive first-pass liver metabolism, resulting in 25 percent bioavailability

Onset: 2 to 5 minutes

Duration: 16 to 18 hours

Indications: Used in the management of hypertension

Contraindications: Known hypersensitivity; should not be given to patients with uncompensated CHF, pulmonary edema, cardiogenic shock, bradycardia, or heart block

Precautions: Use with caution in patients with renal or kidney impairment, pulmonary disease, diabetes mellitus, thyrotoxicosis, or a history of severe allergic reactions.

Route and Dosage

IV (Adult): 20 mg (0.25 mg/kg) initially. Additional doses of 40 to 80 mg may be given every 10 minutes as needed or 2 mg/minute infusion. Maximum total dose should not exceed 300 mg.

How Supplied

Injection: 5 mg/mL

Adverse Reactions and Side Effects

Resp: Bronchospasm, wheezing

CV: ARRHYTHMIAS, BRADYCARDIA, CHF, PULMONARY EDEMA, orthostatic hypotension

CNS: Fatigue, weakness, anxiety, depression, dizziness, drowsiness, insomnia, memory loss, nightmares

EENT: Blurred vision, dry eyes, nasal stuffiness

GI: Constipation, diarrhea, nausea

GU: Erectile dysfunction, decreased libido

Derm: Itching, rashes

Endo: Hyperglycemia or hypoglycemia

Drug Interactions: Verapamil may cause additive myocardial depression. Additive bradycardia may occur with digoxin, verapamil, or diltiazem. Additive hypotension may occur with other antihypertensives.

EMS Considerations: Monitor patient closely for changes in BP, heart rhythm and rate, and respiratory rate. Patients should remain supine during administration, because labetalol may cause orthostatic hypotension.

Lidocaine (LYE-doe-kane)

LidoPen, Xylocaine, 🍁 Xylocard

Classifications: Class IB antiarrhythmic

Pregnancy Class: B

Mechanism of Action: Suppresses automaticity and spontaneous depolarization of the ventricles during diastole by altering the flux of sodium ions across cell membranes with little or no effect on the heart rate

Pharmacokinetics

Absorption: Well absorbed

Onset: Immediate

Duration: 10 to 20 minutes (up to several hours after continuous infusion)

Indications: An alternative to amiodarone in the treatment of cardiac arrest from V-Fib/PVT after successful conversion of perfusing rhythm; stable ventricular tachycardia, wide-complex tachycardias of uncertain origin, and ventricular ectopy in the presence of acute MI.

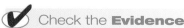

> **Check the Evidence**
>
> Several research studies indicate that amiodarone is superior to lidocaine in the treatment of cardiac arrest due to V-Fib/PVT. Overall, amiodarone seems to have approximately a 33 percent failure rate when treating V-Fib/PVT, while lidocaine has a 91 percent failure rate.

Contraindications: Known hypersensitivity; should not be given to patients in third-degree AV block

Precautions: Use with caution in patients with liver disease or CHF and in patients weighing less than 50 kg (110 lbs.), geriatric patients (reduce bolus or maintenance dose or both), and patients with respiratory depression, shock, or heart block.

> **Check the Evidence**
>
> Patients over the age of 70 have a reduced volume of distribution, which makes it necessary to reduce the IV infusion dosage of lidocaine by 50 percent.

Route and Dosage

IV (Adult): 1 to 1.5 mg/kg bolus. May repeat at 0.5 to 0.75 mg/kg every 5 to 10 minutes up to a total dose of 3 mg/kg. Continuous infusion—1 to 4 mg/minute

ET (Adult): Give 2 to 2.5 times the IV loading dose down the ET tube, followed by 10 mL of a NS flush.

IV (Pediatric): 1 mg/kg bolus (not to exceed 100 mg), followed by a 20 to 50 mcg/kg/minute continuous infusion

> ***effective* Communication**
>
> If there is a delay between the pediatric bolus dose and beginning the continuous infusion, you may repeat a bolus dose at 0.5 to 1 mg/kg.

ET (Pediatric): Give 2 to 3 mg/kg down the ET tube followed by a 5-mL NS flush.

How Supplied

IV injection: 10 mg/mL (1 percent), 20 mg/mL (2 percent)

Premix for IV infusion: 4 mg/mL, 8 mg/mL

Adverse Reactions and Side Effects

Resp: Bronchospasm

CV: CARDIAC ARREST, arrhythmias, bradycardia, heart block, hypotension

CNS: SEIZURES, confusion, drowsiness, blurred vision, dizziness, nervousness, slurred speech

GI: Nausea, vomiting

Misc: ANAPHYLAXIS

Drug Interactions: Concurrent use of lidocaine and beta blockers may cause lidocaine toxicity. Concurrent use with phenytoin, procainamide, propranolol, or quinidine can have additive, antagonistic, or toxic effects.

EMS Considerations: Monitor vital signs and ECG continuously during therapy.

Underline indicates most frequent; CAPITALS indicates life-threatening; 🍁 indicates Canadian drug name. (!) Safety and special populations.

Lisinopril (lyse-IN-oh-pril)

Prinivil, Zestril

Classifications: Antihypertensive, ACE inhibitor

Pregnancy Class: C (first trimester), D (second and third trimesters)

Mechanism of Action: Blocks the conversion of angiotensin I to the vasoconstrictor angiotensin II, resulting in systemic vasodilation

Pharmacokinetics

- *Absorption:* 60 to 70 percent absorbed after PO administration. Absorption is decreased by the presence of food in the stomach.
- *Onset:* 1 hour
- *Duration:* 24 hours

Indications: Used for the management of CHF

Contraindications: Known hypersensitivity; should not be given to patients with a history of angioedema with previous use of ACE inhibitors

Precautions: Use with caution in patients with liver impairment, hypovolemia, or hyponatremia and in patients on concurrent diuretic therapy. ❗ Black patients are at an increased risk of angioedema.

Route and Dosage

PO (Adult): Hypertension—10 mg once daily; CHF—5 mg once daily; Post MI—5 mg once daily

How Supplied

Tablets: 2.5 mg, 5 mg, 10 mg, 30 mg, 40 mg

Adverse Reactions and Side Effects

Resp: Cough, dyspnea

CV: Hypotension, chest pain, edema, tachycardia

CNS: Dizziness, drowsiness, fatigue, headache, insomnia, vertigo, weakness

GI: Taste disturbances, abdominal pain, anorexia, constipation, diarrhea, nausea, vomiting

Derm: Flushing, rashes

Misc: ANGIOEDEMA, fever

Drug Interactions: Excessive hypotension may occur with concurrent use of diuretics and antihypertensives. Antihypertensive response may be decreased by NSAIDs.

EMS Considerations: If possible, correct volume depletion before the initiation of therapy. Monitor vital signs frequently.

Magnesium Sulfate (mag-NEE-zhum SUL-fate)

Classifications: Mineral/electrolyte

Pregnancy Class: D

Mechanism of Action: Essential for the activity of many enzymes; plays an important role in neurotransmission and muscular excitability

Pharmacokinetics

- *Absorption:* Complete bioavailability
- *Onset:* IM—60 minutes; IV—Immediate
- *Duration:* IM—1 to 3 hours; IV—30 minutes

Indications: Used in the treatment and prevention of hypomagnesemia; also used to treat hypertension. Some EMS protocols include magnesium sulfate for the treatment of pediatric torsade de pointes (Fig. 11-6).

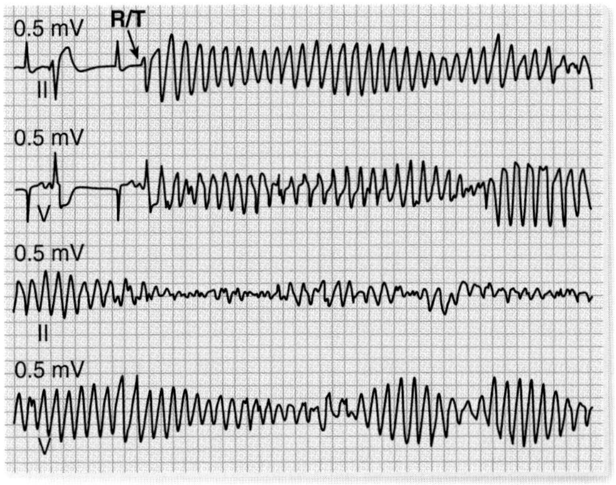

Figure 11-6 Torsade de Pointes.

Contraindications: Known hypersensitivity; should not be given to patients with hypermagnesemia, hypocalcemia, or heart block

Precautions: Use with caution in patients with any degree of renal insufficiency. ❗ Geriatric patients may require a reduced dosage due to age-related decrease in kidney function.

Route and Dosage

IM, IV (Adult): Hypertension—1 g every 6 hours for four doses as needed

IV (Pediatric): Torsade de pointes—25 to 50 mg/kg/dose; maximum dose = 2 g

How Supplied

Injection: 500 mg/mL (50 percent)

Premixed infusion: 1 g/100 mL, 2 g/100 mL, 4 g/50 mL, 4 g/100 mL, 20 g/500 mL, 40 g/1,000 mL

Adverse Reactions and Side Effects

Resp: Decreased respiratory rate

CV: Arrhythmias, bradycardia, hypotension

CNS: Drowsiness

GI: Diarrhea

Derm: Flushing, sweating

Drug Interactions: May potentiate calcium channel blockers and neuromuscular blockers

EMS Considerations: Monitor vital signs frequently during therapy. An overdose of magnesium sulfate may cause respiratory depression and heart block.

effective Communication

To reverse the effects of a magnesium sulfate overdose, ventilate the patient with 100 percent humidified oxygen and give an IV bolus of 10 percent calcium gluconate at 5 to 10 mEq (10 to 20 mL).

Metoprolol (me-TOE-proe-lole)

🍁 Beloc, 🍁 Beloc-Zok, 🍁 Betaloc Dunules, 🍁 Betaloc ZOK, 🍁 Lopressor, 🍁 Lopressor SR, Lopressor, 🍁 Metoprol, 🍁 Novo-Metoprol, 🍁 Seloken ZOK, Toprol-XL

Classifications: Antianginal, antihypertensive, beta blocker

Pregnancy Class: C

Mechanism of Action: Blocks the stimulation of $beta_1$-(myocardial) adrenergic receptors
Pharmacokinetics
Absorption: Well absorbed
Onset: PO—15 minutes; IV—Immediate
Duration: PO—6 to 12 hours; IV—5 to 8 hours
Indications: Used for the prevention of MI and the treatment of hypertension; also used in the management of stable, symptomatic heart failure due to ischemia
Contraindications: Known hypersensitivity; should not be given to patients with uncompensated CHF, pulmonary edema, cardiogenic shock, bradycardia, or heart block
Precautions: Use with caution in patients with renal or liver impairment, pulmonary disease, diabetes mellitus, or a history of severe allergic reactions. (!) Geriatric patients have an increased sensitivity to beta blockers. Therefore, an initial dose reduction may be recommended.

Route and Dosage
PO (Adult): Antihypertensive/antianginal—25 to 100 mg/day as a single dose; MI—25 to 50 mg; Heart failure—12.5 to 25 mg once daily
IV (Adult): MI—5 mg every 2 minutes for three doses, followed by oral dosing

How Supplied
Tablets: 25 mg, 50 mg, 100 mg
Injection: 1 mg/mL

Adverse Reactions and Side Effects
Resp: Bronchospasm, wheezing
CV: BRADYCARDIA, CHF, PULMONARY EDEMA, hypotension, peripheral vasoconstriction
CNS: <u>Fatigue</u>, <u>weakness</u>, anxiety, depression, dizziness, drowsiness, insomnia, memory loss, mental status changes, nervousness, nightmares
EENT: Blurred vision, stuffy nose
GI: Constipation, diarrhea, dry mouth, flatulence, gastric pain, nausea, vomiting
Derm: Rashes
Drug Interactions: IV phenytoin and verapamil may cause increased myocardial depression. Hypotension increases if metoprolol is used with other antihypertensive drugs.
EMS Considerations: Monitor vital signs, ECG, and heart rate every 5 to 15 minutes during therapy.

Milrinone (MILL-ri-none)

Primacor
Pregnancy Class: C
Mechanism of Action: Increases myocardial contractility and decreases preload and afterload by dilating the vascular smooth muscle
Pharmacokinetics
Absorption: Complete bioavailability
Onset: 5 to 15 minutes
Duration: 3 to 4 hours
Indications: Used for the short-term treatment of CHF unresponsive to conventional therapy
Contraindications: Known hypersensitivity; should not be given to patients with severe aortic or pulmonary valvular heart disease
Precautions: Use with caution in patients with a history of arrhythmias, electrolyte abnormalities, or abnormal digoxin levels and in patients having a vascular catheter inserted.

> **Check the Evidence**
> Giving milrinone to patients with the insertion of a vascular catheter may increase the risk of ventricular arrhythmias.

Route and Dosage
IV (Adult): Loading dose—50 mcg/kg followed by an IV infusion; Continuous infusion—0.5 mcg/kg/minute

> ***Understand the Numbers***
> You are ordered to begin a continuous infusion of milrinone for your 150-pound patient. The premixed infusion comes at 20 mg in 100 mL. What is the drip rate using a 60 gtt/mL set?
> 150 lb ÷ 2.2 kg = 68 kg. 0.5 mcg × 68 kg = 34 mcg/minute
> Milrinone concentration = 20 mg ÷ 100 mL = 0.2 mg/mL or 200 mcg/mL
> Volume = 34 mcg ÷ 200 mcg/mL = 0.17 mL
> Infusion rate = 0.17 mL × 60 gtt ÷ 1 minute = 10.2 gtt/minute or 10 gtt/minute

How Supplied
Injection: 1 mg/mL
Premixed infusion: 20 mg/mL, 40 mg/mL

Adverse Reactions and Side Effects
CV: VENTRICULAR ARRHYTHMIAS, angina pectoris, hypotension, supraventricular arrhythmias
CNS: Headache, tremor
Derm: Rashes
Drug Interactions: None significant
EMS Considerations: Monitor ECG and BP continuously during infusion. Arrhythmias are common and may be life threatening.

Morphine (MOR-feen)

Astramorph, Astramorph PF, DepoDur, Duramorph, Embeda, ♣ Epimorph, Infumorph, ♣ M-Eslon, ♣ Morphine HP, ♣ Morphitec, ♣ MOS, MS Contin, Roxanol, Roxanol Rescudose, ♣ Statex
Classification: Opioid analgesic, opioid agonist
Pregnancy Class: C
Mechanism of Action: Binds to the opiate receptors in the CNS, altering the perception of and response to pain
Pharmacokinetics
Absorption: Well absorbed via SubQ, IM, IV, and rectal routes
Onset: SubQ: 20 minutes; IM: 10 to 30 minutes; IV: Rapid-immediate; Rectal: unknown
Duration: SubQ, IM, IV—4 to 5 hours; Rectal: 3 to 7 hours

Indications: Used in the management of severe pain, pulmonary edema, and pain associated with an MI
Contraindications: Known hypersensitivity; should not be given to patients with hypersensitivity to tartrazine, bisulfites, or alcohol
Precautions: Use with caution in patients with head trauma, increased intracranial pressure, undiagnosed abdominal pain, severe renal or liver dysfunction, pulmonary disease, or a history of substance abuse. ! Elderly patients should receive reduced dosages because of increased risk of side effects.
Route and Dosage
Rectal (Adult Less Than 50 kg [less than 110 lbs]): 30 mg
Rectal (Adult & Pediatric More Than 50 kg [more than 110 lbs]): 0.3 mg/kg
IM (Adult More Than 50 kg [more than 110 lbs]): 8 to 15 mg
SubQ, IV (Adult More Than 50 kg [more than 110 lbs]): 4 to 10 mg
SubQ, IM, IV (Adult and Pediatric Less Than 50 kg [less than 110 lbs.]): 0.05 to 0.2 mg/kg; maximum dose = 15 mg
How Supplied
Solution for SubQ, IM, and IV injection: 1 mg/mL, 2 mg/mL, 4 mg/mL, 5 mg/mL, 8 mg/mL, 10 mg/mL, 15 mg/mL, 25 mg/mL, 50 mg/mL
Suppositories: 5 mg, 10 mg, 20 mg, 30 mg
Adverse Reactions and Side Effects
Resp: RESPIRATORY DEPRESSION
CV: Hypotension, bradycardia
CNS: Confusion, sedation, dizziness, euphoria, floating feeling, hallucinations, headache, unusual dreams
EENT: Blurred vision, diplopia, miosis
GI: Constipation, nausea, vomiting
Derm: Flushing, itching, sweating
Misc: Physical dependence, psychological dependence, tolerance
Drug Interactions: Use with extreme caution in patients taking MAO INHIBITORS within 14 days prior to giving morphine due to unpredictable, severe reactions; initial dose of morphine should be reduced to 25 percent of usual dose. There is increased risk of CNS depression if used with other CNS-depressant drugs.
EMS Considerations: ! Do not confuse morphine with hydromorphone or meperidine—errors have resulted in patient deaths. Assess patient vital signs before and frequently during/after administration. Have naloxone available for administration to reverse respiratory depression and overdose.

NICARdipine (nye-KAR-di-peen)

Cardene, Cardene SR, Cardene IV
Classifications: Antianginal, antihypertensive, calcium channel blocker
Pregnancy Class: C
Mechanism of Action: Inhibits the transport of calcium into myocardial and vascular smooth muscle cells
Pharmacokinetics
Absorption: Well absorbed
Onset: PO—20 minutes; IV—within minutes
Duration: PO—8 hours; IV—50 hours following discontinuation
Indications: Used for the management of hypertension, angina pectoris, and vasospastic (Prinzmetal) angina
Contraindications: Known hypersensitivity; should not be given to patients with sick sinus syndrome, second- or third-degree heart block, or a systolic BP lower than 90 mm Hg
Precautions: Use with caution in patients with severe liver or kidney impairment and in patients with a history of serious ventricular arrhythmias or CHF.
Route and Dosage
PO (Adult): 20 mg three times daily initially. Dosage may be increased.
IV (Adult): To replace PO use—0.5 to 2.2 mg/hour continuous IV infusion. For acute hypertension episodes, use 5 mg/hour titrated as needed.
How Supplied
Capsules: 20 mg, 30 mg
Sustained-release capsules: 30 mg, 45 mg, 60 mg
Injection: 2.5 mg/mL
Premixed infusion: 20 mg/200 mL D_5W or 0.9 percent NaCL, 40 mg/200 mL D_5W or 0.9 percent NaCL
Adverse Reactions and Side Effects
Resp: Cough, dyspnea, shortness of breath
CV: ARRHYTHMIAS, CHF, peripheral edema, bradycardia, chest pain, bradycardia, hypotension, palpitations, syncope tachycardia
CNS: Abnormal dreams, anxiety, confusion, dizziness, drowsiness, headache, nervousness, weakness, psychiatric disturbances
EENT: Blurred vision, disturbed equilibrium, epistaxis, tinnitus
GI: Anorexia, constipation, diarrhea, dry mouth, nausea, vomiting
Derm: Dermatitis, erythema, flushing, increased sweating, photosensitivity, rash
Misc: STEVENS-JOHNSON SYNDROME
Drug Interactions: Additive hypotension may occur with other antihypertensives or nitrates. Concurrent use with beta blockers, digoxin, or phenytoin may result in bradycardia, conduction defects, or CHF.
EMS Considerations: Monitor BP and pulse before therapy and frequently throughout therapy.

NIFEdipine (nye-FED-i-peen)

Adalat CC, 🍁 Adalat PA, 🍁 Adalat XL, Afeditab CR, 🍁 Apo-Nifed, Nifedical XL, 🍁 Novo-Nifedin, 🍁 Nu-Nifed, Procardia, Procardia XL
Classifications: Antianginal, antihypertensive, calcium channel blocker
Pregnancy Class: C
Mechanism of Action: Inhibits calcium transport into myocardial and vascular smooth muscles cells
Pharmacokinetics
Absorption: Well absorbed
Onset: PO—20 minutes; PO—PA unknown; PO—CC, PA, XL—unknown
Duration: PO—6 to 8 hours; PO—PA—12 hours; PO—CC, PA, XL—24 hours

Indications: Used for the managemnt of hypertension, angina pectoris, and vasospastic (Prinzmetal) angina
Contraindications: Known hypersensitivity; should not be given to patients with sick sinus syndrome, second- or third-degree heart block, or systolic BP lower than 90 mm Hg or to patients concurrently taking grapefruit juice.

Check the Evidence

Grapefruit juice interferes with the metabolism of nifedipine by inhibiting metabolism and slowing down the rate of gastric emptying.

Precautions: Use with caution in patients with severe liver or renal impairment and in patients with a history of serious ventricular arrhythmias.
Route and Dosage
PO (Adult): 10 to 30 mg three times daily, not to exceed 180 mg/day, or 10 to 20 mg twice daily as immediate-release form, or 30 to 90 mg once daily as sustained-release (CC, XL) form, not to exceed 90to 120 mg/day
How Supplied
Capsules: 🍁 5 mg, 10 mg, 20 mg
Tablets: 🍁 10 mg
Extended-release tablets (Adalat CC, Afeditab CR, Nifedical XL, Procardia XL): 🍁 10 mg, 🍁 20 mg, 30 mg, 60 mg, 90 mg
Adverse Reactions and Side Effects
Resp: Cough, dyspnea, shortness of breath
CV: ARRHYTHMIAS, CHF, peripheral edema, bradycardia, chest pain, hypotension, palpitations, syncope, tachycardia
CNS: Abnormal dreams, anxiety, confusion, dizziness, drowsiness, headache, nervousness, weakness, psychiatric disturbances
EENT: Blurred vision, disturbed equilibrium, epistaxis, tinnitus
GI: Anorexia, constipation, diarrhea, dry mouth, nausea, vomiting
Derm: Dermatitis, erythema, flushing, increased sweating, photosensitivity, rash
Misc: STEVENS-JOHNSON SYNDROME
Drug Interactions: Additive hypotension may occur with other antihypertensives or nitrates. Concurrent use with beta blockers, digoxin, or phenytoin may result in bradycardia, conduction defects, or CHF.
EMS Considerations: Monitor BP and pulse before therapy and frequently throughout therapy.

Nitroglycerin (nye-tro-GLI-ser-in)

Extended-release capsules (Nitro-Time, 🍁 Nitrogard-SR)
Intravenous (Nitro-Bid IV, Tridil)
Translingual spray (Nitrolingual, Nitromist)
Ointment (Nitro-Bid)
Sublingual (Nitrostat, NitroQuick)
Transdermal system (Minitran, Nitrek, Nitro-Dur
Classifications: Antianginal, nitrate
Pregnancy Class: C
Mechanism of Action: Increases coronary blood flow by dilating coronary arteries; produces vasodilation and decreases left ventricular end-diastolic pressure and left ventricular end-diastolic volume (preload); reduces myocardial oxygen consumption
Pharmacokinetics
Absorption: Well absorbed
Onset: SL—1 to 3 minutes; PO—40 to 60 minutes; Ointment—20 to 60 minutes; Patch—40 to 60 minutes; IV—Immediate
Duration: SL—30 to 60 minutes; PO—8 to 12 hours; Ointment—4 to 8 hours; Patch—8 to 24 hours; IV—several minutes
Indications: Translingual and SL—Acute management of angina pectoris; Oral, transdermal—Long-term management of angina pectoris; PO—Adjunct treatment of CHF; IV—Adjunct treatment of acute MI and treatment of CHF associated with acute MI
Contraindications: Known hypersensitivity; should not be given to patients with pericardial tamponade or pericarditis or those who are taking medications for erectile dysfunction (sildenafil, tadalafil, vardenafil)

Check the Evidence

Concurrent use of nitrates in any form with sildenafil, tadalafil, or vardenafil increases the risk of potentially fatal hypotension.

Precautions: Use with caution in patients with head trauma or cerebral hemorrhage, glaucoma, hypertrophic cardiomyopathy (HCM), or severe liver impairment.

***effective* Communication**

Patients requiring cardioversion or defibrillation should have the transdermal patch removed before the procedure.

Route and Dosage
SL (Adult): 0.3 to 0.6 mg; may be repeated every 5 minutes for two additional doses, if necessary
Translingual spray (Adult): 1 to 2 sprays; may be repeated every 5 minutes for two additional doses, if necessary
PO (Adult): 2.5 to 9 mg every 8 to 12 hours
IV (Adult): 5 mcg/minute; may increase dose, if necessary
Transdermal (Adult): Ointment—1 to 2 inches every 6 to 8 hours; Transdermal patch—0.2 to 0.4 mg/hour initially; may titrate to effect, if necessary
How Supplied
Extended-release capsules: 2.5 mg, 6.5 mg, 9 mg
Sublingual tablets: 0.3 mg, 0.4 mg, 0.6 mg
Translingual spray: 400 mcg/spray
Transdermal system: 0.1 mg/hour, 0.2 mg/hour, 0.3 mg/hour, 0.6 mg/hour, 0.8 mg/hour
Transdermal ointment: 2 percent
Injection: 5 mg/mL
Premixed solution: 25 mg/250 mL, 50 mg/250 mL, 50 mg/500 mL, 100 mg/250 mL, 200 mg/500 mL

Adverse Reactions and Side Effects
CV: Hypotension, tachycardia, syncope
CNS: Dizziness, headache, apprehension, restlessness, weakness
EENT: Blurred vision
GI: Abdominal pain, nausea, vomiting
Derm: Contact dermatitis
Drug Interactions: Additive hypotension with antihypertensives, beta blockers, or calcium channel blockers. Concurrent use of nitrates in any form with sildenafil, tadalafil, or vardenafil increases the risk of potentially fatal hypotension.
EMS Considerations: Assess patient's vital signs before and after administration. Nitroglycerin is unstable and may rapidly deteriorate if exposed to the air, light, or temperature extremes.

Nitroprusside (nye-troe-PRUSS-ide)

Nitropress
Classifications: Antihypertensive, vasodilator
Pregnancy Class: C
Mechanism of Action: Produces peripheral vasodilation by a direct action on both venous and arteriolar smooth muscle
Pharmacokinetics
Absorption: Complete bioavailability
Onset: Immediate
Duration: 1 to 10 minutes
Indications: Used for the treatment of hypertensive crisis, cardiac failure, or cardiogenic shock
Contraindications: Known hypersensitivity; should not be given to patients with decreased cerebral perfusion
Precautions: Use with caution in patients with renal or liver disease and in those with hypothyroidism.
Route and Dosage
IV (Adult and Pediatric): 0.3 mcg/kg/minute initially; may be increased as needed up to 10 mcg/kg/minute
How Supplied
Injection: 25 mg/mL
Adverse Reactions and Side Effects
Resp: Dyspnea
CV: Hypotension, palpitations
CNS: Dizziness, headache, restlessness
EENT: Blurred vision, tinnitus
Local: Phlebitis at IV site
Misc: CYANIDE TOXICITY
Drug Interactions: Increased hypotensive effect with antihypertensives. Sympathomimetics may decrease the response to nitroprusside.
EMS Considerations: Monitor vital signs, especially BP, heart rate, and ECG frequently during therapy.

Nitrous Oxide-Oxygen Mixture (NYE-trus-ox-ide)

Nitronox, Entonox
Classifications: Medicinal gas, analgesic
Pregnancy Class: C
Mechanism of Action: Inhalation of a 50 percent mixture of nitrous oxide and oxygen produces CNS depression as well as rapid pain relief. A nitrous oxide-oxygen mixture produces rapid but reversible relief from pain.
Pharmacokinetics
Absorption: Well absorbed
Onset: 2 to 5 minutes
Duration: 2 to 5 minutes after discontinuation
Indications: Nitrous oxide-oxygen mixture is used for the relief of moderate-to-severe pain from any cause.
Contraindications: Known hypersensitivity. Do not administer a nitrous oxide-oxygen mixture if any of the following exist:

1. The patient has a decreased level of consciousness (LOC).
2. The patient has taken any depressant drug.
3. The patient has sustained thoracic trauma.
4. The patient has respiratory compromise from any cause.
5. Cyanosis develops during administration.
6. The patient is unable to follow simple instructions.
7. The patient has sustained abdominal distension or trauma.
8. The patient is pregnant.

Precautions: Monitor the patient closely during administration. Some patients develop severe nausea and may vomit during administration. Also, patients sometimes pass out while receiving this medication.
Route and Dosage
Inhalation (Adult): 20 to 50 percent concentration mixed with oxygen; self-administered by the patient until the pain is relieved
Inhalation (Pediatric): Same as the adult
How Supplied
D and E Cylinders: Blue and green in the United States and blue and white in Canada
Adverse Reactions and Side Effects
CNS: Lightheadedness, drowsiness, decreased respirations
GI: Nausea, vomiting
Drug Interactions: Administration of a nitrous oxide-oxygen mixture in the presence of other drugs that cause CNS depression can produce additive effects.
EMS Considerations: For patients with respiratory compromise, use 100 percent oxygen to prevent nitrous oxide from collecting in dead air spaces and further aggravating chest injuries. For patients with myocardial pain, administer oxygen when the nitrous oxide-oxygen mixture is not being given. If intestinal blockage is present, nitrous oxide may collect in the obstructed space, aggravating the blockage. Do not administer a nitrous oxide-oxygen mixture to patients with abdominal pain unless it is certain that intestinal blockage is not present.

Norepinephrine (NOR-ep-i-nef-rin)

Levophed
Classification: Vasopressor
Pregnancy Class: C
Mechanism of Action: Stimulates alpha-adrenergic receptors located mainly in the blood vessels, causing constriction; also has minor $beta_1$- (myocardial) adrenergic activity
Pharmacokinetics
Absorption: Complete bioavailability
Onset: Immediate
Duration: 1 to 2 minutes

Indications: Produces vasoconstriction and myocardial stimulation required after fluid replacement in the treatment of severe hypotension and shock
Contraindications: Known hypersensitivity; should not be given to patients with vascular, mesenteric, or peripheral thrombosis. Do not give to patients who are hypersensitive to bisulfites.
Precautions: Use with caution in patients with hypertension, patients taking MAO inhibitors or tricyclic antidepressants, and patients with hyperthyroidism or cardiovascular disease.
Route and Dosage
IV (Adult): 0.5 to 1 mcg/minute initially, followed by a maintenance infusion of 2 to 12 mcg/minute titrated to blood pressure

Understand the Numbers
You are asked to begin an IV infusion of norepinephrine at 1 mcg/minute. Your drug comes as 1 mg/mL in a 4-mL ampule, and you are using a 250-mL bag of NS. What is the drip rate/minute using a 60 gtt/mL set?
Concentration = 4 mg ÷ 250 mL = 0.016 mg/mL or 16 mcg/mL
Required Volume = 1 mcg ÷ 16 mcg/mL = 0.0625 mL
Infusion rate = 0.0625 mL × 60 gtt/mL ÷ 1 minute = 3.75 or 4 gtt/minute

How Supplied
Injection: 1 mg/mL in 4-mL ampules
Adverse Reactions and Side Effects
Resp: Dyspnea
CV: Arrhythmias, bradycardia, chest pain, hypertension
CNS: Anxiety, dizziness, headache, insomnia, restlessness, tremor, weakness
Local: Phlebitis at the IV site
Drug Interactions: Use with MAO inhibitors or tricyclic antidepressants may result in severe hypertension. Beta blockers may exaggerate hypertension or block cardiac stimulation.
EMS Considerations: Monitor BP every 2 to 3 minutes until stabilized and every 5 minutes thereafter. Systolic BP is usually maintained at 80 to 100 mm Hg.

Oxygen (OX-ah-gin)

Classification: Medicinal gas
Pregnancy Class: A
Mechanism of Action: Oxygen is required to enable the cells to break down glucose into a usable energy form. Oxygen is a colorless, odorless, tasteless gas essential to respiration. At sea level, oxygen is made up of approximately 10 to 16 percent venous blood and 17 to 21 percent arterial blood. Oxygen is carried from the lungs to the body's tissue by hemoglobin in the red blood cells. The administration of oxygen increases arterial oxygen tension (PaO_2) and hemoglobin saturation. This improves tissue oxygenation when circulation is adequately maintained.
Pharmacokinetics
Absorption: Oxygen is inhaled into the alveoli and then diffuses into the pulmonary capillary bed. The uptake from the lungs is rapid, and carbon dioxide is simultaneously excreted in the expelled air.
Onset: Immediate
Distribution: The delivery of oxygen to the tissues depends on arterial oxygenation, cardiac output, tissue perfusion, and oxygen-delivery systems.
Duration: Approximately 2 minutes
Indications: Oxygen is used: 1) to treat severe chest pain that may be caused by cardiac ischemia, 2) to treat hypoxemia from any cause, and 3) in the treatment of cardiac arrest.
Contraindications: None for out-of-hospital use (See Check the Evidence)

Check the Evidence
Oxygen is contraindicated in patients who are suffering from paraquat poisoning unless they are suffering from severe respiratory distress or respiratory arrest. ❗ Oxygen can increase the toxicity of the paraquat. Paraquat is a toxic chemical used in agriculture to kill certain weeds.

Precautions: If the patient has a history of COPD, begin oxygen administration at a lower flow rate, increasing the rate as necessary.
Route and Dosage
Inhalation (Adult): Low-dose oxygen—1 to 6 L/minute using a nasal cannula giving oxygen concentrations of 24 to 44 percent; Mid-dose oxygen—8 to 10 L/minutes using a simple face mask giving oxygen concentrations of 40 to 60 percent; High-dose oxygen—10 to 15 L/minute using a face mask with oxygen reservoir (nonrebreather) giving oxygen concentrations of almost 100 percent oxygen
Inhalation (Pediatric): Same as the adult
How Supplied
Cylinders in various sizes
Adverse Reactions and Side Effects
There are no adverse reactions or side effects in emergency situations. High concentrations of oxygen *may* cause decreased LOC and respiratory depression in patients with chronic carbon dioxide retention.

***effective* Communication**
Never withhold oxygen from any critically ill patient.

Drug Interactions: None
EMS Considerations: Reassure patients who are anxious about face masks but who require high concentrations of oxygen.

Phenytoin (FEN-i-toyn)

Dilantin, Phenytek
Classifications: Class IB antiarrhythmic, hydantoin
Pregnancy Class: D
Mechanism of Action: Shortens the action potential and decreases automaticity

Pharmacokinetics

Absorption: Absorbed slowly from the GI tract

Onset: 0.5 to 1 hour

Duration: 12 to 24 hours

Indications: Can be used as an antiarrhythmic (unlabeled use) for ventricular arrhythmias associated with digoxin toxicity and in treating prolonged QT interval

Contraindications: Known hypersensitivity; should not be given to patients with sinus bradycardia, sinoatrial block, second- and third-degree heart block, or Stokes-Adams syndrome

Check the Evidence

Stokes-Adams syndrome is a loss of consciousness caused by a decreased flow of blood to the brain.

Precautions: Use with caution in patients with liver or kidney disease and in patients with severe cardiac or respiratory disease. ❗ Phenytoin should be used with caution in all patients; it may increase the risk of suicidal thoughts and behaviors.

Route and Dosage

IV (Adult): 50 to 100 mg every 10 to 15 minutes until arrhythmia is abolished or a total of 15 mg/kg has been given

How Supplied

Injection: 50 mg/mL

Adverse Reactions and Side Effects

CV: Hypotension, tachycardia

CNS: SUICIDAL THOUGHTS, ataxia, agitation, confusion, dizziness, drowsiness, headache, insomnia, weakness

EENT: Diplopia, nystagmus (involuntary movements of the eyes)

GI: Nausea, constipation, vomiting

Derm: Rash

Misc: Allergic reactions including STEVENS-JOHNSON SYNDROME

Drug Interactions: Phenytoin and dopamine may cause additive hypotension. Additive CNS depression can occur with other CNS depressants.

EMS Considerations: ❗ Geriatric patients usually develop toxicity more rapidly. Closely monitor patients for hypotension and for respiratory and cardiac problems.

effective Communication

The slow administration of phenytoin helps prevent toxicity.

Procainamide (proe-KANE-ah-mide)

Classification: Class IA antiarrhythmic

Pregnancy Class: C

Mechanism of Action: Decreases myocardial excitability and slows conduction velocity.

Pharmacokinetics

Absorption: Well absorbed

Onset: Immediate

Duration: 3 to 4 hours

Indications: Used in the treatment of a variety of both ventricular and atrial arrhythmias, including: PACs, premature ventricular contractions (PVCs), ventricular tachycardia (VT), and PAT; also used for maintenance of normal sinus rhythm (NSR) after conversion from atrial fibrillation (A-Fib) or atrial flutter (A-flutter)

Contraindications: Known hypersensitivity; should not be given to patients with AV heart block or myasthenia gravis

Precautions: Use with caution in patients with MI or cardiac glycoside toxicity.

Route and Dosage

IV (Adult): 100 mg every 5 minutes until the arrhythmia is abolished or 1,000 mg have been given. Wait 10 minutes until further dosing or loading infusion of 500 to 600 mg over 30 to 60 minutes, followed by a maintenance infusion of 1 to 4 mg/minute.

effective Communication

The patient should remain supine throughout administration to minimize hypotension.

How Supplied

Injection: 100 mg/mL, 500 mg/mL

Adverse Reactions and Side Effects

CV: ASYSTOLE, HEART BLOCK, VENTRICULAR ARRHYTHMIAS, hypotension

CNS: SEIZURES, confusion, dizziness

GI: Diarrhea, anorexia, bitter taste, nausea, vomiting

Derm: Rashes

Misc: Chills, fever

Drug Interactions: May have additive or antagonist effects with other antiarrhythmics. Antihypertensives and nitrates may potentiate hypotensive effect.

EMS Considerations: Monitor ECG, pulse, and BP continuously. Administration is generally discontinued if any of the following occur: arrhythmia is resolved, QRS complex widens by 50 percent, PR interval is prolonged, blood pressure drops greater than 15 mm Hg, or toxic side effects develop.

Propranolol (proe-PRAN-oh-lole)

🍁 Apo-Propranolol, Inderal, 🍁 Novopranol

Classifications: Antianginal, class II antiarrhythmic, antihypertensive, beta blocker

Pregnancy Class: C

Mechanism of Action: Blocks the stimulation of beta$_1$- (myocardial) and beta$_2$- (pulmonary) adrenergic receptor sites

Pharmacokinetics

Absorption: Well absorbed

Onset: Immediate

Duration: 4 to 6 hours

Indications: Used in the management of hypertension, angina, arrhythmias, and hypertrophic cardiomyopathy (HCM) and in the prevention and management of MI

Contraindications: Known hypersensitivity; should not be given to patients with uncompensated CHF, pulmonary edema, cardiogenic shock, bradycardia, or heart block
Precautions: Use with caution in patients with kidney or liver impairment, pulmonary disease, diabetes mellitus, or a history of severe allergic reactions. (!) Geriatric patients have an increased sensitivity to all beta blockers. Therefore, an initial dose reduction and careful titration is recommended.

Route and Dosage
IV (Adult): 1 to 3 mg; may be repeated after 2 minutes
IV (Pediatric): 10 to 100 mcg (0.01 to 0.1 mg)/kg (up to 1 mg/dose)

> ***Understand the Numbers***
> You are ordered to give 30 mcg (0.03 mg)/kg of propranolol to your 30-pound patient. What is your initial dosage?
> 30 lbs ÷ 2.2 = 13.6 or 14 kg. 14 kg × 0.03 mg = 0.42 mg or 420 mcg

How Supplied
Injection: 1 mg/mL

Adverse Reactions and Side Effects
Resp: Bronchospasm, wheezing
CV: ARRHYTHMIAS, BRADYCARDIA, CHF, PULMONARY EDEMA, orthostatic hypotension, peripheral vasoconstriction
CNS: Fatigue, weakness, anxiety, dizziness, drowsiness, insomnia, memory loss, mental depression
EENT: Blurred vision, dry eyes, nasal stuffiness
GI: Constipation, diarrhea, nausea
GU: Erectile dysfunction, decreased libido
Derm: Itching, rashes
Drug Interactions: IV phenytoin and verapamil may cause additive myocardial depression. Additive bradycardia may occur with digoxin. Additive hypotension may occur with other antihypertensives or nitrates.
EMS Considerations: Vital signs should be assessed frequently during therapy, and continuous ECG monitoring should be done.

> ***effective* Communication**
> **Abrupt withdrawal of procainamide may cause life-threatening arrhythmias, hypertension, or myocardial ischemia.**

Reteplase (RE-te-plase)

Retavase
Classifications: Thrombolytic, plasminogen activator
Pregnancy Class: C
Mechanism of Action: Converts plasminogen to plasmin, which is then able to degrade fibrin present in blood clots
Pharmacokinetics
  Absorption: Complete absorption after IV administration
  Onset: 30 minutes
  Duration: 48 hours
Indications: Used for the treatment of acute MI and acute stroke
Contraindications: Known hypersensitivity; should not be given to patients with a history of stroke, recent intracranial or intraspinal injury or trauma, or intracranial neoplasm or to patients with AV malformation or aneurysm
Precautions: Use with caution in patients with recent major surgery, trauma, GI or GU bleeding, severe liver or renal disease, hemorrhagic ophthalmic conditions, or recent streptococcal infection.

Route and Dosage
IV (Adult): 10 units, followed by an additional 10 units 30 minutes later

How Supplied
Powder for injection: 10.8 units/vial

Adverse Reactions and Side Effects
Resp: Bronchospasm
CV: Hypotension, reperfusion arrhythmias
CNS: INTRACRANIAL HEMORRHAGE
EENT: Epitaxis, gingival bleeding
GI: GI BLEEDING, RETROPERITONEAL BLEEDING, nausea, vomiting
GU: GU TRACT BLEEDING
Local: Phlebitis at IV site
Misc: ANAPHYLAXIS
Drug Interactions: Concurrent use of aspirin and other NSAIDs, warfarin, and heparin may increase the risk of bleeding.
EMS Considerations: (!) Overdosing and underdosing have resulted in patient harm, including death. Monitor vital signs frequently during therapy. Notify medical control if systolic BP higher than 180 mm Hg or diastolic BP higher than 110 mm Hg.

Sotalol (SOE-ta-lole)

Betapace, Sorine, (Canadian) Sotacor
Classification: Class III antiarrhythmic
Pregnancy Class: B
Mechanism of Action: Blocks the stimulation of beta$_1$- (myocardial) and beta$_2$- (pulmonary) adrenergic receptors sites
Pharmacokinetics
  Absorption: Complete bioavailability
  Onset: PO—60 minutes; IV—Within minutes
  Duration: PO and IV 8 to 12 hours
Indications: Used for the management of life-threatening ventricular rhythms and to maintain a NSR in patients with symptomatic atrial fibrillation or atrial flutter
Contraindications: Known hypersensitivity; should not be given to patients with uncompensated CHF, pulmonary edema, asthma, or cardiogenic shock. Do not administer to patients with congenital or acquired long QT syndrome, sinus bradycardia, or second- or third-degree AV block.

> ***effective* Communication**
> **Do not begin sotalol therapy if patient QT interval is longer than 450 msec. If during therapy the QT interval becomes greater than 500 msec, call medical control; the dose may be reduced, the IV infusion may be prolonged, or therapy may be discontinued.**

Underline indicates most frequent; CAPITALS indicates life-threatening; (Canadian leaf) indicates Canadian drug name. (!) Safety and special populations.

Precautions: Use with caution in patients with kidney or liver impairment, in patients with a history of severe allergic reactions, and in patients with diabetes mellitus.

Route and Dosage

IV (Adult): Atrial fibrillation—112.5 mg once or twice daily; Maintenance infusion—112.5 to 150 mg once or twice daily; Atrial flutter—112.5 mg once or twice daily; Maintenance infusion—112.5 to 150 mg once or twice daily; Ventricular arrhythmias—75 mg over 5 hours; Maintenance infusion—75 to 300 mg over 5 hours

How Supplied

Solution for injection: 15 mg/mL

Adverse Reactions and Side Effects

Resp: Bronchospasm, wheezing

CV: ARRHYTHMIAS, BRADYCARDIA, CHF, PULMONARY EDEMA, orthostatic hypotension, peripheral vasoconstriction

CNS: Fatigue, weakness, anxiety, dizziness, drowsiness, insomnia, memory loss, mental depression, mental status changes, nervousness, nightmares

EENT: Blurred vision, dry eyes, nasal stuffiness

GI: Constipation, diarrhea, nausea

GU: Erectile dysfunction, decreased libido

Derm: Itching, rashes

Drug Interactions: IV phenytoin and verapamil may cause additive myocardial depression. Concurrent use with calcium channel blockers may increase the risk of adverse cardiovascular reactions. Additive bradycardia may occur with digoxin. Additive hypotension may occur if used with antihypertensives.

Check the **Evidence**

Concurrent use with class IA antiarrhythmics is not recommended due to the increased risk of developing serious arrhythmias.

EMS Considerations: Monitor vital signs prior to and frequently during therapy. Sotalol may cause life-threatening ventricular tachycardia associated with QT interval prolongation.

Streptokinase (strip-toe-KYE-nase)

Streptase

Classifications: Thrombolytic, plasminogen activator

Pregnancy Class: C

Mechanism of Action: Converts plasminogen to plasmin, which is then able to degrade fibrin present in blood clots

Pharmacokinetics

Absorption: Complete absorption after IV administration

Onset: Immediate

Duration: 4 to 12 hours

Indications: Used for the treatment of acute MI and acute stroke

Contraindications: Known hypersensitivity; should not be given to patients with a history of stroke, recent intracranial or intraspinal injury or trauma, intracranial neoplasm, or AV malformation or aneurysm

Precautions: Use with caution in patients with recent major surgery, trauma, GI or GU bleeding, severe liver or renal disease, hemorrhagic ophthalmic conditions, or recent streptococcal infection.

Route and Dosage

IV (Adult): MI—1.5 million units given as a continuous infusion over 60 minutes

How Supplied

Powder for injection: 250,000 units/vial; 750,000 units/vial; 1,500,000 units/vial

Adverse Reactions and Side Effects

Resp: Bronchospasm

CV: Hypotension, reperfusion arrhythmias

CNS: INTRACRANIAL HEMORRHAGE

EENT: Epitaxis, gingival bleeding

GI: GI BLEEDING, RETROPERITONEAL BLEEDING, nausea, vomiting

GU: GU TRACT BLEEDING

Local: Phlebitis at IV site

Misc: ANAPHYLAXIS

Drug Interactions: Concurrent use of aspirin and other NSAIDs, warfarin, and heparin may increase the risk of bleeding.

EMS Considerations: 🍁 Overdosing and underdosing have resulted in patient harm, including death. Monitor vital signs frequently during therapy. Notify medical control if systolic BP higher than 180 mm Hg or diastolic BP higher than 110 mm Hg.

Tenecteplase (te-NEK-to-plase)

TNKase

Classifications: Thrombolytic, plasminogen activator

Pregnancy Class: C

Mechanism of Action: Converts plasminogen to plasmin, which is then able to degrade fibrin present in blood clots

Pharmacokinetics

Absorption: Complete absorption after IV administration

Onset: Within minutes

Duration: Unknown

Indications: Used for the treatment of acute MI and acute stroke

Contraindications: Known hypersensitivity; should not be given to patients with a history of stroke, recent intracranial or intraspinal injury or trauma, intracranial neoplasm, or AV malformation or aneurysm

Precautions: Use with caution in patients with recent major surgery, trauma, GI or GU bleeding, severe liver or renal disease, hemorrhagic ophthalmic conditions, or recent streptococcal infection.

Route and Dosage

IV [Adult Less Than 60 kg (132 lbs)]: 30 mg

IV [Adult More Than 60 kg (132 lbs) and Less Than 70 kg (154 lbs)]: 35 mg

IV [Adult More Than 70 kg (154 lbs) and Less Than 80 kg (176 lbs)]: 40 mg

IV [Adult More Than 80 kg (176 lbs) and Less Than 90 kg (198 lbs)]: 45 mg

IV [Adult More Than 90 kg (198 lbs)]: 50 mg

How Supplied

Powder for injection: 50 mg/vial

Adverse Reactions and Side Effects
Resp: Bronchospasm
CV: Hypotension, reperfusion arrhythmias
CNS: INTRACRANIAL HEMORRHAGE
EENT: Epitaxis, gingival bleeding
GI: GI BLEEDING, RETROPERITONEAL BLEEDING, nausea, vomiting
GU: GU TRACT BLEEDING
Local: Phlebitis at IV site
Misc: ANAPHYLAXIS
Drug Interactions: Concurrent use of aspirin and other NSAIDs, warfarin, and heparin may increase the risk of bleeding.
EMS Considerations: ❗ Overdosing and underdosing have resulted in patient harm, including death. Monitor vital signs frequently during therapy. Notify medical control if systolic BP higher than 180 mm Hg or diastolic BP higher than 110 mm Hg.

Tirofiban (tye-roe-FYE-ban)

Aggrastat
Classification: Antiplatelet agent
Pregnancy Class: B
Mechanism of Action: Decreases platelet aggregation by reversibly antagonizing the binding of fibrinogen to the glycoprotein IIb/IIIa binding site on platelet surfaces
Pharmacokinetics
Absorption: Complete bioavailability
Onset: Rapid
Duration: Brief
Indications: Used in the treatment of acute coronary syndrome (unstable angina/non-Q wave MI)
Contraindications: Known hypersensitivity; should not be given to patients with active internal bleeding or a history of bleeding within the previous 30 days, to patients who have had a stroke within 30 days, or to patients with severe hypertension
Precautions: Use with caution in patients with severe renal insufficiency.
Route and Dosage
IV (Adult): 0.4 mcg/kg/minute for 30 minutes, then 0.1 mcg/kg/minute
How Supplied
Premixed solution for injection: 5 mg/100 mL (50 mcg/mL) in 100-mL single-dose containers, 12.5 mg/250 mL (50 mcg/mL) in 250-mL single-dose containers
Adverse Reactions and Side Effects
CV: Bradycardia, edema, vasovagal reaction
CNS: <u>Headache</u>, dizziness
Derm: Hives, rash
Drug Interactions: Concurrent use of aspirin, NSAIDs, warfarin, heparin, and heparin-like agents may increase the risk of bleeding.
EMS Considerations: Frequently assess patient vital signs and monitor the patient for any signs of bleeding.

Vasopressin (vay-soe-PRESS-in)

Pitressin, 🍁 Pressyn
Classification: Antidiuretic hormone
Pregnancy Class: C
Mechanism of Action: In high doses, vasopressin acts as a nonadrenergic peripheral vasoconstrictor.
Pharmacokinetics
Absorption: Rapid absorption
Onset: Unknown
Duration: 30 to 60 minutes
Indications: Can be used for the management of pulseless VT/V-Fib unresponsive to initial defibrillation, asystole, or pulseless electrical activity (PEA), according to ACLS guidelines
Contraindications: Known hypersensitivity; should not be given to patients with chronic renal failure or to those who are hypersensitive to beef or pork proteins
Precautions: Use with caution in patients with a history of seizures, asthma, heart failure, migraine headaches and in those with cardiovascular disease or renal impairment.
Route and Dosage
IV (Adult): 40 units as a single dose
IV (Pediatric): 0.4 units/kg after resuscitation and at least two doses of epinephrine

effective **Communication**

Vasopressin should be given rapidly (1 to 2 seconds) during cardiac arrest.

How Supplied
Injection: 20 units/mL in 0.5- and 1-mL ampules and vials
Adverse Reactions and Side Effects
CV: MI, angina
CNS: Dizziness, "pounding" sensation in the head
GI: Abdominal cramps, belching, diarrhea, flatulence, heartburn, nausea, vomiting
Drug Interactions: None significant during resuscitation
EMS Considerations: Monitor BP, HR, and ECG continuously throughout cardiopulmonary resuscitation.

Verapamil (ver-AP-a-mil)

Calan, 🍁 Novo-Veramil, 🍁 Nu-Verap
Classifications: Antianginal, class IV antiarrhythmic, antihypertensive, calcium channel blocker
Pregnancy Class: C
Mechanism of Action: Inhibits the transport of calcium into the myocardial and vascular smooth muscle cells, causing inhibition of excitation-contraction coupling and subsequent contraction; also decreases SA and AV conduction and prolongs the AV node refractory period in conduction tissue
Pharmacokinetics
Absorption: Well absorbed
Onset: 1 to 5 minutes
Duration: 2 hours
Indications: Used in the management of hypertension, angina pectoris, and vasospastic (Prinzmetal) angina; can also be used for the management of supraventricular arrhythmias and rapid ventricular rates in atrial flutter or atrial fibrillation

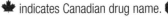

Contraindications: Known hypersensitivity; should not be given to patients with sick sinus syndrome, second- or third-degree AV block, severe ventricular dysfunction, or cardiogenic shock
Precautions: Use with caution in patients with severe liver impairment and in patients with serious ventricular arrhythmias or CHF.

Route and Dosage

IV (Adult): 5 to 10 mg (75 to 150 mcg/kg); may be repeated with 10 mg (150 mcg/kg) after 15 to 30 minutes

How Supplied

Solution for injection: 2.5 mg/mL

Adverse Reactions and Side Effects

Resp: Cough, dyspnea, shortness of breath
CV: ARRHYTHMIAS, CHF, bradycardia, chest pain, hypotension, palpitations, peripheral edema, syncope
CNS: Abnormal dreams, anxiety, confusion, dizziness, drowsiness, headache, nervousness, psychiatric disturbances, weakness
EENT: Blurred vision, epistaxis, tinnitus
GI: Anorexia, constipation, diarrhea, dry mouth, nausea, vomiting
Misc: STEVENS-JOHNSON SYNDROME
Drug Interactions: Additive hypotension may occur with concurrent use of other antihypertensives or nitrates. Concurrent use with beta blockers, digoxin, or phenytoin may result in bradycardia, conduction defects, or CHF.
EMS Considerations: Monitor ECG continuously during therapy. Verapamil may cause a prolonged PR interval.

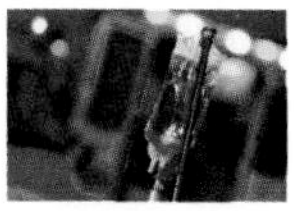

SCENARIO REVISITED

Do you recall the case of Kelvin who had chest pain and trouble breathing? After attaching the ECG leads to Kelvin, you see that he has an underlying sinus rhythm with multifocal PVCs (Fig. 11-7). Multifocal PVCs should be treated immediately. These PVCs are considered malignant, because the ectopic activity causing them originates from more than one area of the ventricles. The fact that the PVCs are multifocal, coupled with Kelvin's presenting signs and symptoms, indicate that the chances are high that the multifocal PVCs will deteriorate to ventricular fibrillation, placing Kelvin in cardiopulmonary arrest.

Let's Recap

This chapter contains some of the most essential and frequently used medications in the out-of-hospital setting. Additionally, it also addresses essential electrical therapy that may be required before medications are used for myocardial stabilization.

The guidelines, dosages, and medications used in cardiovascular emergencies are continually changing. While it is a difficult task, EMS professionals must attain an in-depth knowledge of these medications and remain current on new drugs and guidelines as they evolve.

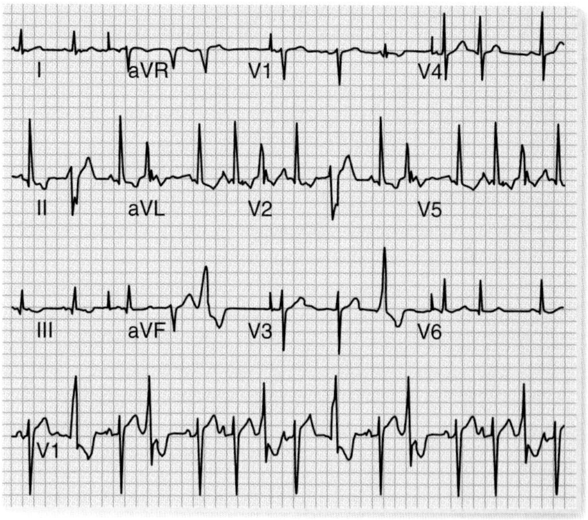

Figure 11-7 Sinus rhythm with multifocal PVCs.

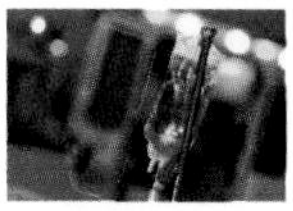

SCENARIO CONCLUSION

After the initial evaluation of Kelvin, the first step in his treatment is reassurance. Reassurance may relieve some of Kelvin's apprehension, which, in turn, may help reduce the frequency of the PVCs. The initial drugs to be considered when treating Kelvin include oxygen, aspirin, nitroglycerin, and possibly morphine.

To begin with, place Kelvin on 6 L of 100 percent humidified oxygen. The oxygen flow can be increased if necessary. Oxygen by itself may aid in controlling PVCs. As Kelvin is short of breath, it may be appropriate to place him in a comfortable position such as sitting or semi-sitting.

Aspirin is given as soon as possible to patients who are experiencing chest pain. It works by decreasing platelet aggregation, thereby decreasing the incidence of an MI. The initial dose of aspirin should be 160 to 325 mg.

The next drug to be considered is nitroglycerin. Nitroglycerin increases myocardial blood flow by dilating coronary arteries and improving collateral flow to ischemic regions of the heart. The dosage of nitroglycerine is 0.3 to 0.4 mg by sublingual spray or tablet every 5 minutes for 15 minutes (three total doses).

If nitroglycerin is ineffective, the next drug to be considered is morphine. Morphine alters the perception of pain and produces generalized CNS depression. It is commonly used for patients who may be experiencing an MI. The dosage for morphine is 4 to 10 mg IV.

It is vital to make the best possible use of treatment time—time is muscle. Whenever appropriate, do as much treatment as possible while en route to the receiving facility.

PRACTICE EXERCISES

1. The correct dosage of atropine to be given to the patient with symptomatic bradycardia is:
   a. 1 to 5 mg by IV initially. This can be repeated every 3 to 5 minutes to a total dose of 20 mg.
   b. 0.5 by IV initially. This may be repeated every 3 to 5 minutes to a total dose of 2.0 mg.
   c. 0.5 mg IV. This may be repeated every 3 to 5 minutes to a total dose of 0.04 mg/kg (3 mg).
   d. 5 mg by IV. Repeat doses may be given at 10 mg by IV bolus.
2. Propranolol is a nonselective beta-adrenergic blocking agent. Its blocking action reduces the rate and force of heart contractions and blood pressure. Which of the following is *not* an adverse reaction or side effect of propranolol?
   a. Coma
   b. Weakness
   c. Congestive heart failure
   d. Bronchospasm, wheezing
3. Which of the following drugs is indicated for the treatment of ventricular fibrillation, ventricular tachycardia, and supraventricular tachycardia?
   a. Lidocaine
   b. Adenosine
   c. Amiodarone
   d. Verapamil
4. Which of the following actions can be attributed to epinephrine when administered during cardiac arrest?
   a. Peripheral vasodilation
   b. Increase in cardiac automaticity
   c. Prolonged refractory period
   d. Decrease in ventricular fibrillation threshold
5. Digoxin:
   a. Is helpful in the treatment of incomplete heart block
   b. Is used in the treatment of bradyarrhythmias
   c. Controls rapid ventricular response caused by atrial fibrillation or atrial flutter
   d. Is used in the treatment of ventricular tachycardia in patients with a pulse who do not respond to more-conventional therapy
6. Potential side effects of diltiazem include all of the following *except*:
   a. AV block
   b. Hypotension
   c. CHF
   d. Tachycardia
7. Morphine is contraindicated in patients with:
   a. Acute cardiogenic pulmonary edema
   b. Severe pain associated with myocardial ischemia
   c. Abnormally rapid respirations
   d. Hypotension
8. Dopamine has dose-dependent effects on adrenergic receptors. A dose of 15 mcg/kg/min would result in:
   a. Improved blood flow to the kidney
   b. Decreased afterload
   c. Increased blood pressure
   d. Decreased cardiac contractility
9. Adenosine is useful in treating which of the following?
   a. Atrial fibrillation
   b. Second-degree AV block
   c. PSVT associated with Wolff-Parkinson-White syndrome
   d. Ventricular tachycardia
10. Nitroglycerin relieves anginal attacks by all of the following actions *except*:
    a. Decrease in ventricular workload
    b. Reduction in myocardial oxygen demand
    c. Increase in coronary blood flow
    d. Increase in heart rate

CASE STUDIES

1. You are called to the home of a man who "feels dizzy and weak." When you arrive, you find your 70-year-old male patient sitting in a chair awake and talking. He states that he does not have any pain or shortness of breath, but, when he gets up to walk, he gets dizzy. You place the patient on 6 L of humidified oxygen and attach the ECG monitor while your partner is taking the patient's blood pressure. The patient's blood pressure is 100/60 mm Hg, and his ECG rhythm is sinus bradycardia with a rate of 44 beats per minute. The treatment for symptomatic bradycardia can include electrical therapy or atropine. Since your patient is alert and talking, you give atropine at 0.5 mg IV bolus. You can repeat this dosage every 5 minutes to a total dose of:
   a. 1 mg
   b. 2 mg
   c. 3 mg
   d. 4 mg

2. You respond to a 46-year-old man who complains of severe substernal chest pain that radiates to his left shoulder and down his left arm. He is short of breath and very apprehensive. The ECG monitor shows a sinus tachycardia at a rate of 110 beats per minute. After assessing vital signs, you note that they are currently within normal limits. Initial treatment should include oxygen, aspirin, reassurance, and:
   a. Nitroglycerin
   b. Amiodarone
   c. Adenosine
   d. Morphine

The Perfect Scenario

It is 6:15 on a Wednesday morning when the patient makes a "funny" noise that awakens his wife, Suzy. Suzy nudges him in hopes that he goes back to sleep. There is no response. She gets up and goes to his side of the bed to shake him, but, again, there is no response. Suzy feels for, and does not find, a pulse. Suzy immediately calls 911 and somehow gets her 215-pound husband off the bed and on to the floor without causing any trauma. Once her husband was on the floor, Suzy began CPR.

EMS arrived at Suzy's home within 4 minutes of her dialing 911. When at the patient's side, the EMS crew attached the defibrillation pads and defibrillated at 200 joules. The ECG immediately converted from ventricular fibrillation to a normal sinus rhythm. The patient also began breathing on his own and attempted to open his eyes. The EMS crew started an IV infusion of amiodarone and transported him to the hospital. No other treatment was needed.

Once at the hospital, the patient was taken for an MRI of the head, which was normal. Then he was taken to the cardiac cath lab where all coronary arteries were found to be clear. The problem was HCM. Apparently, the electrical signal from the AV node had a difficult time moving through a left ventricle that was too thick, causing sudden cardiac arrest. The outcome? The patient now has an implantable cardioverter defibrillator (ICD) and is back playing terrible golf and loving it.

The patient was me—the author of this text. I call this the perfect scenario because everything worked to perfection, just as the textbooks say it should.

- Suzy performed CPR well, probably within a minute of my arrest—my chest hurt for a month. About a month before my arrest, she had updated her CPR skills at work. Suzy has been a nurse for 25 years, and this was the first time she had to perform "real" CPR.
- The EMS crew was there in 4 minutes and immediately defibrillated. The only other treatment I required was oxygen and an IV infusing amiodarone. I was on amiodarone for approximately 24 hours.

The EMS paramedic crew from Williamson Medical Center in Franklin, Tennessee did a perfect job. I met the crew a couple of weeks after the event to thank them. It was an emotional but happy time. We all agreed that, if anyone in EMS begins taking EMS for granted, it is time to move on to another career.

MATH EQUATIONS

1. You are ordered to infuse dopamine at 10 mcg/kg/minute using a 60 gtt/mL IV set. Your patient weighs 205 lbs. The infusion is prepared by adding 800 mg of dopamine in 500 mL of IV solution.
   a. How many kg does your patient weigh?
   b. What is the concentration of the IV solution (mcg/mL)?
   c. What is the infusion rate to give 10 mcg/kg/minute?

2. You are ordered to give an IV bolus of 1.5 mg/kg of lidocaine to your 195 lb patient. This dosage is to be followed by a lidocaine infusion at 3 mg/minute. The IV infusion is prepared by adding 2 g of lidocaine to 500 mL of IV solution.
   a. How many kg does your patient weigh?
   b. How many mg is your initial bolus dosage?
   c. What is the concentration of the IV infusion (mg/mL)?
   d. What is the drip rate/minute using a 60 gtt/mL IV set?

3. You are ordered to begin a norepinephrine infusion at a rate of 0.5 mcg/minute. You prepare the infusion by adding 4 mg of norepinephrine to 250 mL of IV solution.
   a. What is the concentration of the IV infusion (mcg/mL)?
   b. What is the rate of the infusion using a 60 gtt/mL IV set?
4. You are ordered to begin a nitroprusside infusion to your 135-lb patient. The infusion is to initially run at 0.3 mcg/kg/minute. You prepare the infusion by adding 50 mg of nitroprusside to 500 mL of IV solution.
   a. How many kg does your patient weigh?
   b. What is the concentration of the IV infusion (mcg/mL)?
   c. What is the drip rate/minute using a 60 gtt/mL IV set?

REFERENCES

Beck, R. K. (2012). Drugs used to treat cardiovascular emergencies. In *Pharmacology for the EMS provider.* New York, NY: Delmar, Cengage Learning.

Deglin, J. H., Vallerand, A. H., and Sanboski, C. A. (2011). *Davis's drug guide for nurses* (12th ed.). Philadelphia, PA: F. A. Davis Company.

Dorian, P. Amiodarone versus Lidocaine in V-Fib Evaluation (ALIVE) trial in NASPE [CD-ROM]. Presented at: 22nd Annual Scientific Sessions of the North American Society of Pacing and Electrophysiology; May 2–5, 2001; Boston, MA.

Johns Hopkins Medicine. Congestive heart failure. Retrieved June 15, 2014 from http://www.hopkinsmedicine.org/heart_vascular_institute/conditions_treatments/conditions/congestive_heart_failure.html

Kudenchuk, P. T. (1999). Amiodarone for resuscitation after out-of-hospital cardiac arrest due to V-fib., *New England Journal of Medicine, 341*:871.

National Library of Medicine. Congenital heart defects. Retrieved June 15, 2014 from www.nlm.nih.gov/medlineplus/congenitalheartdefects.html

Odou, P., Ferrari, N., Bathélémy, C, et al. (2005). Grapefruit juice-nifedipine interaction: possible involvement of several mechanisms. *Journal of Clinical Pharmacy and Therapeutics, 30,* 153–158. Retrieved June 12, 2014 from www.ncbi.nlm.nih.gov/pubmed/15811168

Venes, D., ed. (2013). *Taber's cyclopedic medical dictionary* (22nd ed.). Philadelphia, PA: F. A. Davis Company.

WebMD LLC. Defibrillation. Retrieved June 10, 2014 from www.emedicine.medscape.com/article/80564-overview#a01

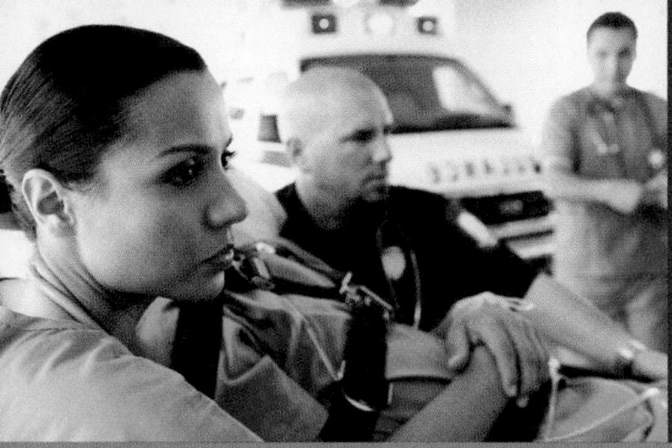

CHAPTER 12

Drugs Used to Treat Disorders of the Eyes, Ears, Nose, and Throat

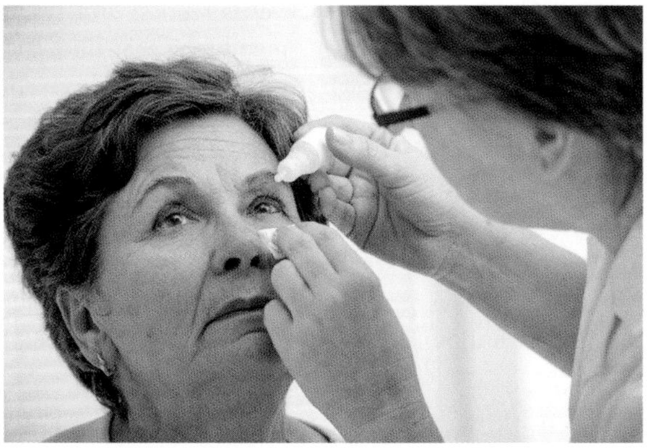

Administering an ophthalmic medication to a patient.
(Photograph © AlexRaths/iStock/Thinkstock)

LEARNING OUTCOMES

- Describe disorders and diseases of the eyes, ears, nose, and throat.
- Discuss the actions, uses, contraindications, precautions, route and dosage, and EMS considerations for the medications used for treating disorders and diseases of the eyes, ears, nose, and throat.
- Be familiar with the medications that are used to treat colds and flu.

KEY TERMS

Aqueous humor
Conjunctivitis
Glaucoma
Ménière disease
Optic nerve
Pharyngitis
Rheumatic fever
Rhinitis
Sinusitis
Sjögren syndrome
Streptococcal pharyngitis
Tinnitus
Tonsillitis
Vertigo

SCENARIO OPENING

You have been assigned to do a clinical rotation in the Emergency Department at Hillside Hospital. During your first four hours, you have started five IVs, given two medications, performed CPR, and did vital signs on several other patients. Just when you are sitting down for lunch, your preceptor says that a mother has brought her 8-year-old son Larry in to be treated for strep throat.

Larry's mom states that Larry was taking penicillin for strep throat for a couple of days. When he began to feel better, Larry stopped taking it. Now Larry feels worse than he did before he first began taking the penicillin. Your initial assessment reveals the following:

- Tachycardia
- Sore throat
- Difficulty swallowing
- Headache
- Fever of 103°F
- Red appearance at the back of Larry's throat
- White pus on Larry's tonsils
- Tender lymph nodes in his neck

Introduction

Eye, ear, nose, and throat (EENT) disorders generally are not life-threatening problems. However, they usually make patients feel uncomfortable and can have serious consequences. Many times, when people experience EENT disorders, they can "weather the storm" and feel better within a week or less. However, sometimes we must rely on medications to help us with the storm. This chapter discusses common EENT disorders and some of the medications that are often administered to treat them.

Pathophysiology of EENT Disorders

Eye Disorders

Dry Eyes

Tears provide constant moisture and lubrication so our eyes can maintain vision and comfort. Tears consist of the following:

- Water, which provides the proper amount of moisture
- Oils, which are used for lubrication
- Mucus, which provides for even spreading of our tears
- Antibodies, which help protect against infection

When tear ducts do not secrete a sufficient amount of tears, or if there is an imbalance in the consistency of tears, dry eyes may develop. Other causes of dry eyes include:

- Dry air from heat or air-conditioning
- The aging process
- Menopause
- Side effects from drugs such as antihistamines and birth control pills
- Diseases that affect the ability to make tears, such as a condition called **Sjögren syndrome (SS)** or rheumatoid arthritis

Dry eyes due to an imbalance of tear consistency or poor tear duct production cannot be cured. However, several treatment options are available. For example, the use of artificial tears is the primary treatment for dry eyes. Most of these medications are available over the counter. Other treatment options may include topical steroids or surgery.

Check the Evidence

In 2002, the U.S. Food and Drug Administration (FDA) approved the prescription eye medication Restasis for the treatment of chronic dry eyes. Restasis helps the eyes increase tear production.

Conjunctivitis

Conjunctivitis (pinkeye) is redness and swelling of the conjunctiva, the mucous membrane that lines the eyelid and eye surface (Fig. 12-1). It is contagious and can spread very easily. However, conjunctivitis is usually not a serious condition and resolves itself in 7 to 10 days without medical treatment. Conjunctivitis is generally caused by infections (viruses or bacteria), dry eyes, chemicals, fumes, smoke, or allergies.

If conjunctivitis is caused by a virus, medications are not usually used. However, if conjunctivitis is caused by bacteria, an antibiotic is usually prescribed to kill the bacteria.

Glaucoma

Glaucoma is a condition that develops when too much fluid **(aqueous humor)** builds up inside of the eye. It causes gradual loss of peripheral vision and ultimately blindness. The increased pressure from the aqueous humor can damage the **optic nerve.** The optic nerve transmits images to the brain. If damage to

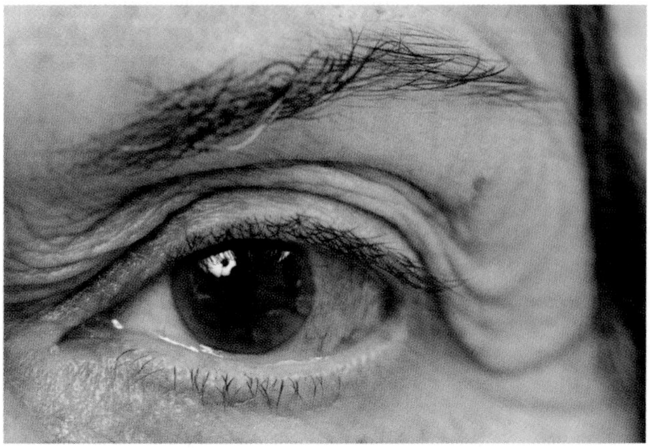

Figure 12-1 Conjunctivitis. *(Photograph © Levent Konuk/iStock/Thinkstock)*

the optic nerve continues, glaucoma leads to blindness. Without treatment, glaucoma can cause total permanent blindness within a few years. For most people, there are usually few or no symptoms of glaucoma. The first sign of glaucoma is often the loss of peripheral vision, which can go unnoticed until late in the disease.

There are three major types of glaucoma:

1. *Narrow- or closed-angle (acute) glaucoma:* Occurs in persons whose eyes are anatomically predisposed to develop glaucoma
2. *Open-angle (chronic) glaucoma:* The structures of the eye appear normal, but fluid in the eye does not flow properly.
3. *Congenital glaucoma:* Occurs in persons who are born with an abnormal fluid drainage angle in their eyes

There are three general treatment options for glaucoma: prescription eyedrops, laser surgery, or microsurgery.

Ear Disorders

Tinnitus

Tinnitus is a ringing, buzzing, or hissing sound in the ear. The most common cause of tinnitus is hearing loss due to aging. However, it can also be caused by working around loud noises, rapid weight loss, excessive earwax, the side effects of some medications such as antibiotics, a dental condition known as temporomandibular joint (TMJ) disorder, Ménière disease, and several other issues.

For some patients, tinnitus is only a minor irritation, but for others it can be disabling. Many medications for treating tinnitus have been studied. For some patients, treatment with antianxiety drugs or antidepressants has helped.

Ménière Disease

Ménière disease is an inner ear disorder that affects hearing and balance. It can affect people of all ages but is most common in those aged 40 to 60. It is thought that Ménière disease may be related to fluids that build up in the inner ear.

Symptoms of Ménière disease can come on quickly. During an attack, patients may experience tinnitus, temporary or permanent hearing loss, **vertigo** (the feeling of surroundings that are spinning), or a sensation of pressure or fullness in the ear. An attack of Ménière disease can last from hours to days. As the disease progresses, attacks generally are more frequent in the beginning and gradually become less frequent.

Medications do not cure Ménière disease but focus on reducing the severity of symptoms such as vertigo. Other medications may be given to help control nausea or vomiting caused by vertigo.

Nose and Sinus Disorders

Sinusitis

Sinusitis is an inflammation of the sinuses. It may be caused by various agents, including viruses, bacteria, or allergies. There are four types of sinusitis:

1. *Acute:* Lasts up to 4 weeks
2. *Subacute:* Lasts 4 to 12 weeks
3. *Chronic:* Lasts more than 12 weeks and can continue for months or even years
4. *Recurrent:* Several attacks may occur within a year.

Treatment for patients with sinusitis may include analgesics to relieve pain, decongestants to shrink the swollen membranes in the nose, or antibiotics to control a bacterial infection.

Rhinitis

Rhinitis is inflammation or irritation of the nasal passages, resulting in runny nose, nasal congestion, or postnasal drainage. Rhinitis is also known as *acute rhinitis*, which is usually a manifestation of the common cold, and *allergic rhinitis*, which is hay fever. Treatment for rhinitis includes rest, adequate fluids, a well-balanced diet, and over-the-counter analgesics and decongestants.

Throat Disorders

Pharyngitis

Pharyngitis is an inflammation of the membranes and tissues of the pharynx. Most people call pharyngitis a sore throat. Pharyngitis is usually caused by viral or bacterial infections. The predominant symptom is throat pain. However, fever, weakness, muscle aches, and painful swallowing can also be present.

The treatment for patients with pharyngitis includes gargling with warm saltwater, analgesic medications, fluids, throat lozenges, or topical anesthetics. A throat culture may be ordered to identify the possibility of bacteria, in which case an antibiotic may be ordered.

Tonsillitis

Tonsillitis is an inflammation of the tonsils. Symptoms of tonsillitis include fever, weakness, and throat pain, especially with swallowing. Patients can also develop runny nose, cough, and diarrhea. Tonsillitis is generally caused by a virus and therefore is treated symptomatically. If tonsillitis is caused by bacteria, an antibiotic is prescribed. If left untreated, bacterial tonsillitis may develop into **rheumatic fever,** a multisystem inflammatory disease that may cause damage to the heart valves.

Streptococcal Pharyngitis (Strep Throat)

Streptococcal (bacterial) pharyngitis or strep throat is an infection of the throat and tonsils (Fig. 12-2). It is caused by the *Streptococcus* bacterium. Although people of all ages can become infected, strep throat is more common in children aged 5 to 13.

Strep throat symptoms are usually more serious than the symptoms of common pharyngitis and may include the following:

- Sudden sore throat
- Loss of appetite
- Painful swallowing

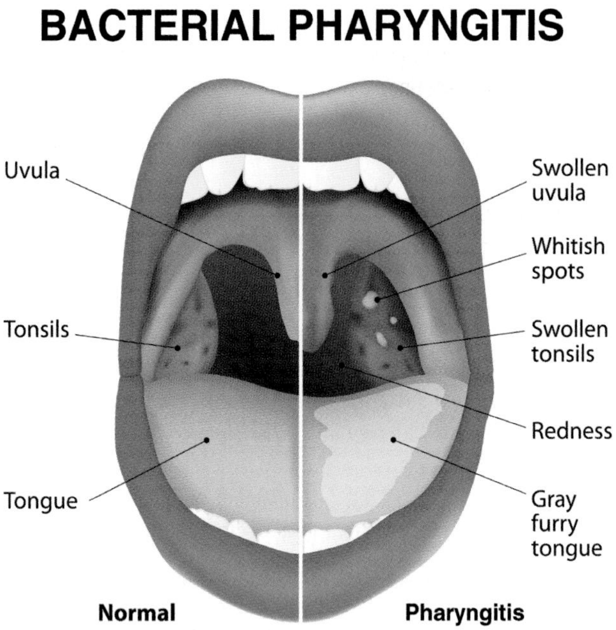

Figure 12-2 Bacterial pharyngitis. *(Photograph © ttsz/iStock/Thinkstock)*

- Red tonsils with white spots
- Fever
- Headache

Strep throat is usually treated with antibiotics as well as over-the-counter pain relievers and fever medications. Strep throat does not usually occur with congestion or a cough.

Pharmacokinetics

Antianxiety Agents

Most antianxiety drugs cause generalized CNS depression. They have no analgesic properties.

Check the Evidence

Prolonged high-dose use of benzodiazepines may lead to psychological or physical dependence.

Antiasthmatics

Antiasthmatics treat airway constriction by causing bronchodilation and decreasing airway inflammation. Adrenergic bronchodilators work by increasing intracellular cAMP, which causes bronchodilation. Corticosteroids act by decreasing airway inflammation. Anticholinergics produce bronchodilation by decreasing intracellular levels of cyclic GMP. Leukotriene receptor antagonist and mast cell stabilizers decrease the release of substances that can contribute to bronchospasm.

Anticholinergics

Anticholinergics competitively inhibit the action of the neurotransmitter acetylcholine (ACh).

Anticonvulsants

Anticonvulsants depress abnormal neuronal discharges in the CNS that may result in seizures. These drugs can work by preventing the spread of seizures, depressing the motor cortex, raising seizure threshold, or altering levels of neurotransmitters.

Antiemetics

Antiemetics can act on the chemoreceptor trigger zone to inhibit nausea and vomiting.

Antiglaucoma Agents

Antiglaucoma drugs treat certain types of glaucoma by either enhancing the outflow of aqueous humor or decreasing its production, or both.

Antihistamines

Antihistamines block the effects of histamine at the H_1 receptor. However, they do not block histamine release, antibody production, or antigen-antibody reactions.

Anti-infectives

Anti-infectives kill bacteria or inhibit the growth of bacteriostatic-susceptible pathogenic bacteria. They are not active against viruses or fungi.

Corticosteroids

Corticosteroids produce varied metabolic effects, in addition to modifying the normal immune response and suppressing inflammation.

Decongestants

Decongestants are sympathomimetic drugs that stimulate the alpha-adrenergic receptors. The decongestant effect is due to vasoconstriction of the blood vessels in the nose, sinuses, and so on. The vasoconstriction effect reduces swelling or inflammation and mucus formation in the nasal passages.

Mydriatics

Mydriatic agents are medicines that cause the pupil of the eye to dilate. Topical mydriatic agents are applied directly to the eye to assist during eye examination and to treat inflammatory eye conditions.

Mucolytics

Mucolytic agents may help thin mucus, improving drainage of mucus from the nose and sinuses in treating sinusitis.

Individual Drugs

AcetaZOLAMIDE (a-seet-a-ZOLE-a-mide)

🍁 Acetazolam, Diamox

Classifications: Antiglaucoma agent, ocular hypotensive
Pregnancy Class: C
Mechanism of Action: Decreases the secretion of aqueous humor

Pharmacokinetics

Absorption: Dose dependent

Onset: 1 to 1.5 hours

Duration: 8 to 12 hours

Indications: Lowers the intraocular pressure in the treatment of glaucoma

Contraindications: Known hypersensitivity; should not be used in patients with liver disease or liver insufficiency; should not be used concurrently with brinzolamide or with dorzolamide; should not be used during the first trimester of pregnancy

Precautions: Use with caution in patients with chronic respiratory disease, gout, kidney disease, or diabetes mellitus.

Route and Dosage

PO (Adult): Open-angle glaucoma—250 to 1,000 mg/day in one to four divided doses (up to 250 mg every 4 hours) or 500 mg extended-release capsules twice daily

PO (Pediatric): Glaucoma—8 to 30 mg/kg in three divided doses

How Supplied

Tablets: 125 mg, 250 mg

Extended-release capsules: 500 mg

Adverse Reactions and Side Effects

CNS: Weakness, depression, drowsiness

EENT: Transient nearsightedness

GI: Anorexia, metallic taste, nausea, vomiting

Derm: STEVENS-JOHNSON SYNDROME

Misc: ANAPHYLAXIS

Drug Interactions: Excretion of barbiturates, aspirin, and lithium is increased and may lead to decreased effectiveness. Excretion of amphetamine, quinidine, procainamide, and tricyclic antidepressants is decreased and may lead to toxicity. Acetazolamide may increase cyclosporine levels.

effective **Communication**

Do not confuse acetazolamide with acetohexamide or Diamox with Diabinese.

EMS Considerations: Monitor vital signs frequently during therapy. Observe patients for signs of hypokalemia (weakness, fatigue, ECG changes, vomiting).

Amoxicillin (a-mox-i-SILL-in)

Moxatag, ♣ Novamoxin

Classification: Anti-infective, aminopenicillin

Pregnancy Class: B

Mechanism of Action: Binds to bacterial cell wall, causing cell death

Pharamcokinetics

Absorption: Well absorbed

Onset: 50 minutes

Duration: 8 to 12 hours

Indication: Used to treat sinusitis and strep throat, as well as other bacterial infections

Contraindications: Known hypersensitivity; should not be used in patients with known hypersensitivity to penicillins (cross-sensitivity exists to cephalosporins)

Precautions: Use with caution in patients with severe kidney insufficiency, infectious mononucleosis, or acute lymphocytic leukemia.

Route and Dosage

PO (Adult): 250 to 500 mg every 8 hours or 500 to 875 mg every 12 hours, not to exceed 2 to 3 g per day

PO (Pediatric older than 3 months): 25 to 50 mg/kg/day in divided doses every 8 hours or 25 to 50 mg/kg/day individual doses

PO (Infants under 3 months and neonates): 20 to 30 mg/kg/day in divided doses

Understand the Numbers

You have been asked to administer 20 mg/kg of amoxicillin to your 3-year-old female patient. When you ask for the child's weight, the baby-sitter does not know, and there is not a working scale in the home. Therefore, how many milligrams will you administer?

The average weight for a 3-year-old girl is between 25 and 38 lbs. The average height is between 35 and 39 inches. Your patient measures 36 inches. Therefore, you estimate your patient weighs 27 lbs.

27 lbs ÷ 2.2 kg = 12.2 kg. 20 mg × 12 lbs = 240 mg.

How Supplied

Chewable tablets: 125 mg, 200 mg, 250 mg, 400 mg

Tablets: 500 mg, 875 mg

Extended-release tablets: 775 mg

Capsules: 250 mg, 500 mg

Suspension: 50 mg/mL, 125, mg/5mL, 200 mg/5mL, 250 mg/5 mL, 400 mg/5mL

Tablets for oral suspension: 200 mg, 400 mg, 600 mg

Route and Dosage

CNS: SEIZURES (high doses)

GI: Diarrhea, nausea, vomiting

Derm: Rash

Misc: ANAPHYLAXIS, superinfection

Drug Interactions: Probenecid decreases kidney excretion and increases blood levels of amoxicillin; may increase the effect of warfarin; may decrease effectiveness of oral contraceptives

EMS Considerations: Monitor patients for any signs of anaphylaxis.

effective **Communication**

Whenever there is a chance for a patient to develop an anaphylactic reaction, have epinephrine, an antihistamine, and resuscitative equipment readily available.

Beclomethasone (be-kloe-METH-a-sone)

QVAR

Classifications: Antiasthmatic, anti-inflammatory (steroidal)
Pregnancy Class: C
Mechanism of Action: Potent, locally acting anti-inflammatory agent
Pharmacokinetics
Absorption: 20 percent absorbed
Onset: Within 24 hours
Duration: Unknown
Indications: Used as an adjunct medication in treating sinusitis
Contraindications: Known hypersensitivity; should not be given to patients having an acute attack of asthma or status asthmaticus
Precautions: Use with caution in patients with diabetes mellitus, glaucoma, or liver dysfunction.

Route and Dosage

Inhalation (Adult and Pediatric over 12 years): 40 to 80 mcg twice daily, not to exceed 320 mcg twice daily
Inhalation (Pediatric 5 to 11 years): 40 mcg twice daily, not to exceed 80 mcg twice daily

How Supplied

Inhalation aerosol: 40 mcg/metered inhalation in 7.3-g canister (delivers 100 metered inhalations), 80 mcg/metered inhalation in 7.3-g canister (delivers 100 metered inhalations)

Adverse Reactions and Side Effects

Resp: BRONCHOSPASM, cough, wheezing
CNS: Headache, agitation, depression, dizziness, restlessness
EENT: Hoarseness, dysphonia, cataracts, nasal congestion, pharyngitis
Misc: ANAPHYLAXIS, LARYNGEAL EDEMA, CHURG-STRAUSS SYNDROME [rare (affecting the respiratory, cardiac, and peripheral nervous systems as well as the musculoskeletal system)]
Drug Interactions: None significant
EMS Considerations: Monitor patients for any signs or symptoms of hypersensitivity reactions.

Budesonide (byoo-DESS-oh-nide)

Rhinocort Aqua

Classifications: Anti-inflammatory (steroidal), corticosteroid (nasal)
Pregnancy Class: B
Mechanism of Action: Potent, locally acting anti-inflammatory
Pharmacokinetics
Absorption: 34 percent absorbed
Onset: 1 to 2 days
Duration: Unknown
Indication: Used for seasonal or perennial allergic rhinitis
Contraindications: Known hypersensitivity; should not be given to patients with known hypersensitivity to alcohol, propylene, or polyethylene glycol
Precautions: Use with caution in patients with active untreated infections, diabetes mellitus, glaucoma, or recent nasal trauma, septal ulcers, or surgery.

Route and Dosage

Intranasal (Adult and Pediatric over 12 years): Spray in each nostril once daily, not to exceed 4 sprays in each nostril once daily.
Intranasal (Pediatric 6 to 11 years): One spray in each nostril once daily

How Supplied

Nasal spray: 32 mcg/metered spray in 8.6-g canister; delivers 120 metered sprays

Adverse Reactions and Side Effects

Resp: Cough, bronchospasm
CNS: Dizziness, headache
EENT: Epistaxis, nasal burning/irritation, nasal congestion, sneezing, tearing eyes
GI: Dry mouth, nausea, vomiting
Misc: ANAPHYLAXIS, ANGIOEDEMA
Drug Interactions: Ketoconazole increases the effects of budesonide.
EMS Considerations: Monitor patients for their degree of nasal stuffiness, amount and color of nasal discharge, and frequency of sneezing. Continually assess patients for developing anaphylaxis and angioedema. Have epinephrine, an antihistamine, and resuscitative equipment readily available.

Cephalexin (sef-a-LEX-in)

Keflex

Classification: Anti-infective, first-generation cephalosporin
Pregnancy Class: B
Mechanism of Action: Binds to bacterial cell wall membrane, causing cell death
Pharmacokinetics
Absorption: Well absorbed
Onset: Rapid
Duration: 12 to 24 hours
Indications: Used to treat streptococcal pharyngitis (strep throat)
Contraindications: Known hypersensitivity; should not be given to patients with known hypersensitivity to cephalosporins or penicillins
Precautions: Use with caution in patients with kidney impairment.

Route and Dosage

PO (Adult): 500 mg every 12 hr
PO (Pediatric): 25–50 mg/kg/day divided every 6–8 hours

How Supplied

Capsules: 250 mg, 333 mg, 500 mg, 750 mg
Tablets: 250 mg, 500 mg
Oral suspension: 100 mg/mL, 125 mg/5 mL, 250 mg/5 mL

Adverse Reactions and Side Effects

CNS: SEIZURES (high doses)
GI: PSEUDOMEMBRANOUS COLITIS, diarrhea, nausea, vomiting, cramps
Derm: STEVENS-JOHNSON SYNDROME, rash
Misc: ANAPHYLAXIS, superinfection
Drug Interactions: Concurrent use of loop diuretics or aminoglycosides may increase the risk of kidney toxicity.
EMS Considerations: Observe patients for anaphylaxis. Keep epinephrine, an antihistamine, and resuscitative equipment available throughout therapy.

Ciclesonide (sys-KLES-oh-nide)

🍁 Drymira, Omnaris, Zetonna

Classifications: Anti-inflammatory (steroidal), corticosteroid (nasal)
Pregnancy Class: C

Mechanism of Action: Potent, locally-acting anti-inflammatory
Indications: Used for seasonal or perennial allergic rhinitis
Contraindications: Known hypersensitivity; should not be given to patients with known hypersensitivity to alcohol, propylene, or polyethylene glycol
Precautions: Use with caution in patients with active untreated infections, diabetes mellitus, glaucoma, or recent nasal trauma, septal ulcers, or surgery.
Route and Dosage
Intranasal (Adult and Pediatric over 6 years): 2 sprays in each nostril once daily
How Supplied
Nasal spray: 50 mcg/metered spray in 12.5-g bottle; delivers 120 metered sprays
Adverse Reactions and Side Effects
Resp: Cough, bronchospasm
CNS: Dizziness, headache
EENT: Epistaxis, nasal burning/irritation, nasal congestion, sneezing, tearing eyes
GI: Dry mouth, nausea, vomiting
Misc: ANAPHYLAXIS, ANGIOEDEMA
Drug Interactions: Ketoconazole use increases the effects of ciclesonide.
EMS Considerations: Monitor the patient's degree of nasal congestion, amount, and color of nasal discharge, and frequency of sneezing. Have epinephrine, an antihistamine, and resuscitative equipment readily available.

Ciprofloxacin (sip-roe-FLOX-a-sin)

Ciloxan
Classification: Fluoroquinolone antibiotic
Pregnancy Class: C
Indications: Stops the growth of bacteria that cause eye infections
Pharmacokinetics
Absorption: Well absorbed
Onset: Rapid
Duration: 12 hours
Indications: Used to treat infections caused by microorganisms that lead to corneal ulcers and conjunctivitis
Contraindications: Known hypersensitivity; should not be given to patients with a history of hypersensitivity to other quinolone-type medications
Precautions: Contact lenses should not be worn during treatment.
Route and Dosage
Topical (Adult and Pediatric over 1 year): Bacterial conjunctivitis—Solution: 1 to 2 drops every 2 hours while awake for 2 days, then every 4 hours while awake for 5 days. Ointment: 1/2-inch ribbon three times daily for 2 days, then twice daily for 5 days. Corneal ulcers—Solution: 1 to 2 drops every 15 min for 6 hours, then every 30 min while awake for the rest of the day, then every 1 hour while awake for the next 24 hours, then every 4 hours while awake for the next 12 hours
How Supplied
Solution: 0.3 percent
Ointment: 1/2-inch ointment strip
Adverse Reactions and Side Effects
CNS: Headache, dizziness
GI: Unpleasant taste sensation
EENT: Burning, redness, tearing, and itching of the eyes; crusting of the eyelid, blurred vision, photophobia
Drug Interactions: The systemic administration of some quinolones has been shown to increase the levels of theophylline and enhance the effects of warfarin.
EMS Considerations: Monitor patients for signs of hypersensitivity: tinnitus, vertigo, hearing loss, rash, and dizziness.

effective **Communication**
Advise patients that ciprofloxacin may cause blurred vision.

ClonazePAM (kloe-NA-ze-pam)

🍁 Clonapam, Klonopin, 🍁 Rivotril
Classification: Anticonvulsant (Schedule IV)
Pregnancy Class: D
Mechanism of Action: Produces sedative effects in the central nervous system (CNS)
Pharmacokinetics
Absorption: Well absorbed
Onset: 20 to 60 minutes
Duration: 6 to 12 hours
Indications: Used as a sedative in the treatment of Ménière disease
Contraindications: Known hypersensitivity; should not be given to patients with severe liver disease or those who are hypersensitive to benzodiazepines
Precautions: ❗ Used with caution in all patients; may increase the risk of suicidal thoughts or behaviors. Use with caution in patients with angle-closure glaucoma or chronic respiratory disease.
Route and Dosage
PO (Adult): 0.5 mg three times daily
PO (Pediatric under 10 years or 30 kg): 0.01–0.03 mg/kg/day given in two to three equally divided doses

Understand the Numbers
You are ordered to give 0.02 mg/kg of clonazepam to your 72-pound patient. How many milligrams will you give?
72 lbs ÷ 2.2 = 32.7 or 33 kg.
33 kg × 0.02 = 0.66 mg.

How Supplied
Tablets: 0.5 mg, 1 mg, 2 mg
Oral disintegrating tablets: 0.125 mg, 0.25 mg, 0.5 mg, 1 mg, 2 mg
Adverse Reactions and Side Effects
Resp: Increased secretions
CV: Palpitations

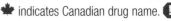

CNS: SUICIDAL THOUGHTS, behavioral changes, drowsiness, slurred speech, sedation
GI: Constipation, diarrhea, weight gain
GU: Urinary retention
Misc: Fever, physical dependence, psychological dependence, tolerance
Drug Interactions: Increased CNS depression if concurrently used with antihistamines, antidepressants, other benzodiazepines, opioid analgesics, or alcohol
EMS Considerations: Monitor patients closely for any changes in behavior.

Cyclosporine (sye-klo-SPORE-een)

Restasis
Classification: Ophthalmic emulsion
Pregnancy Class: C
Mechanism of Action: The exact mechanism of action is not known. However, cyclosporine is an immunosuppressive drug when given systemically.
Pharmacokinetics
Absorption: 15 minutes
Onset: 3 to 6 months
Duration: Unknown
Indications: Used to aid in increased tear production for patients with chronic dry eyes
Contraindications: Known hypersensitivity; should not be administered to patients with active eye infections or uncontrolled hypertension
Precautions: Use with caution in patients with severe liver impairment, renal impairment, or active infection.
Route and Dosage
Topical (Adult): 1 drop of 0.05 percent solution in each eye twice daily
How Supplied
Vial: 0.4 mL/vial
Adverse Reactions and Side Effects
CV: Hypertension
CNS: Headache
EENT: Temporary burning of the eyes, dilated pupils, blurred vision
Drug Interactions: Increased risk of immunosuppression if used with other immunosuppressants
EMS Considerations: Patients should not insert contact lenses until at least 15 minutes after administration. Advise patients that this medication may cause blurred vision.

Diazepam (dye-AZ-e-pam)

Diastat, 🍁 Diazemuls, Valium
Classifications: Antianxiety, sedative/hypnotic (Schedule IV)
Pregnancy Class: D
Mechanism of Action: Depresses the CNS
Pharmacokinetics
Absorption: Rapidly absorbed
Onset: IM—20 minutes; IV—1 to 5 minutes
Duration: IM—unknown; IV—15 to 60 minutes
Indications: Used as adjunct therapy for sedation in treating Ménière disease
Contraindications: Known hypersensitivity; should not be given to patients with preexisting CNS depression, angle-closure glaucoma, severe pulmonary impairment, severe liver dysfunction, uncontrolled pain, myasthenia gravis, or sleep apnea
Precautions: Use with caution in patients with severe kidney impairment or a history of suicide attempt or drug dependence.
Route and Dosage
IM, IV (Adult): 2 to 10 mg, may repeat in 3 to 4 hours as needed
IM, IV (Pediatric over 1 month): 0.04–0.3 mg/kg/dose every 2 to 4 hours to a maximum of 0.6 mg/kg within an 8-hr period, if necessary

> **Check the Evidence**
>
> Diazepam reacts to IV tubing and burns when administered. Therefore, administer diazepam into tubing as close to the insertion site as possible, using the largest vein that is appropriate.

How Supplied
Oral solution: 1 mg/mL, 5 mg/mL
Solution for injection: 5 mg/mL
Adverse Reactions and Side Effects
Resp: RESPIRATORY DEPRESSION
CV: Hypotension
CNS: Dizziness, drowsiness, depression, headache, slurred speech
GI: Constipation, diarrhea, nausea, vomiting
Misc: Physical dependence, psychological dependence, tolerance
Drug Interactions: Additive CNS depression if concurrently used with antidepressants, antihistamines, opioid analgesics, or alcohol
EMS Considerations: Monitor vital signs and ECG frequently during therapy. Assess the IV site frequently, as diazepam may cause phlebitis and venous thrombosis.

Dimenhydrinate (dye-men-HY-drih-nayt)

Dramamine
Classifications: Antihistamine, antiemetic
Pregnancy Class: B
Mechanism of Action: Depresses vestibular (equilibrium) function
Pharmacokinetics
Absorption: Well absorbed
Onset: PO—15 to 30 minutes; IV—immediate
Duration: PO and IV—3 to 6 hours
Indications: Used to treat dizziness and vertigo
Contraindications: Known hypersensitivity
Precautions: ❗ Geriatric patients may be more sensitive to the usual adult dose.
Route and Dosage
PO (Adult): 50 to 100 mg every 4 hours, not to exceed 400 mg per day
IV (Adult): 50 to 100 mg, not to exceed 400 mg in 24 hours, or as directed

Underline indicates most frequent; CAPITALS indicates life-threatening; 🍁 indicates Canadian drug name. ❗ Safety and special populations.

PO (Pediatric 6 to 12 years): 25 to 50 mg every 6 to 8 hours, not to exceed 150 mg per day
PO (Pediatric 2 to 6 years): 12.5–25 mg every 6–8 hours, not to exceed 75 mg per day
How Supplied
Tablet: 25 mg, 50 mg
Chewable tablet: 50 mg
Liquid: 12.5 mg/4 mL, 12.5 mg/5 mL
Solution for injection: Various sizes
Adverse Reactions and Side Effects
CNS: Sedative effect, drowsiness
Drug Interactions: None listed
EMS Considerations: None significant

DiphenhydrAMINE (dye-fen-HYE-dra-meen)

Benadryl (Rx and OTC), 🍁 Benylin
Classification: Antihistamine
Pregnancy Class: B
Mechanism of Action: Depresses the CNS
Pharmacokinetics
Absorption: Well absorbed
Onset: IM—20 to 30 minutes; IV—Rapid
Duration: IM and IV—4 to 8 hours
Indications: Used as an adjunct medication to help control dizziness and vertigo
Contraindications: Known hypersensitivity; should not be used in patients with acute attacks of asthma
Precautions: Use with caution in patients with severe liver disease, angle-closure glaucoma, seizure disorders, or benign prostatic hyperplasia (BPH).
Route and Dosage
IM, IV (Adults): 25 to 50 mg
IM, IV (Pediatric): 1.25 mg/kg
How Supplied
Injection: 50 mg/mL
Adverse Reactions and Side Effects
Resp: Chest tightness, thickened bronchial secretions, wheezing
CV: Hypotension, palpitations
CNS: Drowsiness, headache, dizziness, paradoxical excitation (pediatrics)
EENT: Blurred vision, tinnitus
GI: Dry mouth, anorexia, constipation, nausea
GU: Urinary retention
Drug Interactions: Increased risk of CNS depression if used concurrently with other depressant drugs, such as antihistamines, opioid analgesics, alcohol, and sedative/hypnotics

effective **Communication**

Do not confuse Benadryl with benazepril.

EMS Considerations: Frequently monitor patient vital signs during therapy.

Dipivefrin (dye-pi-VEF-rin)

Propine
Classification: Mydriatic
Pregnancy Class: B
Mechanism of Action: A mydriatic ophthalmic solution that dilates pupils of the eye. It also regulates the flow of intraocular fluid to maintain a normal pressure.
Pharmacokinetics
Absorption: May cause sympathomimetic effects to occur when absorbed
Onset: 30 to 60 minutes
Duration: 12 hours
Indications: Used to treat high pressure inside of the eye due to open-angle glaucoma
Contraindications: Known hypersensitivity; should not be used in patients with narrow-angle glaucoma because any dilation of the pupil may cause an attack of narrow-angle glaucoma
Precautions: Use with caution in patients with active infection.
Route and Dosage
Topical (Adult): 1 drop of 0.1 percent solution in each eye every 12 hours
How Supplied
Vial: 0.1 percent solution in 5 mL, 10 mL, and 15 mL
Adverse Reactions and Side Effects:
CV: Tachycardia, arrhythmias
CNS: Headache
EENT: Blurred vision, dilated pupils
Drug Interactions: None reported
EMS Considerations: Patients should not insert contact lenses until at least 15 minutes after administration. Explain to patients that this medication may cause blurred vision.

Doxycycline (dox-i-SYE-kleen)

🍁 Apprilon, 🍁 Atridox, Doryx, Doxy, 🍁 Doxycin, 🍁 Doxytab, Monodox, Oracea, Periostat, Vibramycin, 🍁 Vibra-Tabs
Classifications: Anti-infective, tetracycline
Pregnancy Class: D
Mechanism of Action: Inhibits bacterial protein synthesis
Pharmacokinetics
Absorption: Well absorbed from the GI tract
Onset: PO—1 to 2 hours; IV—rapid
Duration: PO—12 hours; IV—12 hours
Indications: Used for the treatment of sinusitis
Contraindications: Known hypersensitivity; may contain alcohol or bisulfites; avoid use in patients with known hypersensitivity or intolerance
Precautions: Use with caution in patients with kidney disease or liver impairment.
Route and Dosage
PO (Adult and Pediatric over 8 years and under 45 kg): 100 mg every 12 hours on the first day, then 100 to 200 mg once daily or 50 to 100 mg every 12 hours
PO (Pediatric over 8 years and under 45 kg): 2 to 5 mg/kg/day in one to two divided doses, not to exceed 200 mg/day

IV (Adult and Pediatric over 8 years and under 45 kg): 200 mg once daily or 100 mg every 12 hours on the first day, then 100 to 200 mg once daily or 50 to 100 mg every 12 hours
IV (Pediatric over 8 years and under 45 kg or under 8 years): 4.4 mg/kg once daily or 2.2 mg/kg every 12 hours
How Supplied
Tablets: 20 mg, 50 mg, 75 mg, 100 mg, 150 mg
Delayed-release tablets: 75 mg, 100 mg
Capsules: 50 mg, 100 mg
Delayed-release capsules: 40 mg
Oral suspension: 25 mg/5 mL in 60-mL bottles
Syrup: 50 mg/5 mL in 473-mL bottles
Powder for injection: 100 mg/vial, 200 mg/vial
Adverse Reactions and Side Effects
CNS: Dizziness
GI: <u>Diarrhea</u>, <u>nausea</u>, <u>vomiting</u>, esophagitis
Derm: STEVENS-JOHNSON SYNDROME, rash, pigmentation of skin and mucous membranes
Drug Interactions: May increase the effect of warfarin; may decrease effectiveness of contraceptives. Antacids, calcium, iron, zinc, aluminum, and magnesium decrease the absorption of tetracycline.
EMS Considerations: Periodically check patients for developing rash.

Echothiophate Iodide (eck-oh-THYE-oh-fate EYE-oh-dide)

Phospholine Iodide
Classification: Cholinergic (cholinesterase inhibitor)
Pregnancy Class: C
Mechanism of Action: Stimulates smooth muscle such as the iris of the eye and secretory glands; facilitates the outflow of aqueous humor
Pharmacokinetics
Absorption: Well absorbed
Onset: 10 to 30 minutes
Duration: 1 to 4 weeks
Indications: Controls the intraocular pressure in the treatment of open-angle glaucoma.
Contraindications: Known hypersensitivity; should not be given to patients with active inflammation or to patients with angle-closure glaucoma because of the possibility of increasing angle block
Precautions: Use with caution in patients with preexisting retinal disease because of the possibility of retinal detachment.
Route and Dosage
Topical (Adult): 1 drop one to two times daily
How Supplied
Packaged for reconstitution:

- 1.5-mg package for 0.03 percent
- 3-mg package for 0.06 percent
- 6.25-mg package for 0.125 percent
- 12.5-mg package for 0.25 percent

Adverse Reactions and Side Effects:
CV: ECG irregularities
EENT: Possible retinal detachment, stinging, burning, blurred vision
Drug Interactions: Potentiates other cholinesterase inhibitors
EMS Considerations: Monitor patients for any heart palpitations or if their vision begins to worsen. Advise patients that this medication may cause temporary blurring of vision.

Erythromycin (eh-rith-roe-MYE-sin)

🍁 Ak Mycin, 🍁 Diomycin, Erythrocin
Classification: Anti-infective, macrolide
Pregnancy Class: B
Mechanism of Action: Suppresses protein synthesis-killing bacteria
Pharmacokinetics
Absorption: Minimal after ophthalmic use
Onset: Rapid
Duration: 6 to 12 hours
Indications: Used to treat infections of the eye
Contraindications: Known hypersensitivity; should not be given to patients on concurrent pimozide, procainamide, or amiodarone or to patients with alcohol intolerance; should not be given to patients with a long Q-T interval or to those with a heart rate below 50 beats/minute
Precautions: Use with caution in patients with liver or kidney disease. ❗ Erythromycin may worsen the symptoms of patients with myasthenia gravis.
Route and Dosage
Topical (Adult & Pediatric): 1/2-inch strip two to six times daily
How Supplied
Ophthalmic ointment: 0.5 percent (5 mg/g)
Adverse Reactions and Side Effects
CV: TORSADE DE POINTES, VENTRICULAR ARRHYTHMIAS, QT prolongation
CNS: Seizures (rare)
GI: <u>Nausea</u>, <u>vomiting</u>, abdominal pain, cramping, diarrhea
Derm: Rash
Drug Interactions: Concurrent use with pimozide, diltiazem, verapamil, ketoconazole, itraconazole, nefazodone, and protease inhibitors may increase the risk of serious cardiac arrhythmias.
EMS Considerations: Monitor vital signs frequently during therapy.

Fluticasone (floo-TI-ka-sone)

🍁 Avamys, Flonase, Veramyst
Classifications: Anti-inflammatory (steroidal), corticosteroid (nasal)
Pregnancy Class: C
Mechanism of Action: Potent, locally acting anti-inflammatory
Pharmacokinetics
Absorption: Negligible; action is primarily local after nasal use
Onset: A few days
Duration: Unknown
Indication: Used to treat nonallergic rhinitis
Contraindications: Known hypersensitivity; should not be given to patients with known hypersensitivity to alcohol, propylene, or polyethylene glycol
Precautions: Use with caution in patients with active untreated infections, diabetes mellitus, glaucoma, or recent nasal trauma, septal ulcers, or surgery.

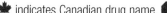

Route and Dosage
Intranasal (Adult and Pediatric over 12 years): Flonase—2 sprays in each nostril once daily or 1 spray in each nostril twice daily; Veramyst—2 sprays in each nostril once daily or 1 spray in each nostril twice daily
Intranasal (Pediatric over 4 years): Flonase—1 spray in each nostril once daily
Intranasal (Pediatric 2 to 4 years): Veramyst—1 spray in each nostril daily; may increase to 2 sprays if no response
How Supplied
Nasal spray (Flonase): 50 mcg/metered spray in 16-g bottle; delivers 120 metered sprays
Nasal spray (Veramyst): 27.5 mcg/spray in a 10-g bottle; delivers 120 metered sprays
Adverse Reactions and Side Effects
Resp: Cough, bronchospasm
CNS: Dizziness, headache
EENT: Epistaxis, nasal burning or irritation, nasal congestion, sneezing, tearing eyes
GI: Dry mouth, nausea, vomiting
Misc: ANAPHYLAXIS, ANGIOEDEMA
Drug Interactions: Ketoconazole increases the effects of fluticasone.
EMS Considerations: Monitor patient's degree of nasal stuffiness, amount and color of nasal discharge, and frequency of sneezing.

Gentamicin (jen-ta-MYE-sin)

🍁 Alcomicin, 🍁 Diogent, 🍁 Garamycin, Genoptic, Gentak
Classification: Anti-infective
Pregnancy Class: C
Mechanism of Action: Inhibits protein synthesis in bacteria
Pharmacokinetics
Absorption: Well absorbed
Onset: Rapid
Duration: N/A
Indications: Used to kill bacteria in the treatment of conjunctivitis
Contraindications: Known hypersensitivity; should not be used in patients hypersensitive to aminoglycosides
Precautions: Use with caution in patients with kidney impairment, hearing impairment, or neuromuscular disease.
Route and Dosage
Topical (Adult and Pediatric): Solution—1 to 2 drops of 0.3 percent solution every 2 to 4 hours; Ointment—1/2-inch ribbon every 8 to 12 hours
How Supplied:
Solution: 0.3 percent
Ointment: 0.1 percent
Adverse Reactions and Side Effects
CNS: Vertigo, headache, dizziness
EENT: Ototoxicity (hearing impairment, tinnitus)
Misc: Rash
Drug Interactions: Inactivated by penicillins and cephalosporins when co-administered to patients with kidney insufficiency
EMS Considerations: Monitor patients for signs of hypersensitivity: tinnitus, vertigo, hearing loss, rash, and dizziness.

GuaiFENesin (gwye-FEN-e-sin)

Alfen Jr, Altarussin, 🍁 Balminil Expectorant, 🍁 Benylin Chest Congestion Extra Strength, Breonesin, 🍁 Bronchophan Expectorant, 🍁 Chest Congestion, 🍁 Cough Syrup Expectorant, Diabetic Tussin, 🍁 Expectorant Syrup, Ganidin NR, Guiatuss, Hytuss, Hytuss-2X, 🍁 Jack & Jill Expectorant, Mucinex, Naldecon Senior EX, Organidin NR, Robitussin, Scot-Tussin Expectorant, Siltussin SA, Siltussin DAS, 🍁 Vicks Chest Congestion Relief, 🍁 Vicks DayQuil Mucus Control
Classification: Mucolytic; allergy, cold, cough remedy; expectorant
Pregnancy Class: C
Mechanism of Action: Reduces viscosity of secretions by increasing respiratory tract fluid
Pharmacokinetics
Absorption: Well absorbed
Onset: 30 minutes
Duration: 4 to 6 hours
Indications: Has been used as an adjunct therapy when treating sinusitis
Contraindications: Known hypersensitivity; should not be given to patients with a known intolerance to alcohol
Precautions: Use with caution in patients with a cough lasting more than 1 week or a cough accompanied by fever, rash, or headache. Diabetic patients should use with caution because most products contain sugar. If available, diabetic patients should use Diabetic Tussin.
Route and Dosage
PO (Adult): 200 to 400 mg every 4 hours, or 600 to 1,200 mg every 12 hours as extended-release product, not to exceed 2,400 mg/day
PO (Pediatric 6 to 12 years): 100 to 200 mg every 4 hours or 600 mg every 12 hours as extended-release product, not to exceed 1,200 mg/day
PO (Pediatric 4 to 6 years): 50 to 100 mg every 4 hours, not to exceed 600 mg/day
How Supplied
Syrup: 100 mg/5 mL (OTC)
Oral solution: 100 mg/5 mL (Rx/OTC), 200 mg/5 mL (OTC)
Capsules: 200 mg (OTC)
Tablets: 100 mg (OTC), 200 mg (Rx/OTC)
Extended-release tablets (Mucinex): 600 mg, 1200 mg
Adverse Reactions and Side Effects
CNS: Dizziness, headache
GI: Nausea, diarrhea, stomach pain, vomiting
Derm: Rash
Drug Interactions: None noted
EMS Considerations: None significant. Do not confuse quaifenesin with guanfacine. Do not confuse Mucinex with Mucomyst.

Levofloxacin (lev-oh-FLOX-a-sin)

Iquix, Quixin
Classification: Fluoroquinolone antibiotic
Pregnancy Class: C
Mechanism of Action: Stops the growth of bacteria that cause eye infections

Pharmacokinetics

Absorption: Well absorbed
Onset: Rapid
Duration: N/A

Indications: Used to treat infections caused by microorganisms that lead to corneal ulcers and conjunctivitis
Contraindications: Known hypersensitivity; should not be given to patients with a history of hypersensitivity to other quinolone-type medications
Precautions: Contact lenses should not be worn during treatment.

Route and Dosage

Topical (Adult and Pediatric over 1 year): Quixin (conjunctivitis)—1 to 2 drops every 2 hours while awake for 2 days (up to eight times/day), then every 4 hours while awake for 5 more days (up to four times/day). Iquix (conjunctival ulcers)—1 to 2 drops every 30 minutes to 2 hours while awake and 4 to 6 hours after retiring for 3 days, then 1 to 2 drops every 1 to 4 hours while awake

How Supplied

Solution: 1.5 percent solution

Adverse Reactions and Side Effects

CNS: Headache, dizziness
GI: Unpleasant taste sensation
EENT: Burning, redness, tearing, and itching of the eyes; crusting of the eyelid, blurred vision, photophobia
Drug Interactions: The systemic administration of some quinolones has been shown to increase the levels of theophylline and enhance the effects of warfarin.
EMS Considerations: Monitor patients for signs of hypersensitivity: tinnitus, vertigo, hearing loss, rash, and dizziness. Advise patients that this medication may cause blurred vision.

Meclizine (MEK-li-zeen)

Antivert, Bonine, Dramamine Less Drowsy Formula

Classification: Antiemetic, antihistamine
Pregnancy Class: B
Classification: Antiemetic, antihistamine
Mechanism of Action: Decreases excitability of the middle ear
Pharmacokinetics

Absorption: Well absorbed
Onset: 1 hour
Duration: 8 to 24 hours

Indications: Used in the management and prevention of vertigo
Contraindications: Known hypersensitivity
Precautions: Use with caution in patients with angle-closure glaucoma or BPH.

Route and Dosage

PO (Adult and Pediatric over 12 years): 25 to 100 mg/day in divided doses

How Supplied

Tablets: 12.5 mg, 25 mg, 50 mg
Chewable tablets: 25 mg

Adverse Reactions and Side Effects

CNS: Drowsiness, fatigue
EENT: Blurred vision
GI: Dry mouth
Drug Interactions: Additive CNS depression when used concurrently with other CNS depressants

effective **Communication**

Do not confuse Antivert (meclizine) with Axert (almotriptan).

EMS Considerations: None significant

Mometasone (moe-MET-a-sone)

Nasonex

Classifications: Anti-inflammatory (steroidal), corticosteroid (nasal)
Pregnancy Class: C
Mechanism of Action: Potent, locally-acting anti-inflammatory
Pharmacokinetics

Absorption: Negligible; action is primarily local after nasal use
Onset: Within 2 days
Duration: Unknown

Indications: Used to treat seasonal or perennial allergic rhinitis
Contraindications: Known hypersensitivity; should not be given to patients with known hypersensitivity to alcohol, propylene, or polyethylene glycol
Precautions: Use with caution in patients with active untreated infections, diabetes mellitus, glaucoma, or recent nasal trauma, septal ulcers, or surgery.

Route and Dosage

Intranasal (Adult and Pediatric over 12 years): 2 sprays in each nostril once daily
Intranasal (Pediatric 2 to 11 years): 1 spray in each nostril once daily

How Supplied

Nasal spray: 50 mcg/metered spray in 17-g bottle; delivers 120 metered sprays

Adverse Reactions and Side Effects

Resp: Cough, bronchospasm
CNS: Dizziness, headache
EENT: Epistaxis, nasal burning or irritation, nasal congestion, sneezing, tearing eyes
GI: Dry mouth, nausea, vomiting
Misc: ANAPHYLAXIS, ANGIOEDEMA
Drug Interactions: Ketoconazole increases the effects of mometasone.
EMS Considerations: Monitor the degree of the patient's nasal congestion, amount and color or nasal discharge, and frequency of sneezing.

Moxifloxacin (mox-ih-FLOX-a-sin)

Moxeza, Vigamox

Classification: Fluoroquinolone antibiotic
Pregnancy Class: C
Mechanism of Action: Stops the growth of bacteria that cause eye infections

Pharmacokinetics

Absorption: Well absorbed

Onset: Rapid

Duration: N/A

Indications: Used to treat infections caused by microorganisms that lead to corneal ulcers and conjunctivitis

Contraindications: Known hypersensitivity; should not be given to patients with a history of hypersensitivity to other quinolone-type medications

Precautions: Contact lenses should not be worn during treatment.

Route and Dosage

Topical (Adult and Pediatric over 1 year): 1 drop three times daily for 7 days

How Supplied

Solution: 0.5 percent solution

Adverse Reactions and Side Effects

CNS: Headache, dizziness

GI: Unpleasant taste sensation

EENT: Burning, redness, tearing, and itching of the eyes; crusting of the eyelid, blurred vision, photophobia

Drug Interactions: The systemic administration of some quinolones has been shown to increase the levels of theophylline and enhance the effects of warfarin.

EMS Considerations: Monitor patients for signs of hypersensitivity: tinnitus, vertigo, hearing loss, rash, and dizziness. Advise patients that this medication may cause blurred vision.

Penicillin (pen-i-SILL-in)

Bicillin L-A, ♣ Crystapen, Permapen

Classification: Anti-infective

Pregnancy Class: B

Mechanism of Action: Binds to the bacterial cell wall, resulting in cell death

Pharmacokinetics

Absorption: Variable absorbed from the GI tract

Onset: Delayed

Duration: 12 hours

Indications: Used to treat streptococcal infections, including streptococcal pharyngitis

Contraindications: Known hypersensitivity

Check the Evidence

Anaphylactic reactions to penicillin cause more deaths than food allergies.

Precautions: Use with caution in patients with severe kidney insufficiency.

Route and Dosage

IM (Adult): 1.2 million units single dose

IM (Pediatric over 27 kg): 900,000 to 1.2 million units, single dose

How Supplied

Suspension for IM injection: 600,000 units/mL

Adverse Reactions and Side Effects

CNS: SEIZURES

GI: PSEUDOMEMBRANOUS COLITIS, diarrhea, epigastric distress, nausea, vomiting

Derm: Rash

Misc: ANAPHYLAXIS, SERUM SICKNESS, superinfection

Drug Interactions: May decrease the effectiveness of oral contraceptive agents. Probenecid decreases kidney excretion.

EMS Considerations: Observe patients for signs or symptoms of anaphylaxis. Have epinephrine, an antihistamine, and resuscitation equipment readily available.

Phenylephrine (fen-ill-EF-rin)

♣ AK-Dilate, ♣ Dionephrine, ♣ Mydfrin, Neo-Synephrine, ♣ Prefrin

Classification: Alpha-adrenergic, mydriatic

Pregnancy Class: C

Mechanism of Action: Acts on alpha receptors, producing vasoconstriction and mydriasis

Pharmacokinetics

Absorption: Complete bioavailability

Onset: 15 to 20 minutes

Duration: 2 to 4 hours

Indications: Used for temporary relief of redness of the eye associated with colds, hay fever, and contact lenses; also used as a vasoconstrictor to treat open-angle glaucoma

Contraindications: Known hypersensitivity; should not be used in patients with severe hypertension or tachycardia

Precautions: Use with caution in patients with bradycardia, heart block, or myocardial disease.

Route and Dosage

Vasoconstriction and pupillary dilation

Topical (Adult): 1 drop of the 2.5 percent or 10 percent solution in each eye

Glaucoma

Topical (Adult): 1 drop of the 10 percent solution in each eye. Both the 2.5 percent and the 10 percent solutions may be used with miotics (agents that constrict pupils) in patients with open-angle glaucoma.

How Supplied

Solution: 0.12 percent, 2.5 percent, and 10 percent solutions

Adverse Reactions and Side Effects

CV: Reflex bradycardia

CNS: Headache

EENT: Blurred vision, rebound miosis

Drug Interactions: May sensitize the heart and cause arrhythmias (rare)

EMS Considerations: Patients should not insert contact lenses until at least 15 minutes after administration. Advise patients that this medication may cause blurred vision. Monitor vital signs and ECG during therapy.

Pilocarpine (pie-low-KAR-peen)

♣ Akarpine, ♣ Diocarpine, Isopto Carpine, Pilopine HS

Classification: Direct-acting cholinergic

Pregnancy Class: C

Mechanism of Action: Stimulates smooth muscle such as the iris of the eye and secretory glands; facilitates the outflow of aqueous humor
Pharmacokinetics
Absorption: Rapidly absorbed
Onset: 10 to 30 minutes
Duration: 4 to 8 hours
Indications: Used to treat open-angle glaucoma or ocular hypertension
Contraindications: Known hypersensitivity
Precautions: Use with caution in patients with asthma, heart disease, low or high blood pressure, or Parkinsonism.
Route and Dosage
Topical (Adult): Solution—1 to 2 drops of 0.5–4 percent solution up to six times daily
How Supplied
Solution: 1 percent in 15-mL bottles, 2 percent in 15-mL bottles, and 4 percent in 15-mL bottles
Adverse Reactions and Side Effects
CNS: Dizziness, headache
GI: Diarrhea, nausea, abdominal pain
EENT: Blurred vision, poor vision in dim light
Drug Interactions: None listed
EMS Considerations: None significant

Scopolamine (scoh-POLL-ah-meen) (Anticolinergic)

Hyoscine
Classification: Anticholinergic
Pregnancy Class: C
Mechanism of Action: Causes pupillary dilation and paralyzes the muscles of the eye
Pharmacokinetics
Absorption: Well absorbed
Onset: 15 to 30 minutes
Duration: Up to 8 hours
Indications: Used to dilate the pupils to determine a patient's refractive error, and paralyze the eye muscles to enable examination of the inner structure of the eye when treating Uveitis, an inflammation of the eye uvea.
Contraindications: Known hypersensitivity; should not be used in pediatric patients under 3 months old who have glaucoma
Precautions: Use with caution in pediatric patients, geriatric patients, and those with diabetes mellitus or hypothyroidism or hyperthyroidism.
Route and Dosage
Topical (Adult): Cycloplegic refraction—1 to 2 drops of the 0.25 percent solution 1 hour prior to procedure. Uveitis—1 drop of a 0.25 percent solution up to 4 times daily.
Topical (Pediatric): 1 drop of the 0.25 percent solution twice a day for 2 days prior to procedure
How Supplied
0.25 percent solution
Adverse Reactions and Side Effects
CV: Tachycardia, palpitations
CNS: Drowsiness, headache
EENT: Blurred vision, increased intraocular pressure, temporary stinging
GI: Dry mouth
Drug Interactions: None noted
EMS Considerations: Patients should not insert contact lenses until at least 15 minutes after administration. Advise patients that this medication may cause blurred vision.

Scopolamine (scoe-POL-a-meen) (Antiemetic)

Transderm-Scop, ♣ Transderm-V
Classification: Antiemetic
Pregnancy Class: C
Mechanism of Action: Corrects the imbalance associated with motion sickness and vertigo
Pharmacokinetics
Absorption: Well absorbed
Onset: Transdermal patch—4 hours
Duration: Transdermal patch—72 hours
Indications: Used as an adjunct medication for patients who experience vertigo
Contraindications: Known hypersensitivity; should not be used in patients with angle-closure glaucoma, prostatic hyperplasia, or tachycardia due to cardiac insufficiency
Precautions: Use with caution in patients with chronic kidney, liver, pulmonary, or cardiac disease.
Route and Dosage
Transdermal (Adult): Apply one patch every 3 days as needed.
How Supplied
Transdermal therapeutic system: A 1.5-mg scopolamine/patch releases 0.5 mg over 3 days.
Adverse Reactions and Side Effects
CV: Tachycardia, palpitations
CNS: Drowsiness, confusion
EENT: Blurred vision, photophobia
GI: Dry mouth, constipation
GU: Urinary retention
Drug Interactions: Increased CNS depression if used concurrently with other CNS depressants such as antihistamines, antidepressants, opioid analgesics, or alcohol
EMS Considerations: None significant

Tobramycin (toe-bra-MYE-sin) AK-Tob, Tobrex

Classification: Anti-infective
Pregnancy Class: C
Mechanism of Action: Inhibits protein synthesis in bacteria
Pharmacokinetics
Absorption: Well absorbed
Onset: Rapid
Duration: N/A
Indications: Used to kill bacteria in the treatment of conjunctivitis
Contraindications: Known hypersensitivity; should not be used in patients hypersensitive to aminoglycosides
Precautions: Use with caution in patients with kidney impairment, hearing impairment, or neuromuscular disease.

Route and Dosage
Topical (Adult and Pediatric over 2 months): Solution—1 to 2 drops of 0.3 percent solution every 1 to 4 hours. Ointment—thin strip every 8 to 12 hours
How Supplied
Solution: 0.3 percent
Ointment: Single-dose thin strips
Adverse Reactions and Side Effects
CNS: Vertigo, headache, dizziness
EENT: Ototoxicity (hearing impairment), tinnitus
Misc: Rash
Drug Interactions: Inactivated by penicillins and cephalosporins when co-administered to patients with kidney insufficiency
EMS Considerations: Monitor patients for signs of hypersensitivity: tinnitus, vertigo, hearing loss, rash, and dizziness.

Triamcinolone (trye-am-SIN-oh-lone)

Nasacort AQ
Classification: Anti-inflammatory (steroidal); corticosteroid (nasal)
Pregnancy Class: C
Mechanism of Action: Potent, locally acting anti-inflammatory
Pharmacokinetics
Absorption: Negligible; action is primarily local after nasal use
Onset: A few days
Duration: Unknown
Indications: Used to treat seasonal or perennial allergic rhinitis
Contraindications: Known hypersensitivity; should not be given to patients with known hypersensitivity to alcohol, propylene, or polyethylene glycol
Precautions: Use with caution in patients with active untreated infections, diabetes mellitus, glaucoma, or recent nasal trauma, septal ulcers, or surgery.
Route and Dosage
Intranasal (Adult and Pediatric over 12 years): 2 sprays in each nostril
Intranasal (Pediatric 2 to 11 years): 1 spray in each nostril once daily
How Supplied
Nasal spray: 55 mcg/metered spray in 16.5-g bottle; delivers 120 metered sprays
Adverse Reactions and Side Effects
Resp: Cough, bronchospasm
CNS: Dizziness, headache
EENT: Epistaxis, nasal burning/irritation, nasal congestion, sneezing, tearing eyes
GI: Dry mouth, nausea, vomiting
Misc: ANAPHYLAXIS, ANGIOEDEMA
Drug Interactions: Ketoconazole increases the effects of triamcinolone.
EMS Considerations: Monitor the patient's degree of nasal stuffiness, amount and color of nasal discharge, and frequency of sneezing.

Trimethoprim/Sulfamethoxazole (trye-METH-oh-prim/sul-fa-meth-OX-a-zole)

Bactrim, 🍁 Protrin DF, Septra, Sulfatrim, TMP/SMX, TMP/SMZ, 🍁 Trisulfa DS, 🍁 Trisulfa S
Classification: Anti-infective, antiprotozoal
Pregnancy Class: C
Mechanism of Action: Inhibits the metabolism of folic acid in bacteria
Pharmacokinetics
Absorption: Well absorbed
Onset: PO—rapid; IV—rapid
Duration: PO, IV—6–12 hours
Indications: Used as a treatment option for sinusitis
Contraindications: Known hypersensitivity; should not be used in patients with severe kidney impairment or with known hypersensitivity to trimethoprim or sulfonamides
Precautions: Use with caution in patients with impaired liver or kidney function.
Route and Dosage
PO, IV (Adult and Pediatric over 2 months): Mild infections—6 to 12 mg/kg/day divided every 12 hours. Severe infections—15 to 20 mg/kg/day divided every 6 to 8 hours
How Supplied
Tablets: 80 mg trimethoprim/400 mg, sulfamethoxazole, 160 mg trimethoprim/800 mg sulfamethoxazole
Oral suspension: 40 mg trimethoprim/200 mg sulfamethoxazole per 5 mL
Solution for injection: 16 mg trimethoprim/80 mg sulfamethoxazole per mL in 5-, 10-, and 30-mL vials
Adverse Reactions and Side Effects
CV: Hypotension
CNS: Fatigue, headache, insomnia, hallucinations
GI: HEPATIC NECROSIS, <u>nausea</u>, <u>vomiting</u>, diarrhea
Derm: STEVENS-JOHNSON SYNDROME, EPIDERMAL NECROSIS, <u>rash</u>
Local: <u>Phlebitis</u> at IV site
Misc: Fever
Drug Interactions: May increase the effects of phenytoin, digoxin, thiopental, and warfarin
EMS Considerations: Frequently assess patients for rash due to the possibility of Stevens-Johnson syndrome. Inspect the IV site frequently; phlebitis is common.

Drugs Used to Treat Colds and Flu

The medications available for colds and flu are too numerous to be presented in this chapter. Therefore, Table 12-1 lists the most-common cold and flu remedies currently available. For more information on these and other cold and flu medications, the following pharmacology reference texts and websites are helpful:

- Physician's Desk Reference (PDR)
- http://www.rxlist.com (RxList)
- http://www.webmd.com (WebMD)

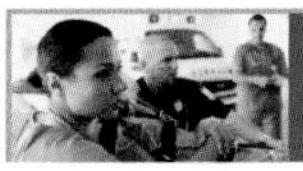

Table 12-1 Common Cold and Flu Medications

Generic Name	Trade Name	Symptoms Treated	Comments
Acetaminophen	Tylenol Children's Tylenol	Fever, aches/pains, sinus pressure, and sore throat	Acetaminophen is the first choice of analgesics for colds and flu.
Aspirin	Anacin Ascriptin Bayer	Fever, aches/pain, sinus pressure, and sore throat	Aspirin should not be given to patients <20 years with cold and flu symptoms because it has been associated with the development of Reye syndrome.
Ibuprofen	Advil Children's Advil Children's Motrin Motrin IB	Fever, aches/pains, sinus pressure, and sore throat	Ibuprofen may worsen asthma.
Pseudoephedrine	Sudafed	Congestion and sinus pressure	N/A
Naphazoline Oxymetazoline Phenylephrine	Privine Afrin Neo-Synephrine	Congestion and sinus pressure	Using nasal sprays for more than 3 days is not recommended. The body gets used to the effects of nasal sprays rapidly, causing them to become less effective.
Brompheniramine Chlorpheniramine Clemastine Diphenhydramine Loratadine	Dimetapp Chlor-Trimeton Tavist-1 Benadryl Claritin	Sinus pressure, runny nose, watery eyes, and cough (except Claritin)	Some antihistamines may be effective as cough suppressants and may also cause drowsiness.
Dextromethorphan	Pertussin DM	Cough	Dextromethorphan is the most widely used nonprescription cough suppressant.
Guaifenesin	Robitussin	Cough	Guaifenesin is an ingredient in many multisymptom cough and cold medications.
Benzocaine Dyclonine Phenol	Cepacol Sucrets Cepastat	Sore throat	Available as throat sprays and lozenges, they provide short-term relief. Lozenges can pose a risk of choking and therefore should not be used by children.
Acetaminophen Pseudoephedrine Dextromethorphan	Tylenol Cold Non-Drowsy Maximum Strength Tylenol Flu	Fever, aches/pain, congestion, sinus pressure, cough, and sore throat	These medications do not cause drowsiness.
Acetaminophen Pseudoephedrine Chlorpheniramine	TheraFlu	Fever, aches/pain, congestion, sinus pressure, runny nose, watery eyes, cough, and sore throat	This medication can cause drowsiness.
Acetaminophen Pseudoephedrine Dextromethorphan Doxylamine	NyQuil	Fever, aches/pain, congestion, sinus pressure, runny nose, watery eyes, cough, and sore throat	This medication can cause drowsiness.
Acetaminophen Caffeine	Aspirin-Free Excedrin	Fever, aches/pain, sinus pressure, and sore throat	Caffeine may be tolerated by some patients.
Ibuprofen Pseudoephedrine	Advil Cold and Sinus	Fever, aches/pain, congestion, and sinus pressure	This medication does not cause drowsiness.
Fexofenadine Pseudoephedrine	Allegra-D	Congestion, sinus pressure, runny nose, and watery eyes	Allegra-D is a prescription medication.

Adapted from WebMD; http://www.webmd.com/cold-and-flu/which-medicine-help.

SCENARIO REVISITED

Do you recall the case of Larry who was brought to the ER by his mother? Larry's mother stated that he had been taking penicillin for strep throat but stopped the medicine when he began feeling better.

Dr. Lawrence ordered a rapid strep test. The test came back indicating that Larry still has strep. Dr. Lawrence ordered an IV of NS due to Larry being dehydrated and cool compresses to help reduce Larry's fever. He also ordered cephalexin at 50 mg/kg (Larry weighs 50 pounds) PO divided every 12 hours for 10 days.

Understand the Numbers

What is the daily dosage of cephalexin for Larry?

50 lbs ÷ 2.2 kg = 22.7 or 23 kg. 23 kg × 50 mg = 1150 mg.

Let's Recap

Eye, ear, nose, and throat disorders can make patients feel very uncomfortable. Fortunately, they have many treatment options available over the counter at their local pharmacy. However, sometimes EMS professionals are needed to treat and transport patients who have an infection that needs to be seen in a health-care facility or those who may have experienced a hypersensitive reaction to their medication.

SCENARIO CONCLUSION

Cephalexin is a first-generation cephalosporin that binds to bacterial cell wall membranes, causing cell death. It is one of the medications used to treat streptococcal pharyngitis (strep throat). Once Larry started taking his penicillin, he should have taken the entire prescription. Stopping an antibiotic before completion can cause serious complications. The infection can continue to spread to anyone with whom Larry comes in contact. It is also possible for strep throat bacteria to spread to other tissues, causing an abscess or more-serious infection. Untreated, strep throat can lead to a more-severe illness such as kidney disease or rheumatic fever (a serious heart condition) that can be fatal.

PRACTICE EXERCISES

1. Whenever there is a chance for a patient to develop an anaphylactic reaction, you should have _________ readily available.
   a. Amiodarone
   b. Epinephrine
   c. Atropine
   d. Vasopressin
2. High doses of cephalexin could cause life-threatening:
   a. Seizures
   b. Anaphylaxis
   c. Superinfection
   d. Stevens-Johnson syndrome
3. A possible life-threatening side effect of diazepam is:
   a. Hypotension
   b. Hypertension
   c. Tachycardia
   d. Respiratory depression
4. Diphenhydramine is classified as a(n):
   a. Direct-acting cholinergic
   b. Anticholinergic
   c. Antihistamine
   d. Sympathomimetic
5. Doxycycline is used in the treatment of:
   a. Rhinitis
   b. Sinusitis
   c. Tinnitus
   d. Dry eye
6. A common GI side effect of erythromycin is:
   a. Diarrhea
   b. Cramping
   c. Vomiting
   d. Abdominal pain
7. A possible life-threatening side effect of penicillin is:
   a. Seizures
   b. Epigastric pain
   c. Superinfection
   d. Stevens-Johnson syndrome
8. Scopolamine is classified as a(n):
   a. Beta blocker
   b. Antihistamine
   c. Anticholinergic
   d. Antiemetic
9. Pilocarpine is a direct-acting cholinergic used to treat:
   a. Closed-angle glaucoma
   b. Open-angle glaucoma
   c. Corneal ulcers
   d. Pinkeye
10. Tobramycin is an anti-infective used in the treatment of:
    a. Conjunctivitis
    b. Tinnitus
    c. Glaucoma
    d. Strep throat

CASE STUDIES

1. You are assigned to the ER for a clinical rotation. A patient arrives complaining of ringing in her ears, headache, and vertigo. After some testing, she is diagnosed as having Ménière disease. The ER doctor tells her to get bedrest and to begin a low-salt diet. A drug that may be prescribed for her vertigo is:
   a. Meclizine
   b. Clonazepam
   c. Pilocarpine
   d. Mometasone

   A drug that can be prescribed for the Ménière disease is:
   a. Meclizine
   b. Clonazepam
   c. Pilocarpine
   d. Mometasone

2. A patient comes in to the ER complaining of painful, itchy, and watery eyes. The eyes look bloodshot, and the patient states the lights are very bright, causing the pain to become more severe. Upon examination, the doctor sees small white patches on each cornea. She diagnoses that the patient with corneal ulcers. The doctor advises that the patient take OTC pain medication and to get some bedrest. A drug that may be prescribed for corneal ulcers is:
   a. Pilocarpine
   b. Scopolamine
   c. Moxifloxacin
   d. Triamcinolone

MATH EQUATIONS

1. You are doing a clinical rotation in the ED. The physician orders you to give 4.4 mg/kg of doxycycline. Your pediatric patient weighs 80 lbs.
   a. How many kg does your patient weigh?
   b. How many mg will you give to this patient?
2. You are ordered to give 0.1 mg/kg of phenylephrine IM to your 120 lb pediatric patient. Phenylephrine has a maximum pediatric dose of 5 mg.
   a. How many kg is your patient?
   b. How many mg do you give your patient?
3. You are transporting a patient from your hospital to a neighboring hospital approximately 25 minutes away. The patient is on 6 L of oxygen/minute. You have an E cylinder with a tank psi of 650 and a safe residual pressure of 200 psi. Do you have enough oxygen to safely transport this patient?
4. You are ordered to give 250 mg/kg of acetazolamine to your 165 lb patient who has closed angle glaucoma. The maximum dose of acetazolamine is 1 g in 24 hours.
   a. How many kg does your patient weigh?
   b. What is the initial dosage of the acetazolamine?
5. Transdermal scopolamine releases 0.5 mg of scopolamine over 72 hours. How many mg are contained in the transdermal scopolamine patch?
6. You are ordered to give 12 mg/kg of trimethoprim to your 125 lb patient. The trimethoprim comes as 16 mg/mL in a 5 mL vial.
   a. How many kg does your patient weigh?
   b. How much volume of the trimethoprim will you give to your patient for the initial dose?

REFERENCES

Allergan Inc. Restasis. Retrieved July 20, 2014 from www.allergan.com/assets/pdf/restasis_pl.pdf

Drugs.com. Antiglaucoma agent, cholinergic, long-acting. Retrieved July 15, 2014 from www.drugs.com/cons/antiglaucoma-agent-cholinergic-long-acting-ophthalmic.html

Drugs.com. Decongestants. Retrieved July 12, 2014 from www.drugs.com/drug-class/decongestants.html

Drugs.com. Mydriatics. Retrieved July 15, 2014 from www.drugs.com/drug/mydriatics

Drugs.com. Phenylephrine. Retrieved July 14, 2014 from www.drugs.com/mtm/phenylephrine.html

Drugs.com. Propine. Retrieved July 13, 2014 from www.drugs.com/monograph/propine.html

Drugs.com. Scopolamine. Retrieved July 17, 2014 from www.drugs.com/monograph/scopolamine.html

U.S. National Library of Medicine. Corneal ulcers and infections. Retrieved July 29, 2014 from www.nlm.nih.gov/medlineplus/ency/article/001032.htm

Vallerand, A. H., Sanboski, C. A., and Deglin, J. H. (2015). *Davis's drug guide for nurses* (14th ed.). Philadelphia, PA: F. A. Davis Company.

Venes, D., ed. (2013). *Taber's cyclopedic medical dictionary* (22nd ed.). Philadelphia, PA: F. A. Davis Company.

WebMD. Mucolytics for sinusitis. Retrieved July 10, 2014 from www.webmd.com/a-to-z-guides/mucolytics-for-sinusitis

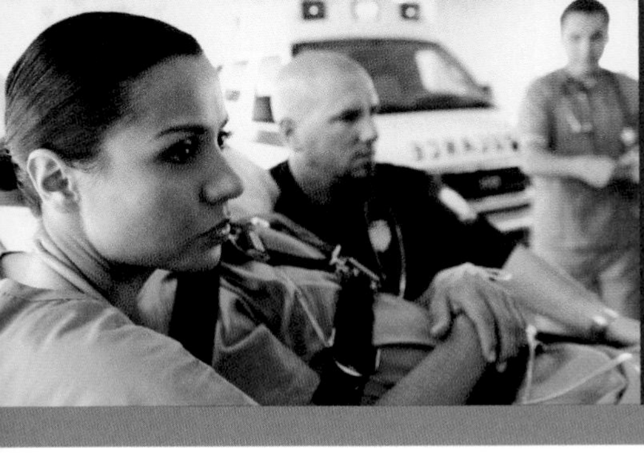

CHAPTER 13

Drugs Used to Treat Metabolic Emergencies

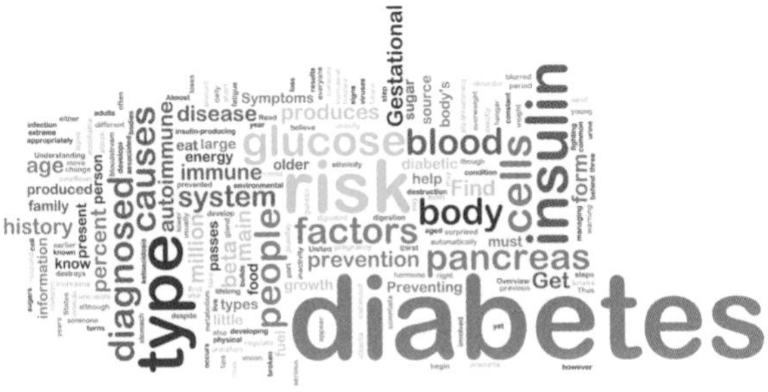

Diabetic word cloud.
(Photograph © Kheng guan Toh/Hemera/Thinkstock)

LEARNING OUTCOMES

- Differentiate and briefly discuss the pathophysiology of type 1 and type 2 diabetes mellitus.
- Briefly discuss the pathophysiology of acute adrenal insufficiency and hyperthyroidism.
- Describe and list the indications, contraindications, route and dosage, and adverse reactions and side effects for dextrose, esmolol, glucagon, hydrocortisone, and thiamine.
- Discuss the effects of insulin in diabetic ketoacidosis.
- Differentiate and briefly discuss hypoglycemia and hyperglycemia.

KEY TERMS

Diabetes mellitus
Diabetic ketoacidosis
Glycogen
Glycosuria
Hyperglycemia
Hyperosmolar hyperglycemic state (HHS)
Hypoglycemia
Ketones
Korsakoff syndrome
Kussmaul breathing
Metabolism
Osmotic diuretic
Polydipsia
Polyphagia
Polyuria
Vitamin
Wernicke encephalopathy

SCENARIO OPENING

You are assigned to Rescue 222 with two paramedic preceptors. While checking out the unit at the beginning of your shift, a call comes in from the residence of an unconscious woman. On arrival, you find a female patient (Margot), about 30 years of age, lying on the bedroom floor. A rapid assessment reveals that the patient's breathing is deep and rapid; she has a weak, rapid pulse and responds only to painful stimuli. While placing the patient on humidified oxygen and connecting the ECG monitor, you notice a MedicAlert bracelet that indicates she has diabetes. There is no evidence of alcohol or drug use.

Additional assessment reveals the following:

Level of consciousness:	unconscious, responds only to pain
Respirations:	Kussmaul breathing, at a rate of 40 breaths/minute
Blood pressure:	112/82 mm Hg
Pulse:	120 beats/minute and weak. ECG shows sinus tachycardia (Fig. 13-1).
Skin:	warm and dry—dehydrated

Introduction

This chapter discusses the most common endocrine emergencies including adrenal insufficiency, diabetic emergencies, and hyperthyroidism (thyrotoxicosis). Adrenal insufficiency is caused by the failure of the adrenal glands to produce sufficient amounts of the hormones cortisol and aldosterone. The lack of cortisol can lead to severe fatigue, chronic exhaustion, depression, loss of appetite, and weight loss. Lack of aldosterone can lead to a drop in blood pressure and to abnormal salt levels in the blood.

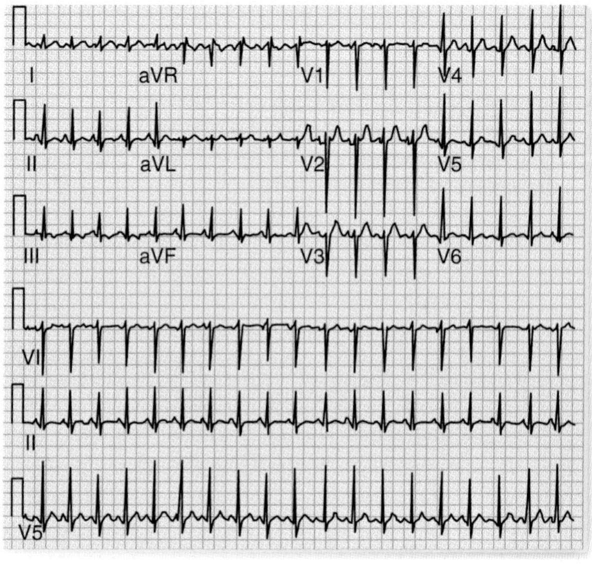

Figure 13-1 Sinus tachycardia (120 beats/minute).

Hypoglycemia and **diabetic ketoacidosis** are two emergencies associated with the metabolic disease **diabetes mellitus.** Diabetes mellitus is a disorder of carbohydrate **metabolism** that results from inadequate production or use of insulin. Insulin is a hormone secreted by beta cells in the islets of Langerhans, which are clusters of specialized cells in the pancreas. Insulin enables the body's cells to receive and metabolize glucose to be used by the body for energy.

Hyperthyroidism is a disease caused by excessive levels of thyroid hormone in the body. It may result from various disorders; however, the most common cause is Graves disease.

Pathophysiology of Endocrine Disorders

Adrenal Insufficiency

Adrenal insufficiency is a disorder that occurs when the adrenal glands do not produce enough of certain hormones. Adrenal insufficiency can be primary or secondary.

Primary adrenal insufficiency is called Addison disease. It occurs when the adrenal glands are damaged and cannot produce enough of the hormone cortisol and often the hormone aldosterone.

Secondary adrenal insufficiency occurs when the pituitary gland fails to produce enough adrenocorticotropin hormone (ACTH), which stimulates the adrenal glands to produce cortisol. If ACTH output is too low, cortisol production drops. Secondary adrenal insufficiency is much more common than Addison disease.

The most important job of Cortisol is to help the body respond to stress by aiding the following:

- Maintaining blood pressure and cardiovascular function
- Slowing the immune system's inflammatory response
- Maintaining levels of glucose in the blood
- Regulating the metabolism of proteins, carbohydrates, and fats

Aldosterone helps maintain blood pressure and water and salt balance in the body by helping the kidneys retain sodium and excrete potassium. When aldosterone production falls too low, the kidneys are not able to regulate water and salt balance, leading to a drop in blood volume, which in turn leads to a drop in blood pressure.

Treatment of adrenal insufficiency involves replacing, or substituting, the hormones that the adrenal glands are not making. Cortisol is replaced with a synthetic glucocorticoid such as hydrocortisone.

Type 1 and Type 2 Diabetes

Diabetes mellitus is classified into two types: type 1 and type 2. Type 1 diabetes mellitus, also known as insulin-dependent diabetes mellitus, typically presents at an early age with an acute onset (Fig. 13-2). Type 1 diabetes is due to the failure of the pancreas to produce insulin. Individuals with type 1

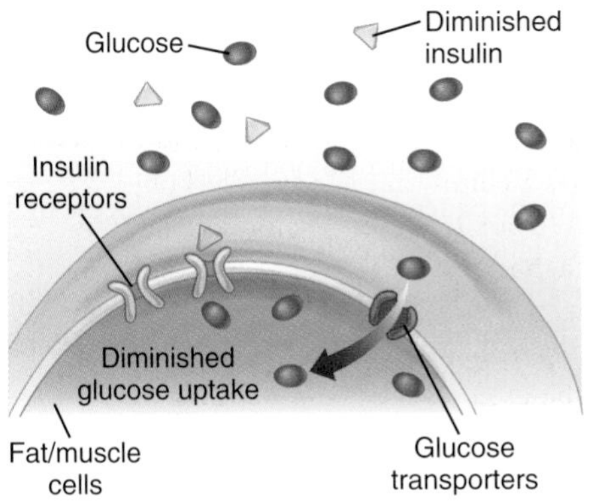

Figure 13-2 Type 1 diabetes.

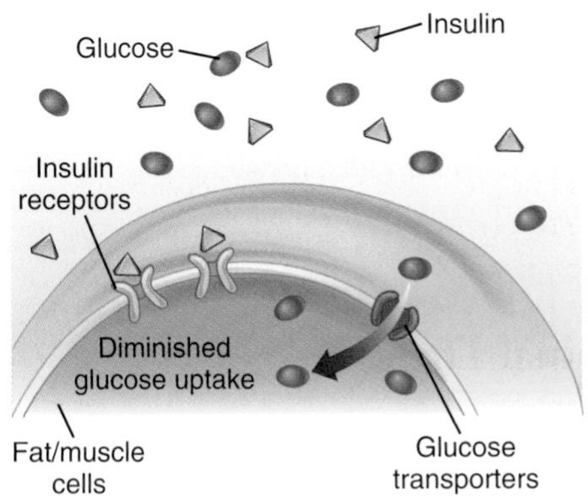

Figure 13-3 Type 2 diabetes.

diabetes mellitus are at risk for ketoacidosis because of their lack of insulin. These patients require the administration of insulin for the remainder of their lives.

Type 2 diabetes mellitus, also known as non-insulin-dependent diabetes mellitus, is caused by tissue resistance to insulin, impaired insulin secretion, and increased hepatic glucose production (Fig. 13-3). Type 2 diabetes mellitus normally develops in individuals who are at least 40 years of age and has a more gradual onset than type 1. Obesity is usually a factor associated with type 2 diabetes mellitus. Treatment of type 2 diabetes mellitus may involve just diet and exercise or oral medications. However, some patients do require insulin administration.

Diabetic ketoacidosis (DKA) occurs when the blood glucose becomes too high **(hyperglycemia).** Hyperglycemia may occur because the insulin dose is too small, the dose is not administered at all, or the amount of carbohydrates taken in is too large. Ketoacidosis may also occur because of physical or emotional stress, such as infection. Signs and symptoms of diabetic ketoacidosis include **polyuria** (excessive urine), **polydipsia** (excessive thirst), **polyphagia** (eating large amounts of food), nausea and vomiting, tachycardia, **Kussmaul breathing** (a deep, repetitive, gasping respiratory pattern), warm and dry skin, dry mucous membranes, a fruity odor to the breath, fever, abdominal pain, hypotension, and coma. Hyperglycemia results in **osmotic diuresis** (excessive urination caused by high blood glucose levels), **glycosuria** (abnormal amount of glucose in the urine), and polyuria. Dehydration occurs as a result of polyuria and vomiting. Polydipsia occurs as the patient becomes dehydrated. Because of the lack of insulin, the body cannot utilize glucose, and the patient develops polyphagia. Fat is metabolized for energy, which results in the production of acids and **ketones** (substances that are made when the body breaks down fat for energy). Ketone production may be detected by a fruity odor on the patient's breath. Kussmaul breathing occurs in an attempt to eliminate excess acid through carbon dioxide excretion. As dehydration worsens, the patient may develop tachycardia, dry skin and mucous membranes, and hypotension. Eventually, diabetic ketoacidosis may progress to coma. Diabetic ketoacidosis progresses slowly, usually over a period of 12 to 48 hours. The out-of-hospital treatment of diabetic ketoacidosis includes making a correct assessment of the disorder. The determination of hyperglycemia can be assisted with the use of a *glucose oxidase reagent strip*. In addition, a tube of blood should be collected prior to administration of any medications for later determination of blood glucose concentration. Fluid administration and supportive care are priorities of the out-of-hospital treatment of diabetic ketoacidosis. Insulin is the definitive treatment for diabetic ketoacidosis.

Hypoglycemia (abnormally low glucose level of the blood) occurs as a result of too much insulin, too little food, or a combination of both. The brain requires glucose for metabolism. If hypoglycemia develops, the lack of glucose reduces brain metabolism and causes neurological and psychiatric symptoms. If hypoglycemia is not corrected, permanent brain damage may occur. Hypoglycemia may develop very rapidly. Signs and symptoms of hypoglycemia include a weak and rapid pulse, cold and clammy skin, weakness and lack of coordination, headache, and irritable or bizarre behavior. Hypoglycemic patients may appear to be intoxicated. In severe cases, patients may develop seizures and coma. The out-of-hospital treatment of hypoglycemia includes a correct assessment of the disorder, which may be assisted with the use of a glucose oxidase reagent strip. A tube of blood should be collected for later determination of the blood glucose concentration. The rapid administration of $D_{50}W$ is necessary to restore adequate blood and brain glucose concentrations. Table 13-1 compares hyperglycemia and hypoglycemia.

Hyperosmolar Hyperglycemic State

Hyperosmolar hyperglycemic state (HHS) is a life-threatening metabolic disorder that occurs in patients with diabetes mellitus. HHS usually presents in older patients who have type 2 diabetes and also have a concurrent illness that leads to reduced fluid intake. The most common preceding illness is infection, but there are several other illnesses that can occur, causing altered mental status, dehydration, or both. Once HHS has developed, it may be difficult to differentiate it from the preexisting illness. HHS is characterized by hyperglycemia, hyperosmolarity, and dehydration without significant ketoacidosis.

Assessment and treatment of the underlying disorder are very critical. Standard care for dehydration and altered mental status is appropriate, including airway management and IV

Table 13-1 Hypoglycemia and Hyperglycemia

	Hypoglycemia	Hyperglycemia
Definition	An abnormally low level of sugar in the blood; develops rapidly, usually within 30–60 minutes	An abnormally high level of sugar in the blood; develops slowly, usually over 12–48 hours
Precipitating factors	1. Insulin overdose 2. Fasting 3. Increased alcohol intake without increased carbohydrate intake 4. Excessive physical activity without sufficient intake of food	1. Low or nonexistent insulin level 2. Infection (respiratory, urinary, or gastroenteritis)
Signs and Symptoms		
History	Recent insulin injection, inadequate food intake, excessive physical activity after insulin	Often acute infection in the diabetic, inadequate intake of insulin, perhaps no history of diabetes
Skin	Pale, sweating	Flushed, dry
Breath	Normal odor (acetone odor rare)	Acetone odor
Thirst	Absent	Intense
Respirations	Shallow	Deep, rapid (Kussmaul breathing)
Pulse	Full, bounding	Rapid, weak
Blood pressure	Normal	Low
Abdominal pain	Absent	Often acute

fluids with crystalloid administration. Many HHS patients respond well to IV fluids alone. However, insulin administration similar to dosages used in DKA can facilitate the correction of hyperglycemia. Insulin used without concurrent IV fluid replacement can increase the risk of shock.

Pharmacokinetics

Dextrose in Water (10 percent, 25 percent, 50 percent)

Dextrose in water increases circulating blood sugar level to normal in cases of hypoglycemia. It also acts briefly as an **osmotic diuretic**. If hypoglycemia is prolonged, serious brain injury may result.

Insulin

Insulin is used in the management of type 1 diabetes mellitus. It may also be used in type 2 diabetes mellitus when diet or oral medications fail to control blood sugar. Insulin is a hormone produced by the pancreas. It lowers blood glucose by increasing transport of glucose into cells and promotes the conversion of glucose to glycogen. Insulin also promotes the conversion of amino acids to proteins in muscle, stimulates triglyceride formation, and inhibits the release of free fatty acids.

Glucagon

Glucagon stimulates liver production of glucose from glycogen stores (glycogenolysis). It also relaxes the musculature of the GI tract, temporarily inhibiting movement. Glucagon has both positive inotropic and chronotropic effects.

Thiamine (Vitamin B_1)

Vitamins serve as components of enzyme systems that cause or accelerate numerous varied metabolic reactions. Thiamine is required for carbohydrate metabolism.

Individual Drugs

Dextrose in Water ($D_{10}W$, $D_{25}W$, $D_{50}W$) (DEX-trohs)

Classifications: Carbohydrate, hyperglycemic (antihypoglycemic)
Pregnancy Class: C
Mechanism of Action: Dextrose in water increases the circulating blood sugar level to normal. It also acts briefly as an osmotic diuretic.

Check the Evidence

The brain requires adequate carbohydrate levels for normal function. Prolonged hypoglycemia can result in serious brain injury.

Pharmacokinetics
Absorption: Rapidly absorbed
Onset: Less than 1 minute
Duration: Varies
Indications: Dextrose in water is used to treat patients in coma caused by hypoglycemia and patients in coma of unknown cause. Patients with an altered level of consciousness whose reagent strip reading indicates less than 45 mg should also be given dextrose in water. Some EMS protocols also recommend giving dextrose in water in certain cardiac arrest situations.
Contraindications: Known hypersensitivity. Do not administer dextrose in water to patients with intracranial pressure or intracranial hemorrhage, because dextrose in water may increase cerebral edema.
Precautions: Use caution in administering dextrose in water to patients with diabetes mellitus or to patients who cannot tolerate carbohydrate agents.

Route and Dosage
IV (Adult): 10 to 50 g of $D_{50}W$ by slow IV bolus. Repeat if necessary.
IV (Pediatric under 2 years): 2 mL/kg of $D_{10}W$, slow IV bolus
IV (Pediatric over 2 years): 2 to 4 mL/kg of $D_{25}W$, slow IV bolus

Understand the Numbers
You are ordered to administer 2 mL/kg of $D_{25}W$ to your 30-pound pediatric patient. How many mLs will you give?
30 lbs ÷ 2.2 kg = 13.6 kg or 14 kg. 2 mL × 14 kg = 28 mL of $D_{25}W$.

Check the Evidence
Research has shown that less-concentrated dextrose solutions ($D_{10}W$ or $D_{25}W$) are just as effective as $D_{50}W$ and do not cause any negative changes or alter blood glucose levels after administration.

How Supplied
Injection: 10 percent, 25 percent, or 50 percent solution in vials or prefilled syringes
Adverse Reactions and Side Effects
CV: May aggravate hypertension and congestive heart failure (CHF) in susceptible patients
CNS: May cause neurological symptoms in the alcoholic patient
Skin: May cause tissue necrosis at the injection site
Drug Interactions: None in the emergency out-of-hospital setting
EMS Considerations: In the emergency setting, there are no contraindications for the patient who is suffering from hypoglycemia. Even if the patient is suffering from ketoacidosis, the administration of $D_{50}W$ will not adversely affect patient outcome. Before establishing an IV line, take a blood sample for glucose analysis. Establish the IV line in the largest vein possible and run the IV wide open during the slow administration of the dextrose solution. Thiamine is necessary for carbohydrate metabolism. Administering dextrose to an alcohol-dependent patient who is deficient in thiamine can cause **Wernick encephalopathy** or **Korsakoff syndrome** (see Thiamine).

***effective* Communication**
It is vital to administer thiamine before dextrose to an alcohol-dependent patient or a patient in a coma of unknown cause that may be alcohol related.

Esmolol (ES-moe-lole)

Brevibloc
Classifications: Class I antiarrhythmic, beta-blocker
Pregnancy Class: C
Mechanism of Action: Blocks the stimulation of beta$_1$-adrenergic (myocardial) receptors; does not usually affect beta$_2$-adrenergic (pulmonary, vascular, or uterine) receptors
Pharmacokinetics
Absorption: IV administration results in complete bioavailability.
Onset: Within minutes
Duration: Up to 20 minutes
Indications: Can be used for the treatment of hyperthyroidism (thyrotoxicosis)
Contraindications: Known hypersensitivity; should not be used in patients with uncompensated CHF, pulmonary edema, cardiogenic shock, or bradycardia or in patients with known alcohol intolerance
Precautions: ! Geriatric patients may develop an increased sensitivity to the effects of beta-blockers. Even though esmolol can be used to treat hyperthyroidism, it can mask its symptoms as well. Esmolol may also mask the symptoms of hypoglycemia. !
OB, Lactation, Pediatric: Safety not yet established. Neonatal bradycardia, hypotension, hypoglycemia, and respiratory depression may occur rarely.
Route and Dosage
IV (Adult): 500 mcg/kg/ over 1 minute, followed by a 50 mcg/kg/minute IV infusion over 4 minutes. Maximum total dose = 200 mcg/kg.
IV (Pediatric): 500 mcg/kg IV over 1 minute, followed by a 25 to 200 mcg/kg/min IV infusion
How Supplied
Solution for Injection (prediluted for use as a loading dose): 10 mg/mL, 20 mg/mL
Premixed Infusion: 2,000 mg/100 mL, 2,500 mg/250 mL
Adverse Reactions and Side Effects
CV: hypotension, peripheral ischemia
CNS: fatigue, agitation, confusion, dizziness, drowsiness, weakness
GI: nausea, vomiting
Derm: sweating
Local: reactions at the injection site
Drug Interactions: Additive hypotension may occur if used with other antihypertensives, alcohol, and nitrates. Additive bradycardia may occur if used with digoxin; may decrease the effects of theophylline
EMS Considerations: Monitor patients for signs of overdose (bradycardia, severe dizziness, fainting, cyanosis, drowsiness, or seizures. IV glucagon can be used in the treatment of esmolol overdose.

Glucagon (GLOO-ka-gon)

GlucaGen
Classification: Hormone
Pregnancy Class: B
Mechanism of Action: Glucagon is a hormone excreted by the alpha cells of the pancreas. When released, glucagon increases the level of circulating blood sugar by stimulating the release of **glycogen** from the liver. The glycogen is quickly broken down to become glucose. Glucagon causes an increase in the plasma glucose levels of the circulating blood, causes smooth muscle relaxation, and has positive inotropic and chronotropic effects on the heart.

Pharmacokinetics
Absorption: Well absorbed by IV, IM, and SubQ administration
Onset: IM and SubQ—within 10 minutes
IV—1 minute
Duration: SubQ—60 to 90 minutes
IM—12 to 27 minutes
IV—9 to 17 minutes
Indications: Acute management of severe hypoglycemia when administration of glucose is not feasible

Check the Evidence

Glucagon has an unlabeled use as an antidote to beta-blockers and calcium channel blockers.

Contraindications: Known hypersensitivity; should not be given to patients with pheochromocytoma (a neuroendocrine tumor that causes hypertension)
Precautions: Use with caution in patients with a history of renal or cardiovascular disease. (!) Safety has not been established in patients who are lactating.
Route and Dosage
IV, IM, SubQ (Adult and Pediatric over 20 kg): 1 mg; may be repeated in 15 minutes, if necessary
IV, IM, SubQ (Pediatric under 20 kg): 0.5 mg or 0.02 to 0.03 mg/kg; may be repeated, if necessary

Understand the Numbers

You are ordered to give your 41-pound patient 0.02 mg/kg of glucagon. How many milligrams of glucagon will you administer?

41 lbs ÷ 2.2 kg = 18.6 kg or 19 kg. 19 kg × 0.02 mg = 0.38 mg.

How Supplied
Powder for Injection: 1-mg (equivalent to 1 unit) vials as an emergency kit for low blood glucose and a diagnostic kit
Adverse Reactions and Side Effects
CV: hypotension
GI: nausea, vomiting
Misc: ANAPHYLAXIS
Drug Interactions: Large doses may enhance the effect of warfarin. Glucagon negates the response to insulin or oral hypoglycemic drugs. (!) Patients on concurrent beta-blocker therapy may have a greater increase in heart rate and blood pressure.
EMS Considerations: In emergency situations, dextrose in water is the drug of choice. Use glucagon only if an IV cannot be started to administer dextrose in water. Before administering glucagon, draw a blood sample for glucose analysis. Assess neurological status throughout therapy.

Hydrocortisone (hye-droe-KOR-ti-sone)

Cortef, Cortenema, Solu-Cortef
Classification: Short-acting corticosteroid
Pregnancy Class: C
Mechanism of Action: Suppresses inflammation as well as the normal immune response. It also replaces steroids that are deficient in adrenal insufficiency.
Pharmacokinetics
Absorption: IV—rapid
IM—slow, but complete
Onset: IM, IV—rapid
Duration: IM—Unknown
IV—variable
Indications: Used in patients for the management of adrenocortical insufficiency
Contraindications: Known hypersensitivity; should not be used in patients with active untreated infections or in patients with known alcohol or bisulfite hypersensitivity
Precautions: Chronic treatment may lead to adrenal suppression. Therefore, the lowest dose for the shortest period of time must be used. Hydrocortisone should be used with caution in patients with hypothyroidism or cirrhosis.
Route and Dosage
IM, IV (Adult): 100 to 500 mg
IM, IV (Pediatric): 0.186 to 0.28 mg/kg/day
How Supplied
Powder for Injection (sodium succinate): 100 mg, 250 mg, 500 mg, 1 g
Adverse Reactions and Side Effects
(Adverse reactions and side effects are more common with high-dose, long-term therapy.)
CV: hypertension
CNS: depression, euphoria, headache, increased intracranial pressure (pediatric)
GI: PEPTIC ULCERATION, anorexia, nausea, vomiting
Derm: acne, decreased wound healing, ecchymoses, fragility, petechiae
Endo: adrenal suppression, hyperglycemia
Hemat: THROMBOEMBOLISM
MS: muscle wasting, osteoporosis, muscle pain
Drug Interactions: Hydrocortisone may cause an increased risk of hypokalemia with the use of a diuretic, may increase the risk of digoxin toxicity, and may increase the risk of GI effects with the concurrent use with NSAIDs, including aspirin.
EMS Considerations: None

Insulin, Regular [short-acting, (injection, concentrated)] (IN-su-lin)

Humulin R, Humulin R U-500 (concentrated), 🍁 Insulin-Toronto, Novolin R
Classifications: Antidiabetic, hormone
Pregnancy Class: B
Mechanism of Action: Lowers blood glucose by stimulating glucose uptake in skeletal muscle and fat and inhibiting liver glucose production
Pharmacokinetics
Absorption: rapidly absorbed by both IM and IV administration
Onset: SubQ—30 to 60 minutes
IV—10 to 30 minutes

Table 13-2 Comparison of Common Insulin Preparations

Insulin	Onset	Peak	Duration
Rapid Acting			
Regular			
Regular Iletin	30 mins–1 hr	2–4 hrs	6–8 hrs
Humulin R*	30 mins–1 hr	2–4 hrs	6–8 hrs
Novolin R	30 mins	2 hrs 30 mins–5 hrs	8 hrs
Prompt Zinc Suspension			
Semilente	1 hr 30 mins	5–10 hrs	16 hrs
Semilente Ilentin I	1–3 hrs	3–8 hrs	10–16 hrs
Lispro	30 mins	30 mins–1 hr 30 mins	3–4 hrs
Intermediate Acting			
Isophane Suspension			
NPH Ilentin	1–4 hrs	6–12 hrs	18–26 hrs
Humulin N*	1–2 hrs	6–12 hrs	18–24 hrs
Insulatard NPH	1 hr 30 mins	4–12 hrs	24 hrs
Novolin N	1 hr 30 mins	4–12 hrs	24 hrs
Zinc Suspension			
Lente Ilentin	2–4 hrs	6–12 hrs	18–26 hrs
Humulin L*	1–3 hrs	6–12 hrs	18–21 hrs
Novolin L	2 hrs 30 mins	7–15 hrs	22 hrs
Long Acting			
Protamine Zinc Suspension			
Protamine Zinc Iletin	4–8 hrs	14–24 hrs	28–36 hrs
Extended Zinc Suspension			
Ultralente	4 hrs	10–30 hrs	36 hrs
Glargine	4 hrs	Peakless	24 hrs

*Humulin insulins have a slightly more rapid onset and a shorter duration of action than animal-derived insulins.

Duration: SubQ—5 to 7 hours
IV—30 to 60 minutes

Indications: Control of hyperglycemia in patients with type 1 or type 2 diabetes. Can be used to treat diabetic ketoacidosis.
Concentrated insulin U-500—only for use in patients with insulin requirements more than 200 units/day

Contraindications: Known hypersensitivity; should not be given to patients with hypoglycemia

Precautions: Use with caution in patients who have an infection (may increase insulin requirements) or in patients with renal/hepatic impairment (may decrease insulin requirements).
(!) Pregnancy may temporarily increase insulin requirements.

Route and Dosage

(Dose depends on the patient's blood glucose, response, and many other factors.)

Ketoacidosis—Regular insulin only (100 units/mL)
IV (Adult): 0.1 unit/kg/hr as a continuous infusion
IV (Pediatric): loading dose = 0.1 unit/kg, then a maintenance continuous infusion of 0.05 to 0.2 unit/kg/hr
Maintenance Therapy
SubQ (Adult & Pediatric): 0.5 to 1 unit/kg/day

How Supplied

Insulin Injection (regular insulin): 100 units/mL in 10-mL vials and 3-mL disposable delivery devices (OTC)
Regular (concentrated) insulin injection: 500 units/mL in 20-mL vials

Adverse Reactions and Side Effects

Endo: HYPOGLYCEMIA
Local: erythema, pruritis, swelling
Misc: ANAPHYLAXIS *Drug Interactions:* Some of the signs and symptoms of hypoglycemia may be masked by beta-adrenergic blocking drugs. Corticosteroids and thiazide diuretics can cause increases in the insulin required. Table 13-2 compares some of the common insulin preparations.

EMS Considerations: Only regular insulin can be administered intravenously. When administering insulin by IV bolus, administer each 50 U over 1 minute. Assess the patient constantly for signs of hypoglycemia. Keep dextrose available.

Thiamine (THYE-a-min)

🍁 Betaxin, 🍁 Bewon, Biamine, vitamin B_1
Classification: Water-soluble vitamin
Pregnancy Class: A

Mechanism of Action: Required for the metabolism of carbohydrates and fats. It is necessary for the freeing of energy and the oxidation of pyruvic acid. Without enough thiamine, the cells of the body cannot use most of the energy usually available in glucose. The organ most sensitive to thiamine deficiency is the brain. Administering thiamine when deficiency exists restores the body's supply of the **vitamin.**

Pharmacokinetics

Absorption: Well absorbed from the GI tract and from IM and IV sites

Onset: IM, IV—1 hour

Duration: IM, IV—day to weeks

Indications: Used for the treatment of thiamine deficiencies (beriberi), for the prevention of Wernicke encephalopathy and Korsakoff syndrome, or for patients in a coma of unknown cause

Contraindications: Known hypersensitivity; should not be given to patients with known alcohol intolerance or bisulfite hypersensitivity

Precautions: Use with caution in patients with Wernicke encephalopathy because it may worsen unless thiamine is administered before glucose.

Wernicke encephalopathy is an acute and reversible disorder associated with chronic alcoholism. It is characterized by poor voluntary muscle coordination, eye muscle weakness, and mental derangement.

Korsakoff syndrome is a frequent result of chronic alcoholism. It is characterized by disorientation, illusions, hallucinations, and painful extremities. In addition, the patient may have bilateral footdrop.

Route and Dosage

IM, IV (Adult): 5 to 100 mg

IM, IV (Pediatric): 10 to 25 mg

How Supplied

Injection: 100 mg/mL in 1-mL ampules and prefilled syringes and 1-, 2-, 10-, and 30-mL vials

Adverse Reactions and Side Effects

Resp: pulmonary edema, respiratory distress

CV: VASCULAR COLLAPSE, hypotension, vasodilation

GI: bleeding, nausea

EENT: tightness of the throat

Misc: ANGIOEDEMA

effective Communication

Adverse reactions and side effects are extremely rare and are usually associated with IV administration or extremely large doses.

Drug Interactions: None significant

EMS Considerations: Thiamine is necessary for carbohydrate metabolism. The administration of dextrose to an alcohol-dependent patient who is deficient in thiamine may cause Wernicke encephalopathy or Korsakoff syndrome. Therefore, it is important to administer thiamine before administering dextrose to an alcohol-dependent patient.

SCENARIO REVISITED

Did you consider the case of Margot? As you recall, Margot is lying unconscious on her bedroom floor. She is wearing a MedicAlert bracelet indicating that she is a diabetic. Differentiating between diabetic ketoacidosis and hypoglycemia can be difficult in the out-of-hospital setting. Therefore, management of the unconscious diabetic patient is generally directed toward treating hypoglycemia, which is the more severe condition. Out-of-hospital management of Margot should proceed as follows:

- Maintain a patent airway; be prepared to intubate and to assist ventilation, if necessary.
- Attempt to draw a blood sample for glucose analysis at the hospital.
- Measure her glucose level using a glucose reagent strip. However, this may not be accurate. A reading of less than 45 mg indicates a need for further treatment.

Once you have performed an appropriate assessment, you should proceed using a critical thinking approach to medication administration.

Step 1: Determine signs and symptoms to be treated.

Step 2: Consider both the risks and benefits of treating or not treating Margot.

Step 3: Choose the medication that provides the best possible outcome.

Step 4: Remember the drug's indications, contraindications, and precautions.

Step 5: Decide the best route for administering the medication for the best outcome.

Step 6: Administer the medication(s) according to the Seven Patient Rights.

1. The right patient
2. The right drug
3. The right drug amount
4. The right time
5. The right route
6. The right documentation
7. The right of the patient to accept or refuse the medication(s)

Step 7: Reevaluate the patient for the desired and undesired effects.

- If possible, begin an IV at a keep-open rate.
- Administer 25 g of $D_{50}W$ by slow IV bolus. $D_{50}W$ is a hyperglycemic drug that increases circulating blood sugar levels in the hypoglycemic patient.
- If an IV line cannot be established, administer 0.5 to 1 mg of glucagon IM. Glucagon elevates blood sugar levels by stimulating the release of glycogen from the liver. Glucagon does not produce results as quickly as $D_{50}W$. $D_{50}W$ can show immediate results, while glucagon may take as long as 20 minutes.

- Monitor vital signs and cardiac rhythm closely.
- Transport the patient to the nearest appropriate hospital.

Let's Recap

Patients suffering from metabolic disorders can exhibit many different signs and symptoms. Treatment for the diabetic patient depends on an accurate assessment. Correct, timely treatment is vital. For example, the brain relies on glucose for its metabolism. If a patient becomes severely hypoglycemic, the brain cannot function properly. If the hypoglycemia is left untreated for an extended period, permanent brain damage could result.

A patient found in a coma needs a rapid, accurate assessment. Drug treatment for these patients is diagnostic in nature as well as potentially life saving. Treatment can include thiamine, glucose, and naloxone (see chapter 17).

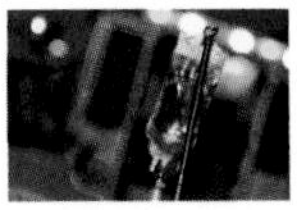

SCENARIO CONCLUSION

Depending on the circumstances at the scene, management can usually take place while Margot is being transported. In this case, Margot's condition does not change during transport. Margot is trying to compensate for metabolic acidosis by creating respiratory alkalosis through Kussmaul breathing. After arrival at the hospital, treatment will include decreasing serum glucose levels with insulin.

Check the **Evidence**

Diabetic ketoacidosis starves red blood cells of glucose and also produces a low pH.

How would Margot be managed if she were in a coma of unknown cause with no available previous history? After the airway has been appropriately managed, blood drawn, and an IV started, the following treatment should take place:

- If Margot is suspected of being alcohol dependent, administer 100 mg of thiamine by slow IV bolus.
- Administer 25 g of $D_{50}W$ by slow IV bolus.
- If the previous treatment is not successful, consider giving naloxone. Naloxone is a narcotic antagonist sometimes used in comas of unknown cause if narcotic drugs are suspected or to rule out narcotic drugs. Chapter 17 has a detailed discussion of naloxone.
- Transport Margot to the nearest appropriate hospital. Depending on the circumstances at the scene, management can usually take place while en route to the hospital.

PRACTICE EXERCISES

1. The pancreas is responsible for the production of insulin. Without insulin:
a. Hypoglycemia will result.
b. Glucose cannot pass into the body's cells.
c. Starches cannot be metabolized into glucose.
d. A buildup of carbon dioxide produces acidosis.

2. The organ most sensitive to the effects of thiamine deficiency is the:
a. Liver
b. Heart
c. Brain
d. Kidney

3. Insulin is indicated for the treatment of:
a. Hypoglycemia
b. Hyperglycemia
c. Metabolic acidosis
d. Coma of unknown cause

4. Though extremely rare, a possible life-threatening adverse reaction to thiamine may be:
a. Hypotension
b. Angioedema
c. Pulmonary edema
d. Vascular collapse

5. Esmolol blocks the stimulation of:
a. $Beta_1$ adrenergic receptors
b. $Beta_2$ adrenergic receptors
c. $Alpha_1$ receptors
d. $Alpha_2$ receptors

6. Hydrocortisone suppresses inflammation. It is contraindicated in patients with:
a. Adrenocortical insufficiency
b. Untreated infection
c. Hypothyroidism
d. Hypoglycemia

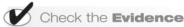

7. Thiamine is also known as:
   a. Vitamin B_1
   b. Vitamin B_{12}
   c. Vitamin C
   d. Vitamin D

8. Too-rapid administration of thiamine may cause:
   a. Dyspnea
   b. Hypotension
   c. Hypertension
   d. Cardiac arrhythmias

9. The initial adult dose of $D_{50}W$ is:
   a. 25 g
   b. 50 g
   c. 100 g
   d. 150 g

10. Before giving dextrose in water to your patient, you should first:
   a. Dilute 1:1 with sterile water
   b. Monitor cardiac rhythm
   c. Take a blood sample
   d. Start an IV

CASE STUDIES

1. You respond to an unconscious, unresponsive man who was found lying in his car. There is nothing to indicate that trauma has occurred. The patient has a patent airway, vital signs are within normal limits, and there are no apparent physical injuries. Several empty beer cans are found on the floor of the car. What is the first drug that medical control might order after you complete your assessment?
   a. $D_{50}W$
   b. Insulin
   c. Thiamine
   d. Glucagon

2. You respond to the home of an unconscious, unresponsive male patient. Initial assessment finds the patient presenting with Kussmaul breathing at 40 breaths/minute. The ECG monitor shows sinus tachycardia at a rate of 120 beats/minute. Skin is warm and dry, and the patient has a fruity odor in his breath. His blood pressure is low. This patient is presenting with classic signs and symptoms of:
   a. Ketoacidosis
   b. Insulin overdose
   c. Metabolic alkalosis
   d. Respiratory acidosis

3. After initial assessment, treatment for the patient in question 2 should include:
   a. IV and $D_{50}W$
   b. IV, $D_{50}W$, and insulin
   c. IV, thiamine, and $D_{50}W$
   d. IV for volume replacement and insulin

MATH EQUATIONS

1. You have been ordered to give 0.03 mg/kg of glucagon to your 16 lb pediatric patient.
   a. How many kg does your patient weigh?
   b. What is the initial dose of glucagon for this patient?
2. While you are working in the ED, the physician orders 0.1 unit/kg/hr of regular insulin as a continuous infusion to be given to a 170 lb patient. The insulin comes as 1 unit/mL in a 5 mL ampule.
   a. What is the concentration of the IV solution after adding 5 mL of the insulin to 500 mL of solution?
   b. How many kg does your patient weigh?
   c. Using a 60 gtt/mL IV set, what is the drip rate to deliver the required dosage?
3. You have been ordered to give 0.3 mg of thiamine to your pediatric patient. The thiamine comes as 1 mg in 1 mL. How much of the thiamine will you give to your patient?
4. While you are working in the ED, the physician orders esmolol to treat a patient with hyperthyroidism. The patient weighs 145 lbs. She orders a loading dose of 500 mcg/kg over 1 minute initially, followed by 50 mcg/kg/minute infusion for 4 minutes. The esmolol comes pre-diluted for the loading as 20 mg/mL in 5 mL vials, and the pre-mixed infusion comes as 2,500 mg/250 mL.
   a. How many kg does the patient weigh?
   b. How much of the esmolol will be given for the loading dose?
   c. How many gtt/minute will be administered for the infusion using a 60 gtt IV set?

■ REFERENCES

Beck, R. K. (2012). Drugs used to treat gastrointestinal emergencies. In *Pharmacology for the EMS Provider.* New York: Delmar, Cengage Learning.

Deglin, J. H., Vallerand, A. H., and Sanboski, C. A. (2011). *Davis's drug guide for nurses* (12th ed.). Philadelphia, PA: F. A. Davis Company.

Diabetes Health Center: ketones. Retrieved January 4, 2014 from http://www.webmd.com/diabetes/ketones-14241

Hemphill, R. R. Hyperosmolar hyperglycemic state. Retrieved January 4, 2014 from http://.emedicine.medscape.com/article/1914705-overview

National Endocrine and Metabolic Diseases Information Service (NEMDIS). Retrieved January 3, 2014 from www.endocrine.niddk.nih.gov/index.aspx

Osmotic diuresis. Retrieved January 8, 2014 from http://www.nlm.nih.gov/medlineplus/ency/article/001266.htm

Venes, D., ed. (2013). *Taber's cyclopedic medical dictionary* (22nd ed.). Philadelphia, PA: F. A. Davis Company.

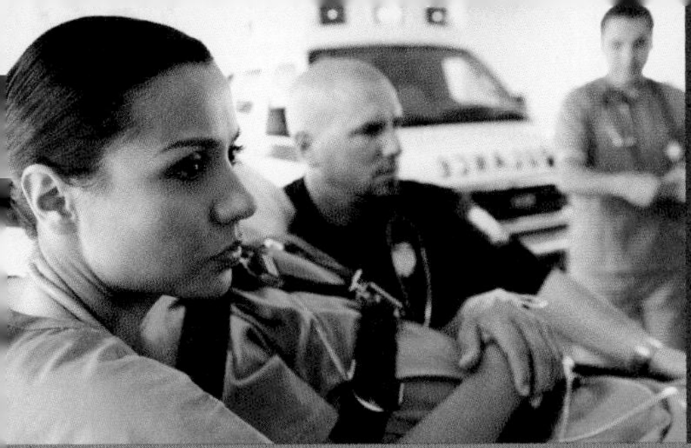

CHAPTER 14

Drugs Used to Treat Neurological Emergencies

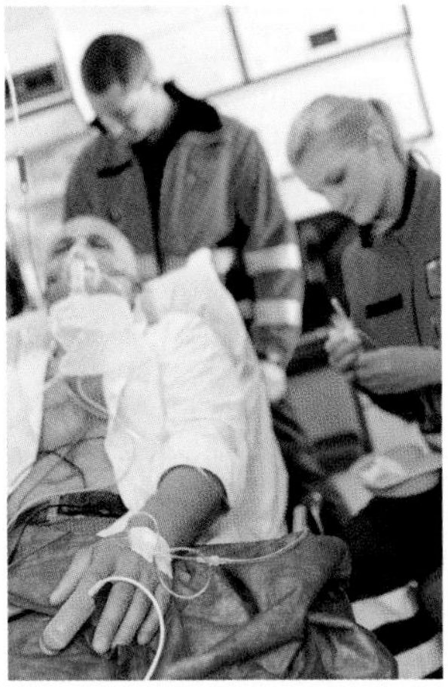

Paramedics assessing a patient with a possible stroke. *(Photograph © CandyBox Images/iStock/Thinkstock)*

LEARNING OUTCOMES

- Explain the assessment and treatment of a patient suspected of a stroke.
- Explain the assessment and treatment of the seizure patient.
- Briefly discuss the pathophysiology of stroke and seizures.
- Describe and list the indications, contraindications, precautions, route and dosages, and adverse reactions and side effects for the following:
  - the anticonvulsants diazepam, fosphenytoin, lorazepam, phenobarbital, and phenytoin
  - the antihypertensive labetalol
  - the nonopioid analgesic acetylsalicylic acid (aspirin).
  - the osmotic diuretic mannitol
  - the thrombolytic drug alteplase
  - the vasodilator nitroprusside

KEY TERMS

Anticonvulsant
Epilepsy
Generalized motor seizure
Seizure
Status epilepticus
Stevens-Johnson syndrome
Stroke

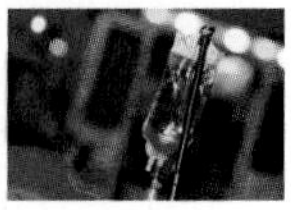

SCENARIO OPENING

You have been assigned to Rescue 14 for one of your field-internship rides. During lunch, Rescue 14 gets a call to respond to the home of a man "having a seizure." On arrival, you find Norman, who appears to be approximately 40, experiencing active seizures. Norman's extremities are outstretched, his jaw is clenched, and he is drooling. As you approach Norman, seizure activity appears to be slowing down. However, just as Norman is placed on humidified oxygen, seizures begin again. Norman's wife states that he has been going from one seizure to another.

Norman is experiencing **status epilepticus.** Status epilepticus is considered a major emergency because of the possibility of aspiration, hypoxia, fracturing of long bones including the spinal column, or sustaining myocardial damage caused by cardiac ischemia. Hyperthermia, exhaustion, and possibly death can also result from prolonged seizure activity.

Introduction

Neurological emergencies are often very difficult to manage. Frequently, patients experiencing a neurological emergency show signs and symptoms that are very subtle, ranging from a headache to a coma. The status of a patient experiencing a neurological emergency may change rapidly; a patient may initially respond appropriately but then become comatose within minutes. These factors can greatly complicate the out-of-hospital treatment of the patient experiencing a neurological emergency.

Pathophysiology of Neurological Disorders

Stroke

Stroke is a sudden loss of neurological function, caused by reduced blood flow to an area of the brain. There are two types of strokes (Fig. 14-1): ischemic and hemorrhagic.

Ischemic Stroke

There are two classifications of ischemic stroke as follows.

- *Embolic Stroke (embolus):* In an embolic stroke, a blood clot forms somewhere in the body and travels to the brain. Once the clot is in the brain, it eventually travels to a blood vessel small enough to block its passage. The clot lodges there, blocking the blood vessel and causing a stroke.
- *Thrombotic Stroke:* In a thrombotic stroke, blood flow is impaired because of a blockage to one or more of the arteries supplying blood to the brain. Thrombotic strokes can also occur due to unhealthy blood vessels clogged with a buildup of fatty deposits and cholesterol.

Hemorrhagic Stroke

Strokes caused by the rupture of a blood vessel in the brain are called hemorrhagic strokes. Hemorrhages can be caused by a number of disorders that affect the blood vessels, including long-standing high blood pressure and cerebral aneurysms. Aneurysms develop over a number of years and usually do not cause detectable problems until they rupture. There are two types of hemorrhagic stroke: subarachnoid and intracerebral.

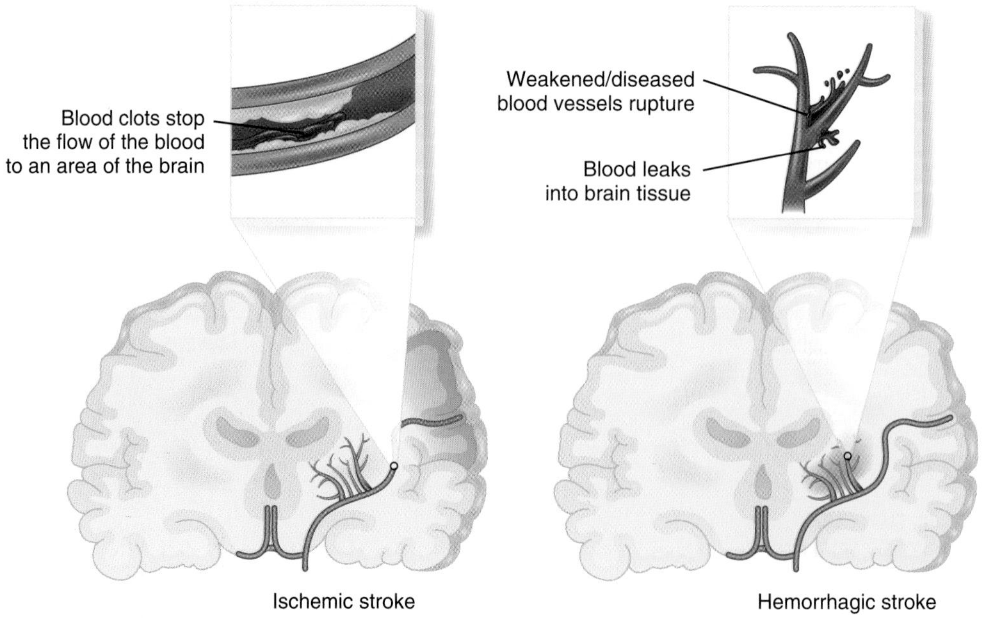
Blood clots stop the flow of the blood to an area of the brain
Weakened/diseased blood vessels rupture
Blood leaks into brain tissue
Ischemic stroke
Hemorrhagic stroke

Figure 14-1 Ischemic vs. hemorrhagic stroke.

In an intracerebral stroke, bleeding occurs from vessels within the brain itself. Hypertension is the primary cause of this type of hemorrhage. In a subarachnoid stroke, an aneurysm ruptures in a large artery on or near the thin, delicate membrane surrounding the brain. Blood spills into the area around the brain, which is filled with a protective fluid, causing the brain to be surrounded by blood-contaminated fluid.

Acute ischemic stroke can be treated with thrombolytic drugs such as alteplase if the stroke is recognized in the first 90 to 180 minutes and intracerebral hemorrhage has been ruled out. Therefore, once EMS has determined the patient may be having an ischemic stroke, the patient must be rapidly transported to the closest appropriate facility for treatment.

Table 14-1 lists the risk factors and warning signs of stroke.

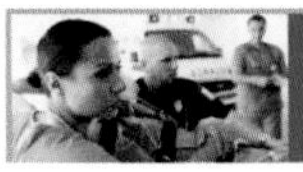

Table 14-1 Risk Factors and Warning Signs of Stroke

Stroke Risk Factors	Stroke Warning Signs
Advanced age (over 65 years old)	Sudden weakness or numbness of the face, arm, or leg
Atherosclerosis of the aortic arch	Sudden loss of vision
Atrial fibrillation	Double vision
Carotid artery disease	Dimming of vision in one or both eyes
Cigarette use	Sudden difficulty in speaking or understanding speech
Excessive alcohol use (more than 5 drinks/day)	Sudden severe headache
Heart failure	Sudden falling, gait disturbance, or dizziness
Hyperlipidemia	
Hypertension	
History of MI	
Diabetes mellitus	
Male gender	
Nonwhite race	
Peripheral vascular disease	
Physical inactivity	
Pregnancy	
Immediate post-partum	
Obesity	
Using combination hormonal contraception	
Recent TIA	

Seizures

A **seizure** is a convulsion or other clinical event caused by a sudden discharge of electrical activity in the brain (Fig. 14-2). There are several classifications of seizures:

- *Absence seizure*: A sudden, brief lapse of consciousness, usually for less than 20 seconds. Patients (usually children) generally show a blank facial expression that may be accompanied by repeated eye blinking or lip-smacking. There are no convulsions or falls that accompany an absence seizure.
- *Breakthrough seizure*: A seizure that occurs despite the use of current therapeutic medications
- *Complex seizure*: A seizure in which the patient loses consciousness
- *Jacksonian seizure*: A form of epilepsy with spasms that are confined to one group of muscles
- *Nonepileptic seizure*: A seizure that results in loss of consciousness due to inadequate perfusion to the brain (for example, a seizure caused by a sudden drop in blood pressure or a seizure caused by hypoglycemia)

Epilepsy

Epilepsy is a disease marked by recurrent seizures due to repetitive abnormal electrical discharges within the brain. Epilepsy is categorized as partial, **generalized**, or drug-resistant, or it may be unclassified.

Partial seizures generally begin with local or focal discharges in one part of the brain. On occasion, the discharges may become generalized. When patients remain awake during a seizure, the seizure is referred to as simple and partial. If loss of consciousness occurs after a focal seizure, the seizure is called partial and complex. Drug-resistant epilepsy is a failure of current medications to control seizures. Table 14-2 lists some of the common causes of seizures.

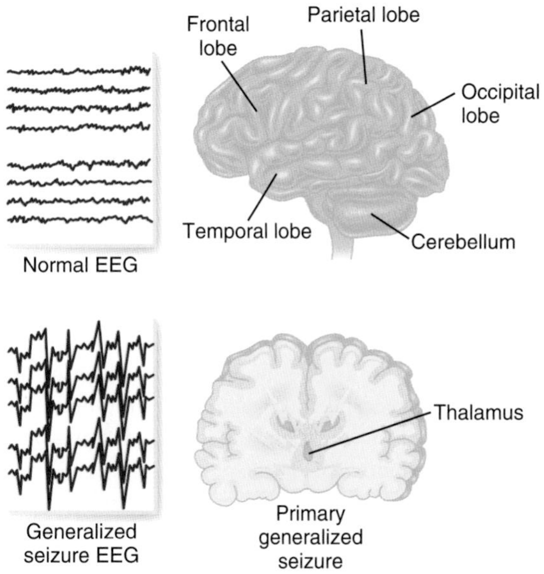

Figure 14-2 Discharge of electrical activity during a seizure.

Table 14-2 Common Causes of Seizures

Common Causes of Seizures
Genetic factors
Congenital conditions
Metabolic imbalances
Fever/infection
Neurological disorders
Alzheimer disease
Alcohol/drugs
Head trauma
Stroke
Brain tumors
Progressive brain diseases
Drug withdrawal
Medications
Unknown reasons

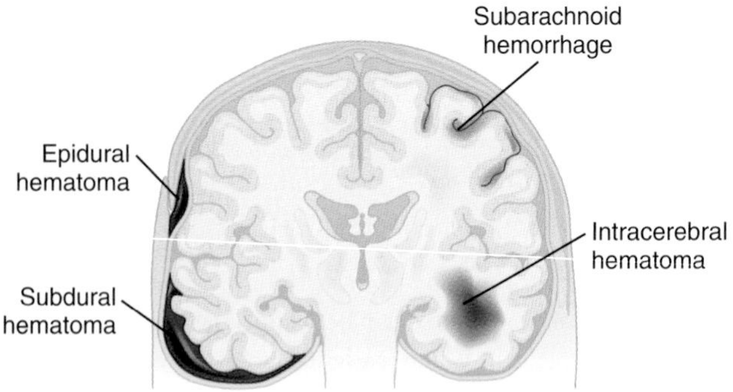

Figure 14-3 Traumatic brain injuries.

Traumatic Brain Injury

Traumatic brain injury (TBI) is a form of brain injury that occurs when a sudden trauma causes damage to the brain (Fig. 14-3). TBI can result when the head hits an object or when an object pierces the skull and enters brain tissue. Symptoms of a TBI can be mild, moderate, or severe, depending on the extent of the damage to the brain.

Symptoms of mild TBI can include headache, confusion, lightheadedness, dizziness, blurred vision, ringing in the ears, bad taste in the mouth, fatigue, a change in sleep patterns, behavioral changes, and trouble with memory, concentration, or attention. A person with a moderate or severe TBI may show these same symptoms but may also have a headache that gets worse or does not go away; repeated vomiting or nausea; seizures; an inability to awaken from sleep; dilation of one or both pupils; slurred speech; weakness or numbness in the extremities; loss of coordination; and increased confusion, restlessness, or agitation.

Because little can be done to reverse the initial brain damage caused by trauma, EMS professionals must try to stabilize the patient with TBI and focus on preventing further injury. Primary concerns include insuring proper oxygenation to the brain, maintaining adequate circulation, and controlling blood pressure while rapidly transporting the patient to the nearest appropriate hospital. Though rarely used, mannitol may be included in some EMS protocols. Mannitol is an osmotic diuretic that can be useful in reducing brain edema.

Pharmacokinetics

Anticonvulsants

Anticonvulsants are used to decrease the incidence and severity of seizures. They include a variety of drugs, all capable of depressing abnormal neuronal discharges in the CNS. Anticonvulsants work by preventing the spread of seizure activity, depressing the motor cortex, raising the seizure threshold, or altering levels of neurotransmitters.

Antihypertensives

Antihypertensive medications are used to lower blood pressure to a normal level (lower than 90 mm Hg diastolic) or to the lowest level tolerated. Hypertensive therapy is designed to prevent end-organ damage. Antihypertensive medications are classified into groups according to their site of action.

Nonopioid Analgesics

Most nonopioid analgesic medications inhibit prostaglandin synthesis peripherally for analgesic effect and centrally for antipyretic effect. Aspirin also decreases platelet aggregation.

Osmotic Diuretics

Diuretics are used to enhance the selective excretion of various electrolytes and water by affecting renal mechanisms for tubular secretion and reabsorption. Osmotic diuretics are used in the management of cerebral edema.

Thrombolytics

Thrombolytic medications convert plasminogen to plasmin, which then degrades fibrin in clots. Alteplase is a thrombolytic used in the management of acute ischemic stroke.

Individual Drugs

Aspirin (AS-pir-in)

🍁 Apo-ASA, 🍁 Arthrinol, 🍁 Arthrisin, 🍁 Artria S.R., ASA, 🍁 Asaphen, Ascriptin, Aspercin, Aspergum, Aspirtab, 🍁 Astrin, Bayer Aspirin, Bufferin, 🍁 Coryphen, Easprin, Ecotrin, 🍁 Entrophen, Genacote, Halfprin, 🍁 Headache Tablets, Healthprin, 🍁 Novasen, 🍁 PMS-ASA, 🍁 Rivasa, St. Joseph Adult Chewable Aspirin, ZORprin

Classifications: Antipyretic, nonopioid analgesic, salicylate

Pregnancy Class: D (first trimester)

Mechanism of Action: Produces analgesia and reduces inflammation and fever by inhibiting the production of prostaglandins; decreases platelet aggregation

Pharmacokinetics

Absorption: Well absorbed from the upper small intestine. Absorption from enteric-coated aspirin is unreliable. Rectal absorption is slow and variable.

Onset: PO—5 to 30 minutes

Rectal—1 to 2 hours

Duration: PO—3 to 6 hours

Rectal—7 hours

Indications: Used as a prophylaxis of transient ischemic attacks

Contraindications: Known hypersensitivity; should not be given to patients with bleeding disorders

***effective* Communication**

Aspirin should not be given to children or adolescents with viral infections due to the risk of developing Reye syndrome.

Precautions: Use with caution in patients with a history of GI bleeding or ulcer disease, in patients with chronic alcohol use or severe renal disease, and in patients with severe liver disease.

Route and Dosage

PO (Adult): 50 to 325 mg once daily

How Supplied (All OTC)

Tablets: 81 mg, 162.5 mg, 325 mg, 500 mg, 650 mg, 🍁 975 mg

Chewable tablets: 🍁 80 mg, 81 mg

Chewing gum: 227 mg

Dispersible tablets: 325 mg, 500 mg

Enteric-coated (delayed-release) tablets: 80 mg, 165 mg, 🍁 600 mg, 650 mg, 975 mg

Extended-release tablets: 🍁 325 mg, 650 mg, 800 mg

Delayed-release capsules: 🍁 325 mg, 🍁 500 mg

Suppositories: 60 mg, 120 mg, 125 mg, 130 mg, 🍁 150 mg, 🍁 160 mg, 195 mg, 200 mg, 300 mg, 🍁 320 mg, 325 mg, 600 mg, 🍁 640 mg, 650 mg, 1.2 g

Adverse Reactions and Side Effects

EENT: Tinnitus

GI: GI BLEEDING, <u>dyspepsia</u>, <u>epigastric distress</u>, <u>nausea</u>, abdominal pain, anorexia, vomiting

Hemat: Anemia, increased bleeding time

Misc: ANAPHYLAXIS, LARYNGEAL EDEMA

Drug Interactions: Aspirin may increase the risk of bleeding when taken with thrombolytic medications. There is increased risk of GI irritation when taken with NSAIDs.

EMS Considerations: Aspirin should be administered as soon as possible if a TIA or stroke is suspected.

Check the Evidence

Patients who have asthma, allergies, and nasal polyps or who are hypersensitive to tartrazine are at an increased risk for developing hypersensitive reactions.

Alteplase (AL-te-plase)

Activase, 🍁 Activase rt-PA, Cathflo Activase, tissue plasminogen activator, t-PA

Classifications: Thrombolytic, plasminogen activator

Pregnancy Class: C

Mechanism of Action: Converts plasminogen to plasmin, which is then able to degrade fibrin present in clots. Alteplase directly activates plasminogen.

Pharmacokinetics

Absorption: complete absorption after IV administration

Onset: 30 minutes

Duration: unknown

Indications: Used for acute ischemic stroke

Contraindications: Known hypersensitivity; should not be given to patients with active internal bleeding, a history of stroke, an intracranial neoplasm, or severe uncontrolled hypertension

Precautions: Use with caution in patients with a recent history of trauma, recent GI or GU bleeding, and severe liver or renal disease.

***effective* Communication**

Use extreme caution when giving alteplase to patients receiving concurrent anticoagulant therapy because of an increased risk of intracranial bleeding.

Route and Dosage

IV (Adult): 0.9 mg/kg (not to exceed 90 mg), given as an IV infusion over 1 hour, with 10 percent of the dose given as an IV bolus over the first minute

Understand the Numbers

You are ordered to give alteplase to your 240-pound patient. How much of this dose should be given as a bolus over the first minute?

240 lbs ÷ 2.2 kg = 109 kg. 0.9 mg × 109 kg = 98 mg. 10% of 90 mg (max. dose) = 9 mg given by IV bolus over 1 minute

How Supplied

Powder for injection: 2 mg/vial, 50 mg/vial, 100 mg/vial

Adverse Reactions and Side Effects

Resp: Bronchospasm

CV: Hypotension, reperfusion arrhythmias

CNS: INTRACRANIAL HEMORRHAGE

GI: GI BLEEDING, RETROPERITONEAL BLEEDING

Derm: Ecchymoses, flushing, urticaria

Hemat: BLEEDING

Local: Hemorrhage at the injection sites, phlebitis at the IV site

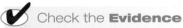

MS: Musculoskeletal pain
Misc: ANAPHYLAXIS, fever
Drug Interactions: Concurrent use of aspirin, other NSAIDs, or direct thrombin inhibitors may increase the risk of bleeding.
EMS Considerations: Assess vital signs every 15 minutes. ECG should be continuously monitored. Assess patient frequently for signs of bleeding; if the patient deteriorates, stop the infusion immediately. ❗ Overdosing and underdosing have resulted in patient harm or death. Have a second person independently check the original order, dosage calculations, and infusion pump settings. Do not confuse the abbreviation *t-PA* for alteplase with the abbreviation *TNK t-PA* for tenecteplase and *r-PA* for reteplase. You should clarify orders that contain any of these abbreviations.

Diazepam (dye-AZ-e-pam)

🍁 Apo-Diazepam, Diastat, 🍁 Diazemuls, 🍁 Novo-Dipam, 🍁 PMS-Diazepam, Valium, 🍁 Vivol
Classifications: Benzodiazepine, anticonvulsant
Pregnancy Class: D
Mechanism of Action: Depresses the CNS by potentiating GABA, an inhibitory neurotransmitter; produces skeletal muscle relaxation; has anticonvulsant properties due to enhanced presynaptic inhibition
Pharmacokinetics
Absorption: Rapidly absorbed form the GI tract, with 90 percent absorbed from the rectal mucosa. Absorption from IM sites may be slow and unpredictable.
Onset: IM—within 30 minutes
IV—1 to 5 minutes
Rectal—2 to 10 minutes
Duration: IM—unknown
IV—15 to 60 minutes
Rectal—4 to 12 hours
Indications: Used to treat seizure activity including status epilepticus or uncontrolled seizures; can be used as a skeletal muscle relaxant
Contraindications: Known hypersensitivity; should not be given to patients with severe pulmonary impairment, severe liver dysfunction, uncontrolled severe pain, angle-closure glaucoma, or preexisting CNS depression
Precautions: Use with caution in patients with severe renal impairment and in patients with a history of suicide attempt or drug dependence.
Route and Dosage
Seizure Activity
IV (Adult): 5 to 10 mg; may be repeated every 10 to 15 minutes to a total dose of 30 mg

> *effective* **Communication**
> An IM route may be used if an IV route is unavailable; however, larger doses may be required.

Rectal (Adult and Pediatric over 12 years): 0.2 mg/kg
Rectal (Pediatric 6 to 11 years): 0.3 mg/kg
Rectal (Pediatric 2 to 5 years): 0.5 mg/kg
IM, IV (Pediatric over 5 years): 0.05 to 0.3 mg/kg/dose given over 3 to 5 minutes; may be repeated every 15 to 30 minutes to a total dose of 10 mg
IM, IV (Pediatric 1 m to *5 years):* 0.05 to 0.3 mg/kg/dose given over 3 to 5 minutes; may be repeated every 15 to 30 minutes to a total dose of 5 mg
Skeletal Muscle Relaxant
IM, IV (Adult): 2 to 10 mg
IM, IV (Pediatric over 5 years): 5 to 10 mg
IM, IV (Pediatric 1 mo to *5 years):* 1 to 2 mg
How Supplied
Solution for injection: 5 mg/mL
Rectal gel delivery system: 2.5 mg, 10 mg, 20 mg
Adverse Reactions and Side Effects
Resp: Respiratory depression
CV: Hypotension (IV only)
CNS: Dizziness, drowsiness, depression, hangover, ataxia, slurred speech, headache, paradoxical excitation
GI: Constipation, diarrhea, nausea, vomiting
EENT: Blurred vision
Derm: Rashes
Local: Pain (IM), phlebitis (IV)
Drug Interactions: Concurrent use of other CNS depressants may cause additive CNS depression.
EMS Considerations: Diazepam may cause respiratory arrest if given too rapidly or in excess. Do not mix diazepam with any other drug. Diazepam may react with the IV tubing; to minimize this, administer at the IV site, not higher in the tubing. Thoroughly flush the IV line before administering diazepam if other drugs have already been given through the line. Assess the patient's vital signs continuously.

Fosphenytoin (foss-FEN-i-toyn)

Cerebyx
Classification: Anticonvulsant
Pregnancy Class: D
Mechanism of Action: Limits seizure activity by altering ion transport; may also decrease synaptic transmission
Pharmacokinetics
Absorption: Rapidly converted to phenytoin after IV administration and completely absorbed after IM administration
Onset: IM—unknown
IV—15 to 45 minutes
Duration: IM and IV—up to 24 hours
Indications: Used for the short-term management of generalized motor seizures and status epilepticus
Contraindications: Known hypersensitivity; should not be used in patients with sinus bradycardia, sinoatrial block, second- or third-degree heart block, or Adams-Stokes syndrome
Precautions: Use with caution in patients with liver or renal disease due to the increased risk of adverse reactions. ❗ Safety has not been established during lactation.

Route and Dosage (Note: dose is expressed as phenytoin sodium equivalent [PE]).

***effective* Communication**

Adjustments in the recommended dose should not be made when substituting fosphenytoin for phenytoin sodium or vice versa.

IV (Adult): 15 to 20 mg PE/kg given at a rate of 100 to 150 mg PE/min. Dilute fosphenytoin in solution to make a concentration of 1.5 to 25 mg PE/mL.
How Supplied
Injection: 50 mg PE/mL
Adverse Reactions and Side Effects
CV: Hypotension (with rapid administration)
CNS: Dizziness, drowsiness, nystagmus (involuntary movements of the eyes), agitation, headache stupor, vertigo
GI: Dry mouth, nausea, taste perversion, vomiting
EENT: Deafness, diplopia, tinnitus
Derm: Pruritus, rash, STEVENS-JOHNSON SYNDROME
MS: Back pain
Drug Interactions: Phenytoin levels and risk of toxicity are increased by acute ingestion of alcohol, amiodarone, cimetidine, and diazepam.
EMS Considerations: Monitor respirations, ECG, and blood pressure frequently. ❗ Do not confuse fosphenytoin (Cerebyx) with celocoxib (Celebrex) or citalopram (Celexa).

Labetalol (la-BET-a-lole)

Trandate
Classifications: Beta-blocker, antihypertensive
Pregnancy Class: C
Mechanism of Action: Blocks the stimulation of beta$_1$-, beta$_2$-, and alpha$_1$-adrenergic receptor sites
Pharmacokinetics
Absorption: Well absorbed
Onset: 2 to 5 minutes
Duration: 16 to 18 hours
Indication: Used to treat hypertension in stroke patients
Contraindications: Known hypersensitivity; should not be given to patients with uncompensated CHF, pulmonary edema, cardiogenic shock, bradycardia, or heart block
Precautions: Use with caution in patients with renal or liver impairment, pulmonary disease, or diabetes mellitus. ❗ Labetalol may cause fetal bradycardia, hypotension, hypoglycemia, or respiratory depression.
Route and Dosage
IV (Adult): 20 mg initially. Additional doses of 40 to 80 mg may be given every 10 minutes as needed up to a total dose of 300 mg.
How Supplied
Injection: 5 mg/mL
Adverse Reactions and Side Effects
Resp: Bronchospasm, wheezing
CV: ARRHYTHMIAS, BRADYCARDIA, CHF, PULMONARY EDEMA, orthostatic hypotension
CNS: Fatigue, weakness, anxiety, depression, dizziness, drowsiness, insomnia, memory loss, nightmares
GI: Constipation, diarrhea, nausea
GU: Erectile dysfunction, decreased libido
EENT: Blurred vision, dry eyes, nasal stuffiness
Endo: Hyper- or hypoglycemia
MS: Back pain, muscle cramps
Drug Interactions: Additive hypotension may occur if used with other antihypertensives. Additive bradycardia may occur with digoxin, verapamil, or diltiazem.
EMS Considerations: Monitor patient vital signs and ECG continuously.

Lorazepam (lor-AZ-e-pam)

🍁 Apo-Lorazepam, Ativan, 🍁 Novo-Lorazem, 🍁 Nu-Loraz
Classifications: Anticonvulsant, antianxiety
Pregnancy Class: D
Mechanism of Action: Depresses the CNS by potentiating GABA, an inhibitory neurotransmitter
Pharmacokinetics
Absorption: Rapidly and completely absorbed following IV administration
Onset: 15 to 30 minutes
Duration: 8 to 12 hours
Indications: Used to decrease anxiety and seizure activity (unlabeled)
Contraindications: Known hypersensitivity; should not be given to patients with preexisting CNS depression, uncontrolled severe pain, angle-closure glaucoma, and severe hypotension
Precautions: Use with caution in patients with severe liver, renal, or pulmonary impairment, in patients with a history of suicide attempt or drug abuse, or in patients with COPD.
Route and Dosage (Anticonvulsant)
IV (Adult): 50 mcg (0.05 mg)/kg up to 4 mg; may be repeated after 10 to 15 minutes but not to exceed 8 mg/12 hours

Understand the Numbers

You are ordered to give 50 mcg/kg to your 300-pound patient. Will this dosage exceed the maximum dose of 4 mg? 300 lbs ÷ 2.2 kg = 136 kg. 50 mcg (0.05 mg) × 136 kg = 6800 mcg or 6.8 mg. Therefore, the dose for this patient should be 4,000 mcg or 4 mg, the maximum initial dose.

Check the Evidence

Administer lorazepam at a rate not to exceed 2 mg/minute or 0.05 mg/kg over 2 to 5 minutes. Rapid administration may result in apnea, hypotension, bradycardia, or cardiac arrest.

How Supplied
Injection: 2 mg/mL, 4 mg/mL
Adverse Reactions and Side Effects
Resp: Respiratory depression
CV: APNEA, CARDIAC ARREST *(rapid IV only.*
CNS: Dizziness, drowsiness, lethargy, hangover, headache, ataxia, slurred speech, confusion, forgetfulness

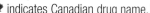

GI: Constipation, diarrhea, nausea, vomiting
EENT: Blurred vision
Derm: Rashes
Drug Interactions: Additive CNS depression if used with other CNS depressants
EMS Considerations: Assess patient vital signs continuously. Thoroughly flush the IV line before administering lorazepam if other drugs have already been given.

Mannitol (MAN-i-tol)

Osmitrol, Resectisol
Classification: Osmotic diuretic
Pregnancy Class: C
Mechanism of Action: Increases the osmotic pressure inhibiting reabsorption of water and electrolytes. Mannitol causes excretion of water, sodium, potassium, chloride, calcium, phosphorus, magnesium, urea, and uric acid.
Pharmacokinetics
 Absorption: IV administration produces complete bioavailability.
 Onset: 50 to 60 minutes
 Duration: 6 to 8 hours
Indications: Used to treat increased intracranial or intraocular pressure
Contraindications: Known hypersensitivity; should not be given to dehydrated patients or to patients with known active intracranial bleeding
Precautions: Use cautiously in the OB patient; safety has not been established.
Route and Dosage
IV (Adult): 0.25 to 2 g/kg as a 15 to 25 percent solution over 30 to 60 minutes

> **Check the Evidence**
>
> Mannitol solution occasionally contains small crystals, especially at temperatures below 45 degrees Fahrenheit (7.22 degrees Celsius). Therefore, IV administration should include an in-line filter to remove any crystals.

How Supplied
IV injection: 5 percent, 10 percent, 15 percent, 20 percent
Adverse Reactions and Side Effects
Resp: Pulmonary edema
CV: Transient volume expansion, chest pain, CHF, tachycardia
CNS: Confusion, headache
EENT: Blurred vision, rhinitis
GI: Nausea, thirst, vomiting
GU: Renal failure, urinary retention
F and E: Dehydration, hyperkalemia, hypernatremia, hypokalemia, hyponatremia
Local: Phlebitis at IV site
Drug Interactions: Hypokalemia increases the risk of digoxin toxicity.
EMS Considerations: Monitor patients closely for any signs of dehydration (hypotension, thirst, decreased skin turgor, dry skin and mucous membranes). Use a slow infusion if signs of pulmonary edema occur (dyspnea, cyanosis, rales, or frothy sputum).

Midazolam (mid-AY-zoe-lam)

Versed
Classifications: Benzodiazepine, antianxiety, sedative/hypnotic
Pregnancy Class: D
Mechanism of Action: Acts on the CNS to produce generalized CNS depression. The effects are mediated by GABA, an inhibitory neurotransmitter.
Pharmacokinetics
 Absorption: Rapidly absorbed by nasal administration; well absorbed followed by IM administration; IV administration results in complete bioavailability
 Onset: IN—5 minutes
 IM—15 minutes
 IV—1.5 to 5 minutes
 Duration: IN—30 to 60 minutes
 IM and IV—2 to 6 hours
Indications: Used as a premedication before painful procedures, such as cardioversion; can also be used as an anticonvulsant
Contraindications: Known hypersensitivity; should not be given to patients with preexisting CNS depression, uncontrolled severe pain, or angle-closure glaucoma
Precautions: Use with caution in geriatric patients; in patients with pulmonary disease, CHF, renal impairment, or liver impairment; and in patients who are obese.

> **Check the Evidence**
>
> Patients over 70 years old are generally more susceptible to cardiorespiratory depressant effects. Therefore, the dosage of midazolam may have to be reduced.

> *effective* **Communication**
>
> Patients who are obese should have the midazolam dosage calculated on the basis of ideal body weight.

Route and Dosage (Note: The dosage of midazolam must be individualized. Typically, the initial dosage is given on the basis of ideal body weight and increased as necessary. The average adult dose of midazolam is 5 mg. Many health-care facilities give children midazolam by mouth or intranasally. Check your protocols for the dosing of midazolam).
IM (Adult): 0.07 to 0.08 mg/kg, initially
IV (Adult): 1 to 2.5 mg, initially
How Supplied
Injection: 1 mg/mL, 5 mg/mL
Adverse Reactions and Side Effects
Resp: APNEA, LARYNGOSPASM, RESPIRATORY DEPRESSION, bronchospasm, coughing
CV: CARDIAC ARREST, arrhythmias
CNS: Agitation, drowsiness, excess sedation, headache
EENT: Blurred vision

GI: Hiccups, nausea, vomiting
Derm: Rashes
Local: Phlebitis at the IV site, pain at the IM site
Drug Interactions: Increased CNS depression if used with other CNS depressant drugs; increased risk of hypotension if used with other antihypertensive drugs

effective Communication

If midazolam is used concurrently with other CNS depressant drugs, the dosage of midazolam may have to be reduced by 30 to 50 percent.

EMS Considerations: Monitor blood pressure, pulse, and respirations continuously during administration. Oxygen and resuscitative equipment should be immediately available.

Nitroprusside (nye-troe-PRUSS-ide)

Nitropress
Classifications: Antihypertensive, vasodilator
Pregnancy Class: C
Mechanism of Action: Produces peripheral vasodilation by direct action on both the arteriolar and venous smooth muscle
Pharmacokinetics
- *Absorption:* Complete bioavailability
- *Onset:* Immediate
- *Duration:* 1 to 10 minutes

Indication: Control hypertension in acute stroke
Contraindications: Known hypersensitivity; should not be given to patients with decreased cerebral perfusion
Precautions: Use with caution in patients with renal disease, liver disease, hypothyroidism, and hyponatremia.

Check the Evidence

Patients with liver disease who are given nitroprusside have an increased risk of cyanide accumulation, which can lead to deadly cyanide toxicity.

Route and Dosage
IV (Adult): 0.3 mcg/kg/minute initially; may be increased, as needed, up to 10 mcg/kg/minute; should not exceed 10 minutes of therapy at 10 mcg/kg/minute infusion
(Note: The usual dose is 3 mcg/kg/minute.)

effective Communication

Once the nitroprusside infusion is prepared, the IV bag must be wrapped with aluminum foil or with a brown plastic bag during infusion.

How Supplied
Injection: 25 mg/mL
Adverse Reactions and Side Effects
Resp: Dyspnea
CV: Hypotension, palpitations
CNS: Dizziness, headache, restlessness
EENT: Blurred vision, tinnitus
GI: Abdominal pain, nausea, vomiting
Misc: CYANIDE TOXICITY
Drug Interactions: Additive hypotension if used with other antihypertensives
EMS Considerations: Monitor vital signs and ECG continuously during infusion. If hypotension occurs, decrease or discontinue the infusion.

Phenobarbital (fee-noe-BAR-bi-tal)

✤ Ancalixir, Luminal, Solfoton
Classifications: Anticonvulsant, barbiturate
Pregnancy Class: D
Mechanism of Action: Produces generalized CNS depression; decreases motor activity and alters cerebellar function; inhibits transmission in the nervous system and raises the seizure threshold
Pharmacokinetics
- *Absorption:* Absorption is slow but up to 90 percent complete.
- *Onset:* 5 minutes
- *Duration:* 4 to 6 hours

Indications: Used as an anticonvulsant in grand mal, partial, and febrile seizures in pediatrics
Contraindications: Known hypersensitivity; should not be given to patients with preexisting CNS depression, severe respiratory disease, or uncontrolled severe pain
Precautions: Use with caution in patients with liver dysfunction or severe renal impairment and in patients with a history of suicide attempt or drug abuse. (!) The initial dose should be reduced for geriatric patients.
Route and Dosage
Status Epilepticus
IV (Adult and Pediatrics over 1 month): 15 to 18 mg/kg in a single dose or divided doses. The maximum loading dose is 20 mg/kg.
Maintenance Anticonvulsant
IV (Adult and Pediatric over 12 years): 1 to 3 mg/kg/day as a single dose or 2 double doses
IV (Pediatric 5 to 12 years): 4 to 6 mg/kg/day in 1 to 2 divided doses
IV (Pediatric 1 to 5 years): 6 to 8 mg/kg/day in 1 to 2 divided doses
How Supplied
Injection: 30 mg/mL in 1-mL prefilled syringes; 60 mg/mL in 1-mL prefilled syringes; 65 mg/mL in 1-mL vials; 130 mg/mL in 1-mL prefilled syringes, 1-mL vials, and 1-mL ampules
Adverse Reactions and Side Effects
Resp: Respiratory depression, LARYNGOSPASM, bronchospasm
CV: Hypotension
CNS: Hangover, delirium, depression, drowsiness, excitation, vertigo
GI: Constipation, diarrhea, nausea, vomiting
Derm: Photosensitivity, rashes, urticaria
Misc: Hypersensitivity reactions including ANGIOEDEMA and SERUM SICKNESS
Drug Interactions: Additive CNS depression if used with other CNS depressants
EMS Considerations: Monitor respiratory status, pulse, and blood pressure frequently. Equipment for resuscitation should be readily

available. Geriatric patients may react to phenobarbital with marked excitement, depression, and confusion.

Phenytoin (FEN-i-toyn)

Dilantin, Phenytek

Classification: Anticonvulsant

Pregnancy Class: D

Mechanism of Action: Limits seizure activity by altering ion transmission; may also decrease synaptic transmission

Pharmacokinetics

Absorption: Absorbed slowly from the GI tract

Onset: 0.5 to 1 hour

Duration: 12 to 24 hours

Indications: Used in the treatment and prevention of grand mal seizures and complex partial seizures

Contraindications: Known hypersensitivity; should not be given to patients with alcohol intolerance, to patients with sinus bradycardia or high-degree AV heart block, or to patients with Stokes-Adams syndrome

Precautions: Use with caution in patients with liver or renal disease or in patients with severe cardiac or respiratory disease. Phenytoin increases the risk of suicidal thoughts and behaviors in all patients.

Route and Dosage

IV (Adult): Loading dose of 15 to 20 mg/kg at a rate not to exceed 25 to 50 mg/minute

IV (Pediatric): Loading dose of 15 to 20 mg/kg at 1 to 3 mg/kg/minute

effective Communication

IM administration of phenytoin is not recommended due to the erratic absorption and pain on injection. IV administration should occur in a large vein, if possible. Avoid using veins in the patient's hands.

Check the **Evidence**

NS is the fluid of choice when giving phenytoin. If phenytoin comes in contact with dextrose, a precipitate will form.

How Supplied

Injection: 50 mg/mL

Adverse Reactions and Side Effects

CV: Hypotension, tachycardia

CNS: SUICIDAL THOUGHTS, ataxia, agitation, confusion, dizziness, drowsiness, headache, insomnia, weakness

EENT: Diplopia, nystagmus

Misc: Hypersensitivity reactions including STEVENS-JOHNSON SYNDROME, fever

Drug Interactions: Additive CNS depression if used with other CNS depressant drugs

EMS Considerations: Slow administration of phenytoin helps prevent toxicity. Elderly patients may develop toxic effects more rapidly than younger patients.

SCENARIO REVISITED

Do you recall the case of Norman who is experiencing status epilepticus?

Patients experiencing status epilepticus are very difficult to manage. This can easily become a life-threatening emergency, so rapid treatment is essential.

Maintain Norman's airway with the administration of high-flow humidified oxygen. Assist ventilations if necessary and monitor cardiac function. It may be difficult to keep the ECG leads attached or to record an accurate strip because of the seizure activity. If possible, establish an IV of normal saline. Normal saline is the fluid of choice in case phenytoin is administered. Phenytoin is not compatible with dextrose because a precipitate forms when phenytoin comes in contact with dextrose. Phenytoin causes an increase in the transport of sodium out of motor cortex cell neurons to limit cell depolarization, thus preventing the spread of seizure activity. The suggested route and dosage of phenytoin is 15 to 20 mg/kg by slow IV bolus.

Let's Recap

The neurological emergencies presented in this chapter are frequently encountered in the out-of-hospital setting. In cases of acute head injury, EMS protocols may include the administration of mannitol in reducing cerebral edema. However, medication therapy is secondary to cervical spine stabilization and airway management with the use of supplemental oxygen.

It is common for EMS professionals to respond to patients experiencing possible stroke or seizure activity. Symptoms of seizure activity may vary from alterations in consciousness to tonic-clonic convulsions of the entire body. Stroke involves the disruption of blood flow within the brain. The signs and symptoms of stroke are subtle and often go unrecognized. Immediate recognition of a stroke and initiation of treatment can reduce the amount of disability and death.

Drug therapy used for neurological emergencies plays a secondary role to initial stabilization, rapid transport, detailed assessment of patients, and early notification of the receiving facility.

SCENARIO CONCLUSION

Once an IV has been established, medical control orders diazepam as the drug of choice for Norman. Diazepam is a CNS depressant with anticonvulsant properties. The suggested route and dosage for diazepam in this case is 5 to 10 mg by slow IV bolus initially, repeated if necessary, but not to exceed a total dose of 30 mg.

Status epilepticus is a true emergency. Rapid transport to the nearest appropriate facility is essential.

PRACTICE EXERCISES

1. A contraindication for the use of phenytoin is:
a. Headache
b. Heart block
c. Elderly patients
d. Respiratory problems

2. All of the following are possible life-threatening adverse reactions to aspirin, *except*:
a. GI bleeding
b. Hepatotoxicity
c. Laryngeal edema
d. Stevens-Johnson syndrome

3. A contraindication for the use of alteplase is:
a. History of stroke
b. Severe liver disease
c. Severe renal disease
d. Recent GI or GU bleeding

4. The initial recommended adult dosage of diazepam for a patient experiencing status epilepticus is:
a. 2 to 5 mg by slow IV bolus
b. 5 to 10 mg by slow IV bolus
c. 10 to 20 mg by slow IV bolus
d. 20 to 30 mg by slow IV bolus

5. You are ordered to administer 15 mg PE/kg of fosphenytoin to your 235-pound patient. How many mg should you administer?
a. 1,505 mg
b. 1,550 mg
c. 1,605 mg
d. 1,650 mg

6. A contraindication and possible life-threatening adverse reaction of labetalol is:
a. Bradycardia
b. Hypoglycemia
c. Diabetes mellitus
d. Pulmonary disease

7. A frequent CNS side effect of lorazepam is:
a. Dizziness
b. Headache
c. Confusion
d. Slurred speech

8. Mannitol has a pregnancy class of:
a. B
b. C
c. D
d. X

9. The average adult dose of midazolam is:
a. 5 mg
b. 10 mg
c. 15 mg
d. 20 mg

10. Nitroprusside is contraindicated in patients with:
a. Liver disease
b. Renal disease
c. Hypothyroidism
d. Decreased cerebral perfusion

CASE STUDIES

1. You respond to the home of a woman "unable to walk and speak." On arrival, you find a 70-year-old woman sitting in a chair at the kitchen table. She is conscious, and her eyes follow movements in the room, which indicate she is aware of her surroundings. However, she cannot stand to walk, and she cannot speak. The initial assessment reveals the following:
Level of consciousness: Conscious, appears aware of surroundings, but unable to communicate
Respirations: 16 breaths/minute
Pulse: 90 beats/minute, irregular. ECG shows atrial fibrillation (Fig.14-4).
Blood pressure: 152/112 mm Hg
Skin: Normal
HEENT: Pupils equal and reactive, slight drooling
Paralysis: Affecting only the left side of her body

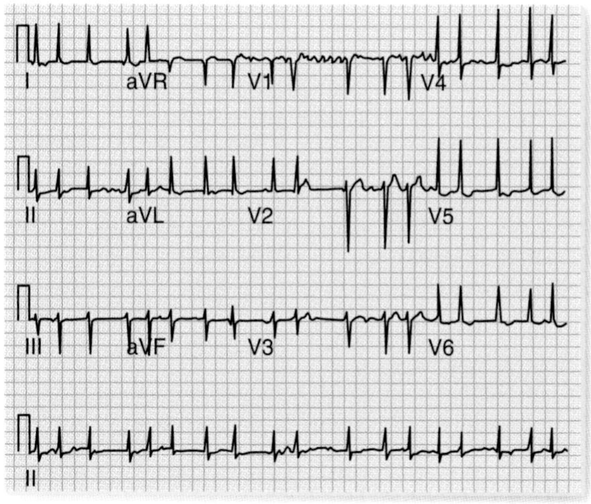

Figure 14-4 Atrial fibrillation.

The patient's husband states that his wife is currently being treated for high blood pressure, and she has a history of heart disease. His wife appeared normal about 1 hour ago. Immediate treatment for this patient should include:

- IV line, rapid transport
- Humidified oxygen, rapid transport
- IV line, verapamil bolus, rapid transport
- Humidified oxygen, precautionary IV line, rapid transport

2. You respond to an alley where you find a man, approximately 50 years old, passed out. There are several beer cans and wine bottles in the area. There is no indication that trauma is a factor. Your assessment reveals the following:
Level of consciousness: Unconscious, responds to pain
Respirations: 20 breaths/minute, no respiratory difficulty, breath smells of alcohol
Pulse: 50 beats/minute, irregular. ECG monitor shows a second-degree heart block, type 2 (Fig. 14-5).
Blood pressure: 196/94 mm Hg
Skin: Cool, clammy

You start an IV of normal saline. As soon as the IV is established, the patient begins to experience seizure activity. The drug of choice to control his seizure activity is:
a. Phenytoin
b. Diazepam
c. Lorazepam
d. Midazolam

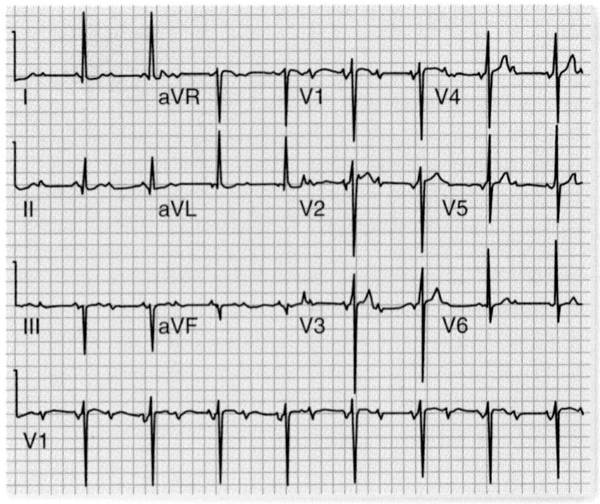

Figure 14-5 Second-degree heart block type 2.

MATH EQUATIONS

1. You have been ordered to give 0.3 mg/kg of labetalol to your 45 lb pediatric patient.
   a. How many kg does your patient weigh?
   b. How many mg of the labetalol will you administer?
2. You are ordered to give 0.05 mg/kg of lorazepam to your 270 lb patient. You are not to exceed 4 mg.
   a. How many kg does your patient weigh?
   b. How many mg of the lorazepam will you administer?
3. You are ordered to infuse 0.3 mcg/kg/minute of nitroprusside to your 160 lb patient. You have dissolved 50 mg of nigroprusside in 250 mL of IV solution.
   a. How many kg does your patient weigh?
   b. What is the concentration of the IV solution (mcg/mL)?
   c. What is the drip rate of your infusion using a 60 gtt IV set?
4. You are ordered to give 340 mg of ASA to your 75 lb pediatric patient. You have aspirin tablets at 81 mg each. How many aspirin tablets will you give this patient?

REFERENCES

Beck, R. K. (2012). Drugs used to treat neurologic emergencies. In *Pharmacology for the EMS Provider.* New York, NY: Delmar, Cengage Learning.
Deglin, J. H., Vallerand, A. H., and Sanboski, C.A. (2011). *Davis's drug guide for nurses* (12th ed.). Philadelphia, PA: F. A. Davis Company.
Drugs.com. (2014). Fosphenytoin dosage. Retrieved February 8, 2014 from www.drugs.com/dosage/fosphenytoin.html.
Food and Drug Administration. (2011). Parenteral Dilantin® (Phenytoin sodium injection, USP). Retrieved February 17, 2014 from http://www.accessdata.fda.gov/drugsatfda_docs/label/2011/010151s036lbl.pdf
Johns Hopkins Medicine. (2014). Causes of a seizure. Retrieved February 8, 2014 from www.hopkinsmedicine.org/neurology_neurosurgery/specialty_areas/epilepsy/seizures/causes
Mistovich, J. J., Krost, W. S., and Limmer, D. L., for *EMS World.* (2006). Prehospital assessment and care of the stroke patient. Retrieved February 8, 2014 from www.emsworld.com/article/10323034/prehospital-assessment-and-care-of-the-stroke-patient
National Institute of Neurological Disorders and Stroke. (2013). NINDS traumatic brain injury information page. Retrieved February 1, 2014 from www.ninds.nih.gov/disorders/tbi/tbi.htm
National Stroke Association. (2014). Types of stroke. Retrieved February 3, 2014 from www.stroke.org/site/PageServer?pagename=type
Venes, D., ed. (2013). *Taber's cyclopedic medical dictionary* (22nd ed.). Philadelphia, PA: F. A. Davis Company.
WebMD, LLC. (2011). Epilepsy Health Center: Seizures: topic overview. Retrieved January 29, 2014 from www.webmd.com/epilepsy/tc/seizures-topic-overview

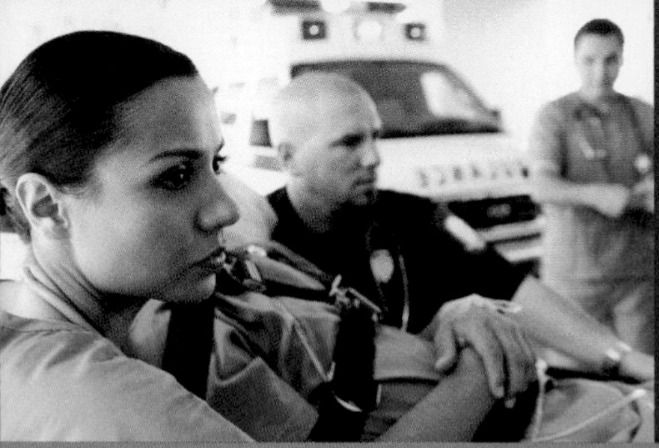

CHAPTER 15

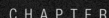

Drugs Used to Treat Gastrointestinal Emergencies

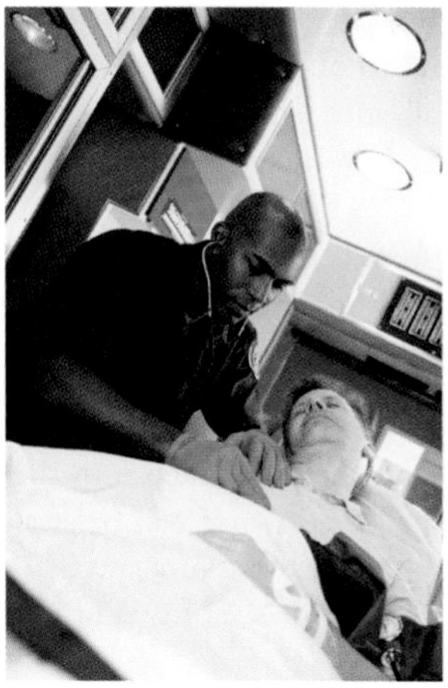

Paramedics performing an abdominal assessment. *(Photograph © Monkey Business Images/Monkey Business/Thinkstock)*

LEARNING OUTCOMES

- List and briefly describe the components of the alimentary canal within the gastrointestinal (GI) system.
- List and briefly describe the accessory organs within the GI system.
- Discuss the antidote activated charcoal as it relates to GI emergencies.
- Describe the use of the anticholinergic hydroxyzine for GI emergencies.
- Discuss the antiemetics dolasetron, metoclopramide, ondansetron, prochlorperazine, and promethazine for GI emergencies.

KEY TERMS

Adsorbent, antidote
Anticholinergic
Antiemetic
Antihistamine
Chemoreceptor trigger zone (CTZ)
Neuroleptic malignant syndrome

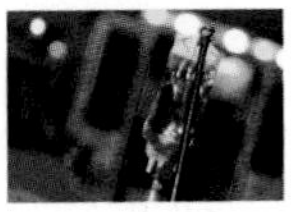

SCENARIO OPENING

As you study this chapter, consider this scenario for Ms. Odessa Owens.

You and your partner respond to a 23-year-old female complaining of vomiting approximately every 2 hours for the past 24 hours. Upon questioning, Ms. Owens reveals that she is 6 weeks pregnant. Physical examination reveals the following:

Level of consciousness:	alert and oriented
Respirations:	24/minute
Blood pressure:	110/70 mm Hg
Pulse:	regular with a rate of approximately 110 beats/minute (Fig. 15-1)
Skin:	dry, poor turgor

Further questioning about Ms. Owen's medical history reveals that she has a history of seizures.

You and your partner should think about the following:

1. What do you think the diagnosis will be for Ms. Owens?
2. What are the goals of your treatment?
3. What steps will you take to help Ms. Owens?
4. What is your rationale for choosing your treatment options for Ms. Owens?
5. How will you know if the treatment choices are working?

effective Communication

These five questions are a few suggestions for you and your partner. You may have other relevant questions as well. Also, priorities within this scenario must be established. For example, dehydration, pregnancy, and seizure history must be prioritized while treatment goals are established. To assist in the establishment of your priorities and treatment options, attempt to establish communication with any family members, friends, or anyone else who may be of assistance. Remember to continue communicating with the patient throughout treatment.

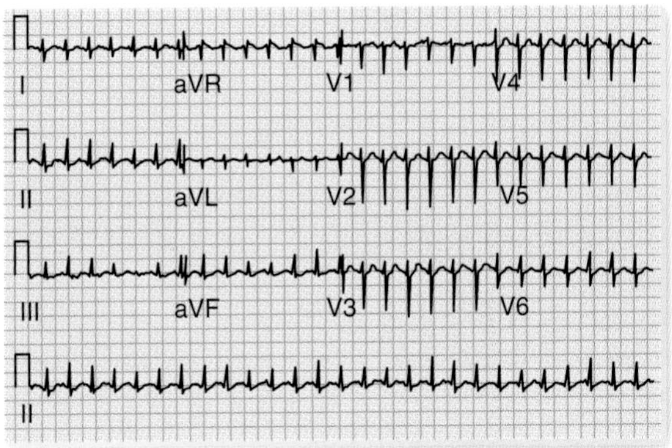

Figure 15-1 Sinus tachycardia (110 beats/minute).

Introduction

There are many gastrointestinal (GI) emergencies that may be encountered in the EMS out-of-hospital setting. These may include traumatic injuries and nontraumatic illnesses. Traumatic GI injuries may include blunt or penetrating trauma. The primary responsibility of EMS professionals in traumatic GI emergencies is stabilization and rapid transport to the appropriate health-care facility.

The majority of nontraumatic GI emergencies (such as aortic aneurysm, GI bleeding, appendicitis, peptic ulcer, pancreatitis, and peritonitis) are managed in the out-of-hospital setting with stabilization and transport to the appropriate health-care facility. Few GI emergencies require drug therapy in the out-of-hospital setting. Drug therapy discussed in this chapter is for the management of nausea and vomiting caused by a variety of conditions.

Pathophysiology of the Gastrointestinal System

The GI system (also called the digestive system) consists of the alimentary canal (mouth or oral cavity, pharynx, esophagus, stomach, small intestine, and large intestine) and the accessory organs (teeth, tongue, salivary glands, liver, and pancreas (Fig. 15-2).

The digestive system is the process by which food is broken down in the GI tract and converted into absorbable forms. It is responsible for taking foods and turning them into nutrients and energy. There are six primary processes in digestion:

1. **Ingestion of food:** Food is taken into the mouth and chewed into small pieces so it can be swallowed down into the stomach.

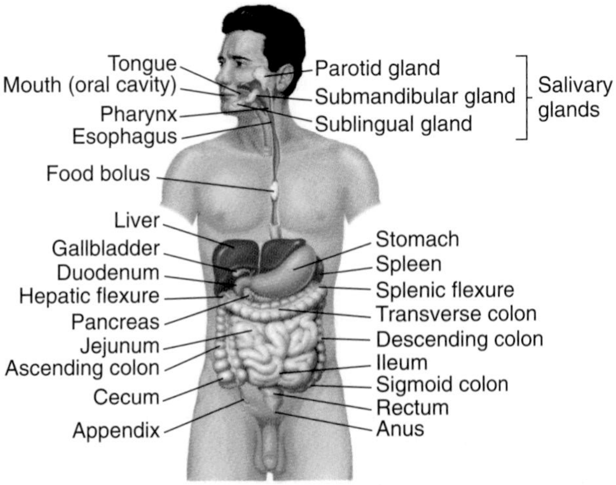

Figure 15-2 The digestive system. *(From: Venes, D., ed. (2013).* Taber's cyclopedic medical dictionary. *Philadelphia, PA: F.A. Davis Company.)*

2. **Secretion of fluids and digestive enzymes:** The GI system secretes saliva, mucus, hydrochloric acid, enzymes, and bile.
3. **The movement of food and wastes throughout the body:** The GI system uses the following three processes for food movement.
   - *Swallowing*: Muscles of the mouth, tongue, and pharynx are used to push food out of the mouth, into the esophagus, and down to the stomach.
   - *Peristalsis*: This is a muscular wave that travels the length of the GI tract.
   - *Segmentation*: The small intestine contracts to help the absorption of nutrients.
4. **Digestion of food:** This is the process of turning large pieces of food into its component chemicals. Digestion begins in the mouth with the saliva.
5. **Absorption of nutrients:** Once food has been reduced to its nutrients, it becomes absorbed by the body.
6. **Excretion of wastes:** Indigestible substances are then removed from the body.

Pharmacokinetics

Anticholinergics

Anticholinergic medications block the neurotransmitter acetylcholine in the nervous system, inhibiting parasympathetic nerve impulses. Selected nerve fibers of the parasympathetic nervous system are responsible for the involuntary movement of smooth muscle in the GI tract. Anticholinergics can reduce the amount of stomach acid and slow movement in the bowel. Some anticholinergics are used to prevent nausea and vomiting and also to prevent motion sickness.

Antihistamines

Antihistamine medications block the effects of histamine at the H_2 receptor site. Most antihistamines also have anticholinergic properties, making some of these drugs effective in preventing nausea and vomiting, as well as treating motion sickness.

Antiemetics

Antiemetic medications are used to manage nausea and vomiting. They act on the Chemoreceptor trigger zone (CTZ) to inhibit nausea and vomiting. The CTZ is an area of the brain that receives input from blood-borne drugs or hormones and communicates with the vomiting center to inhibit vomiting.

Individual Drugs

Activated Charcoal (CHAR-kole)

Acta-Char Liquid-A, Actidose-Aqua, 🍁 Charac-50, CharcoAid 2,000, 🍁 Aqueous Charcodote, Insta-Char, Insta-Char Aqueous Suspension, Liqui-Char, SuperChar Aqueous

Classifications: **Antidote—**A substance that neutralizes poisons or their effects; **adsorbent—**a substance that draws other substances out of solution.

Pregnancy Class: C

Mechanism of Action: Adsorbs toxic substances or irritants, inhibiting GI absorption. Sorbitol is added to some formulations to cause hyperosmotic laxative action and promote elimination of the toxic substance.

Pharmacokinetics

Absorption: well absorbed (90 percent)
Onset: immediate
Duration: continual while in the GI tract

Indications: May be considered if a patient has ingested a potentially toxic amount of a poison up to 1 hour previously, following emesis or lavage

Contraindications: Known hypersensitivity. Activated charcoal is contraindicated in patients who do not have an intact or protected airway. Otherwise, there are no known contraindications.

Precautions: Activated charcoal may cause vomiting, which is hazardous in petroleum distillate and caustic ingestions. Therefore, use with caution in poisonings due to cyanide, corrosives, ethanol, methanol, petroleum distillates, organic solvents, mineral acids, or iron.

Route and Dosage

Adult: PO or NG tube, 25 to 100 g (may be repeated every 4 to 6 hours)

Pediatric (under 1 year): PO or NG tube, 1 g/kg (may be repeated every 4 to 6 hours)

Pediatric (1 to 12 years): PO or NG tube, 25 to 50 g (may be repeated every 4 to 6 hours)

How Supplied

25 g/125 mL bottle (200 mg/mL)
50 g/240 mL bottle (200 mg/mL)
Most products come premixed with water or with sorbitol.

Adverse Reactions and Side Effects

GI: Black stools, constipation, diarrhea, vomiting

Drug Interactions: Do not administer with syrup of ipecac. Milk, ice cream, or sherbet will decrease the ability of activated charcoal to adsorb other agents.

EMS Considerations: Activated charcoal binds with syrup of ipecac, rendering it ineffective.

Check the Evidence

There are studies suggesting that there is no evidence that the administration of activated charcoal improves clinical outcome. Activated charcoal is considered a less commonly used drug.

Dolasetron (dol-A-se-tron)

Anzemet

Classification: **Antiemetic—**A drug that is used to manage nausea and vomiting.

Pregnancy Class: B

Mechanism of Action: Blocks the effects of serotonin at the receptor sites located in the vagal nerve terminals and in the CTZ in the central nervous system (CNS)

Underline indicates most frequent; CAPITALS indicate lifethreatening; 🍁 indicates Canadian drug name.

Pharmacokinetics

Absorption: Well absorbed but rapidly metabolized
Onset: Unknown for both PO and IV
Duration: Up to 24 hours

Indications: Used in the prevention of nausea and vomiting
Contraindications: Known hypersensitivity
Precautions: Use with caution in patients with risk factors for prolongation of cardiac conduction intervals. Safe use during pregnancy or lactation has not been established.

Route and Dosage
PO (Adults): 100 mg
PO (Pediatric 2 to 16 years): 1.2 mg/kg, up to 100 mg
IV (Adults): 12.5 mg
IV (Pediatric 2 to 16 years): 0.35 mg/kg, up to 12.5 mg

How Supplied
Tablets: 50 mg, 100 mg
Injection: 12.5 mg/0.625 mL ampules, 20 mg/mL in 5 mL vials

Adverse Reactions and Side Effects
CNS: <u>Headache</u>, dizziness, fatigue, syncope
CV: Bradycardia, ECG changes, hyper- or hypotension, tachycardia
GI: Diarrhea
Miscellaneous: Chills, fever, pain
Drug Interactions: An increased risk of conduction abnormalities may occur when concurrently used with diuretic or antiarrhythmic therapy.
EMS Considerations: Vital signs should be monitored closely after administration. IV administration may be followed by severe hypotension, bradycardia, and syncope.

effective **Communication**

Make sure that you document the ECG for any indication of prolongation of cardiac conduction.

Hydroxyzine (hy-DROX-ih-zeen)

🍁 Apo-Hydroxyzine, Atarax, Hyzine-50, 🍁 Multipax, 🍁 Novo-Hydroxyzin, Vistaril

Classifications: **Anticholinergic—**A drug that blocks parasympathetic nerve impulses; antiemetic; **antihistamine—**a drug that opposes the effects of histamine.
Pregnancy Class: C
Mechanism of Action: Has anticholinergic, antihistamine, and antiemetic properties; acts as a CNS depressant
Pharmacokinetics

Absorption: Well absorbed
Onset: PO, IM—15 to 30 minutes
Duration: PO, IM—4 to 6 hours

Indications: Can be used for the treatment of anxiety and to decrease nausea and vomiting
Contraindications: Known hypersensitivity; potential for congenital defects; safety not established in lactation
Precautions: Dosage reduction is recommended in elderly patients because of increased susceptibility to adverse effects. Use with caution in patients with severe liver disease.

Route and Dosage
IM (Adult): 25 to 100 mg every 6 hours as needed
IM (Pediatric): 0.5 to 1 mg/kg/dose every 6 hours as needed

How Supplied
Tablets: 10 mg, 25 mg, 50 mg, 100 mg
Capsules: 🍁 10 mg, 25 mg, 50 mg, 100 mg
Syrup: 10 mg/5 mL
Oral suspension: 25 mg/5 mL
Injection: 25 mg/mL, 50 mg/mL

Adverse Reactions and Side Effects
Respiratory: Wheezing
CNS: <u>Drowsiness</u>, agitation, ataxia, dizziness, headache, weakness
GI: <u>Dry mouth</u>, bitter taste, constipation, nausea
GU: Urinary retention
Derm: Flushing
Local: <u>Pain</u> at IM site, abscesses at IM site
Drug Interactions: Additive CNS depression when used with other CNS depressants; additive anticholinergic effects when used with other drugs having anticholinergic properties
EMS Considerations: Hydroxyzine should not be administered via IV in the out-of-hospital setting.

Understand the Numbers

The physician orders you to administer 1 mg/kg of hydroxyzine to your 68-pound pediatric patient. How many milligrams will you give?
68 lbs ÷ 2.2 kg = 30.9 kg or 31 kg
You will administer 31 mg of hydroxyzine to your patient.

Metoclopramide (met-oh-KLOE-pra-mide)

🍁 Apo-Metoclop, 🍁 Emex, 🍁 Maxeran, Metozolv ODT, Reglan

Classification: Antiemetic
Pregnancy Class: B
Mechanism of Action: Blocks dopamine receptors in the CTZ of the CNS; stimulates motility of the upper GI tract
Pharmacokinetics

Absorption: Well absorbed from the GI tract
Onset: PO—30 to 60 min.
IM—10 to 15 min.
IV—1 to 3 min.
Duration: PO, IM, IV—1 to 2 hours

Indications: Used for the prevention of nausea and vomiting
Contraindications: Known hypersensitivity; possible GI obstruction or hemorrhage; history of seizures, pheochromocytoma, or Parkinson disease
Precautions: Use with caution in patients with a history of depression, diabetes, and kidney impairment.

Route and Dosage
IM, IV (Adults and Pediatric over 14 years): 10 mg; may be repeated in 6 to 8 hours
IM, IV (Pediatric under 14 years): 0.1 to 0.2 mg/kg/dose; may be repeated in 6 to 8 hours

How Supplied
Injection: 5 mg/mL
Adverse Reactions and Side Effects
CV: Arrhythmias (SVT, bradycardia), hyper- or hypotension
CNS: Drowsiness, extrapyramidal reactions, restlessness, NEUROLEPTIC MALIGNANT SYNDROME (a potentially fatal syndrome marked by hyperthermia), anxiety, depression, irritability, tardive dyskinesia
GI: Constipation, diarrhea, dry mouth, nausea
Drug Interactions: Additive CNS depression when used with other CNS depressants. Use cautiously with MAO inhibitors, due to the release of catecholamines.
EMS Considerations: None

Ondansetron (on-DAN-se-tron)

Zofran, Zofran ODT
Classification: Antiemetic
Pregnancy Class: B
Mechanism of Action: Blocks the effects of serotonin located in the CTZ in the CNS.
Pharmacokinetics
Absorption: 100 percent
Onset: PO, IV—15 to 30 minutes
IM—40 minutes
Duration: PO, IV—4 to 8 hours
IM—unknown
Indications: Prevention of nausea and vomiting
Contraindications: Known hypersensitivity
Precautions: Use with caution in patients with liver impairment.
Route and Dosage
PO (Adults and Pediatric over 11 years): 8 mg
PO (Pediatric 4 to 11 years): 4 mg
IV (Adults): 0.15 mg/kg
IM (Adults): 4 mg
IV (Pediatric 6 months–18 years): 0.15 mg/kg
Liver Impairment: PO, IM, IV (Adults): not to exceed 8 mg
How Supplied
Oral disintegrating tablets: 4 mg, 8 mg
Oral tablets: 4 mg, 8 mg, 24 mg
Oral solution: 4 mg/5 mL
Solution for injection: 2 mg/mL
Premixed infusion: 32 mg/50 mL D5W
Adverse Reactions and Side Effects
CNS: Headache, dizziness, drowsiness, fatigue, weakness
GI: Constipation, diarrhea, abdominal pain, dry mouth, increased liver enzymes
Drug Interactions: May be affected by drugs that alter the activity of liver enzymes
EMS Considerations: For orally disintegrating tablets, do not attempt to push through foil backing. Use dry hands to peel back and remove tablet. Then, immediately place the tablet under the patient's tongue; it will dissolve in seconds. Then the patient should swallow with saliva. The administration of liquid is not necessary.

Check the Evidence

Studies have concluded that ondansetron is safe and effective for out-of-hospital treatment of nausea and vomiting when administered by paramedics via the IV, IM, or the oral route. When available to paramedics, ondansetron is used frequently.

Prochlorperazine (proe-klor-PAIR-a-zeen)

Compazine, Compro, ✦ Stemetil
Classification: Antiemetic
Pregnancy Class: C
Mechanism of Action: Depresses the CTZ in the CNS
Pharmacokinetics
Absorption: PO absorption is variable; well absorbed after IM administration
Onset: PO—30 to 40 minutes
Rectal—60 minutes
IM—10 to 20 minutes
IV—rapid
Duration: PO, Rectal, IM, IV—3 to 4 hours
Indication: Management of nausea and vomiting
Contraindications: Known hypersensitivity; severe cardiovascular or liver disease; hypersensitivity to bisulfites or benzyl alcohol
Precautions: Use with caution in patients with respiratory disease, diabetes mellitus, benign prostatic hypertrophy (BPH), and epilepsy.
Route and Dosage
PO (Adults and Pediatric over 12 years): 5 to 10 mg 3 to 4 times daily. Do not exceed 40 mg/day.
IM (Adults and Pediatric over 12 years): 5 to 10 mg every 3 to 4 hours as needed
IV (Adults and Pediatric over 12 years): 2.5 to 10 mg. Do not exceed 40 mg/day.
Rectal (Adults): 25 mg twice daily
How Supplied
Tablets: 5 mg, 10 mg
Syrup: ✦ 5 mg/5mL
Solution for injection: 5 mg/mL; ✦ 5 mg/mL
Suppositories: 25 mg
Adverse Reactions and Side Effects
CV: ECG changes, hypotension, tachycardia
CNS: NEUROLEPTIC MALIGNANT SYNDROME, extrapyramidal reactions, sedation, tardive dyskinesia
EENT: Blurred vision, dry eyes
GI: Constipation, dry mouth, anorexia
GU: Pink or reddish-brown urine, urinary retention
Dermatological: Photosensitivity, pigment changes, rashes
Drug Interactions: Additive hypotension when used with antihypertensives, nitrates, or acute ingestion of alcohol; additive CNS depression when used with other CNS depressants
EMS Considerations: None

Promethazine (proe-METH-a-zeen)

🍁 Histantil, Phenergan, Promethacon

Classifications: Antiemetic, antihistamine

Pregnancy Class: C

Mechanism of Action: Has inhibitory effect on the CTZ in the brain; blocks the effects of histamine

Pharmacokinetics

Absorption: Well absorbed after PO and IM administration. Rectal administration is less reliable.

Onset: PO, IM, Rectal—20 minutes

IV—3 to 5 minutes

Duration: PO, IM, Rectal, IV—4 to 12 hours

Indications: Treatment and prevention of nausea and vomiting

Contraindications: Known hypersensitivity; should not be given to patients with BPH or angle-closure glaucoma or to those who are comatose

Precautions: Use with caution in patients with hypertension, cardiovascular disease, impaired liver function, BPH, or asthma. IV administration may cause severe tissue injury.

Route and Dosage

PO (Adults): 25 mg

Rectal, IM, IV (Adults): 12.5 to 25 mg

PO, Rectal, IM, IV (Pediatric over 2 years): 0.25 to 1 mg/kg, not to exceed 25 mg

How Supplied

Tablets: 12.5 mg, 25 mg, 🍁 25 mg(OTC), 50 mg, 🍁 50 mg(OTC)

Syrup: 6.25 mg/5 mL, 🍁 10 mg/5 mL(OTC)

Injection: 25 mg/mL, 50 mg/mL

Suppositories: 12.5 mg, 25 mg, 50 mg

Adverse Reactions and Side Effects

CV: Bradycardia, hyper- or hypotension, tachycardia

CNS: NEUROLEPTIC MALIGNANT SYNDROME, confusion, disorientation, sedation, dizziness, extrapyramidal reactions, fatigue, insomnia, nervousness

EENT: Blurred vision, diplopia, tinnitus

GI: Constipation, dry mouth

Derm: Photosensitivity, severe tissue necrosis upon infiltration at IV site, rashes

Drug Interactions: Additive CNS depression when used with other CNS depressants; neuroleptic malignant syndrome can occur when used concurrently with antipsychotics; additive anticholinergic effects when used with other drugs containing anticholinergic properties

EMS Considerations: Do not administer to pediatric patients less than 2 years of age.

effective Communication

During your patient assessment, make sure that you ask about BPH and narrow-angle glaucoma to prevent adverse reactions.

SCENARIO REVISITED

Did you consider the case of Odessa Owen? As you recall, your patient is 23 years old, has been vomiting every 2 hours for the past 24 hours, and is 6 weeks pregnant. Once a thorough assessment has been completed and a treatment protocol has been decided, you should proceed using a critical thinking approach to medication administration.

Step 1: Determine signs and symptoms to be treated.

Step 2: Consider both the risks and benefits of treating or not treating your patient.

Step 3: Choose the medication that provides the best possible outcome.

Step 4: Remember the drug's indications, contraindications, and precautions.

Step 5: Decide the best route for administering the medication for the best outcome.

Step 6: Administer the medication(s) according to the Seven Patient Rights.

1. The right patient
2. The right drug
3. The right drug amount
4. The right time
5. The right route
6. The right documentation
7. The right of the patient to accept or refuse the medication(s)

Step 7: Reevaluate the patient for the desired and undesired effects.

Let's Recap

Very few GI emergencies require medications in the out-of-hospital setting. Most of the GI emergencies require paramedics to provide supportive care, manage possible life threats, and transport the patient to an appropriate health-care facility. However, EMS professionals should be familiar with the drugs necessary to treat patients who are experiencing severe nausea and vomiting or who may require the emergency adsorbent activated charcoal. This chapter has presented the common drugs used by EMS professionals for these conditions.

SCENARIO CONCLUSION

Ms. Owens appears to be dehydrated because of excessive vomiting over a prolonged time period and due to the lack of oral intake. The initial management for Ms. Owens should include initiation of IV access with the administration of normal saline to provide rehydration. An antiemetic should be administered to prevent further vomiting and loss of fluids. The most appropriate antiemetic to administer is ondansetron at a dose of 4 mg by IM or IV.

Underline indicates most frequent; CAPITALS indicate lifethreatening; 🍁 indicates Canadian drug name.

Understand the Numbers
Ondansetron comes in a 2 mg/mL solution for injection. Therefore, you will give 2 mL to achieve a 4 mg dose.

Ondansetron has a pregnancy classification of B. Although safety has not been fully established in pregnancy, ondansetron has been used safely in pregnant patients. Other antiemetics are not indicated for Ms. Owens. For example, hydroxyzine is contraindicated during pregnancy, metoclopramide is contraindicated in patients with a history of seizures, and both prochlorperazine and promethazine are to be used with caution in patients with a history of seizures.

PRACTICE EXERCISES

1. Activated charcoal should not be administered for which of the following ingestions?
   a. Aspirin
   b. Gasoline
   c. Phenobarbital
   d. Acetaminophen
2. You receive an order for ondansetron at 0.15 mg/kg to be administered intravenously. Your patient weighs 150 pounds. You determine the dosage of ondansetron to be:
   a. 4 mg
   b. 8 mg
   c. 10.2 mg
   d. 22.5 mg
3. Ondansetron should be used cautiously in patients with:
   a. Kidney impairment
   b. Liver impairment
   c. Nausea
   d. CHF
4. Hydroxyzine is contraindicated in patients with:
   a. Kidney dysfunction
   b. Liver dysfunction
   c. Pregnancy
   d. CHF
5. The most frequent CNS side effect for hydroxyzine is:
   a. Headache
   b. Dizziness
   c. Agitation
   d. Drowsiness
6. Promethazine should not be given to patients with:
   a. Angle-closure glaucoma
   b. A history of seizures
   c. Hypertension
   d. Asthma
7. Your patient is 8 years old, and you are ordered to give her promethazine at 0.25 mg/kg, not to exceed:
   a. 10 mg
   b. 15 mg
   c. 20 mg
   d. 25 mg
8. A possible life-threatening side effect of prochlorperazine is:
   a. Neuroleptic malignant syndrome
   b. Tardive dyskinesia
   c. Photosensitivity
   d. Tachycardia
9. A contraindication for the use of metoclopramide is:
   a. History of depression
   b. History of seizures
   c. Kidney impairment
   d. Diabetes mellitus
10. The common initial adult IM dose of metoclopramide is:
    a. 10 mg
    b. 15 mg
    c. 20 mg
    d. 25 mg

CASE STUDIES

1. You and your partner respond to an overdose of acetaminophen. Your patient is a 29-year-old male who ingested a bottle of acetaminophen approximately 15 minutes prior to his wife calling 911. He is fully conscious. After your assessment, what is the appropriate action to take?
   a. Administer syrup of ipecac, 30 mL PO followed by 240 mL of water to cause vomiting.
   b. Administer activated charcoal to adsorb the acetaminophen.
   c. Administer promethazine, 12.5 mg IM to prevent vomiting.
   d. Administer ondansetron, 8 mg IV to prevent vomiting.
2. En route to the hospital, your patient has vomited several times, and you believe the contents of his stomach appear to be emptied. The most appropriate action to take at this time is to administer:
   a. A second dose of syrup of ipecac
   b. A second dose of activated charcoal
   c. Promethazine
   d. Ondansetron

MATH EQUATIONS

1. You have been ordered to give 0.35 mg/kg of dolasetron to your 55-lb pediatric patient. The maximum dosage for dolasetron is 12.5 mg.
   a. How many kg does your patient weigh?
   b. How many mg will you administer to your patient?
2. You are ordered to give 10 mg of metoclopramide to your 150-lb patient. The total dose should not exceed 0.5 mg/kg in a day.
   a. How many kg does your patient weigh?
   b. How many mg will you administer to your patient?
3. You are ordered to give 0.15 mg/kg of ondansetron to your 185-lb patient. The maximum dose for ondansetron is 16 mg.
   a. How many kg does your patient weigh?
   b. How many mg will you give to your patient?
4. You are ordered to give 12.5 mg IV of promethazine to your patient. You have 50 mg in 2 mL. How much of the promethazine (mL) will you administer?
5. You are ordered to give 0.1 mg/kg of metoclopramide to your 10-lb pediatric patient, preceded by 1.25 mg/kg of diphenhydramine.
   a. How many kg does your patient weigh?
   b. How many mg of the diphenhydramine will you administer?
   c. How many mg of the metoclopramide will you administer?

REFERENCES

Beck, R. K. (2012). Drugs used to treat gastrointestinal emergencies. In *Pharmacology for the EMS provider.* New York: Delmar, Cengage Learning.

Bhargava, K. P., and Dixit, K. S. (1968). Role of chemoreceptor trigger zone in histamine-induced emesis. *British Journal of Pharmacology, 34*(3), 508–518.

Chyka, P. A., Seger, D., Krenzelok, E. P., and Vale, J. A., for the American Academy of Clinical Toxicology; European Association of Poisons Centres and Clinical Toxicologists. (2005). Position paper: Single-dose activated charcoal. *Clinical Toxicology (Philadelphia), 43*(2), 61–87.

Deglin, J. H., Vallerand, A. H., and Sanboski, C. A. (2011). *Davis's drug guide for nurses* (12th ed.). Philadelphia, PA: F.A. Davis Company.

Olsen, K. R. Activated charcoal for acute poisoning. Retrieved September 12, 2013 from http://www.asiatox.org/9th%20apamt/OP/ACTIVATED%20CHARCOAL%20FOR%20ACUTE%20POISONING.pdf

Salvicci, A., Squire, B., Burdick, M., Luoto, M., Brazzel, D., and Vaezazizi, R. (2011). Ondansetron is safe and effective for prehospital treatment of nausea and vomiting by paramedics. *Prehospital Emergency Care, 15*(1), 34–38.

Taylor, T. (1999). The digestive system. Retrieved August 12, 2013 from http://www.innerbody.com

Venes, D., ed. (2013). *Taber's cyclopedic medical dictionary* (22nd ed.). Philadelphia, PA: F. A. Davis Company.

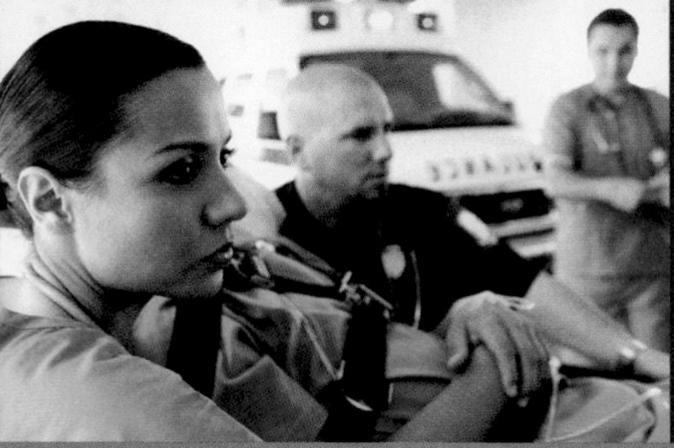

CHAPTER 16

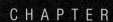

Drugs Used to Treat Obstetric and Gynecologic Emergencies

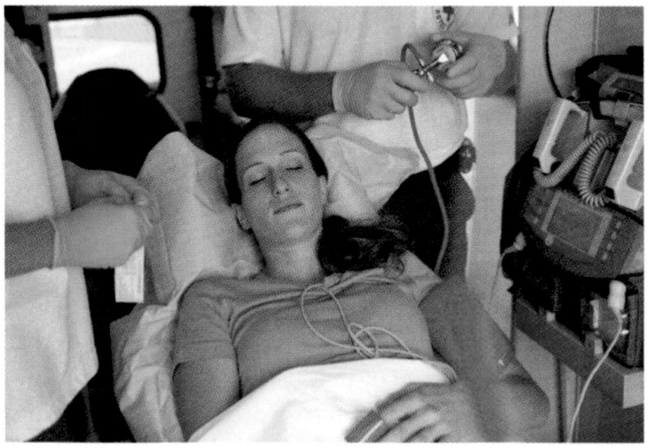

Paramedics assessing a pregnant patient. *(Photograph © Jochen Sand/Digital Vision/Thinkstock)*

LEARNING OUTCOMES

- Describe the out-of-hospital management of a patient experiencing preterm labor, postpartum hemorrhage, and preeclampsia and eclampsia.
- Describe the actions, indications, contraindications, dosage, and adverse reactions and side effects of the anticonvulsant drugs diazepam and magnesium sulfate.
- Describe the actions, indications, contraindications, dosage, and adverse reactions and side effects of the antihypertensive drug hydralazine.
- Describe the actions, indications, contraindications, dosage, and adverse reactions and side effects of the oxytocic drug oxytocin.
- Describe the actions, indications, contraindications, dosage, and adverse reactions and side effects of the tocolytic drug terbutaline.

KEY TERMS

Eclampsia
Oxytocic
Preeclampsia
Pregnancy-induced hypertension
Preterm labor
Postpartum hemorrhage
Toxemia of pregnancy
Uterine atony

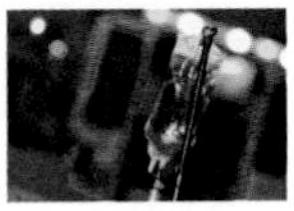

SCENARIO OPENING

You are assigned to Rescue 225 at fire station #1. While sitting down for coffee after completing the initial vehicle and equipment check, you are dispatched to a "woman in labor." On arrival, a 32-year-old patient, Patty, is found experiencing strong uterine contractions every 2 minutes, each lasting approximately 1 minute. Patty tells you that this is her second child, but it is not due for another 3 weeks. On visual examination, you notice that the baby's buttocks are visible, which indicates that delivery is imminent. Preparations for delivery are made quickly. You place Patty on 100 percent humidified oxygen. If delivery complications arise, it is important to increase oxygen content and oxygen delivery to the tissues.

As the baby emerges, the buttocks and legs come out smoothly, but the head remains in the birth canal. In this situation, an adequate airway must be provided, because the baby may attempt to begin spontaneous respirations. You form an airway at the bottom of the birth canal, but there is no evidence of respirations. After approximately 2 minutes, the baby's head delivers. Initial assessment of the baby reveals the following:

Level of consciousness:	unconscious
Respirations:	none
Pulse:	none

Effective Communication

While wearing gloves, fingers are inserted into the birth canal to form a space, making a temporary airway for the baby.

Introduction

For most EMS professionals, the opportunity to assist in the delivery of a baby is one of the most exciting and fulfilling events in their careers. Most out-of-hospital deliveries occur without complications. During and after delivery, treatment for both mother and infant is usually supportive. In some cases, however, EMS providers encounter a potentially fatal obstetric emergency, such as **preterm labor, postpartum hemorrhage,** and **preeclampsia** or **eclampsia.**

Whenever you respond to a pregnant patient, remember that not only are you responding to the mother, you have the fetus, or fetuses, to consider as well. EMS treatment protocols appropriately focus on the mother. However, if medications are given to the mother, you must also consider how these medications may affect the fetus. Remember you are actually treating multiple patients simultaneously.

During pregnancy, the mother's heart rate, cardiac output, and blood volume all increase. This increase in the mother's physiology may alter the therapeutic effects of many medications on the mother and, at the same time, be potentially harmful to the fetus. Giving medications to pregnant patients is oftentimes very necessary. Remember to consider the risk-benefit ratio when giving medications to pregnant patients. When medications are necessary for the pregnant patient, carefully follow your treatment protocols and always remember that you have medical control to assist when needed.

Pathophysiology of OB/GYN Disorders

Preeclampsia

Preeclampsia is a **toxemia of pregnancy** characterized by an increase in blood pressure (exceeding 140/90), headaches, proteinuria (loss of proteins in the urine), and edema during pregnancy (Fig. 16-1). It may progress rapidly from mild to severe. If untreated, preeclampsia can progress to eclampsia.

The cause of preeclampsia is unknown. However, it occurs more frequently in first pregnancies, smokers, and overweight or diabetic patients. Preeclampsia generally develops between the 20th week of gestation and the end of the first postpartum week. Other symptoms of preeclampsia include sudden weight gain, disturbances in vision, epigastric or abdominal pain, high blood pressure, and generalized presacral and facial edema.

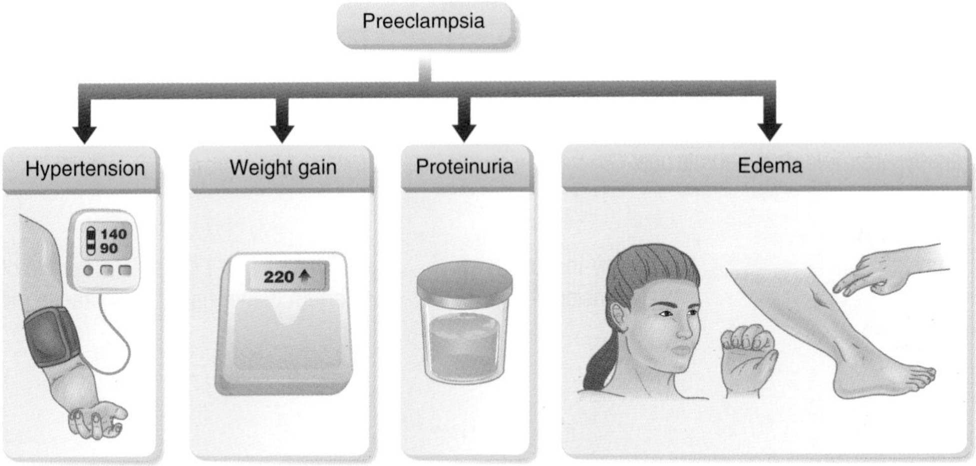

Figure 16-1 Preeclampsia.

HELLP Syndrome

HELLP syndrome is a life-threatening complication considered a variation of preeclampsia. Both preeclampsia and HELLP syndrome usually occur in the later stages of pregnancy. HELLP stands for:

- H—hemolysis
- EL—elevated liver enzymes
- LP—low platelet count

The most common causes of severe illness or death of a patient are liver rupture or stroke. Table 16-1 compares the signs and symptoms of preeclampsia and HELLP.

Eclampsia

Eclampsia is a severe hypertensive disorder of pregnancy characterized by convulsions and coma (Fig. 16-2). It typically occurs between 20 weeks' gestation and the end of the first postpartum week. Eclampsia is the most serious complication of **pregnancy-induced hypertension.**

The cause of eclampsia is unknown. However, vasospasm is one of the underlying mechanisms. Some of the risk factors for eclampsia include nulliparity (the woman has not given birth previously), advanced maternal age, maternal hypertension, renal disease, and diabetes mellitus. The symptoms of eclampsia include high blood pressure, severe headache, changes in vision, nausea and vomiting, abdominal pain, and edema. Patients may suffer seizures without warning. The drugs used for the out-of-hospital treatment of eclampsia are magnesium sulfate and diazepam.

Preterm Labor

Preterm labor occurs between the beginning of the 21st week and the end of the 37th week of pregnancy. Preterm labor

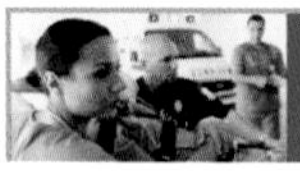

Table 16-1 Comparison of the Signs/Symptoms of Preeclampsia vs. HELLP

Preeclampsia	HELLP Syndrome
Sudden weight gain	Headache
Severe headache	Nausea or vomiting with pain after eating
Visual disturbances	Epigastric pain
Abdominal pain	Tender right-upper quadrant
Presacral and facial edema	Bleeding
Increased blood pressure	Visual disturbances
Proteinuria	Increased blood pressure
	Swelling
	Proteinuria

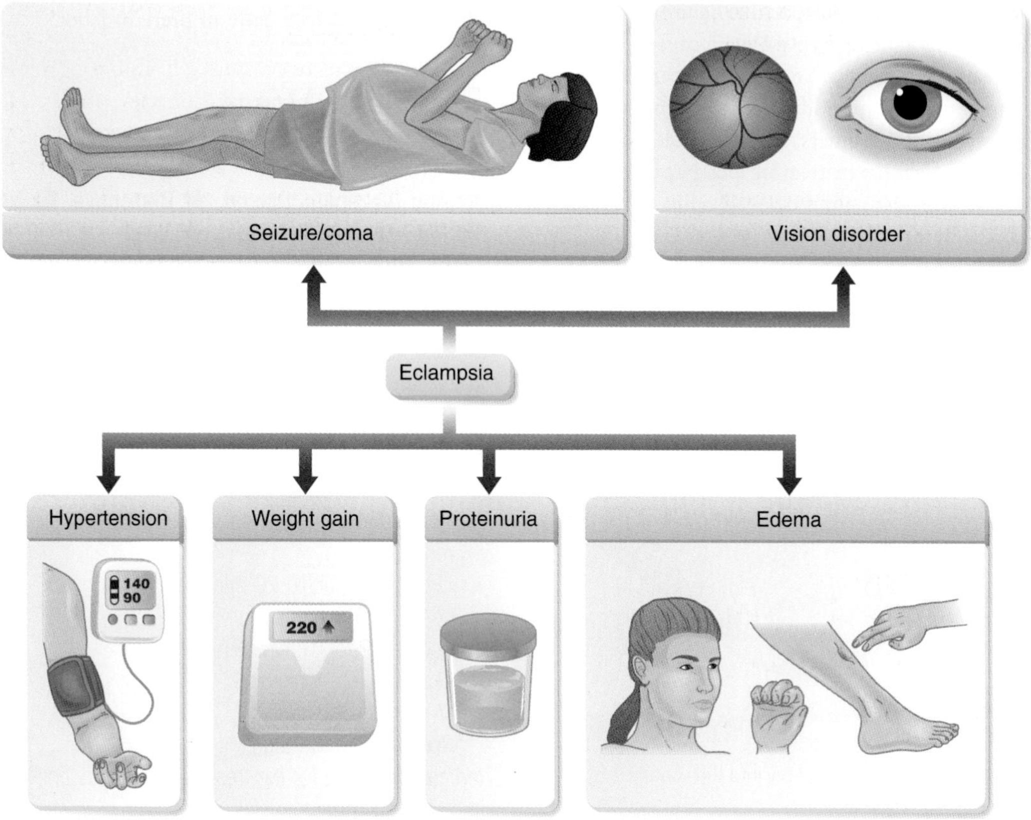

Figure 16-2 Eclampsia.

occurs in approximately 5 to 15 percent of pregnancies and is the most common complication that occurs during the 3rd trimester. The exact cause of preterm labor is unknown in the majority of cases, but it may be initiated by an underlying maternal, fetal, or placental problem. **Tocolytics,** such as terbutaline, are used to decrease or inhibit uterine contractions. The goal is to extend the pregnancy until the fetus is mature enough to survive outside the womb. The following criteria are used to determine if tocolytic therapy is appropriate: the fetus is alive with a gestational age of less than 35 weeks, the fetal weight is less than 2,500 g, the membranes are unruptured, cervical dilation is less than 4 cm, effacement is less than 80 percent complete, and there are no maternal or fetal problems that require immediate delivery. Terbutaline is very effective in terminating preterm labor and decreasing the mortality and morbidity associated with preterm birth.

Postpartum Hemorrhage

Postpartum hemorrhage is the loss (by the mother) of more than 500 mL of blood within 24 hours after delivery (Fig. 16-3). Generally, hemorrhage occurs within the first few hours after delivery, but it can happen up to 24 hours after delivery.

Causes of postpartum hemorrhage can include incomplete contraction of the uterine muscle fibers, retained pieces of placenta or membranes in the uterus, or vaginal or cervical tears sustained during delivery. A risk factor associated with postpartum hemorrhage is **uterine atony** (lack of uterine tone). It is important to frequently assess the patient's clinical appearance and vital signs in order to determine blood loss. The initial treatment for severe postpartum hemorrhage is the same as for anyone experiencing hypovolemia caused by hemorrhage. This treatment includes maintaining an adequate airway, using supplemental humidified oxygen, and administering intravenous volume expanders. If pharmacologic therapy is needed, the drug of choice in treating postpartum hemorrhage is oxytocin. If this treatment is delayed, a life-threatening situation could rapidly develop.

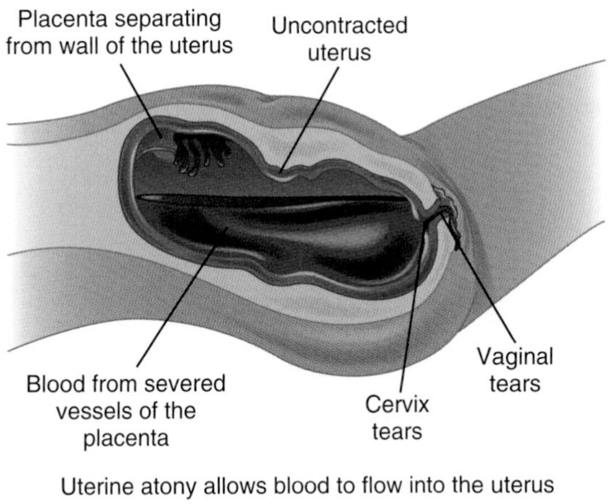

Figure 16-3 Postpartum hemorrhage.

Pharmacokinetics

Anticonvulsants

Anticonvulsants are used to decrease the incidence and severity of seizures due to various etiologies. These drugs are capable of depressing abnormal neuronal discharges in the central nervous system (CNS) that may result in seizures. Anticonvulsants work by preventing the spread of seizure activity, depressing the motor cortex, raising seizure threshold, or altering levels of neurotransmitters.

Antihypertensives

Antihypertensives are used to lower blood pressure to a normal level (lower than 90 mm Hg diastolic) or to the lowest level tolerated. The goal of antihypertensive therapy is the prevention of end-organ damage. Anithypertensives are classified into groups according to their site of action. Hydralazine is a hypertensive that is a direct-acting peripheral arteriolar vasodilator.

Oxytocic

An oxytocic is a drug that stimulates the uterine smooth muscle, producing uterine contractions similar to those of spontaneous labor. In the out-of-hospital setting, an oxytocic (oxytocin) is used for the postpartum control of bleeding after the delivery of the placenta.

Tocolytic

Tocolytic agents inhibit uterine contractions and suppress preterm labor. They can delay labor and give more time for fetal growth and for the fetal lungs to mature. They are most effective when given early in preterm labor.

Individual Drugs

Diazepam (dye-AZ-e-pam)

🍁 Apo-Diazepam, Diastat, 🍁 Diazemuls, 🍁 Novo-Dipam, 🍁 PMS-Diazepam, Valium, 🍁 Vivol

Classifications: Anticonvulsant, benzodiazepine

Pregnancy Class: D

Mechanism of Action: Depresses the CNS by potentiating gamma-aminobutyric acid (GABA), an inhibitory neurotransmitter; has anticonvulsant properties due to enhanced presynaptic inhibition

Pharmacokinetics

Absorption: Rapidly absorbed from the GI tract. Absorption from IM sites may be slow and unpredictable. Well absorbed from rectal mucosa.

Onset: IM—within 20 minutes
IV—1 to 5 minutes
Rectal—2 to 10 minutes

Duration: IM—unknown
IV—15 to 60 minutes
Rectal—4 to 12 hours

Indications: Used for the treatment of status epilepticus or uncontrolled seizures.

Contraindications: Known hypersensitivity; should not be given to patients with myasthenia gravis, severe pulmonary impairment, sleep apnea, severe liver dysfunction, or preexisting CNS depression; increases the risk of congenital malformation in OB patients
Precautions: Use with caution in patients with severe kidney impairment and in patients with a history of suicide attempts or drug dependence. Long-acting benzodiazepines cause prolonged sedation in the elderly.
Route and Dosage
IV (Adult): 5 to 10 mg; may be repeated every 10 to 15 minutes to a total dose of 30 mg

Effective Communication

The IM route may be used if the IV route is unavailable, but larger doses may be required.

IM, IV (Pediatric over 5 years): 0.05 to 0.3 mg/kg/dose given over 3 to 5 minutes every 15 to 30 minutes to a total dose of 10 mg
IM, IV (Pediatric 1 mo to 5 years): 0.05 to 0.3 mg/kg/dose given over 3 to 5 minutes every 15 to 30 minutes to a total dose of 5 mg
Rectal (Adult & Pediatric over 12 years): 0.2 mg/kg
Rectal (Pediatric 6 to 11 years): 0.3 mg/kg
Rectal (Pediatric 2 to 5 years): 0.5 mg/kg

Understand the Numbers

You are ordered to administer diazepam at 0.05 mg/kg to your 4-year-old patient who weighs 55 pounds. How much of the drug will you give?
55 pounds ÷ 2.2 kg = 25 kg. 0.05 mg × 25 kg = 1.25 mg.

How Supplied
Solution for Injection: 5 mg/mL
Rectal Gel Delivery System: 2.5 mg, 10 mg, 20 mg
Adverse Reactions and Side Effects
Resp: respiratory depression
CV: hypotension (IV only)
CNS: dizziness, drowsiness, lethargy, depression, hangover, slurred speech, headache, paradoxical excitation
EENT: blurred vision
GI: constipation, diarrhea, nausea, vomiting
Derm: rashes
Local: pain (IM), phlebitis (IV), venous thrombosis
Misc: physical dependence, psychological dependence, tolerance
Drug Interactions: Additive CNS depression may occur if diazepam is administered with other CNS depressants.
EMS Considerations: Diazepam may cause respiratory arrest if administered too rapidly or in excess. Do not mix diazepam with any other drug. Diazepam may react with the IV tubing; to minimize this, administer diazepam at the IV site, not higher in the tubing. Thoroughly flush the IV line before administering diazepam if other drugs have already been administered through the line. Assess the patient's vital signs continuously.

HydrALAZINE (hye-DRAL-a-zeen)

Apresoline, Novo-Hylazin
Classifications: Antihypertensive, vasodilator
Pregnancy Class: C
Mechanism of Action: Direct-acting peripheral arteriolar vasodilator
Pharmacokinetics
Absorption: Well absorbed from IM sites
Onset: IM—10 to 30 minutes
IV—5 to 20 minutes
Duration: IM—3 to 8 hours
IV—2 to 6 hours
Indication: Moderate-to-severe hypertension (with a diuretic)
Contraindications: Known hypersensitivity; should not be given to patients with known intolerance to tartrazine
Precautions: Use with caution in patients with cardiovascular, cerebrovascular, and severe renal and hepatic disease.
Route and Dosage
IM, IV (Adult): Hypertension—5 to 40 mg, repeated as needed. Eclampsia—5 mg every 15 to 20 minutes
How Supplied
Injection: 20 mg/mL
Adverse Reactions and Side Effects
CV: tachycardia, angina, arrhythmias, edema, orthostatic hypotension
CNS: dizziness, drowsiness, headache
GI: diarrhea, nausea, vomiting
Derm: rashes
Drug Interactions: There may be an increased chance of hypotension if used with other antihypertensives, nitrates, or MAO inhibitors.
EMS Considerations: Monitor vital signs closely during therapy. Do not confuse hydralazine with hydroxyzine.

Magnesium sulfate (mag-NEE-zhum SUL-fate)

Classifications: Mineral and electrolyte replacement, anticonvulsant
Pregnancy Class: D
Mechanism of Action: Essential for the activity of many enzymes; plays an important role in neurotransmission and muscular excitability
Pharmacokinetics
Absorption: IV administration results in complete bioavailability. Well absorbed from IM sites.
Onset: IM—60 minutes
IV—immediate
Duration: IM—3 to 4 hours
IV—30 minutes
Indications: Anticonvulsant associated with severe eclampsia and preeclampsia

Check the Evidence

An unlabeled use of magnesium sulfate is for patients in preterm labor. ***Check local protocols.***

Contraindications: Known hypersensitivity; should not be given to patients with hypermagnesemia, hypocalcemia, or anuria or in patients with heart block
Precautions: Use with caution in patients with any degree of renal insufficiency.
Route and Dosage
IM, IV (Adult): 4 to 5 g by IV infusion, concurrently with up to 5 g IM in each buttock
How Supplied
Injection: 500 mg/mL (50 percent)
Premixed infusion: 1 g/100 mL, 2 g/100 mL, 4 g/50 mL, 4 g/100/mL, 20 g/500 mL, 40 g/1,000 mL
Adverse Reactions and Side Effects
Resp: decreased respiratory rate
CV: arrhythmias, bradycardia, hypotension
GI: diarrhea
MS: muscle weakness
Derm: flushing, sweating
Metab: hypothermia
Drug Interactions: May potentiate calcium channel blockers and neuromuscular blocking agents
EMS Considerations: ❗ Accidental overdose of IV magnesium sulfate has resulted in serious respiration depression and, in some cases, even death due to cardiac arrest. Constant monitoring of the patient's vital signs is extremely important.

Check the Evidence

To reverse the effects of an IV overdose, you can administer an IV bolus of 10 percent calcium gluconate at 5 to 10 mEq (10 to 20 mL).

Oxytocin (ox-i-TOE-sin)

Pitocin, 🍁 Syntocinon
Classifications: Hormone, oxytocic
Pregnancy Class: X
Mechanism of Action: Stimulates uterine smooth muscle, producing uterine contractions similar to those in spontaneous labor
Pharmacokinetics
Absorption: Well absorbed at the IM sites. IV administration results in 100 percent bioavailability.
Onset: IM—3 to 5 minutes
IV—Immediate
Duration: IM—30 to 60 minutes
IV—1 hour
Indication: Postpartum control of bleeding after delivery of the placenta
Contraindications: Known hypersensitivity
Precautions: Use with caution in patients with hypertension or cardiac arrhythmias and in patients with decreased renal function.
Route and Dosage
IM (Adult): 10 units after delivery of the placenta
IV (Adult): 10 units infused at 20 to 40 milliunits/minute after delivery of the placenta
How Supplied
Solution for injection: 10 units/mL
Adverse Reactions and Side Effects (Noted for IV administration only)
CV: hypotension
CNS: COMA, SEIZURES
GI: nausea, vomiting
F and E: hypochloremia, hyponatremia, water intoxication
Misc: painful uterine contractions
Drug Interactions: Concurrent use with vasoconstrictors may cause severe hypertension.
EMS Considerations: If possible, place the newborn at the mother's breast. The baby's sucking action promotes the secretion of oxytocin, which will also aid in controlling postpartum hemorrhage. 🍁 Do not confuse Pitocin (oxytocin) with Pitressin (vasopressin).

***Effective* Communication**

Magnesium sulfate should be available for administration to relax the uterus in the event of tetanic (continuous) uterine contractions.

Terbutaline (ter-BYOO-ta-leen)

Classifications: Bronchodilator, adrenergic, tocolytic
Pregnancy Class: B
Mechanism of Action: Terbutaline is selective for beta$_2$ (pulmonary)-adrenergic receptor sites, with less effect on beta$_1$ (cardiac)-adrenergic receptors.
Pharmacokinetics
Absorption: Well absorbed after SubQ administration
Onset: SubQ—Within 15 minutes
IV—Immediate
Duration: SubQ—1.5 to 4 hours
IV—Unknown
Indications: Can be used in the management of preterm labor (unlabeled use)
Contraindications: Known hypersensitivity; should not be used in patients with hypersensitivity to adrenergic amines
Precautions: Use with caution in patients with cardiac disease, hypertension, hyperthyroidism, diabetes, or glaucoma. ❗ The elderly are more susceptible to adverse reactions, which may require reduced dosing.
Route and Dosage (Unlabeled—refer to protocols and medical control)
IV (Adult): 2.5 to 10 mcg/minute IV infusion. Increase rate by 5 mcg/minute every 10 minutes until contractions stop (not to exceed 30 mcg/minute). After contractions have stopped for 30 minutes, decrease the infusion rate to the lowest effective amount and maintain this rate for 4 to 8 hours.

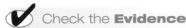

Effective Communication

The IV concentration is 1 mg/mL undiluted. If possible, use an infusion pump to ensure accurate dosing.

How Supplied

Injection: 1 mg/mL

Adverse Reactions and Side Effects

CNS: nervousness, restlessness, tremor, headache, insomnia

CV: angina, arrhythmias, hypertension, tachycardia

GI: nausea, vomiting

Endo: hyperglycemia

Drug Interactions: Use with caffeine-containing products increases the stimulating effect. Concurrent use with other adrenergic agonists will have additive adrenergic side effects. Beta-adrenergic blockers may make terbutaline less effective.

EMS Considerations: Monitor maternal and fetal vital signs continuously. Notify medical control if contractions persist or increase in frequency or duration or if symptoms of maternal or fetal distress occur.

Understand the Numbers

You are mixing terbutaline in 250 mL of NS. What is the resulting concentration (mcg/mL)? The terbutaline comes packaged 1 mg/mL in a 2-mL vial.

C = 2 mg ÷ 250 mL = 0.008 mg/mL.

0.008 mg = 0.008 × 1000 = 8.0 mcg/mL.

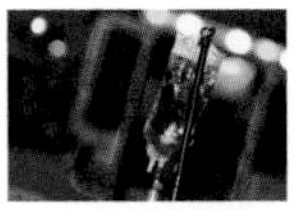

SCENARIO REVISITED

Did you consider the case of Patty? As you recall, Patty has just given birth, but the baby has no respirations or pulse.

Immediately use suction to clear the baby's airway and ventilate with 100 percent humidified oxygen using a bag-valve mask and chest compressions. There is a risk (rare) that 100 percent oxygen will have toxic effects on the baby's lungs and eyes, but oxygen should never be withheld from an infant during an emergency.

Assessment of ventilations reveals good breath sounds over the chest and gastric area. It is now a good idea to place an ET tube in the baby for airway protection and administration of emergency drugs, if necessary. Vascular access in a newborn is difficult at best, so in most cases ET access for drug administration is preferable. The ECG monitor shows asystole.

Check the **Evidence**

Intubation attempts are often unsuccessful in the newborn. Successful ET attempts frequently take longer than 30 seconds. Newborns frequently deteriorate during intubation attempts. Follow your local protocols and medical control.

Once you have performed an appropriate assessment, you should proceed using a critical thinking approach to medication administration.

Step 1: Determine signs and symptoms to be treated.

Step 2: Consider both the risks and benefits of treating or not treating your patient.

Step 3: Choose the medication that provides the best possible outcome.

Step 4: Remember the drug's indications, contraindications, and precautions.

Step 5: Decide the best route for administering the medication for the best outcome.

Step 6: Administer the medication(s) according to the seven Patient Rights.

1. The right patient
2. The right drug
3. The right drug amount
4. The right time
5. The right route
6. The right documentation
7. The right of the patient to accept or refuse the medication(s)

Step 7: Reevaluate the patient for the desired and undesired effects.

Once the ET tube is in place and adequate ventilations are achieved, administer approximately 0.1 mg (0.04 mL) epinephrine in a 1:1000 solution down the ET tube. The dosage of epinephrine is 0.01 mg/kg IV of a 1:10000 solution or 0.1 mg/kg of a 1:1000 solution via the ET tube.

Effective Communication

The average birth weight of a newborn is 4 to 5 kg. When giving epinephrine ET, it is best to dilute the drug with normal saline (NS) solution.

Epinephrine is a natural catecholamine that stimulates both alpha-adrenergic and beta-adrenergic receptors. It elevates perfusion pressure during cardiac compressions, improves cardiac contractions, and stimulates spontaneous contractions in asystole. In this case, the newborn responds to the epinephrine and ventilations with a heart rate beginning at 40 beats/minute and gradually increasing to a normal sinus rhythm. In the newborn, a heart rate less than 80 beats/minute is considered bradycardia, and it does not produce adequate perfusion. Therefore, chest compressions are necessary until the epinephrine and ventilation gradually increase the newborn's heart rate to normal.

Let's Recap

Most out-of-hospital OB/GYN emergencies do not require pharmacologic intervention. EMS professionals can manage the majority of these emergencies by maintaining an adequate airway, using supplemental oxygen, and administering IV volume expanders, if needed. If out-of-hospital pharmacologic intervention is needed in preterm labor, terbutaline should be used. If out-of-hospital pharmacologic intervention is needed to treat severe cases of postpartum hemorrhage, the drug of choice is oxytocin; to treat preeclampsia, the drug of choice is magnesium sulfate; to treat seizures caused by eclampsia, diazepam and magnesium sulfate should be used.

In treating out-of-hospital OB/GYN emergencies, medical control may order other drugs in place of or in addition to the drugs presented in this chapter. For example, the physician may order an antihypertensive drug to treat hypertension associated with the OB patient. Other obstetric and gynecologic out-of-hospital emergencies may call for other kinds of flexibility in treatment. It is important that EMS professionals be knowledgeable about local protocols to that they are ready to carry out treatment orders from medical control.

SCENARIO CONCLUSION

The key to successful resuscitation of a newborn is adequate airway maintenance and ventilation using supplemental oxygen. Medical control may call for medications if the patient does not respond to ventilation and chest compressions. In this case, the newborn now has a sinus rhythm rate of 144 beats/minute, with a good pulse and adequate respirations.

While attention is focused on the baby, another member of the team begins having problems with Patty. She complained of severe abdominal pain after delivery of the placenta and soon began hemorrhaging.

Hemorrhage after delivery calls for several out-of-hospital management techniques. Immediately, one member of the team begins massaging Patty's fundus, while another team member starts an IV of NS. Patty should remain on high-flow 100 percent humidified oxygen. If massaging the fundus does not control hemorrhage, the drug of choice for hemorrhage control is oxytocin. Oxytocin is a hormone secreted by the pituitary gland that stimulates uterine contractions. In this emergency, oxytocin is used to contract uterine blood vessels, thus reducing postpartum hemorrhaging. If possible, the newborn should be placed at Patty's breast. The sucking action of the baby will promote the secretion of oxytocin, also aiding in controlling hemorrhage. However, in this case the baby should be closely monitored while en route to the emergency department because of its potentially unstable condition. The oxytocin dosage is 10 to 20 units added to the IV at a rate adjusted to the severity of the hemorrhage. By the way, Patty named her new baby Emma.

PRACTICE EXERCISES

1. The out-of-hospital indication for oxytocin is for the:
   a. Control of seizures
   b. Treatment of hypertension
   c. Control of postpartum hemorrhage
   d. Treatment of severe bronchospasm
2. A major concern in a patient with eclampsia is seizures. The out-of-hospital drug of choice in the treatment of severe eclampsia is:
   a. Labetalol
   b. Oxytocin
   c. Diazepam
   d. Magnesium sulfate
3. One of the most frequent CNS side effects for the use of terbutaline is:
   a. Restlessness
   b. Headache
   c. Insomnia
   d. Hypertension
4. The maximum adult dose of hydralazine for the treatment of eclampsia is:
   a. 5 mg
   b. 10 mg
   c. 15 mg
   d. 20 mg
5. Magnesium sulfate is contraindicated in patients with:
   a. Heart block
   b. Preterm labor
   c. Severe renal function
   d. Congestive heart failure
6. The initial adult dosage of magnesium sulfate for eclampsia is:
   a. 1 to 2 g by IV infusion
   b. 2 to 4 g by IV infusion
   c. 4 to 5 g by IV infusion
   d. 5 to 6 g by IV infusion

7. Oxytocin is used in the out-of-hospital setting for:
a. Induction of labor
b. Preeclampsia
c. Facilitation of abortion
d. Postpartum hemorrhage

8. A possible life-threatening adverse reaction of oxytocin is:
a. Seizures
b. Hypotension
c. Hyponatremia
d. Hypochloremia

9. When used in the management of preterm labor, terbutaline is classified as a:
a. Beta-blocker
b. Bronchodilator
c. Adrenergic
d. Tocolytic

10. An overdose of magnesium sulfate could cause respiratory depression and heart block. To reverse these effects, oxygenate the patient with 100 percent oxygen and give an IV bolus of:
a. Hydralazine
b. Sodium chloride
c. Calcium chloride
d. Calcium gluconate

CASE STUDIES

1. You are dispatched to the home of a "woman having chest pain." On arrival, you find a 24-year-old patient who says that she is 8 months pregnant. She also reports that she has had a headache for the past 2 days and today has developed chest pain. Further history and physical examination identify the chest pain as epigastric pain. Initial assessment reveals the following:

Level of consciousness: alert, oriented
Respirations: 18 breaths/minute, lungs clear bilaterally
Pulse: 96 beats/minute, regular
Blood pressure: 164/110 mm Hg
Skin: pale, edematous

The patient says that this is her first pregnancy. She has no history of high blood pressure or any other illness.

All signs and symptoms indicate this patient is preeclamptic. Preeclampsia can lead to true eclampsia. Do not delay transport to the emergency department. Headache and epigastric pain in this situation could be signs of impending seizure activity. The drug of choice for the prevention of seizure activity in the preeclampsia patient is:
a. Diazepam
b. Oxytocin
c. Mannitol
d. Magnesium sulfate

2. You are called to the home of a woman "having seizures." On arrival, you find a woman in her late twenties who is experiencing active seizures. The patient's mother states that her daughter is 7 months pregnant. She also reports this is her daughter's second seizure since she called for help. Earlier in the day, the patient had complained of severe headache, dizziness, nausea, chest pain, and spots before her eyes. Seizure control for this patient should begin with:
a. Diazepam
b. Calcium gluconate
c. Magnesium sulfate
d. Oxytocin

MATH EQUATIONS

1. You are ordered to give 0.3 mg/kg/dose of diazepam over 3 minutes every 15 minutes to a total dose of 10 mg. Your patient weights 60 lbs.
   a. How many kg does your patient weigh?
   b. What is the initial dosage for your patient?
   c. How many doses will need to be administered to reach a total dose of 10 mg?
2. You are ordered to give 0.2 mg/kg of hydralazine to your 70 lb patient. The maximum dose for this patient is 20 mg.
   a. How many kg does your patient weigh?
   b. How many mg will you give this patient?
3. You are ordered to infuse 1 g/hour of magnesium sulfate to your patient. The pre-mix magnesium solution comes as 2 g/100 mL. How many gtt/minute will you run the IV using a 60 gtt IV set?
4. You are ordered to infuse 5 mcg/minute of terbutaline to your patient. You prepare the IV solution by adding 2 mg of terbutaline to 250 mL of solution.
   a. What is the concentration of the IV solution?
   b. What is the drip rate to administer 5 mcg/minute using a 60 gtt IV set?

REFERENCES

Beck, R. K. (2012). Drugs used to treat gastrointestinal emergencies. In *Pharmacology for the EMS provider.* New York: Delmar, Cengage Learning.

Deglin, J. H., Vallerand, A. H., and Sanboski, C. A. (2011). *Davis's drug guide for nurses* (12th ed.). Philadelphia, PA: F. A. Davis Company.

DNA Learning Center. Gamma-aminobutyric acid (GABA). Retrieved January 20, 2014 from www.dnalc.org/view/485-GABA-Neurotransmitter

Drugs.com. Magnesium sulfate. Retrieved January 19, 2014 from www.drugs.com/pro/magnesium-sulfate.html. American Academy of Pediatrics. (2010).

Drugs.com. Tocolytic agents. Retrieved January 20, 2014 from www.drugs.com/drug-class/tocolytic-agents.html

O'Donnell, C. P., Kamlin, C. O., Davis, P. G., Morley, C. J. (2006). Endotracheal intubation attempts during neonatal resuscitation: Success rates, duration, and adverse effects. *Pediatrics, 117,* e16–e21. Retrieved January 20, 2014 from www.ncbi.nlm.nih.gov/pubmed/16396845

Preeclampsia Foundation. HELLP syndrome: What is HELLP syndrome? Retrieved January 22, 2014 from www.preeclampsia.org/health-information/hellp-syndrome?gclid=CK13jNWNkrwCFaZAMgodogMAYw

Special report—Neonatal resuscitation: 2010 American Heart Association Guidelines for Cardiopulmonary Resuscitation and Emergency Cardiovascular Care. *Pediatrics, 126,* e1400–e1413.

Venes, D., ed. (2013). *Taber's cyclopedic medical dictionary* (22nd ed.). Philadelphia, PA: F. A. Davis Company.

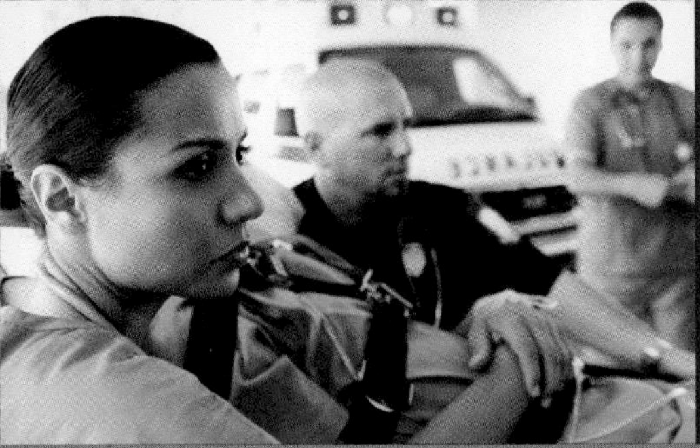

CHAPTER 17

Drugs Used to Treat Toxicological Emergencies

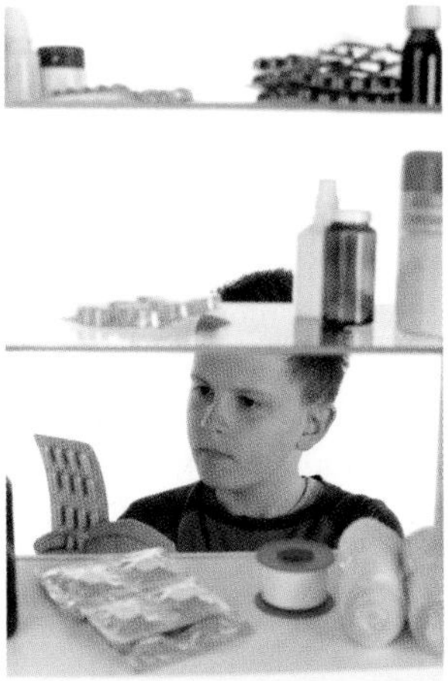

Child reaching into a medicine cabinet for "candy." *(Photograph © Marek Tarabura/iStock/Thinkstock)*

LEARNING OUTCOMES

- Describe the standard of care of the suspected poisoned patient.
- Explain the ways of contacting the poison control centers.
- Describe the indications, contraindications, precautions, route and dosages, and adverse reactions and side effects of the following:
  - The alkalinizing agent sodium bicarbonate
  - The alpha-adrenergic blocker phentolamine
  - The anticholinergic atropine
  - The anticonvulsant diazepam
  - The antidotes acetylcysteine, activated charcoal, flumazenil, naloxone, and pralidoxime
  - The cyanide antidotes amyl nitrite, hydroxocolbalamin, sodium nitrite, and sodium thiosulfate
  - The hormone glucagon

KEY TERMS

Adsorbent
Anticholinergic
Anticholinesterase
Antidote
Coagulation necrosis
Overdose
Poison
Poisoning
Withdrawal symptoms

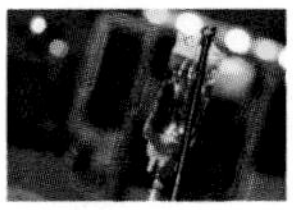

SCENARIO OPENING

You and your partner have been dispatched to a "possible overdose." On arrival, an anxious mother directs you to her 17-year-old son's room. Quinton is found on the bedroom floor; his level of consciousness is depressed, and he is unable to speak coherently. His mother says that she has not noticed anything unusual concerning her son lately. In a rapid survey of Quinton's room, you notice four empty beer bottles and an empty medication bottle labeled "Tofranil-PM, 50 mg. Take two tablets at bedtime." Initial assessment of Quinton reveals the following:

Level of consciousness:	conscious, disoriented, slurred speech
Resp:	16/minute, shallow
Pulse:	120 beats/minute with occasional PVCs (Fig. 17-1)
Blood pressure:	118/64
Skin:	warm, dry
Pupils:	equal, do not respond to light

Check the **Evidence**

Tofranil-PM (imipramine) is a tricyclic antidepressant prescribed for various forms of depression, often in conjunction with psychotherapy. Tofranil-PM is often used in suicide attempts. Adverse reactions and side effects of Tofranil-PM include drowsiness, hypotension, confusion, hallucinations, ECG changes, and ARRHYTHMIAS.

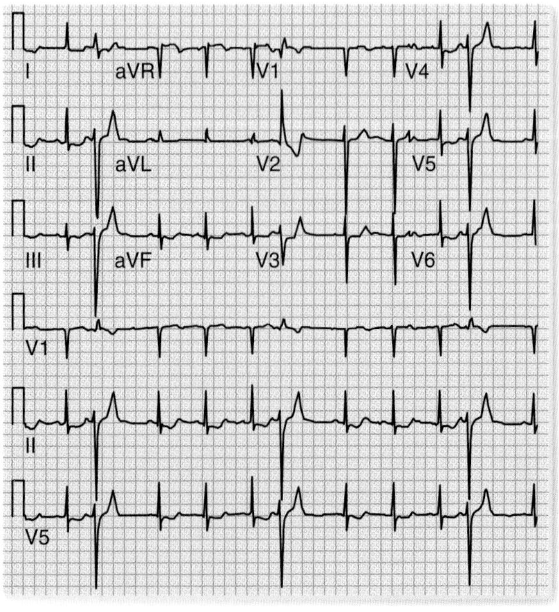

Figure 17-1 Sinus tachycardia with occasional PVCs.

Introduction

Out-of-hospital toxicological emergencies include the management of overdoses and poisonings. An **overdose** is the intake of a drug in sufficient quantity to cause harm to the body. The drugs involved in overdoses are commonly drugs of abuse but may also consist of prescription medications, over-the-counter medications, herbals, or home remedies. Acute reactions from overdoses may range from excessive excitement to coma and may progress to death. A **poison** is any substance that irritates, damages, or impairs the activity of the body's tissues. Poisons may be absorbed through the skin, inhaled, or ingested. A wide variety of substances are potential poisons. Out-of-hospital management of toxicological emergencies includes immediate stabilization of the patient, identifying the substance, attempting to slow or stop the absorption of the substance, and administering an **antidote**. The drugs used in the treatment of toxicological emergencies include specific antidotes, emetics, drug antagonists, oxygen, anticonvulsants, and alkalinizing agents.

The standard care of the poisoned patient begins with immediate stabilization of the patient's airway, breathing, circulation, and neurological status if these are compromised. Further assessment should include unusual skin color (that is, cherry red skin with carbon monoxide poisoning) and assessment of patient's breath for odors that may indicate what substance was involved in the poisoning (that is, bitter almonds with cyanide poisoning). Obtaining a history of the poisoning should help to determine what substance and how much was involved in the poisoning, when the poisoning occurred, what attempts were made to treat the poisoning, whether the poisoning was accidental or a suicide attempt, and any significant medical history of the patient. Signs and symptoms should be continually assessed to assist in identifying the poison.

If the poison can be identified, refer to texts, call the poison control center, and, of course, contact medical control in order to determine specific antidotes or treatments. Decontamination of the gastrointestinal (GI) tract includes activated charcoal if the patient has ingested a drug or chemical to which the charcoal can bind.

Check the **Evidence**

Inducing vomiting, formerly relied on in poisonings, is now rarely used because it has not been shown to improve outcome and may cause complications such as aspiration pneumonia.

To contact a Regional Poison Control Center in the United States, call the American Association of Poison Control Centers (AAPCC) at 1-800-222-1222, or go to www.aapcc.org. The AAPCC supports the nation's 56 poison centers in their efforts to treat poison exposures. However, unlike the United States, the Canadian Poison Control Centre does not have a national poison control centre phone number. So, in Canada, you can find the closest poison control centre by going to www.safetyxchange.org/health-safety/canadian-poison-centres-contact-information. It is important that every EMS service have the contact information readily available for the closest poison control center.

Pathophysiology of Poisoning

Poisoning is any illness caused by a toxic substance (poison) introduced into the body. Virtually any substance can be poisonous if consumed in sufficient quantity. The extent of illness, or damage, depends on the pH of the poison, the amount consumed into the body, the form of the poison, and the length of exposure.

Acids produce **coagulation necrosis**, a type of accidental cell death typically caused by ischemia or infarction. Coagulation necrosis changes the molecular composition of proteins when the poison contacts tissues. The mechanism of action of toxic inhalants is unknown. However, toxic inhalants act on the central nervous system (CNS) similarly to a very potent anesthetic. Hydrocarbons produced by the toxic inhalants sensitize the myocardial tissue and allow the tissue to be sensitive to catecholamines, which can cause arrhythmias and possibly death. Table 17-1 lists common Medical Emergencies for Poisons and Poisoning.

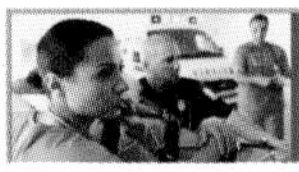

Table 17-1 Medical Emergencies for Poisons and Poisoning

Agent	Pathology	Signs and Symptoms	EMS Treatment
Acetaminophen	Production of toxic intermediate metabolite	Anorexia, nausea, vomiting	Supportive care including careful monitoring Activated charcoal
Acids	Immediate destruction and necrosis of tissues on contact	Burning pain on contact, abdominal pain, nausea, GI perforation, shock, death	Airway patency, aggressive volume resuscitation, irrigation of exposed tissues
Amphetamines	Excessive stimulation of the CNS, peripheral alpha- and beta-receptor sites	Excitement, nausea, vomiting, palpitations, arrhythmias, hypertension, seizures, coma, death	Supportive care including airway and cardiac monitoring, activated charcoal, and benzodiazepines for seizures Possible vasodilators and beta-blockers
Antidepressants (SSRIs)	CNS depression, excessive stimulation of serotonin receptors	Confusion, diaphoresis, tremor, agitation, nausea, vomiting, seizures, coma	Maintenance of ABCs, activated charcoal, supportive care
Antidepressants (Cyclic)	Toxic cardiovascular and CNS effects	Confusion, dizziness, hypotension, tachycardia, prolonged QRS complex, cardiac dysrhythmias, seizures	Cardiac monitoring with 12-lead ECG, activated charcoal, supportive care
Barbiturates	Depressed CNS, hypotension, inhibition of cardiac contractility	Drowsiness, confusion, vertigo, slurred speech, shallow respirations, thread pulse, hypotension, CV collapse, respiratory arrest	ABCs, treatment of hypotension, activated charcoal
Benzodiazepines	Generalized CNS depression	Confusion, dizziness, hypotension, respiratory and cardiovascular depression	ABCs, activated charcoal. For patients with no history of chronic use, give flumazenil.
Calcium channel blockers	Prevention of calcium entry into cells, resulting in decreased cardiac contractility and blockage of the SA and AV nodes; also causes peripheral vasodilation	Nausea, vomiting, dizziness, confusion, hypotension, bradycardia, seizures, coma, death	ABCs, fluids and vasopressors for hypotension, multiple-dose activated charcoal, atropine for bradycardia
Carbon monoxide	Hemoglobin binding preventing delivery of oxygen to cells	Headache, fatigue, nausea, vomiting, confusion, syncope convulsions, death from respiratory arrest	ABCs with 100 percent oxygen, IV fluids, cardiac monitoring
Cocaine	CNS stimulation, depressed conduction and myocardial contractility	Anxiety, delirium, hypertension, tachycardia, seizures, ECG abnormalities, stroke, coma, death	ABCs, cardiac monitoring, activated charcoal, benzodiazepines

Continued

Table 17-1 Medical Emergencies for Poisons and Poisoning-cont'd

Agent	Pathology	Signs and Symptoms	EMS Treatment
Cyanide	Binds to cytochrome oxidase of cells, blocking oxygen use	Nausea, vomiting, abdominal pain, almond odor on breath, headache, confusion, syncope, convulsions, coma, cardiovascular collapse, death	ABCs, activated charcoal, inhalation of amyl nitrite pearls until antidote is available—amyl and sodium nitrites and sodium thiosulfate. Vitamin B_{12} may be helpful.
Digoxin and digitalis	Excessive excitability, cardiac conduction disturbances, AV block	Nausea, vomiting, headache, drowsiness, electrolyte disturbances, confusion, delirium, bradycardia, AV block, ventricular fibrillation	Cardiac monitoring, activated charcoal, lidocaine or phenytoin for ventricular irritability
Ethanol	CNS depression; additive effects if combined with other CNS depressants	Impaired coordination, slurred speech, tachycardia, nausea, vomiting, stupor, coma, hypotension, vascular collapse, respiratory failure	Supportive care, IV fluids, thiamine
Iron salts	Corrosive effects on GI mucosa, cardiovascular compromise, metabolic acidosis	Nausea, vomiting, diarrhea, tachypnea, tachycardia, hypotension, convulsions, coma, shock, or death	ABCs, supportive care, IV fluids
Isopropyl alcohol	Potent CNS depressant	Nausea, vomiting, abdominal pain, hypotension, weakness, respiratory and myocardial depression, coma, death	ABCs, supportive care. Do not induce emesis.
Lithium	Disturbances in the GI system, kidneys, and the CNS	Nausea, vomiting, confusion, tremors, ECG abnormalities, stupor, seizures, renal failure, coma, death	ABCs and supportive care. Activated charcoal is not effective because it does not bind to metals.
Methanol	Metabolism to formaldehyde and formic acid	Dizziness, blurred vision, headache, nausea, vomiting, abdominal pain, delirium, shallow respirations, weak or rapid pulse, blindness, metabolic acidosis, death	Activated charcoal, IV ethanol to inhibit toxic metabolites
Nicotine	Binding to cholinergic nicotine receptors Neuromuscular blockade	Nausea, vomiting, abdominal pain, salivation, tachycardia, hypertension, confusion, hypotension, shock muscle paralysis, coma, death	ABCs, activated charcoal, thorough washing of exposed skin. Treat for seizures, hypertension and hypotension, and arrhythmias.
Nitroglycerine, nitrates, nitrites	Vasodilation causing hypotension	Headache, hypotension, syncope, nausea, cardiac ischemia, seizures secondary to hypotension	Activated charcoal, IV fluids, anticonvulsant medications
Nonsteroidal anti-inflammatory agents	Can result in acute renal failure	Nausea, vomiting, GI distress and bleeding, CNS depression, respiratory depression, acute renal failure, seizures	Activated charcoal, IV fluids, supportive care
Opioids and opiates	Excessive stimulation of CNS opiate receptors causing sedation and respiratory failure	Drowsiness, nausea, bradycardia, respiratory depression, hypotension, weak pulse, apnea, death	ABCs, naloxone as an antidote; activated charcoal may adsorb recently ingested pills.
Organophosphates	Excessive acetylcholine stimulation of muscarinic and nicotinic receptors	Nausea, vomiting, abdominal pain, excessive salivation, dehydration, bradycardia, weakness, shock, death due to respiratory paralysis	ABCs, atropine or pralidoxime for anticholinergic crisis; diazepam for seizures; use standard antiarrhythmic protocols for ventricular disturbances
Phenothiazines and neuroleptics	Prominent CV and CNS toxicity	Sedation, stupor, tachycardia, dysrhythmias, extrapyramidal symptoms, coma, seizures, death	ABCs; follow ACLS protocols for cardiac rhythm disturbances; give diphenhydramine for dystonias
Salicylates	Interfere with the Krebs cycle; stimulate the respiratory center and alter platelet function	Nausea, vomiting, tachypnea, delirium, acid-base disturbances, electrolyte imbalance, cerebral edema, convulsions, CV collapse	ABCs, activated charcoal, correction of acid-base abnormalities
Xanthine derivatives	Antagonism of adenosine activity and release of catecholamines	Nausea, vomiting, hypotension, metabolic acidosis, ventricular dysrhythmias, seizures, CV collapse	Activate charcoal. Treat seizures with benzodiazepines or barbiturates and cardiac rhythm with standard ACLS protocols.

Pharmacokinetics

Adsorbent

An adsorbent is a substance (for example, activated charcoal) that draws other substances out of the body or out of solution.

Alpha-Adrenergic Blocker

This is a drug that interferes with the transmission of stimuli that normally allow sympathetic nervous stimuli to be effective.

Antianginal

This is any drug used to relieve angina pectoris (chest pain). Drugs in this class include long- and short-acting nitrates, beta-blockers, aspirin, and oxygen.

Antianxiety or Anticonvulsant

These drugs control CNS overstimulation and produce skeletal muscle relaxation by inhibition of spinal pathways. They also decrease seizure activity caused by enhanced presynaptic inhibition.

Antidote

An antidote is a remedy to counteract the effects of a poison or toxin. It may work by directly neutralizing the poison, preventing the absorption of the poison, inactivating the poison, or keeping the poison from binding to a receptor, blocking its action.

Benzodiazepine Antagonist

This drug antagonizes the effects of benzodiazepines by inhibiting their action at the benzodiazepine receptor.

Cholinesterase Reactivator

This drug is used to reverse the inactivation of cholinesterase caused by organophosphates. It reverses respiratory depression and skeletal muscle paralysis.

Hydrogen Ion Buffer

A buffer neutralizes excess acid to assist returning the blood to a physiological pH, in which normal metabolic processes work more effectively.

Hormones

These are substances that have a specific effect on target tissue. Hormones differ greatly in their effects, depending on the individual agent and function of the target tissue.

Narcotic Antagonist

This drug combines with narcotic receptors to block or reverse the action of narcotic analgesics.

Sedatives or Hypnotics

These drugs cause generalized CNS depression. They can be used to decrease seizure activity caused by enhanced presynaptic inhibition.

Individual Drugs

Acetylcysteine (a-se-teel-SIS-teen)

Acetadote, 🍁 Mucomyst, 🍁 Parvolex

Classification: Antidote (acetaminophen toxicity)

Pregnancy Class: B

Mechanism of Action: PO, IV—decreases the buildup of a hepatotoxic metabolite in acetaminophen overdose. *Inhalation*—degrades mucus, allowing easier mobilization and expectoration

Pharmacokinetics

Absorption: Absorbed from the GI tract following oral administration. Action is local following inhalation. The remainder may be absorbed from pulmonary epithelium.

Onset: PO, IV—unknown

Duration: PO, IV—4 hours

Indications: PO—antidote for the management of potentially hepatotoxic overdose of acetaminophen (administer within 24 hours of ingestion). IV—antidote for the management of potentially hepatotoxic overdose of acetaminophen (administer within 8–10 hours of ingestion)

Contraindications: Known hypersensitivity

Precautions: Use with caution in patients with severe respiratory insufficiency or asthma, in patients with a history of bronchospasm, or in patients with a history of GI bleeding (oral only).

Route and Dosage

PO (Adult & Pediatric): 140 mg/kg

IV (Adult & Pediatric): 150 mg/kg over 15 minutes as a loading dose, followed by 50 mg/kg over 4 hours

How Supplied

Oral solution: 10 percent in 4-, 10-, and 30-mL vials; 20 percent in 4-, 10-, 30-, and 100-mL vials

Solution for injection: 20 percent in 30-mL vials

Adverse Reactions and Side Effects

Resp: bronchospasm, bronchial/tracheal irritation, chest tightness, increased secretions

CV: Vasodilation

CNS: Drowsiness

GI: Nausea, vomiting

Derm: Rash, clamminess

Misc: Hypersensitivity (primarily IV), which includes ANAPHYLAXIS, ANGIOEDEMA, chills, or fever

Drug Interactions: Activated charcoal may adsorb orally administered acetylcysteine and decrease its effectiveness as an antidote.

EMS Considerations: The odor of the solution is very unpleasant. Be prepared for vomiting. Acetylcysteine increases secretions. Monitor respiratory status.

Effective **Communication**

Explain to your patients that acetylcysteine has a very unpleasant odor that will dissipate as treatment progresses.

Activated Charcoal (CHAR-kole)

Acta-Char Liquid-A, Actidose-Aqua, 🍁 Charac-50, CharcoAid 2,000, 🍁 Charcodoat, Insta-Char, Insta-Char Aqueous Suspension, Liqui-Char, SuperChar Aqueous

Classifications: **Antidote**—a substance that neutralizes poisons or their effects; **adsorbent**—a substance that draws other substances out of solution

Pregnancy Class: C

Mechanism of Action: Adsorbs toxic substances or irritants, inhibiting GI absorption. Sorbitol is added to some formulations to cause hyperosmotic laxative action and promote elimination of the toxic substance.

Pharmacokinetics

- *Absorption:* Well absorbed (90 percent)
- *Onset:* Immediate
- *Duration:* Continual while in the GI tract

Indications: May be considered if a patient has ingested a potentially toxic amount of a poison up to 1 hour previously, following emesis or lavage.

Contraindications: Known hypersensitivity. Activated charcoal is contraindicated in patients who do not have an intact or protected airway. Otherwise, there are no known contraindications.

Precautions: Activated charcoal may cause vomiting, which is hazardous in petroleum distillate and caustic ingestions. Therefore, use with caution in poisonings due to cyanide, corrosives, ethanol, methanol, petroleum distillates, organic solvents, mineral acids, or iron.

Route and Dosage

Adult: PO or NG tube, 25 to 100 g (may be repeated every 4 to 6 hr)

Pediatric (under 1 year): PO or NG tube, 1 g/kg (may be repeated every 4 to 6 hr)

Pediatric (1 to 12 years): PO or NG tube, 25 to 50 g (may be repeated every 4 to 6 hr)

How Supplied

25 g/125 mL bottle (200 mg/mL)

50 g/240 mL bottle (200 mg/mL)

Most products come premixed with water or with sorbitol.

Adverse Reactions and Side Effects

GI: Black stools, constipation, diarrhea, vomiting

Drug Interactions: Do not administer with syrup of ipecac. Milk, ice cream, or sherbet will decrease the ability of activated charcoal to adsorb other agents.

EMS Considerations: Activated charcoal binds with syrup of ipecac, rendering it ineffective.

Check the **Evidence**

There are studies suggesting that there is no evidence that the administration of activated charcoal improves clinical outcome. Activated charcoal is considered a less commonly used drug.

Amyl Nitrite (AM-ill-NY-tryt)

Classification: Cyanide poisoning antidote

Pregnancy Class: X

Mechanism of Action: Converts hemoglobin into methemoglobin. Methemoglobin reacts with cyanide and chemically binds it, which prevents it from having any toxic effect.

Pharmacokinetics

- *Absorption:* Rapid
- *Onset:* 10 to 30 seconds
- *Duration:* 3 to 5 minutes

Indication: Immediate treatment of cyanide poisoning

Contraindications: Known hypersensitivity. Otherwise, there are no contraindications for cyanide poisoning.

Precautions: Use with caution in patients with head trauma, cerebral hemorrhage, increased intracranial pressure, hypotension, or glaucoma.

Route and Dosage

Inhalation (Adult): 1 to 2 ampules crushed. Inhale for 15 to 30 seconds of each minute until sodium nitrite is prepared or administer for 30 to 60 seconds every 5 minutes until the patient is conscious.

Inhalation (Pediatric): 1 ampule crushed. Inhale for 15 to 30 seconds of each minute until sodium nitrite is prepared or administer for 30 to 60 seconds every 5 minutes until the patient is conscious.

How Supplied

Ampules for inhalation: 0.3 mL

Effective Communication

Amyl nitrite inhalants are part of a Cyanide Antidote Package. Other drugs contained in the package include sodium nitrite solution for IV use and sodium thiosulfate for IV use.

Adverse Reactions and Side Effects

Resp: Shortness of breath

CV: Hypotension, tachycardia

CNS: Headache, dizziness, syncope, weakness

Derm: Cyanosis of the lips, fingernails, or palms (indicates methemoglobinemia)

Drug Interactions: Additive hypotension may occur with antihypertensive drugs, acute ingestion of alcohol, phenothiazines, or beta-blockers.

EMS Considerations: Assess vital signs frequently. Patients should remain lying or sitting down during and after amyl nitrite administration because of the potential of hypotension to develop. Amyl nitrite is the first step in a three-step treatment protocol for cyanide poisoning. After the administration of amyl nitrite, administer sodium nitrite, followed by sodium thiosulfate.

Check the **Evidence**

Amyl nitrite should be kept locked up with narcotics. It is one of the major drugs used as a "popper." Poppers are inhaled for recreational purposes, especially as an aphrodisiac.

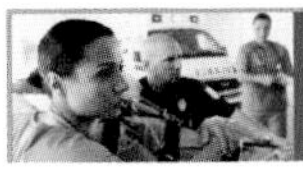

Table 17-2 Common Organophosphate Pesticides

Azamethiphos
Azinphos-methyl
Chlorpyrifos
Diazinon
Dichlorvos
Fenitrothion
Malathion
Methyl parathion
Parathion
Phosmet
Tetrachlorvinphos

Atropine (AH-troh-peen)

Atro-Pen

Classification: **Anticholinergic**; an agent that blocks parasympathetic nerve impulses

Pregnancy Class: C

Mechanism of Action: Blocks the action of acetylcholine in the parasympathetic nervous system, aiding in the treatment of anticholinesterase poisoning from organophosphate pesticides. Table 17-2 lists some of the common organophosphate pesticides with which an individual may come in contact.

Pharmacokinetics

Absorption: Well absorbed following IM administration

Onset: IM—Rapid

IV—Immediate

Duration: IM and IV—4 to 6 hours

Indication: Treatment of **anticholinesterase** (organophosphate pesticide) poisoning.

Contraindications: Known hypersensitivity. Do not give to patients with angle-closure glaucoma, to patients with tachycardia secondary to cardiac insufficiency or acute hemorrhage, or to patients with obstructive disease of the GI tract.

Precautions: Use with caution in patients with chronic kidney, liver, pulmonary, or cardiac disease. Children may have increased susceptibility to adverse reactions. Infants with Down syndrome have increased sensitivity to cardiac effects.

Route and Dosage

IM (Adult): 2 mg initially, then 2 mg every 10 minutes as needed up to 3 times total

IV (Adult): 1 to 2 mg/dose every 10 to 20 minutes until effects are observed

IM (Pediatric more than 10 years, 90 lbs): 2 mg

IM (Pediatric 4 to 10 years, 40 to 90 lbs): 1 mg

IM (Pediatric 6 months to 4 years, 15 to 40 lbs): 0.5 mg

IV (Pediatric): 0.02 to 0.05 mg/kg every 10 to 20 minutes until effects are observed

Understand the Numbers

You are ordered to administer 0.02 mg/kg of atropine IV to your 130-pound pediatric patient. What is the correct dosage for this patient?

130 lb ÷ 2.2 kg = 59 kg. Therefore, 0.02 mg/kg × 59 kg = 1.18 mg.

How Supplied

Injection: 0.05 mg/mL, 0.1 mg/mL, 0.4 mg/mL, 1 mg/mL, 0.5 mg/0.7 mL Auto-injector; 1 mg/0.7 mL Auto-injector; 2 mg/0.7 mL Auto-injector

Adverse Reactions and Side Effects

Resp: Tachypnea, pulmonary edema

CV: Tachycardia, palpitations, arrhythmias

CNS: Drowsiness, confusion

GI: Dry mouth, constipation, impaired GI motility

GU: Urinary hesitancy, urinary retention, impotency

Misc: Flushing, decreased sweating

Drug Interactions: Increases anticholinergic effects if used with other anticholinergics. Antacids decrease the absorption of anticholinergics. Anticholinergics may alter the response to beta-blockers.

EMS Considerations: Initial stabilization should include obtaining and maintaining a patent airway, administering humidified oxygen, and obtaining IV access. Assess the patient frequently for adverse effects and monitor vital signs and ECG continuously.

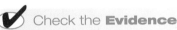

Check the **Evidence**

Severe cases of organophosphate poisoning may require the administration of pralidoxime in addition to atropine.

Diazepam (dye-AZ-e-pam)

🍁 Apo-Diazepam, Diastat, 🍁 Diazemuls, 🍁 Novo-Dipam, 🍁 PMS-Diazepam, Valium, 🍁 Vivol

Classifications: Antianxiety agent, anticonvulsant, sedative/hypnotic, skeletal muscle relaxant, benzodiazepine

Pregnancy Class: D

Mechanism of Action: Depresses the CNS by potentiating GABA, an inhibitory neurotransmitter; produces skeletal muscle relaxation by inhibiting spinal polysynaptic afferent pathways; has anticonvulsant properties due to enhanced presynaptic inhibition

Pharmacokinetics

Absorption: Rapidly absorbed from the GI tract. Absorption from IM sites may be slow and unpredictable; well absorbed (90 percent) from rectal mucosa

Onset: PO—30 to 60 minutes

IM—within 20 minutes

IV—1 to 5 minutes

Rectal—2 to 10 minutes

Duration: PO—up to 24 hours

IM—unknown

IV—15 to 60 minutes

Rectal—4 to 12 hours

Underline indicates most frequent; CAPITALS indicates life-threatening; 🍁 indicates Canadian drug name.

Indications: Prevention or treatment of seizures caused by poisoning or overdoses from various substances; control of advancing CNS overstimulation caused by cocaine overdose
Contraindications: Known hypersensitivity. Do not give diazepam to patients hypersensitive to benzodiazepines or propylene glycol. Do not give to patients with preexisting CNS depression or acute narrow-angle glaucoma or to those who are pregnant or who are lactating.
Precautions: Use with caution in patients with severe kidney impairment, patients with a history of suicide attempt, or patients with a history of drug dependence.

Route and Dosage

IV (Adult): 5 to 10 mg. May be repeated every 10 to 15 minutes to a total dose of 30 mg
IM, IV (Pediatric over 5 years): 0.05 to 0.3 mg/kg/dose over 3 to 5 minutes every 15 to 30 minutes to a total dose of 10 mg

How Supplied

Solution for injection: 5 mg/mL

Adverse Reactions and Side Effects

Resp: Respiratory depression
CV: Hypotension (IV only)
CNS: <u>Dizziness</u>, <u>drowsiness</u>, <u>lethargy</u>, depression, hangover, slurred speech, headache, paradoxical excitation
GI: Constipation, diarrhea, nausea, vomiting
Derm: Rashes
Local: Pain (IM), phlebitis (IV)
Misc: Physical or psychological dependence, tolerance
Drug Interactions: Additive CNS depression if concurrently used with other CNS depressants such as antihistamines, antidepressants, opioid analgesics, or alcohol
EMS Considerations: Monitor blood pressure, pulse, and respiratory rate prior to administration and frequently after IV administration.

Flumazenil (flu-MAZ-e-nil)

🍁 Anexate, Romazicon

Classifications: Antidote, benzodiazepine
Pregnancy Class: C
Mechanism of Action: Antagonizes the CNS depressant effects of benzodiazepines

Check the Evidence

Flumazenil has no effect on CNS depression from other causes, including opioids, alcohol, or barbiturates.

Pharmacokinetics

Absorption: IV administration results in complete bioavailability.
Onset: IV—1 to 2 minutes
Duration: IV—1 to 2 hours

Indications: Used in the management of intentional or accidental overdose of benzodiazepines
Contraindications: Known hypersensitivity. Do not give to patients receiving benzodiazepines for life-threatening medical problems, including status epilepticus or increased intracranial pressure.
Precautions: Use with caution in patients with a history of seizures, head injury, or severe liver impairment.

Route and Dosage

IV (Adult): 0.2 mg. Additional 0.3 mg may be given 30 seconds later. Further doses of 0.5 mg may be given at 1-minute intervals, if necessary, to a total dose of 3 mg.

Effective Communication

Administer each dose of flumazenil 15 to 30 seconds into a free-flowing IV in a large vein.

How Supplied

Injection: 0.1 mg/mL in 5- and 10-mL vials

Adverse Reactions and Side Effects

CV: Arrhythmias, chest pain, hypertension
CNS: SEIZURES, <u>dizziness</u>, agitation, confusion, drowsiness, headache
GI: <u>Nausea</u>, <u>vomiting</u>, hiccups
Derm: Flushing, sweating
Local: Pain, injection-site reactions
Drug Interactions: None significant
EMS Considerations: If the patient has not responded 5 minutes after receiving a cumulative dose of 3 mg, the major cause of sedation is probably not from benzodiazepines. The duration of the effect of a benzodiazepine may exceed that of flumazenil. Therefore, observe closely for resedation and redose if needed. Be prepared for patients attempting to remove airway or IV access while awakening.

Glucagon (GLOO-ka-gon)

GlucaGen

Classification: Hormone
Pregnancy Class: B
Mechanism of Action: Glucagon is a hormone excreted by the alpha cells of the pancreas. When released, glucagon increases the level of circulating blood sugar by stimulating the release of glycogen.

Pharmacokinetics

Absorption: Well absorbed
Onset: IV—1 minute
Duration: IV—60 to 90 minutes

Indications: Can be used as an antidote for beta-blocker and calcium channel-blocker overdose
Contraindications: Known hypersensitivity; should not be given to patients with pheochromocytoma—a catecholamine-secreting tumor
Precautions: Use with caution in patients who are fasting or who have adrenal insufficiency or chronic hypoglycemia.

Route and Dosage
IV (Adult, beta-blocker overdose): 50 to 150 mcg (0.05 to 0.15 mg)/kg loading dose, followed by 1 to 5 mg/hr IV infusion
IV (Adult, calcium channel-blocker overdose): 2 mg; may require additional dosing
How Supplied
Powder for injection: 1 mg vials
Adverse Reactions and Side Effects
CV: Hypotension
GI: Nausea, vomiting
Misc: ANAPHYLAXIS
Drug Interactions: Large doses may enhance the effect of warfarin. Glucagon negates the response to insulin or oral hypoglycemic agents.
EMS Considerations: Assess for signs of hypoglycemia (sweating, weakness, headache, dizziness, tremor, irritability, tachycardia, anxiety) prior to and frequently during treatment.

Hydroxocobalamin (hye-drox-oh-koe-BAL-a-min)

CYANOKIT
Classification: Vitamin B_{12} preparation, cyanide poisoning antidote
Pregnancy Class: C
Mechanism of Action: A necessary coenzyme for metabolic processes, including fat and carbohydrate metabolism and protein synthesis; required for cell production

Check the Evidence

Hydroxocobalamin neutralizes cyanide without interfering with cellular oxygen use. It is conducive with EMS use due to its tolerability and safety profiles.

Pharmacokinetics
Absorption: Well absorbed
Onset: Rapid
Duration: Unknown
Indications: Used to reverse the symptoms of cyanide toxicity
Contraindications: Known hypersensitivity
Precautions: Use with caution in patients with kidney dysfunction. The safety and effectiveness have not been established in pediatrics.
Route and Dosage
IV (Adult): 5 g over 15 minutes. Another 5 g dose may be infused over 15 to 120 minutes depending upon severity of the poisoning. The maximum cumulative dose is 10 g.
How Supplied
Powder for injection: 2.5 g/vial (2 vials in each kit)
Adverse Reactions and Side Effects
Resp: Dyspnea
CV: Hypertension, chest pain, tachycardia
CNS: Dizziness, memory impairment, restlessness
GI: Abdominal discomfort, nausea, vomiting
GU: Red urine
Drug Interactions: None
EMS Considerations: If any other drugs are administered, they should be given through a separate IV line.

Naloxone (nal-OX-one)

Narcan
Classification: Antidote (opioids)
Pregnancy Class: B
Mechanism of Action: Blocks the effects of opioids, including CNS and respiratory depression, without producing any opioid-like effects.
Pharmacokinetics
Absorption: Well absorbed
Onset: IM, SubQ—2 to 5 minutes
IV—1 to 2 minutes
Duration: IM, SubQ—more than 45 minutes
IV—45 minutes
Indication: Used for the reversal of CNS and respiratory depression because of suspected opioid overdose
Contraindications: Known hypersensitivity
Precautions: Use with caution in patients with cardiovascular disease and in patients physically dependent on opioids, because naloxone may cause **withdrawal symptoms**, irritability, autonomic hyperactivity, hallucinations, or other phenomena resulting from opiates.
Route and Dosage
SubQ, IM, IV (Adult not suspected of being opioid dependent): 0.4 mg (10 mcg/kg); may be repeated every 2 to 3 minutes (IV route is preferred)
SubQ, IM, IV (Adult suspected to be opioid dependent): 0.1 to 0.2 mg every 2 to 3 minutes; may also be given by IV infusion at a rate adjusted to patient's response

Understand the Numbers

For IV infusion, dilute 2 mg of naloxone in 500 mL of 0.9 percent NS or D5W. This will give you a concentration of 4 mcg/mL (2 mg ÷ 500 mL = 0.004 mg/mL = 4.0 mcg/mL).

SubQ, IM, IV (Pediatric over 5 years or more than 20 kg): 2 mg/dose; may be repeated every 2 to 3 minutes
SubQ, IM, IV (Pediatric up to 5 years or 20 kg): 0.1 mg/kg; may be repeated every 2 to 3 minutes
How Supplied
Injection: 0.4 mg/mL, 1 mg/mL
Adverse Reactions and Side Effects
CV: VENTRICULAR ARRHYTHMIAS, hypertension or hypotension
GI: Nausea, vomiting
Drug Interactions: Can precipitate withdrawal in patients physically dependent on opioid analgesics
EMS Considerations: The duration of action of naloxone is shorter than that of narcotics. Therefore, repeat doses of naloxone may be necessary. Monitor vital signs and ECG continuously.

Phentolamine (fen-TOLE-a-meen)

OraVerse, Regitine, ♣ Rogitine
Classifications: Alpha-adrenergic blocker, antihypertensive
Pregnancy Class: C
Mechanism of Action: Produces vasodilation by blocking alpha-adrenergic receptors
Pharmacokinetics
Absorption: Well absorbed following IM and IV administration
Onset: IM—unknown
IV—immediate
Duration: IM—30 to 45 minutes
IV—15 to 30 minutes
Indications: Used to treat hypertensive emergencies caused by pheochromocytoma or cocaine-induced vasospasm of the coronary arteries
Contraindications: Known hypersensitivity; should not be given to patients with coronary or cerebral arteriosclerosis, or to patients with kidney impairment
Precautions: Use with caution in patients with peptic ulcer disease.
Route and Dosage
IV (Adult): 5 mg; may be repeated if necessary
How Supplied
Powder for injection: 5 mg/vial

Effective Communication

Reconstitute each 5 mg of phentolamine with 1 mL of sterile water for injection or 0.9 percent NS. Properly discard unused portion.

Adverse Reactions and Side Effects
CV: HYPOTENSION, MI, angina, arrhythmias, tachycardia
CNS: CEREBROVASCULAR SPASM, dizziness, weakness
GI: Abdominal pain, diarrhea, nausea, vomiting
EENT: Nasal stuffiness
Derm: Flushing
Drug Interactions: Antagonizes the effects of alpha-adrenergic stimulants. Severe hypotension may occur with the concurrent use of epinephrine.
EMS Considerations: Monitor blood pressure, pulse, and ECG frequently until the patient is stable.

Check the **Evidence**

If a hypotensive crisis occurs, epinephrine is contraindicated because it may cause paradoxical further decrease in blood pressure. Norepinephrine may be used.

Pralidoxime (pra-li-DOKS-eem)

2-PAM, Protopam
Classifications: Antidote (organophosphate poisoning), anticholinesterase inhibitor
Pregnancy Class: C
Mechanism of Action: Reactivates cholinesterase that has been inactivated by organophosphate poisoning or anticholinesterase overdose; results in the reversal of respiratory paralysis and paralysis of skeletal muscles
Pharmacokinetics
Absorption: Well absorbed
Onset: IM, IV; varies
Duration: IM, IV; approximately 3 hours
Indications: Use after atropine in severe cases of organophosphate poisoning and for the treatment of anticholinesterase overdose.
Contraindications: Known hypersensitivity; should not be given to patients who have been poisoned by inorganic phosphates
Precautions: Use with caution in patients with myasthenia gravis because it may precipitate a myasthenic crisis. Dosage reduction may be necessary for patients with impaired kidney function; pralidoxime may accumulate to toxic concentrations.
Route and Dosage
IV (Adult, organophosphate poisoning): 1 to 2 g IV infusion over 30 to 60 minutes after atropine administration. Give 600 mg IM if IV access cannot be obtained.
IV (Adult, anticholinesterase overdose): 1 to 2 g IV infusion over 30 to 60 minutes; then give 250 mg every 5 minutes as needed

Understand the Numbers

You are ordered to administer 2 g of pralidoxime by IV infusion over 30 minutes. You add the pralidoxime to 250 mL of NS. What is the resulting concentration (in mg) of drug in the IV bag? Concentration = 2 g = 2,000 mg ÷ 250 mL = 8 mg/mL

How Supplied
Powder for injection: 1 g/20mL vial
Auto-injector (IM use): 600 mg/2mL
Adverse Reactions and Side Effects
Resp: Laryngospasm, hyperventilation
CV: Tachycardia
CNS: Dizziness, drowsiness, headache
GI: Nausea
Derm: Rash
HEENT: Blurred vision, double vision
Misc: Muscle rigidity, muscle weakness
Drug Interactions: Do not use concurrently with succinylcholine, morphine, aminophylline, theophylline, and respiratory depressants.
EMS Considerations: Draw a blood sample before drug administration. Rapid administration may cause tachycardia, laryngospasm, or muscle rigidity.

Sodium Bicarbonate (SOE-dee-um bye-KAR-boe-nate)

Classification: Alkalinizing agent
Pregnancy Class: C

Mechanism of Action: Buffers excess acid to assist returning the blood to a physiological pH, in which normal metabolic processes work more effectively. Sodium bicarbonate is excreted in the urine, resulting in an alkalinized pH of the urine that causes increased urinary elimination of some drugs, such as barbiturates and aspirin.

Pharmacokinetics

Absorption: Well absorbed

Onset: IV—immediate

Duration: IV—unknown

Indications: Used in the treatment of metabolic acidosis in certain poisonings or overdoses, such as ethylene glycol (antifreeze), aspirin, and methanol; promotes urinary excretion of some drugs taken in overdoses such as barbiturates and aspirin

Contraindications: Known hypersensitivity; should not be given to patients with metabolic or respiratory alkalosis, hypocalcemia, or excessive chloride loss; as an antidote following ingestion of strong mineral acids; or in patients who cannot tolerate high sodium loads

Precautions: Use with caution in patients with CHF and kidney insufficiency and in those who are concurrently using corticosteroid therapy.

Route and Dosage

IV (Adult & Pediatric): 1 mEq/kg slow IV; may be repeated at 0.5 mEq in 10 minutes

How Supplied

Vials/prefilled syringe: 8.4 percent (1 mEq/kg) in 10- and 50-mL vials and prefilled syringes

Adverse Reactions and Side Effects

CV: Edema

Local: Irritation at IV site

Fluids and electrolytes: Metabolic alkalosis, hypocalcemia, hypokalemia, sodium and water retention

Drug Interactions: Sodium bicarbonate may inactivate catecholamines and will form a precipitate with calcium agents.

EMS Considerations: Monitor patients closely for the possible development of fluid overload (rales, peripheral edema, pink and frothy sputum).

Sodium Nitrite (SO-dee-um NY-tryt)

Classification: Cyanide poisoning adjunct

Pregnancy Class: X

Mechanism of Action: Sodium nitrite reacts with hemoglobin to form methemoglobin. Methemoglobin reacts with cyanide, causing the cyanide to be chemically bound, which prevents it from having any toxic effect.

Pharmacokinetics

Absorption: Well absorbed

Onset: 2 to 6 minutes

Duration: Unknown

Indications: Sodium nitrite is the second of a three-step treatment protocol for cyanide poisoning. It should be preceded by amyl nitrite and followed by sodium thiosulfate.

Effective Communication

An IV can be started for the sodium nitrite and the sodium thiosulfate while the patient is inhaling the amyl nitrite.

Contraindications: Known hypersensitivity

Precautions: Sodium nitrite is a strong vasodilator. If administered too rapidly, it could cause significant hypotension.

Route and Dosage

IV (Adult): 300 mg over 5 minutes after amyl nitrite inhalation

Understand the Numbers

You can also infuse the sodium nitrite by diluting 300 mg in 50 to 100 mL of NS, infusing slowly.

IV (Pediatric): 0.15 to 0.33 mL/kg slow IV

How Supplied

Injection: 3 percent (300 mg/10 mL) solution

Drug Interactions: Not applicable

EMS Considerations: Monitor blood pressure during administration. Excessive doses of sodium nitrite may cause methemoglobinemia and death. Signs of methemoglobinemia include cyanosis, vomiting, shock, and coma.

Sodium Thiosulfate (SO-dee-um thye-oh-SUL-fate)

Classification: Cyanide poisoning adjunct

Pregnancy Class: C

Mechanism of Action: Sodium thiosulfate converts cyanide to the less toxic thiocyanate. Thiocyanate is then excreted in the urine, and the body is detoxified.

Pharmacokinetics

Absorption: Well absorbed

Onset: 2 to 5 minutes

Duration: Unknown

Indication: Sodium thiosulfate is the third of a three-step treatment protocol for cyanide poisoning. It should be preceded by amyl nitrite and sodium nitrite.

Contraindication: Known hypersensitivity

Precautions: None

Route and Dosage

IV (Adult): 12.5 g slow IV bolus

IV (Pediatric): 1.65 mL/kg slow IV bolus

How Supplied

Injection: 25 percent (12.5 g/50 mL solution)

Adverse Reactions and Side Effects

GI: Nausea, vomiting

Drug Interactions: Not applicable

EMS Considerations: If the clinical response to treatment is inadequate, administer a second dose of both sodium nitrite and sodium thiosulfate at half the initial doses, 30 minutes after the initial doses.

SCENARIO REVISITED

Did you consider the case of Quinton?

As you recall, Quinton, 17, is the patient with a possible (Tofranil-PM, tricyclic antidepressant [TCA]) overdose. Tricyclic antidepressants are often used in suicide attempts. Adverse reactions and side effects of Tofranil-PM include sedation, drowsiness, confusion, hypotension, convulsions, life-threatening arrhythmias, and coma. The evidence of alcohol ingestion in conjunction with a TCA overdose means that this is truly an emergency situation. It is important to maintain a patent airway, give humidified oxygen, establish an IV, and monitor Quinton's ECG.

You place Quentin in the ambulance and continue treatment while en route to the emergency department (ED).

On the way to the ED, Quinton develops seizure activity. Your protocol states that the drug of choice in this situation is diazepam, a benzodiazepine. While en route, medical control orders 5 mg of diazepam.

Check the **Evidence**

Benzodiazepines, such as diazepam, are recommended for TCA-associated convulsions. However, flumazenil, a benzodiazepine derivative, is not recommended for patients with TCA poisoning. Flumazenil is indicated for the management of benzodiazepine overdose.

Once you have performed an appropriate assessment, you should proceed using a critical thinking approach to medication administration.

Step 1: Determine signs and symptoms to be treated.
Step 2: Consider both the risks and benefits of treating or not treating your patient.
Step 3: Choose the medication that provides the best possible outcome.
Step 4: Remember the drug's indications, contraindications, and precautions.
Step 5: Decide the best route for administering the medication for the best outcome.
Step 6: Administer the medication(s) according to the seven Patient Rights.

1. The right patient
2. The right drug
3. The right drug amount
4. The right time
5. The right route
6. The right documentation
7. The right of the patient to accept or refuse the medication(s)

Step 7: Reevaluate the patient for the desired and undesired effects.

Let's Recap

Toxicological emergencies are becoming more and more common in out-of-hospital emergency care. Patients who are experiencing either poisoning or overdose emergencies should be treated symptomatically. The initial out-of-hospital management of toxicological emergencies should include management of the ABCs, the administration of humidified oxygen, the establishment of an IV, and placement of the patient on a cardiac monitor.

Management of poisoning emergencies includes identifying the poison, attempting to slow or stop the absorption process, and administering an antidote. Management of overdose emergencies is aimed at stabilizing the ABCs and, in some cases, giving antidotes.

SCENARIO CONCLUSION

After you give the 5 mg of diazepam, the seizure activity subsides. However, when you assess Quinton's ECG, you notice he has a rate of 100 beats/minute with a widening of the QRS complex. A widening of the QRS complex is an indication that metabolic acidosis may be developing (Fig. 17-2). Therefore, medical control may order sodium bicarbonate at a dosage of 1 to 2 mEq/kg. Finally, the lack of improvement in Quinton's overall condition could be caused by his blood alcohol level, the possible ingestion of another drug, or hypoglycemia. It would be appropriate to give Quinton 25 g (50 mL) of $D_{50}W$ to reverse possible hypoglycemia while still en route to the ED.

Out-of-hospital treatment of TCA overdose is symptomatic. Toxic syndromes such as cardiac arrhythmias, seizures, and CHF can occur rapidly. Treatment protocols may also include advanced cardiovascular life support (ACLS) guidelines. Patients must be transported rapidly to the ED.

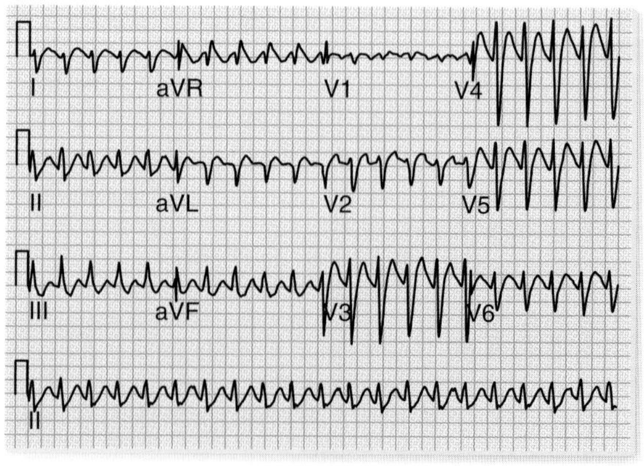

Figure 17-2 ECG indicating possible TCA overdose.

PRACTICE EXERCISES

1. Amyl nitrite is indicated in the treatment of:
   a. Narcotic overdose
   b. Cyanide poisoning
   c. Anticholinergic poisoning
   d. Organophosphate poisoning
2. Naloxone is classified therapeutically as a(n):
   a. Cholinesterase poisoning antidote
   b. Cyanide poisoning adjunct
   c. Narcotic antagonist
   d. Emetic
3. Your patient has overdosed on an unknown amount of cocaine. She is experiencing severe chest pain. The physician orders you to give her phentolamine. The initial dose is:
   a. 15 mg SubQ
   b. 15 mg IV
   c. 5 mg SubQ
   d. 5 mg IV
4. Flumazenil is used in the treatment of:
   a. Benzodiazepine overdose
   b. Phenobarbital overdose
   c. Narcotic overdose
   d. Aspirin overdose
5. The initial IM adult dose of atropine for organophosphate poisoning is:
   a. 1 mg
   b. 2 mg
   c. 3 mg
   d. 4 mg
6. Sodium thiosulfate is one of the drugs used in the treatment of:
   a. Cocaine overdose
   b. Cyanide poisoning
   c. Aspirin overdose
   d. Opioid overdose
7. The initial dose of hydroxocobalamin for the treatment of cyanide poisoning is:
   a. 5 mcg
   b. 15 mg
   c. 15 g
   d. 5 g
8. A cardiovascular life-threatening adverse reaction of phentolamine is:
   a. Tachycardia
   b. Hypotension
   c. Arrhythmias
   d. Angina
9. In severe cases of organophosphate poisoning, pralidoxime should be given after:
   a. Naloxone
   b. Atropine
   c. Amyl nitrite
   d. Sodium bicarbonate
10. A contraindication for the use of diazepam is:
    a. Preexisting CNS depression
    b. Liver dysfunction
    c. Drug addiction
    d. Psychosis

CASE STUDIES

1. You and your partner are dispatched to a farm, and upon arrival you are directed to the cotton field. A male patient is found lying on the ground, shivering. The patient's son says that his father was spraying malathion on the cotton crop when he started "acting funny" just before he collapsed. Initial assessment of the patient reveals the following:
   Level of consciousness: Depressed, responds to pain, in obvious distress
   Resp: 36/minute, shallow
   Pulse: 42 beats/minute, regular
   Blood pressure: 60 systolic
   Skin: Diaphoretic
   Eyes: Watering, constricted pupils

   The patient is also salivating and has a watering nose. His shivering is caused by virtually all of his skeletal muscles twitching simultaneously.

   This patient is probably suffering from:
   a. Narcotic overdose
   b. Cyanide poisoning
   c. Stroke
   d. Organophosphate poisoning

   Pharmacologic treatment for this patient will probably include:
   a. Amyl nitrite and sodium nitrite
   b. Naloxone and pralidoxime
   c. Atropine and diazepam
   d. Atropine and pralidoxime

2. You and your partner respond to the home of a 21-year-old male known cocaine abuser. On arrival, the patient is found lying unresponsive in a closet. He has a pair of panty hose tied around his right arm. There are obvious "tracks" on both arms. The patient's roommate says the patient had been high on cocaine and suddenly became unconscious. Further assessment reveals the following:
Level of consciousness: Unconscious; responds to painful stimuli by occasional tonic and clonic jerking movements and incoherent speech
Resp: 28/minute, shallow
Pulse: 124 beats/minute, irregular
Blood pressure: 190/102
Skin: Warm and moist
Pupils: Dilated, slow to react

Medical control instructs you to start an IV of normal saline (NS). The first drug ordered in this case will probably be:
   a. Pralidoxime
   b. Naloxone
   c. Atropine
   d. Diazepam

MATH EQUATIONS

1. You are ordered to infuse 150 mg/kg of acetylcysteine to your patient over 1 hour. Your patient weighs 195 lbs.
   a. How many kg does your patient weigh?
   b. How many gtts/minute will you infuse the acetylcysteine using a 60 gtt/mL IV set?
2. You are ordered to give 0.01 mg/kg of flumazenil to your 95 lb pediatric patient. The maximum dose of flumazenil for this patient is 0.2 mg.
   a. How many kg does your patient weigh?
   b. How many mg of flumazenil will you administer?
3. You are ordered to give 10 mcg/kg of naloxone to your patient, repeating every 2 to 3 minutes as needed. The maximum dosage is 2 mg. Your patient weighs 145 lbs.
   a. How many kg does your patient weigh?
   b. How many doses of the naloxone will it take to equal 2 mg?
4. You are ordered to give 0.15 mL/kg of sodium nitrate to your 85 lb pediatric patient. You have sodium nitrate as 300 mg/10 mL.
   a. How many kg does your patient weigh?
   b. How many mL is required for this patient to receive 0.15 mL/kg?
5. You are ordered to administer 2 g of pralidoxime by IV infusion over 30 minutes. You add the pralidoxime to 250 mL of NS. What is the resulting concentration (mg/mL) of drug in the IV solution?

REFERENCES

American Association of Poison Control Centers. (2013). www.aapcc.org

Beck, R. K. (2012). Drugs used to treat gastrointestinal emergencies. In *Pharmacology for the EMS provider.* New York, NY: Delmar, Cengage Learning.

Canadian Poison Control Centres. (2013). Canadian Poison Control Centres contact information. www.safetyxchange.org/health-safety/canadian-poison-control-centres-contact-information

Deglin, J. H., Vallerand, A. H., and Sanboski, C. A. (2011). *Davis's drug guide for nurses* (12th ed.). Philadelphia, PA: F. A. Davis Company.

Leybell, I., and Tarabar, A. Cyanide toxicity medication. (2013). Retrieved September 29, 2013 from http://emedicine.medscape.com/article/814287-medication.

Venes, D., ed. (2013). *Taber's cyclopedic medical dictionary* (22nd ed.). Philadelphia, PA: F. A. Davis Company.

Vivian, T. (2012). Tricyclic antidepressant toxicity and management. Retrieved October 5, 2013 from http://emedicine.medscape.com/article/819204-treatment

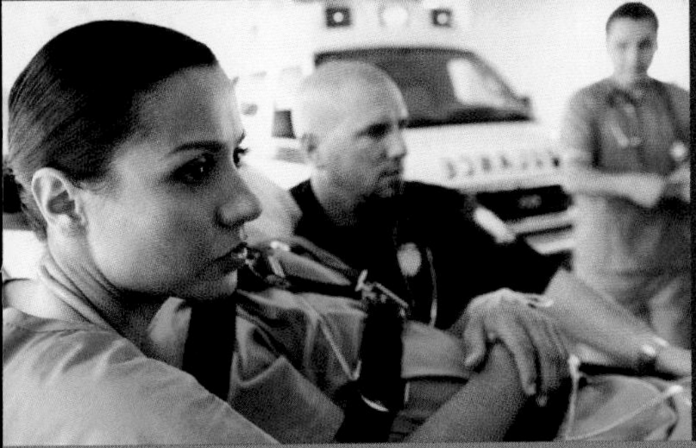

CHAPTER 18

Drugs Used to Treat Behavioral Emergencies

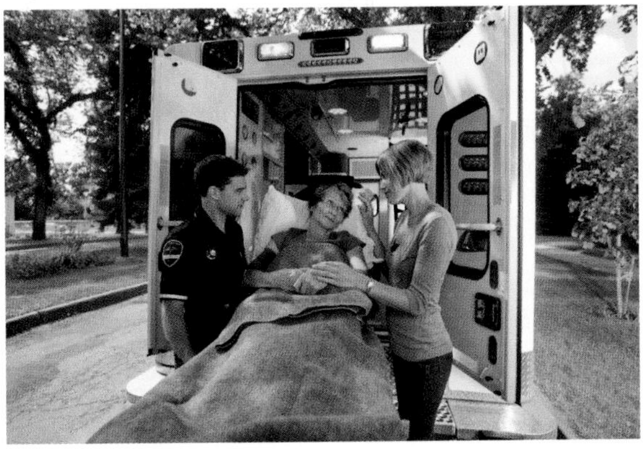

Paramedic assessing a patient with a possible behavioral disorder. *(Photograph © tyler olson/iStock/Thinkstock)*

LEARNING OUTCOMES

- Describe the basic principles to follow when treating a patient with a behavioral emergency.
- Describe and list the indications, contraindications, precautions, route, dosage, and side effects for the following:
  - The antihistamine diphenhydramine
  - The antianxiety drugs diazepam, hydroxyzine, lorazepam, and midazolam
  - The antipsychotic drugs chlorpromazine, haloperidol, olanzapine, and ziprasidone
  - The sedative and hypnotic drug droperidol

KEY TERMS

Antipsychotic
Anxiety
Behavior
Behavioral emergency
Chemical restraint
Psychosis

SCENARIO OPENING

You and your partner respond to a local warehouse for a "man acting bizarre." While en route, it is requested that the police also respond.

On arrival, the warehouse foreman tells you that the patient, Ron Reilly, is an excellent employee and has never before caused problems. However, today he has been very loud, has broken several pieces of equipment, and has been rude to several of his fellow workers. He is now sitting quietly at a table in the corner. His wife is in the foreman's office, confused and scared.

Before approaching Mr. Reilly, you go and talk with his wife in an attempt to determine what may be going on in his life that may have triggered today's problem. Mr. Reilly's wife, Rachelle, states that her husband has been under a lot of stress at work lately because of increased project deadlines. He is 40 years old, in good health, takes no medications, and has no history of psychiatric disorders.

You approach Mr. Reilly slowly, in a peaceful manner. You calmly explain to Mr. Reilly why you and your partner were called and assure him that you are there to help in any way that you can. So far, Mr. Reilly has exhibited no aggressive behavior and has permitted you and your partner to take his vital signs; they are as follows:

Level of consciousness:	alert, disoriented
Respirations:	16 breaths/minute and regular
Pulse:	82 beats/minute, regular (Fig. 18-1)
Blood pressure:	156/96

There are no other obvious signs of trauma or medical problems.

You and your partner should be thinking about the following questions:

1. What do you think the diagnosis will be for Mr. Reilly?
2. What are the goals for your treatment?
3. What steps will you take to help Mr. Reilly?
4. What is your rationale for choosing your treatment options for Mr. Reilly?
5. How will you know if the treatment choices are working?

These five questions are suggestions. You may have other relevant questions as well.

effective **Communication**

Approach the patient with a suspected mental disorder in a slow, calm, deliberate manner. Calmly explain why you were called and assure him that you are there to help in any way that you can.

It is very difficult for an EMS professional to eliminate probable causes of patients who have a possible behavioral emergency. It is not appropriate to draw any definite conclusions based solely on information gathered from the patient's history, which is only suggestive at best.

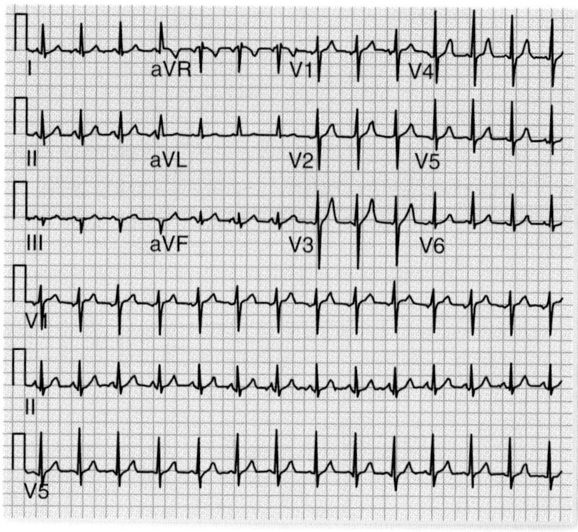

Figure 18-1 Normal sinus rhythm.

It can be frustrating to try to communicate with this type of patient, who may not be dealing with reality. A commonsense approach to the patient, combining reassurance with reinforcement of factual information, is recommended.

Introduction

Many EMS professionals feel most uncomfortable and unprepared when treating patients in behavioral emergencies. As a result, many EMS professionals are uncertain when faced with behavioral emergencies. This uncertainty stems in part from the lack of behavior protocols for out-of-hospital use and in part from the knowledge that the outcome of a behavioral emergency is not as predictable as that of trauma or other medical emergencies. The behavioral emergency presents us with the most unpredictable scenarios and patient outcomes.

One of the medical definitions of **behavior** is the actions or reactions of individuals under specific circumstances. For example, most of us get excited when our favorite team wins, and we get a little nervous when we go to the dentist or when we have to see the boss for our annual evaluation. There are common reactions that most of us consider the "norm." We experience these in our everyday lives.

A **behavioral emergency** goes beyond the norm, causing a change in the patient's mood or behavior that cannot be tolerated, and it requires immediate attention. Specific causes for behavioral disorders are not known; however, most behavioral emergencies are related to biological, psychosocial, or sociocultural influences (Table 18-1).

There are no definite presenting signs or symptoms for individuals with a behavioral disorder. Basically, a behavioral "emergency" call is a result of anxiety on the part of the patient, the patient's family, or bystanders. **Anxiety** is a feeling of apprehension caused by the anticipation of danger. The source

Table 18-1 Common Influences of Behavioral Emergencies

Biological	Psychosocial	Sociocultural
Prenatal factors	Childhood trauma	Relationships
Genetic factors	Childhood abuse	Unstable family
Chemical imbalance in the brain	Dysfunctional family	Economic status
Altered neurotransmission	Biological disorders	Social values
		Work situation
		Personal values

of the anxiety is often nonspecific or unknown to the patient. The problem for EMS is that abnormal behavior may stem from mental illness or some other condition.

effective Communication

Your EMS call can come in as "bizarre behavior" indicating a possible behavioral emergency, but, while preforming your assessment, do not rule out the possibility of drug or alcohol abuse, stroke, infection, or a metabolic disorder that can appear to indicate a behavioral or mental problem.

These are the basic principles to follow when treating an individual who shows signs of a psychological or emotional disorder.

1. Clearly identify yourself, being as calm and direct as possible.
2. If possible, interview the patient alone, letting the individual tell his own story.
3. Provide honest reassurance, maintaining a nonjudgmental attitude.
4. Take a definite plan of action. This will help to relieve the patient's anxiety.
5. Never leave the patient alone and never assume it is impossible to talk with the patient unless you have tried.

Only rarely do the most progressive EMS systems use pharmacologic interventions when treating behavioral emergencies. Patient management is generally directed at supportive measures and the attempt to give the patient a feeling of friendly and secure surroundings. However, there may be times when a patient must be restrained either physically or with the use of drugs. The term **chemical restraint** refers to administering specific drugs to a patient for the purpose of providing sedation.

Check the **Evidence**

When chemical restraint is used, there is a decrease in patient agitation. Paramedics are most likely to use chemical sedation drugs for life or limb threats to facilitate assessment after an assault on the EMS team, as well as for the most agitated patients.

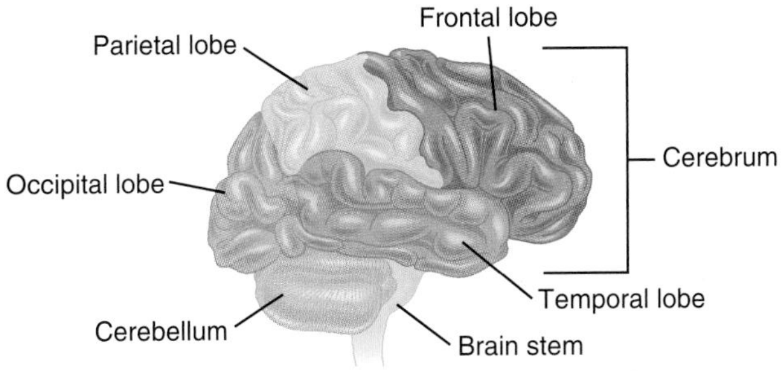

Figure 18-2 The brain.

Ten drugs that some out-of-hospital systems use to treat patients with behavioral emergencies are covered in this chapter: chlorpromazine, diazepam, diphenhydramine, droperidol, haloperidol, hydroxyzine, lorazepam, midazolam, olanzapine, and ziprasidone.

Pathophysiology of the Brain

The brain is a soft, compact organ responsible for consciousness, planned neural programs, and cognition. There are three primary areas of the brain; the cerebrum, the brain stem, and cerebellum (Fig. 18-2).

Cerebrum

The cerebrum consists of two hemispheres, each containing four lobes.

Frontal Lobes

- Perform high-level cognitive functions such as reasoning, concentration, and control.
- Provide information storage.
- Control voluntary eye movement.
- Influence somatic motor control of activities such as respiration, GI activity, and blood pressure regulation.
- Perform motor control of speech.
- Controls voluntary motor function.
- Contain the motor association areas that are involved with generalized movement.

Parietal Lobes

- Interpret sensory information to define size, weight, shape, consistency, texture, and awareness of body parts.

Temporal Lobes

- Contain the primary auditory areas.
- Involved with auditory, visual, olfactory, and somatic perception and integration.

Occipital Lobes

- Contain the primary visual cortex and visual association areas.

Brain Stem

The brain stem consists of three areas: the midbrain, the pons, and the medulla.

Midbrain

- The midbrain processes visual stimuli, integrates visual and auditory motor reflexes, and relays auditory information.

Pons

- The pons is the bridge between the midbrain and the medulla. It connects higher cerebral regions with the lower regions of the nervous system.

Medulla

- The medulla transmits information for the coordination of head and eye movement, contains cardiac, vasomotor, and respiratory centers.

Cerebellum

The cerebellum controls fine movement, coordinates muscle groups, and maintains balance. Table 18-2 gives an overview of the pathophysiology of the brain.

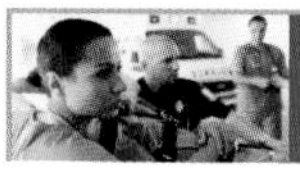

Table 18-2 Overview of the Pathophysiology of the Brain

Frontal Lobe
• Emotions
• Short-term memory
• Voluntary movement
• Expressive language
• Social functioning
Parietal Lobe
• Sensation
• Comprehension of speech and reading
• Production of writing and calculation
• Awareness of size and shape
Temporal Lobe
• Hearing
• Smell
• Long-term memory
• Musical awareness
Occipital Lobe
• Visual perception
Brain Stem
• Appetite, chewing, taste, swallowing
• Smell
• Vision, eye, and eyelid muscle movement
• Pulse, respiration, and blood pressure regulation
• Hearing and balance
• Wakefulness
• Upper GI peristalsis
• Facial sensation
• Neck muscle movement
Cerebellum
• Balance
• Coordination

Pharmacokinetics

Antianxiety Drugs

Most antianxiety drugs cause generalized CNS depression. Benzodiazepines may produce tolerance with long-term use and thus have the potential for dependence. Antianxiety drugs are used in the management of various forms of anxiety, including generalized anxiety disorder.

Antihistamines

Antihistamines block the effects of histamine at the H_1 receptor. Most antihistamines have anticholinergic properties and may cause constipation, dry eyes, dry mouth, and blurred vision. This chapter will present diphenhydramine due to its effects on extrapyramidal side effects of some drugs used for behavioral disorders.

Antipsychotics

Antipsychotics block dopamine receptors in the brain. Peripheral effects include anticholinergic properties and alpha-adrenergic blockade. Antipsychotics are used in the treatment of acute and chronic psychoses (plural of psychosis), particularly when accompanied by increased psychomotor activity. **Psychosis** is a mental disorder in which there is severe loss of contact with reality, evidenced by delusions, hallucinations, disorganized speech patterns, and bizarre or catatonic behavior. Selected antipsychotics are also used as antihistamines or antiemetics.

Sedatives and Hypnotics

Sedatives and hypnotics cause generalized CNS depression. They may produce tolerance with chronic use and thus have the potential for dependence. These classes of drugs have no analgesic properties. Sedatives are used to provide sedation, while hypnotics are used to manage insomnia. Some of these drugs are used as anticonvulsants, and some are used as adjuncts in the management of alcohol withdrawal syndrome.

Individual Drugs

ChlorproMAZINE (klor-PROH-mah-zeen)

🍁 Chlorpromanyl, 🍁 Largactil, 🍁 Novo-Chlorpromazine, Thorazine

Classifications: Antipsychotic, antiemetic

Pregnancy Class: C

Mechanism of Action: Alters the effects of dopamine in the CNS; has significant anticholinergic and alpha-adrenergic blocking activity

Pharmacokinetics

Absorption: PO—Variable
IM—Well absorbed

Onset: PO—30 to 60 minutes
IM—unknown
IV—rapid

Duration: PO and IM—4 to 8 hours
IV—unknown

Indications: Used as second-line treatment for schizophrenia and psychoses after failure with atypical antipsychotics; can also be given for the treatment of mild alcohol withdrawal
Contraindications: Known hypersensitivity; should not be given to patients who are hypersensitive to sulfites, patients with severe liver disease, or patients with severe cardiovascular disease; should not be given to patients concurrently with pimozide

effective Communication

It is important that you do a medication assessment with your patient. If your patient is currently taking pimozide and you also give chlorpromazine, the patient has an increased risk of potentially serious cardiovascular reactions.

Precautions: Use with caution in patients with diabetes, respiratory disease, prostatic hyperplasia, epilepsy, or intestinal obstruction.

Route and Dosage

PO (Adult): 10 to 25 mg
PO (Pediatric): 0.55 mg/kg
IM (Adult): 25 to 50 mg
IM (Pediatric): 0.55 mg/kg

How Supplied

Tablets: 10 mg, 25 mg, 50 mg, 100 mg, 200 mg
Injection: 25 mg/mL

Adverse Reactions and Side Effects

CV: Hypotension, tachycardia
CNS: NEUROLEPTIC MALIGNANT SYNDROME, sedation, extrapyramidal reactions, tardive dyskinesia

Check the **Evidence**

Extrapyramidal reactions are neuromuscular effects that can be caused by some antipsychotic drugs. Reactions include Parkinson-like symptoms, akathisia, dystonias, and tardive dyskinesia. If this occurs, a common EMS medication that can be given for treatment is diphenhydramine (page 248).

GI: Constipation, dry mouth, anorexia, priapism
GU: Urinary retention
EENT: Blurred vision, dry eyes
Metab: Hyperthermia
Drug Interactions: Concurrent use with pimozide increases the risk of potentially serious cardiovascular reactions. Additive CNS depression may occur if chlorpromazine is given with antidepressants, antihistamines, MAO inhibitors, opioid analgesics, or sedatives/hypnotics or if the patient recently ingested alcohol.
EMS Considerations: Monitor blood pressure, pulse, and respiratory rate prior to and after administration.

Diazepam (dye-AZ-eh-pam)

🍁 Apo-Diazepam, Diastat, 🍁 Diazemuls, 🍁 Novo-Dipam, 🍁 PMS-Diazepam, Valium, 🍁 Vivol

Classifications: Antianxiety, anticonvulsant, sedative/hypnotic, skeletal muscle relaxant
Pregnancy Class: D
Mechanism of Action: Depresses the CNS by potentiating gamma-aminobutyric acid (GABA), an inhibitory neurotransmitter; produces skeletal muscle relaxation by inhibiting spinal polysynaptic afferent pathways; has anticonvulsant properties due to enhanced presynaptic inhibition
Pharmacokinetics
Absorption: Rapidly absorbed from the GI tract. Absorption from IM sites may be slow and unpredictable. Well absorbed (90 percent) from rectal mucosa.
Onset: PO—30 to 60 minutes
IM—within 20 minutes
IV—1 to 5 minutes
Rectal—2 to 10 minutes
Duration: PO—up to 24 hours
IM—unknown
IV—15 to 60 minutes
Rectal—4 to 12 hours
Indications: Used as an adjunct in the management of anxiety disorder; can also be given for the treatment of status epilepticus, as a skeletal muscle relaxant, and for the management of the symptoms of alcohol withdrawal
Contraindications: Known hypersensitivity; should not be given to patients with myasthenia gravis, severe pulmonary impairment, sleep apnea, severe liver dysfunction, preexisting CNS depression, uncontrolled severe pain, and angle-closure glaucoma
Precautions: Use with caution in patients with severe kidney impairment, patients with a history of suicide attempt, or patients with a history of drug dependence.

Route and Dosage

PO (Adult, Antianxiety): 2–10 mg
IV (Adult, Seizures/Status epilepticus): 5 to 10 mg
PO (Adult, Skeletal Muscle Relaxation): 2 to 10 mg
IM, IV (Adult, Skeletal Muscle Relaxation): 5 to 10 mg
IM, IV (Adult Geriatric or Debilitated, Skeletal Muscle Relaxation): 2 to 5 mg
PO, IM, IV (Adult, Alcohol Withdrawal): 10 mg
PO (Pediatric over 6 months, Antianxiety): 1 to 2.5 mg
IM, IV (Pediatric over 1 month, Antianxiety): 0.04 to 0.3 mg/kg/dose
IM, IV (Pediatric over 5 years, Seizures/Status epilepticus): 0.05 to 0.3 mg/kg/dose given over 3 to 5 minutes

Understand the Numbers

The physician has ordered a 0.05 mg/kg IV of diazepam to be given to your pediatric patient to control seizure activity. Your patient weighs 60 pounds. What is the required dose?
Pt. Wt. = 60 lb ÷ 2.2 kg = 27.27 kg, rounded down to 27 kg
27 kg × 0.05 mg = 1.35 mg of diazepam to be given to your patient

Rectal (Adult and Pediatric over 12 years, Seizures/Status epilepticus): 0.2 mg/kg
How Supplied
Tablets: 2 mg, 5 mg, 10 mg
Oral solution: 1 mg/mL, 5 mg/mL
Solution for injection: 5 mg/mL
Rectal gel delivery system: 2.5 mg, 10 mg, 20 mg
Adverse Reactions and Side Effects
Resp: Respiratory depression
CV: Hypotension (IV only)
CNS: Dizziness, drowsiness, lethargy, depression, hangover, slurred speech, headache, paradoxical excitation
GI: Constipation, diarrhea, nausea, vomiting
Derm: Rashes
Local: Pain (IM), phlebitis (IV)
Misc: Physical or psychological dependence, tolerance
Drug Interactions: Additive CNS depression if concurrently used with other CNS depressants such as antihistamines, antidepressants, opioid analgesics, or alcohol
EMS Considerations: Monitor blood pressure, pulse, and respiratory rate prior to administration and frequently after IV administration.

Diphenhydramine (dye-fen-HYE-dra-meen)

Benadryl
Classification: Antihistamine
Pregnancy Class: B
Mechanism of Action: Significant CNS depressant and anticholinergic properties
Pharmacokinetics
Absorption: Well absorbed
Onset: PO—15 to 60 minutes
IM—20 to 30 minutes
IV—rapid
Duration: PO, IM, IV—4 to 8 hours
Indication: Relief of acute dystonic reactions
Contraindications: Known hypersensitivity. Do not administer to patients with acute attacks of asthma.
Precautions: Use with caution in patients with severe liver disease, angle-closure glaucoma, seizure disorders, prostatic hyperplasia, or peptic ulcer. Diphenhydramine may cause paradoxical excitation in pediatric patients.
Route and Dosage
IM, IV (Adult): 25 to 50 mg
IM, IV (Pediatric): 1.25 mg/kg
How Supplied
Injection: 10 mg/mL, 50 mg/mL
Adverse Reactions and Side Effects
Resp: Chest tightness, thickened bronchial secretions, wheezing
CV: Hypotension, palpations
CNS: Drowsiness, dizziness, headache, paradoxical excitation (pediatrics)
GI: Anorexia, dry mouth, constipation, nausea
GU: Dysuria, urinary retention
Derm: Photosensitivity
Local: Pain at IM site
Drug Interactions: Increased risk of CNS depression if used with other CNS depressant drugs. Increased anticholinergic effects with tricyclic antidepressants, quinidine, or disopyramide. MAO inhibitors prolong the anticholinergic effects of antihistamines.
EMS Considerations: Assess patients for any movement disorders before and after administration. Do not confuse Benadryl (diphenhydramine) with Benylin (dextromethorphan).

Droperidol (droe-PER-i-dole)

Inapsine
Classifications: Sedative or hypnotic
Pregnancy Class: C
Mechanism of Action: Alters the action of dopamine in the CNS—similar to haloperidol
Pharmacokinetics
Absorption: Well absorbed
Onset: IM, IV—3 to 10 minutes
Duration: IM, IV—2 to 4 hours
Indications: Use for the treatment of acute psychotic episodes. Is also used for the treatment of severe anxiety.
Contraindications: Known hypersensitivity; should not be given to patients with angle-closure glaucoma, CNS depression, severe liver or cardiac disease, or known or suspected QT prolongation (Fig. 18-3).
Precautions: Use with caution in patients with diabetes, respiratory insufficiency, prostatic hyperplasia, or intestinal obstruction. Droperidol may lower the seizure threshold in patients with a seizure history.

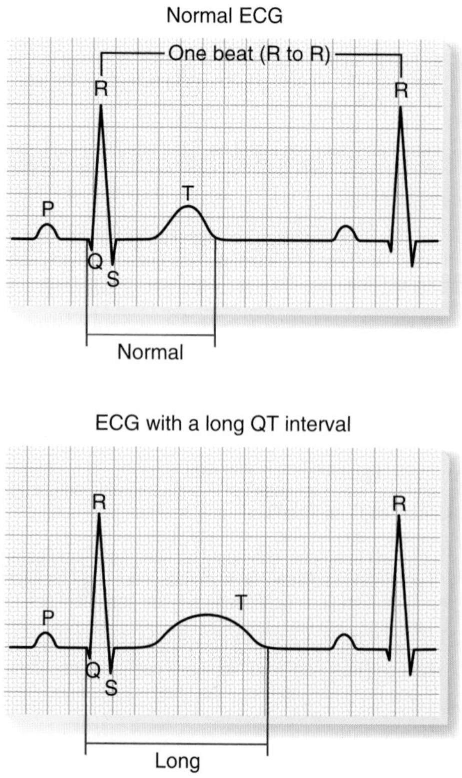

Figure 18-3 QT prolongation.

Route and Dosage
IM, IV (Adult): 2.5 mg initially
How Supplied
Injection: 2.5 mg/mL
Adverse Reactions and Side Effects
Resp: Bronchospasm, laryngospasm
CV: ARRHYTHMIAS (including torsade de pointes), hypotension, tachycardia, QT prolongation, tachycardia
CNS: SEIZURES, extrapyramidal reactions, abnormal electroencephalogram (EEG), anxiety, confusion, dizziness, excessive sedation, hallucinations, restlessness, tardive dyskinesia
GI: Constipation, dry mouth
Misc: Chills, facial sweating, shivering
Drug Interactions: Additive hypotension if used with other antihypertensives or nitrates; additive CNS depression if used with other CNS depressants
EMS Considerations: Assess 12-lead ECG in all patients prior to administration to determine if prolonged QT interval is present. Observe patients for extrapyramidal symptoms throughout therapy; have diphenhydramine readily available.

Haloperidol (ha-loe-PER-i-dole)

🍁 Apo-Haloperidol, Haldol, 🍁 Haldol LA, 🍁 Novo-Peridol, 🍁 Peridol, 🍁 PMS Haloperidol
Classification: Antipsychotic
Pregnancy Class: C
Mechanism of Action: Alters the effects of dopamine in the CNS; also has anticholinergic and alpha-adrenergic blocking activity
Pharmacokinetics
Absorption: Well absorbed
Onset: PO—2 hours
IM—20 to 30 minutes
Duration: PO—8 to 12 hours
IM—4 to 8 hours; however, effect may last for several days
Indications: Acute and chronic psychotic disorders including schizophrenia, manic states, and drug-induced psychoses. It is also useful in managing aggressive or agitated patients.
Contraindications: Known hypersensitivity; should not be given to patients with angle-closure glaucoma, CNS depression, or severe liver or cardiovascular disease that includes QT prolongation
Precautions: Use with caution in patients with cardiac disease, diabetes, respiratory insufficiency, prostatic hyperplasia, or intestinal obstruction.
Route and Dosage
PO (Adult): 0.5 to 5 mg 2 to 3 times daily
PO [Pediatric, 3 to 12 years or 15 to 40 kg (33 to 88 lb)]: 50 mcg/kg/day in 2 to 3 divided doses
IM (Adult): 2 to 5 mg
IV (Adult): 0.5 to 5 mg
How Supplied
Tablets: 0.5 mg, 1 mg, 2 mg, 5 mg, 10 mg, 20 mg
Oral concentrate: 2 mg/mL
Injection: 50 mg/mL, 100 mg/mL

Adverse Reactions and Side Effects
Resp: Respiratory depression
CV: Hypotension, tachycardia
CNS: SEIZURES, extrapyramidal reactions, confusion, drowsiness, restlessness, tardive dyskinesia

effective **Communication**

Wherever there is a possibility of the patient developing a life-threatening seizure during treatment, have diazepam (or medication as per protocol) readily available.

GI: Constipation, dry mouth, anorexia
GU: Urinary retention
Derm: Photosensitivity, rashes
Misc: NEUROLEPTIC MALIGNANT SYNDROME
Drug Interactions: Risk of increased hypotension with the concurrent use of antihypertensives; risk of increased anticholinergic effects with concurrent use of other drugs with anticholinergic properties; risk of increased CNS depression with the concurrent use of other CNS depressants
EMS Considerations: Monitor blood pressure (sitting, standing, lying) and pulse before and during therapy. Haloperidol may cause QT interval changes on the ECG.

Hydroxyzine (hye-DROX-i-zeen)

🍁 Apo-Hydroxyzine, Atarax, Hyzine-50, 🍁 Multipax, 🍁 Novo-Hydroxyzin, Vistaril
Classifications: Antianxiety, antihistamine, sedative/hypnotic
Pregnancy Class: C
Mechanism of Action: Acts as a CNS depressant at the subcortical level of the CNS
Pharmacokinetics
Absorption: Well absorbed
Onset: PO, IM—15 to 30 min
Duration: PO, IM—4 to 6 hr
Indications: Used for the treatment of anxiety
Contraindications: Known hypersensitivity; potential for congenital defects; safety not established in lactation
Precautions: Dosage reduction is recommended in elderly patients because of increased susceptibility to adverse effects. Use with caution in patients with severe liver disease.
Route and Dosage
IM (Adult): 25 to 100 mg
IM (Pediatric): 0.5 to 1 mg/kg/dose
How Supplied
Tablets: 10 mg, 25 mg, 50 mg, 100 mg
Capsules: 🍁 10 mg, 25 mg, 50 mg, 100 mg
Syrup: 10 mg/5 mL
Oral suspension: 25 mg/5 mL
Injection: 25 mg/mL, 50 mg/mL
Adverse Reactions and Side Effects
Resp: Wheezing
CNS: Drowsiness, agitation, ataxia, dizziness, headache, weakness
GI: Dry mouth, bitter taste, constipation, nausea

Underline indicates most frequent; CAPITALS indicates life-threatening; 🍁 indicates Canadian drug name.

GU: Urinary retention
Derm: Flushing
Local: Pain at IM site, abscesses at IM site
Drug Interactions: Additive CNS depression when used with other CNS depressants; additive anticholinergic effects when used with other drugs having anticholinergic properties
EMS Considerations: Hydroxyzine should not be administered IV in the out-of-hospital setting.

Lorazepam (lor-AZ-e-pam)

🍁 Apo-Lorazepam, Ativan, 🍁 Novo-Lorazem, 🍁 Nu-Loraz
Classifications: Antianxiety, sedative/hypnotic
Pregnancy Class: D
Mechanism of Action: Depresses the CNS by potentiating GABA, an inhibitory neurotransmitter
Pharmacokinetics
Absorption: Well absorbed following oral administration; rapidly and completely absorbed following IM administration. Sublingual absorption is more rapid than oral and is similar to IM.
Onset: PO—15 to 60 minutes
IM—30 to 60 minutes
IV—15 to 30 minutes
Duration: PO, IM, IV—8 to 12 hours
Indications: Used for the treatment of anxiety disorder; can also be used for premedication before cardioversion
Contraindications: Known hypersensitivity; should not be given to patients with preexisting CNS depression, angle-closure glaucoma, or severe hypotension
Precautions: Use with caution in patients with severe liver/kidney/respiratory impairment, depression, a history of suicide attempt or drug abuse, COPD, or myasthenia gravis.

Route and Dosage
PO (Adult): 1 to 3 mg
PO (Pediatric): 0.02 to 0.1 mg/kg/dose, not to exceed 2 mg
SL (Adult and Adolescent): 2 to 3 mg in divided doses, not to exceed 6 mg

How Supplied
Tablets: 0.5 mg, 1 mg, 2 mg
Concentrated oral solution: 0.5 mg/5 mL, 2 mg/mL
SL tablets: 🍁 0.5 mg, 🍁 1 mg, 🍁 2 mg
Injection: 2 mg/mL, 4 mg/mL

Adverse Reactions and Side Effects
Resp: Respiratory depression
CV: APNEA, CARDIAC ARREST (rapid IV), bradycardia, hypotension

effective **Communication**

If you are in an EMS system that permits IV administration of lorazepam, have resuscitation equipment readily available.

CNS: Dizziness, drowsiness, lethargy, hangover, headache, slurred speech, confusion, mental depression, paradoxical excitation
GI: Constipation, diarrhea, nausea, vomiting
Derm: Rashes
Misc: Physical or psychological dependence, tolerance
Drug Interactions: Additive CNS depression when used with other CNS depressant drugs
EMS Considerations: IV rate; administer lorazepam at a rate not to exceed 2 mg/minute or 0.05 mg/kg over 2 to 5 minutes. Rapid IV administration may result in apnea, hypotension, bradycardia, or cardiac arrest. Do not confuse Ativan (lorazepam) with Atarax (hydroxyzine).

Midazolam (mid-AY-zoe-lam)

Versed
Classifications: Antianxiety, sedative/hypnotic
Pregnancy Class: D
Mechanism of Action: Acts at many levels of the CNS to produce generalized CNS depression
Pharmacokinetics
Absorption: Rapidly absorbed
Onset: IM—15 min
IV—1.5 to 5 minutes
Duration: IM, IV—2 to 6 hours
Indications: Used for the purpose of sedation and amnesia for anxiety, sedation before cardioversion, and for status epilepticus
Contraindications: Known hypersensitivity; should not be given to patients in shock or to those with preexisting CNS depression, uncontrolled severe pain, or acute angle-closure glaucoma
Precautions: Use with caution in patients with pulmonary disease, CHF, kidney impairment, or severe liver impairment as well as obese pediatric patients. Older patients (over 70 years) are more susceptible to cardiorespiratory depressant effects.

effective **Communication**

The dose of midazolam for obese pediatric patients should be calculated on the basis of ideal body weight.

Route and Dosage
Note: Dose must be individualized, taking caution to reduce the dose in geriatric patients and those who are already sedated.
PO (Pediatric, 6 months to 16 years): 0.25 to 0.5 mg/kg initially
IM (Adult, healthy and over 60 years): 0.07 to 0.08 mg/kg. Usual dose is 5 mg.
IM (Adult, under 60 years): 0.02 to 0.03 mg/kg. Usual dose is 1 to 3 mg.
IM (Pediatric): 0.1 to 0.15 mg/kg up to 0.5 mg/kg
IV (Adult and Pediatric over 12 years and under 60 years): 1 to 2.5 mg initially. Dosage may be increased as needed.
IV (Adult over 60 years): 1 to 1.5 mg initially. Dosage may be increased as needed.
IV (Pediatric, 6 months to 5 years): 0.05 mg/kg initially
IV (Pediatric, 6 to 12 years): 0.025 to 0.05 mg/kg initially

Understand the Numbers

The physician has ordered you to give midazolam to your 6-year-old male patient. The patient's mother states her son weighs approximately 80 pounds. What is the dosage of midazolam to be given to your patient when ordered at 0.025 mg/kg?

Do not make the mistake of figuring this problem using the patient weight of 80 pounds. Remember, the initial dose of midazolam for obese pediatric patients is the ideal body weight, not the actual weight. The ideal body weight for a 6-year-old male is approximately 46 pounds. Therefore, 46 lbs ÷ 2.2 kg = 20.9, or 21 kg. At 0.025 mg/kg, 21 kg × 0.025 mg = 0.525 mg or 0.53 mg.

How Supplied

Injection: 1 mg/mL, 5 mg/mL
Syrup: 2 mg/mL

Adverse Reactions and Side Effects

Resp: APNEA, LARYNGOSPASM, RESPIRATORY DEPRESSION, bronchospasm, coughing
CV: CARDIAC ARREST, arrhythmias
CNS: Agitation, drowsiness, headache
GI: Hiccups, nausea, vomiting
Derm: Rashes
Local: Phlebitis at IV site, pain at IM site

Drug Interactions: Increased risk of CNS depression if used concurrently with antihistamines, opioid analgesics, and other sedatives or hypnotics; decrease dose by 30 to 50 percent; increased risk of hypotension if used with antihypertensives, opioid analgesics, or nitrates

EMS Considerations: Monitor blood pressure, pulse, and respirations continuously. Oxygen and resuscitative equipment should be immediately available. If overdose occurs, monitor pulse, respirations, and blood pressure continuously. Maintain patient's airway and assist ventilations as needed. If hypotension occurs, treatment includes IV fluids, repositioning, and vasopressors. The effects of midazolam can be reversed with flumazenil (Romazicon).

Olanzapine (oh-LAN-za-peen)

Zyprexa, Zyprexa Zydis

Classification: Antipsychotic
Pregnancy Class: C
Mechanism of Action: Antagonizes dopamine and serotonin type 2 in the CNS; also has anticholinergic, antihistaminic, and anti-alpha$_1$-adrenergic effects

Pharmacokinetics

Absorption: Well absorbed but rapidly metabolized, resulting in 60 percent bioavailability
Onset: PO—unknown
IM—rapid
Duration: PO—unknown
IM—2 to 4 hours

Indications: Acute and maintenance treatment of schizophrenia; acute treatment of manic episodes associated with bipolar I disorder

Contraindications: Known hypersensitivity; should not be used if patient is lactating. If so, olanzapine should be discontinued or the child should be bottle-fed.

Precautions: Use with caution in patients with liver impairment, cardiovascular or cerebrovascular disease, a history of seizures, a history of attempted suicide, diabetes, prostatic hyperplasia, or angle-closure glaucoma.

Route and Dosage

PO (Adult): 5 to 10 mg
IM (Adult): 5 to 10 mg

How Supplied

Tablets: 2.5 mg, 5 mg, 7.5 mg, 10 mg, 15 mg, 20 mg
Orally disintegrating tablets (Zydis): 5 mg, 10 mg, 15 mg, 20 mg
Powder for injection: 10 mg/vial

Adverse Reactions and Side Effects

Resp: Cough, dyspnea
CV: Orthostatic hypotension, tachycardia, chest pain
CNS: NEUROLEPTIC MALIGNANT SYNDROME, SEIZURES, SUICIDAL THOUGHTS, agitation, dizziness, headache, restlessness, weakness, insomnia, mood changes, personality disorder, speech impairment, tardive dyskinesia
GI: Constipation, dry mouth, abdominal pain, nausea
GU: Decreased libido, urinary incontinence
EENT: Amblyopia, rhinitis, increased salivation, pharyngitis
Derm: Photosensitivity
Misc: Fever, flu-like syndrome

Drug Interactions: Effects may be decreased by concurrent use of carbamazepine, omeprazole, or rifampin. Increased hypotension may occur with concurrent use of other antihypertensives. Increased CNS depression may occur if olanzapine is concurrently used with other CNS depressants.

EMS Considerations: Assess patient mood, orientation, and behavior before and during therapy. Monitor blood pressure (sitting, standing, lying), ECG, pulse, and respiratory rate before and frequently during therapy.

Ziprasidone (zi-PRA-si-done)

Geodon

Classification: Antipsychotic
Pregnancy Class: C
Mechanism of Action: Effects mediated by antagonism of dopamine type 2 and serotonin type 2

Pharmacokinetics

Absorption: 60 percent absorbed following oral administration;
100 percent absorbed from following IM administration
Onset: PO—Within hours
IM—Rapid
Duration: PO, IM—Unknown

Indications: Used in the treatment of schizophrenia and bipolar mania (acute manic and manic/mixed episodes)

Contraindications: Known hypersensitivity; should not be used in patients with QT prolongation or with other drugs known to prolong the QT interval; should not be given to patients who have had a recent MI

Precautions: Use with caution in patients experiencing diarrhea, those with hypotension, and patients with a history of cardiovascular or cerebrovascular disease.

Route and Dosage

PO (Adult): 20 mg

IM (Adult): 10 to 20 mg

How Supplied

Capsules: 20 mg, 40 mg, 60 mg, 80 mg

Lyophilized powder for injection: 20 mg/vial

Adverse Reactions and Side Effects

Resp: Cough/runny nose

CV: PROLONGED QT INTERVAL, orthostatic hypotension

CNS: NEUROLEPTIC MALIGNANT SYNDROME, seizures, dizziness, drowsiness, restlessness, extrapyramidal reactions, syncope, tardive dyskinesia

GI: Constipation, diarrhea, nausea

Derm: Rashes, urticaria

Drug Interactions: The concurrent use of any drug that prolongs the QT interval may result in potentially life-threatening adverse drug reactions. Additive CNS depression may occur with the concurrent use of other CNS depressant drugs.

EMS Considerations: Monitor the patient's orientation, mood, and behavior prior to and during therapy. Monitor blood pressure (sitting, standing, lying) prior to and frequently during therapy.

SCENARIO REVISITED

Did you consider the case of Ron Reilly?

As you recall, you were called because Mr. Reilly was acting "bizarre." When you and your partner arrived, you were able to gather some history from Mrs. Reilly and perform an assessment on Mr. Reilly who has exhibited no aggressive behavior. Therefore, you decide to take Mr. Reilly to the ambulance for transport to the hospital.

While Mr. Reilly is being taken to the ambulance, he suddenly goes into a grand mal seizure. The immediate course of action should be to protect Mr. Reilly from injuring himself and to protect his airway. The seizure is clonic and subsides after approximately 2 minutes. Mr. Reilly remains unconscious. At this point, you place him in the ambulance and administer humidified oxygen.

While en route to the hospital, Mr. Reilly goes into another seizure, which also lasts approximately 2 minutes. Your EMS system protocol states that you start an IV of NS at a keep-open rate and 5 mg of diazepam by slow IV bolus. If necessary, another 5 mg can be given. Once you have performed an appropriate assessment, you should proceed using a critical thinking approach to medication administration.

Step 1: Determine signs and symptoms to be treated.
Step 2: Consider both the risks and benefits of treating or not treating your patient.
Step 3: Choose the medication that provides the best possible outcome.
Step 4: Remember the drug's indications, contraindications, and precautions.
Step 5: Decide the best route for administering the medication for the best outcome.
Step 6: Administer the medication(s) according to the seven Patient Rights.

1. The right patient
2. The right drug
3. The right drug amount
4. The right time
5. The right route
6. The right documentation
7. The right of the patient to accept or refuse the medication(s)

Step 7: Reevaluate the patient for the desired and undesired effects.

Let's Recap

Patients who present with irrational behavior may do so because of disease or injury process, not because of mental illness. For example, head injury, drug abuse, or a severe diabetic episode can lead to behavior suggestive of a psychotic disorder. If possible, the patient who presents with psychotic behavior should be assessed for other medical or physical causes. For example, giving an antipsychotic drug to an individual suffering from an overdose of crack cocaine would not help and could be harmful.

It is more appropriate to give antipsychotic drugs in the hospital setting, which is a more controlled environment. However, there may be occasions when out-of-hospital antipsychotic drug therapy is ordered before transport to an emergency facility is complete. As with any emergency situation, you must follow your protocols and medical control.

SCENARIO CONCLUSION

Patients with mental disorders are rarely sedated in the out-of-hospital setting. In this case, the diazepam is primarily to help control seizure activity. Diazepam depresses the CNS, causing seizure activity to subside.

Check the Evidence

The efficacy of IV diazepam for the treatment of seizure activity is well recognized, with termination of episodes in some 80 percent of cases.

During transport, monitor Mr. Reilly closely, being alert for any changes. Mr. Reilly is still unconscious. His reflexes are normal, his vital signs are stable, and his pupils are equal and reactive.

Underline indicates most frequent; CAPITALS indicates life-threatening; ♣ indicates Canadian drug name.

Patients with mental disorders are usually difficult to manage. The role of the EMS professional is primarily supportive. Occasionally, these patients exhibit aggressive behavior and may perceive you as a threat to their safety or an ally of their enemies. A calm, nonthreatening approach can work toward patient confidence, regardless of whether the patient is behaving aggressively or passively. Expressing a desire to help frequently produces positive results.

Patients who experience severe psychotic episodes in the out-of-hospital setting may require antipsychotic drugs such as chlorpromazine or haloperidol. These drugs block dopamine receptors in the brain associated with behavior and mood. The adult dose of chlorpromazine is 25 to 50 mg IM, and the adult dose of haloperidol is 2 to 5 mg, also IM. Although it is rare for these drugs to be administered in the out-of-hospital setting, it is important for you to be familiar with them, because you may administer them while working in the hospital setting.

In most cases when a mental disorder is suspected, quiet transport to the emergency department is called for. The siren can be disturbing for the patient, and it should not be used unless a life-threatening emergency exists.

PRACTICE EXERCISES

1. Extrapyramidal reactions are neuromuscular effects that can be caused by some antipsychotic drugs. A common EMS medication that can be given for the treatment of extrapyramidal reactions is:
   a. Diphenhydramine
   b. Diazepam
   c. Dopamine
   d. Droperidol
2. A common CV side effect of chlorpromazine is:
   a. Bradycardia
   b. Hypotension
   c. Blurred vision
   d. Cardiac arrest
3. In behavioral-emergency protocols, diphenhydramine can be used to treat:
   a. Seizures
   b. Anxiety
   c. Hallucinations
   d. Acute dystonic reactions
4. A significant contraindication for droperidol is:
   a. Diabetes
   b. QT prolongation
   c. Prostatic hyperplasia
   d. Respiratory insufficiency
5. The adult IV dose of droperidol is:
   a. 0.25 mg
   b. 25 mg
   c. 2.5 mg
   d. 0.025 mg
6. Haloperidol is classified as a(n):
   a. Sedative/hypnotic
   b. Antihistamine
   c. Antianxiety
   d. Antipsychotic
7. The adult IM dose of hydroxyzine is:
   a. 2.5 to 10 mg
   b. 2.5 to 50 mg
   c. 25 to 100 mg
   d. 50 to 100 mg
8. A frequent CNS side effect of lorazepam is:
   a. Drowsiness
   b. Headache
   c. Confusion
   d. Paradoxical excitation
9. You are ordered to give 0.25 mg/kg of midazolam to your 75-lb 6-year-old patient. Your dose for this patient should be:
   a. 18.75 mg
   b. 10.50 mg
   c. 8.5 mg
   d. 5.5 mg
10. A possible CNS life-threatening adverse reaction to olanzapine is:
    a. Tardive dyskinesia
    b. Agitation
    c. Tachycardia
    d. Seizures

CASE STUDIES

1. At 5:30 a.m., you are called to the home of a man "not breathing." On arrival, it is determined that the individual has been down too long, and resuscitative efforts should not be initiated. When his wife is told, she becomes hysterical. Attempts are made to calm her down, but nothing seems to help. After calming efforts fail, medical control is called, and you explain the situation. The physician orders sedation and transport. What drug should the physician order for sedation?
   a. Chlorpromazine
   b. Hydroxyzine
   c. Haloperidol
   d. Diazepam

2. You are called to the home of an individual who has previously experienced psychotic episodes and seizures. On arrival, the patient is displaying bizarre and aggressive behavior. The more attempts are made to calm him down, the more aggressive he seems to become. Medical control is familiar with this patient and instructs you to give 25 mg of chlorpromazine to treat his psychosis. In this situation, what other drug should be readily available?
   a. Haloperidol
   b. Hydroxyzine
   c. Diazepam
   d. $D_{50}W$

MATH EQUATIONS

1. You are ordered to give 0.55 mg/kg of chlorpromazine 65 lb patient. The maximum dose of chlorpromazine for this patient is 75 mg. You have chlorpromazine tablets in 10 mg and 25 mg doses.
   a. How many kg is your patient?
   b. What is the dosage of chlorpromazine for this patient?
   c. How many tablets are required to equal the correct dosage?
2. The physician has ordered a 0.05 mg/kg IV of diazepam to be given to your pediatric patient. Your patient weighs 60 pounds.
   a. How many kg does your patient weigh?
   b. What is the required dosage for this patient?
3. You are ordered to give 0.5 mg/kg of hydroxyzine to your 45 lb pediatric patient. The hydroxyzine comes packaged as 25 mg in 1 mL.
   a. How many kg does your patient weigh?
   b. What is the correct dosage (mg) of the hydroxyzine for this patient?
   c. What is the correct volume of hydroxyzine to equal the correct dosage?
4. The physician has ordered you to give midazolam to your 6-year-old male patient. The patient's mother states her son weighs approximately 80 pounds.
   a. How many kg does your patient weigh?
   b. What is the dosage of midazolam to be given to your patient when ordered at 0.025 mg/kg?

REFERENCES

Beck, R. K. (2012). Drugs used to treat gastrointestinal emergencies. In *Pharmacology for the EMS provider.* New York, NY: Delmar, Cengage Learning.

Better Medicine. Behavioral disorders: causes. Retrieved September 19, 2013 from www.localhealth.com/article/behavioral-disorders/causes

Deglin, J. H., Vallerand, A. H., and Sanboski, C. A. (2011). *Davis's drug guide for nurses* (12th ed.). Philadelphia, PA: F. A. Davis Company.

Holloman, L. C., and Marder, S. R. (1997). Management of acute extrapyramidal effects influenced by antipsychotic drugs. *American Journal of Health-System Pharmacy. 54,* 2461–2477.

Taskar, R. C. (1998). Emergency treatment of acute seizures and status epilepticus. *Archives of Disease in Childhood. 79,* 78–83.

Venes, D., ed. (2013). *Taber's cyclopedic medical dictionary* (22nd ed.). Philadelphia, PA: F. A. Davis Company.

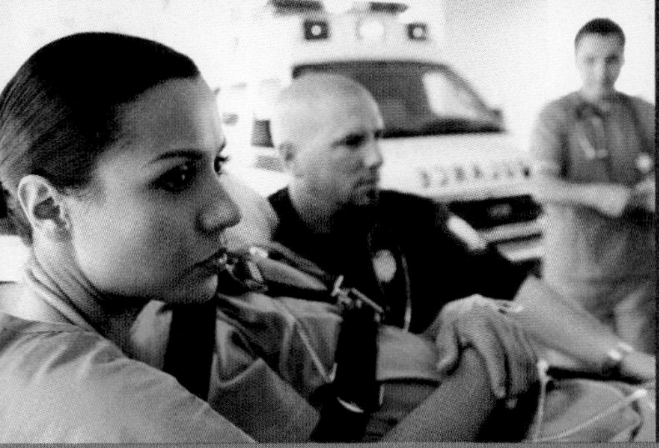

CHAPTER 19

Drugs Used for Pain Management and Sedation

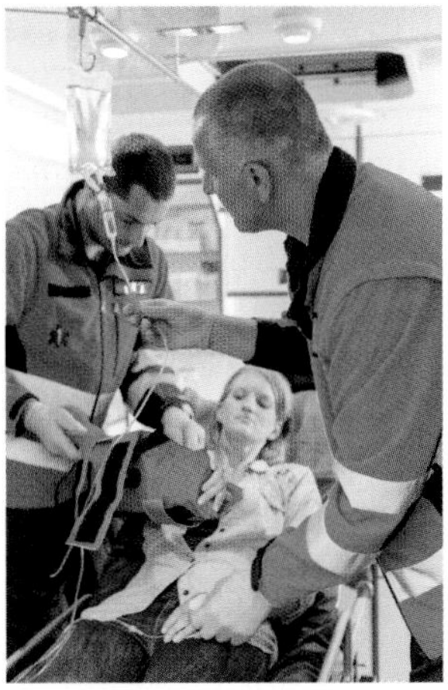

Paramedics administering an analgesic medication to a patient. *(Photograph © CandyBox Images/iStock/Thinkstock)*

LEARNING OUTCOMES

- Discuss the pros and cons of pain management in the out-of-hospital setting.
- Discuss the role of sedation in the out-of-hospital setting.
- List and discuss the indications, contraindications, precautions, route and dosage, and adverse reactions and side effects of the following drugs:
  - The nonopioid analgesics acetaminophen, aspirin, ibuprofen, ketamine, and ketorolac
  - The opioid analgesics butorphanol, fentanyl, hydromorphone, morphine, and nalbuphine
  - The sedative or hypnotic drugs etomidate, lorazepam, midazolam, and promethazine
  - The medicinal gas nitrous oxide

KEY TERMS

Analgesic
Nociception
Nociceptive impulse
Nociceptor
Nonopioid analgesic
Opioid analgesic
Pain
Prostaglandins

SCENARIO OPENING

You are assigned to Rescue 44, which is assigned to your local county hospital. After the equipment and vehicle are checked, you are told to report to the ER where you will be assigned to a nurse preceptor. While you are being oriented to the ER, a call comes in for Rescue 44 to respond to a local high school gym.

Upon arrival at the high school, you are directed to the weight room where you find a gym teacher in severe pain with a towel wrapped around his left foot. As it turns out, the teacher, Mr. Smyth, dropped a 50-pound weight on his foot. On examination, the foot has obvious deformity, swelling, and bruising. Vital signs are as follows:

Level of Consciousness:	alert and in severe pain
Respirations:	24 breaths/minute
Pulse:	120 beats/minute and regular (Fig.19-1)
Blood pressure:	190/92 mm Hg
Skin:	warm and damp

Mr. Smyth states that he weighs 215 pounds.

On a pain scale of 0 to 10, Mr. Smyth says, "12. Please give me something for pain."

Introduction

Pain is probably the most common patient complaint encountered by EMS professionals. It is defined by the International Association for the Study of Pain (IASP) as an unpleasant sensory and emotional experience arising from actual or potential tissue damage or described in terms of such damage. Pain includes not only the perception of an uncomfortable stimulus but also the response to that perception. Figure 19-2 illustrates the Pain Relief Ladder as developed by the World Health Organization (WHO) originally for cancer patients.

In recent years, pain management was not the initial priority in EMS patient care. However, now pain management is an important aspect of patient management. Pain is an unpleasant sensation that disturbs a patient's comfort, thought, sleep, or normal daily activity. Pain is caused by an underlying disorder. Pain is now considered the fifth vital sign. However, it is the most difficult to assess because of its subjective nature. A patient's presentation of pain and the manner in which the pain is handled vary widely. Some patients may be in a great deal of pain but not exhibit significant symptoms, while others may be very anxious and emotional. Pain may greatly affect the anxiety level of the patient and result in physical symptoms such as tachypnea, tachycardia, and hypertension. Pain management must be individualized for each patient based on the patient's reporting of pain and the symptoms exhibited, as well as the occurrence of adverse reactions. EMS professionals must have an understanding of the importance of pain management and its effect on the overall condition of the patient.

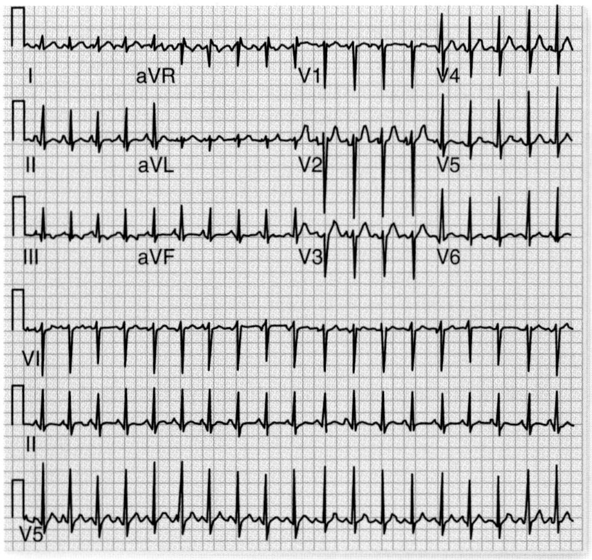

Figure 19-1 Sinus tachycardia (120 beats/minute).

Pathophysiology of Pain

Pain generation is a complicated interaction that involves all parts of the nervous system. As we know, if we cut our finger, we feel the sensation of pain due to stimuli transferred to our brain. These stimuli are transferred to our brain from nerve endings located throughout the skin, bones, connective tissues, and organs by way of the somatic nervous system.

A **nociceptor** is a free nerve ending that is a receptor for painful stimuli. The impulse we feel giving rise to the sensation of pain is called a **nociceptive impulse**. Finally, **nociception** is the stimulus-response process involving the stimulation of peripheral pain-carrying nerve fibers and the transmission of impulses along peripheral nerves to the CNS where the stimulus is perceived as pain (Fig. 19-3).

When we cut our finger, a nociceptive stimulus is sent to the spinal cord and then on to the brain. Simultaneously, a

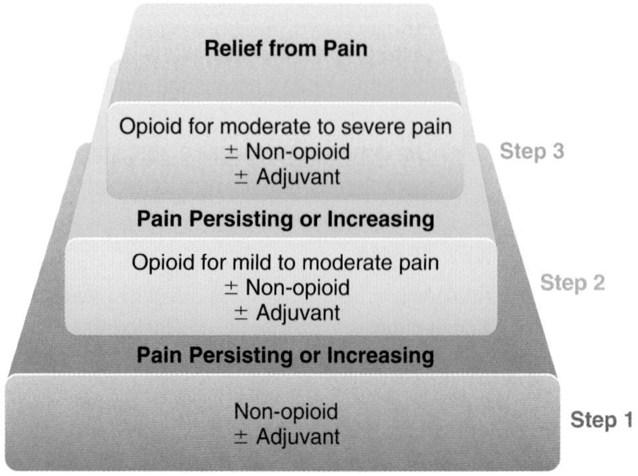

Figure 19-2 The WHO pain relief ladder.

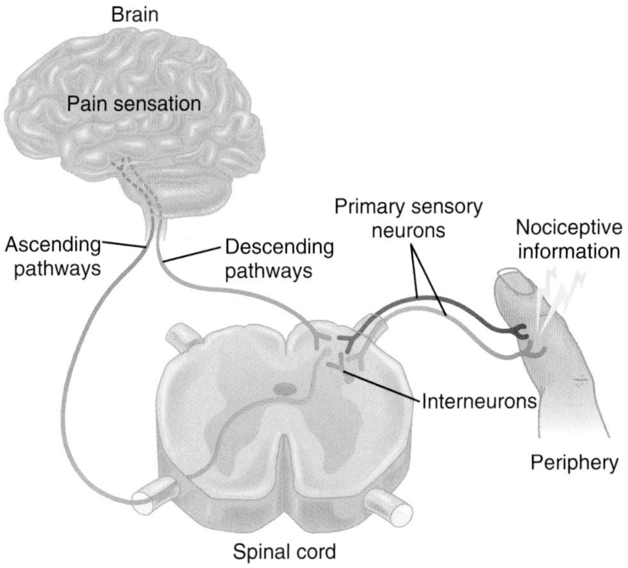

Figure 19-3 Pathophysiology of pain.

local sensitization takes place, releasing certain chemicals from the nerve endings that cause inflammation and the beginning of the repair process. This inflammation causes the swelling, redness, and warmth that the injury ultimately produces.

Pharmacokinetics

Nonopioid Analgesics

Nonopioid analgesics are used to control moderate pain or fever. These drugs inhibit prostaglandin synthesis peripherally for their analgesic effect and centrally for their antipyretic effect. **Prostaglandins** are the primary mediators of inflammation and pain.

Opioid Analgesics

Opioid analgesics are used in the management of moderate-to-severe pain. They bind to opiate receptors in the CNS, resulting in alteration to the perception of and the response to pain. Opioid antagonists compete with opioid agonists for receptor sites and reverse the effects of the opioid agonist, including sedation, respiratory depression, and hypotension.

Some opioids possess both agonist and antagonist properties. These agents act as agonist at some receptors and antagonist at other receptors. Opioid agonists and antagonists have less potential for overdose than do agonists alone; however, they do have potential to cause opioid withdrawal in patients physically dependent on opioids. The opioid antagonist naloxone must be readily available for administration should symptoms of opioid overdose occur. The dosages of opioid analgesics are compared in Table 19-1.

Sedatives and Hypnotics

Sedatives are used to provide sedation, usually prior to procedures, and hypnotics are used to manage insomnia. Some

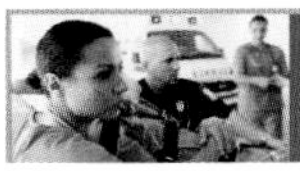

Table 19-1 Dosages of Opioid Analgesics

Drug	Routes	Adult Dosages	Duration
Butorphanol	IM IV	2 mg 1 mg	3 to 4 hours 2 to 4 hours
Fentanyl	IV	0.5 to 1 mcg/kg	0.5 to 1 hour
Hydromorphone	SubQ, IM, IV Rectal	1.5 mg 3 mg	SubQ, IM 4 to 5 hours IV 2 to 3 hours Rectal 4 to 5 hours
Meperidine	PO, SubQ, IM IV	50 mg 15 to 35 mg	PO, SubQ, IM 2 to 4 hours IV 2 to 3 hours
Morphine	SubQ, IV IM Rectal	4 to 10 mg 8 to 15 mg 30 mg	SubQ, IM, IV 4 to 5 hours 3 to 7 hours
Nalbuphine	SubQ, IM, IV	10 mg	SubQ, IM, IV 3 to 6 hours

selected drugs are used as anticonvulsants, some are used as skeletal muscle relaxants, and some are used as amnestics. Sedatives and hypnotics cause generalized CNS depression. They may produce tolerance with chronic use and have potential for psychological or physical dependence. Sedatives and hypnotics have no analgesic properties.

Individual Drugs

Acetaminophen (a-seet-a-MIN-oh-fen)

♣ Abenol, Acephen, Aceta, Aminofen, Apacet, APAP, ♣ Apo-Acetaminophen, Aspirin Free Anacin, Aspirin Free Pain Relief, Children's Pain Reliever, Dapacin Feverall, Extra Strength Dynafed E.X., Extra Strength Dynafed (Billups, P.J.) Genapap, Genebs, Halenol, Infant's Pain Reliever, Liquiprin, Mapap, Maranox, Meda, Neopap, ♣ Novo-Gesic, Oraphen-PD, Panadol, Redutemp, Ridenol, Silapap, Tapanol, Tempra, Tylenol, Uni-Ace

Classifications: Nonopioid analgesic, antipyretic

Pregnancy Class: B

Mechanism of Action: Inhibits the synthesis of prostaglandins that may serve as mediators of pain and fever; does not have any significant anti-inflammatory properties

Pharmacokinetics

Absorption: Well absorbed following oral administration. Rectal administration is variable.

Onset: PO—0.5 to 1 hour
Rectal—0.5 to 1 hour

Duration: PO—3 to 8 hours, depending on the dose
Rectal—3 to 4 hours

Indications: Used for patients with mild pain or fever
Contraindications: Known hypersensitivity; should not be given to patients with a hypersensitivity to alcohol, aspartame, saccharin, sugar, or tartrazine (FDC yellow dye #5)
Precautions: Use with caution in patients with liver or kidney disease and in patients with chronic alcohol use.

Route and Dosage

PO (Adult and Pediatric over 12 years): 325 to 650 mg every 4 to 6 hours, or 1 g 3 to 4 times daily or 1,300 mg every 8 hours (do not exceed 4 g or 2.5 g/24 hours in patients with liver or renal impairment)
PO (Pediatric 1 to 12 years): 10 to 15 mg/kg/dose every 4 to 6 hours (do not exceed 5 doses/24 hours)
PO (Infants): 10 to 15 mg/kg/dose every 4 to 6 hours (do not exceed 5 doses/24 hours)
PO (Neonates): 10 to 15 mg/kg/dose every 6 to 8 hours as needed
Rectal (Adult and Pediatric over 12 years): 325 to 650 mg every 4 to 6 hours as needed or 1 g 3 to 4 times/day (do not exceed 4 g/24 hours)
Rectal (Pediatric 1 to 12 years): 10 to 20 mg/kg/dose every 4 to 6 hours as needed
Rectal (Infants): 10 to 20 mg/kg/dose every 4 to 6 hours as needed
Rectal (Neonates): 10 to 15 mg/kg/dose every 6 to 8 hours as needed

Understand the Numbers

You are ordered to give 15 mg/kg of acetaminophen rectally to your 87-pound, 7-year-old patient. How many mg will you give?
87 lbs ÷ 2.2 kg = 39.5 or 40 kg.
15 mg × 40 kg = 600 mg.

How Supplied (All OTC)

Chewable tablets: 80 mg, 160 mg
Tablets: 160 mg, 325 mg, 500 mg, 650 mg
Caplets: 325 mg, 500 mg
Solution: 100 mg/mL
Liquid: 160 mg/5 mL, 500 mg/15 mL
Elixir: 160 mg/5 mL
Drops: 100 mg/mL
Suspension: 🍁 100 mg/mL, 🍁 160 mg/5 mL
Syrup: 160 mg/5 mL
Suppositories: 80 mg, 120 mg, 325 mg, 650 mg

Adverse Reactions and Side Effects

GI: LIVER FAILURE, HEPATOTOXICITY (overdose)
GU: Renal failure (high doses/chronic use)
Derm: Rash, urticaria
Drug Interactions: Chronic high-dose acetaminophen may increase the risk of bleeding with warfarin. Concurrent NSAIDs increase the risk of adverse renal effects.
EMS Considerations: PO doses can be given with food or on an empty stomach. Acetaminophen should be taken with a full glass of water.

Aspirin (AS-pir-in)

🍁 Apo-ASA, 🍁 Arthrinol, 🍁 Arthrisin, 🍁 Artria S.R., ASA, 🍁 Asaphen, Ascriptin, Aspercin, Aspergum, Aspirtab, 🍁 Astrin, Bayer Aspirin, Bufferin, 🍁 Coryphen, Easprin, Ecotrin, 🍁 Entrophen, Genacote, Halfprin, 🍁 Headache Tablets, Healthprin, 🍁 Novasen, 🍁 PMS-ASA, 🍁 Rivasa, St. Joseph Adult Chewable Aspirin, ZOR-prin

Classifications: antipyretic, nonopioid analgesic, salicylate
Pregnancy Class: D (first trimester)
Mechanism of Action: Produces analgesia and reduces inflammation and fever by inhibiting the production of prostaglandins; decreases platelet aggregation
Pharmacokinetics
Absorption: Well absorbed from the upper small intestine. Absorption from enteric-coated aspirin is unreliable. Rectal absorption is slow and variable.
Onset: PO; 5 to 30 minutes
Rectal; 1 to 2 hours
Duration: PO; 3 to 6 hours
Rectal; 7 hours
Indications: Used as a prophylaxis of transient ischemic attacks
Contraindications: Known hypersensitivity; should not be given to patients with bleeding disorders

***effective* Communication**

Aspirin should not be given to children or adolescents with viral infections due to the risk of developing Reye syndrome.

Precautions: Use with caution in patients with a history of GI bleeding or ulcer disease, in patients with chronic alcohol use or severe renal disease, and in patients with severe liver disease.

Route and Dosage

PO (Adult): 50 to 325 mg once daily

How Supplied (All OTC)

Tablets: 81 mg, 162.5 mg, 325 mg, 500 mg, 650 mg, 🍁 975 mg
Chewable tablets: 🍁 80 mg, 81 mg
Chewing gum: 227 mg
Dispersible tablets: 325 mg, 500 mg
Enteric-coated (delayed-release) tablets: 80 mg, 165 mg, 🍁 600 mg, 650 mg, 975 mg
Extended-release tablets: 🍁 325 mg, 650 mg, 800 mg
Delayed-release capsules: 🍁 325 mg, 🍁 500 mg
Suppositories: 60 mg, 120 mg, 125 mg, 130 mg, 🍁 150 mg, 🍁 160 mg, 195 mg, 200 mg, 300 mg, 🍁 320 mg, 325 mg, 600 mg, 🍁 640 mg, 650 mg, 1.2 g

Adverse Reactions and Side Effects

EENT: Tinnitus
GI: GI BLEEDING, dyspepsia, epigastric distress, nausea, abdominal pain, anorexia, vomiting
Hemat: Anemia, increased bleeding time
Misc: ANAPHYLAXIS, LARYNGEAL EDEMA

Drug Interactions: Aspirin may increase the risk of bleeding when taken with thrombolytic medications. There is increased risk of GI irritation when taken with NSAIDs.
EMS Considerations: Aspirin should be administered as soon as possible if a TIA or stroke is suspected.

Check the Evidence

Patients who have asthma, allergies, and nasal polyps or who are hypersensitive to tartrazine are at an increased risk for developing hypersensitive reactions.

Butorphanol (byoo-TOR-fa-nole)

Stadol, Stadol NS
Classification: Opioid analgesic, opioid agonist/antagonist
Pregnancy Class: C
Mechanism of Action: Binds to opiate receptors in the CNS; alters the perception of and response to painful stimuli while producing generalized CNS depression
Pharmacokinetics
Absorption: Well absorbed from nasal mucosa, IM and IV sites
Onset: IM—Within 15 minutes
IV—Within minutes
Intranasal—Within 15 minutes
Duration: IM—3 to 4 hours
IV—2 to 4 hours
Intranasal—4 to 5 hours
Indication: Used for the management of moderate-to-severe pain
Contraindications: Known hypersensitivity; should not be given to patients physically dependent on opioids
Precautions: Use with caution in patients with severe renal, liver, or pulmonary disease; in patients with head trauma or increased intracranial pressure; and in patients with undiagnosed abdominal pain. (!) Decrease dosage by 50 percent in geriatric patients.
Route and Dosage
IM (Adult): 2 mg every 3 to 4 hours as needed
IV (Adult): 1 mg every 3 to 4 hours as needed
IM, IV (Geriatric): 1 mg every 4 to 6 hours; increase dosage as necessary
Intranasal (Adult): 1 mg (1 spray in 1 nostril initially). An additional dose may be given 60 to 90 minutes later.

effective **Communication**

If the pain is severe, an initial dose of 2 mg (1 spray in each nostril) may be given.

Intranasal (Geriatric): 1 mg (1 spray in 1 nostril) initially. An additional dose may be given 90 to 120 minutes later.
How Supplied
Injection: 1 mg/mL, 2 mg/mL
Intranasal solution: 10 mg/mL, in 2.5-mL metered-dose spray pump (14 to 15 doses; 1 mg spray)
Adverse Reactions and Side Effects
Resp: Respiratory depression
CV: Hypertension or hypotension, palpitations
CNS: Confusion, dysphoria, hallucinations, sedation, euphoria, floating feeling, headache, unusual dreams
GI: Nausea, constipation, dry mouth, vomiting
GU: Urinary retention
EENT: Blurred vision, diplopia, miosis (high doses)
Derm: Sweating, clammy feeling
Misc: Physical dependence, psychological dependence, tolerance
Drug Interactions: Concurrent use of kava-kava, valerian, chamomile, or hops can increase CNS depression.
EMS Considerations: Use extreme caution in patients receiving MAO INHIBITORS; may produce severe, potentially fatal reactions—reduce the initial dose of butorphanol to 25 percent of the usual dose. Concurrent use with alcohol, antidepressants, antihistamines, and sedatives or hypnotics may cause additive CNS depression.

Etomidate (e-TOM-i-date)

Amidate
Classification: Sedative/hypnotic
Pregnancy Class: C
Mechanism of Action: The exact mechanism of action of etomidate is unknown. However, it is believed to enhance gamma-aminobutyric acid (GABA) neurotransmission.
Pharmacokinetics
Absorption: Well absorbed via IV
Onset: Within 1 minute
Duration: 4 to 15 minutes
Indications: Used as a premedication before tracheal intubation or cardioversion
Contraindications: Known hypersensitivity; should not be given to patients in labor
Precautions: Use with caution in patients with severe hypotension, severe asthma, or severe cardiovascular disease.
Route and Dosage
IV (Adult): 0.2 to 0.4 mg/kg over 30 to 60 seconds
IV (Pediatric over 10 years): 0.2 to 0.4 mg/kg over 30 to 60 seconds; maximum dose = 20 mg

Understand the Numbers

You are ordered to administer 0.4 mg/kg of etomidate to your 110-pound, 13-year-old patient. How many milligrams should you administer?
122 lbs ÷ 2.2 kg = 55 kg. 55 kg × 0.4 = 22 mg. However, the maximum dose is 20 mg for pediatric patients. Therefore, your dose is 20 mg.

How Supplied
Vials: 2 mg/mL
Adverse Reactions and Side Effects
Resp: Apnea, laryngospasm
CV: Hypertension or hypotension, tachycardia or bradycardia
GI: Nausea, vomiting
MS: Involuntary muscle movement

Drug Interactions: When administered concurrently with verapamil, it may increase the risk of respiratory depression and apnea.
EMS Considerations: Patient vital signs must be constantly monitored.

Fentanyl (FEN-ta-nil)

Sublimaze
Classification: Opioid analgesic, opioid agonist
Pregnancy Class: C
Mechanism of Action: Binds to opiate receptors in the CNS, altering the response to and the perception of pain
Pharmacokinetics
Absorption: Immediate
Onset: IV—1 to 2 minutes
Duration: IV—0.5 to 1 hour
Indications: Used for patients in severe pain and as maintenance of analgesia in tracheal intubation
Contraindications: Known hypersensitivity
Precautions: Use with caution in patients with diabetes; severe renal, pulmonary, liver, or cardiac disease; increased intracranial pressure; or undiagnosed abdominal pain.
Route and Dosage
IV (Adult and Pediatric over 12 years): 0.5 to 1 mcg/kg
IV (Pediatric 1 to 12 years): Bolus—1 to 2 mcg/kg; continuous infusion—1 to 5 mcg/kg/hour following bolus dose
How Supplied
Injection: 0.05 mg/mL
Adverse Reactions and Side Effects
Resp: APNEA, LARYNGOSPASM, bronchospasm, respiratory depression
CV: Arrhythmias, bradycardia, circulatory depression, hypotension
CNS: Confusion, paradoxical excitation, drowsiness
EENT: Blurred or double vision
GI: Nausea, vomiting
Derm: Facial itching
MS: Skeletal and thoracic muscle rigidity (rapid infusion)
Drug Interactions: Avoid use in patients who have received MAO INHIBITORS within 14 days, because potentially fatal reactions may occur. Additive CNS depression may occur if used with other CNS depressant drugs.
EMS Considerations: Patient vital signs must be constantly monitored. Opioid antagonist drugs, oxygen, and resuscitative equipment should be readily available during the administration of fentanyl.

Hydromorphone (hye-droe-MOR-fone)

Dilaudid
Classification: Opioid analgesic, opioid agonist
Pregnancy Class: C
Mechanism of Action: Binds to opiate receptors in the CNS, altering the perception of and response to pain
Pharmacokinetics
Absorption: Well absorbed following rectal, SubQ, IM, and IV administration
Onset: SubQ and IM—15 minutes
IV—10 to 15 minutes
Rectal—15 to 30 minutes
Duration: SubQ and IM—4 to 5 hours
IV—2 to 3 hours
Rectal—4 to 5 hours
Indications: Used for moderate-to-severe pain, alone and in combination with nonopioid analgesics
Contraindications: Known hypersensitivity; (!) should not be used during pregnancy or lactation
Precautions: Use with caution in patients with head trauma, increased intracranial pressure, and severe renal, liver, or pulmonary disease. (!) Geriatric patients may be more susceptible to side effects. Therefore, a dose reduction may be ordered.
Route and Dosage (doses depend on the level of pain and patient tolerance)
SubQ, IM, IV (Adult over 50 kg [over 110 lbs]): 1.5 mg initially. Dosage may be increased.
SubQ, IM, IV (Adult and Pediatric under 50 kg [under 110 lbs]): 0.015 mg/kg initially. Dosage may be increased.
Rectal (Adult): 3 mg initially; may be repeated as needed

effective Communication

Rapid administration may lead to an increased risk of respiratory depression, hypotension, and CIRCULATORY COLLAPSE.

How Supplied
Injection: 1 mg/mL, 2 mg/mL, 4 mg/mL, 10 mg/mL
Suppositories: 3 mg
Adverse Reactions and Side Effects
Resp: Respiratory depression
CV: Hypotension, bradycardia
CNS: Confusion, sedation, dizziness, euphoria, floating feeling, hallucinations, headache, unusual dreams
GI: Constipation, dry mouth, nausea, vomiting
EENT: Blurred vision, diplopia, miosis
Derm: Flushing, sweating
Misc: Physical dependence, psychological dependence, tolerance
Drug Interactions: Use extreme caution with MAO INHIBITORS because of the risk of unpredictable reactions; reduce the initial dose of hydromorphone to 25 percent of the usual dose. Use with other CNS depressant drugs increases the risk of CNS depression.
EMS Considerations: Assess blood pressure, pulse, and respirations before and frequently during administration. (!) If respiratory rate falls below 10 breaths/minute, the dose may need to be decreased by 25 to 50 percent.

Ibuprofen Injection (eye-byoo-PROE-fen)

Caldolor
Classifications: Nonopioid analgesic, nonsteroidal anti-inflammatory

Pregnancy Class: C (up to 30-week gestation), D (beginning at 30-week gestation)

Check the Evidence

Giving ibuprofen injection after 30-week gestation may cause premature closure of the fetal ductus arteriosus.

Mechanism of Action: Inhibits prostaglandin synthesis, decreasing pain and inflammation

Pharmacokinetics

Absorption: Well absorbed—complete bioavailability

Onset: within 2 hours

Duration: 6 hours

Indications: Used in the management of mild-to-moderate pain and fever

Contraindications: Known hypersensitivity; cross-sensitivity may also exist if used with other NSAIDs, including aspirin; should not be given to patients with active GI bleeding or ulcer disease; should not be given to *aspirin triad* patients (asthma, nasal polyps, and aspirin intolerance) because of the risk of fatal ANAPHYLAXIS

Precautions: Use with caution in patients with cardiovascular disease and in patients with renal or liver disease.

Route and Dosage

IV (Adult): Analgesic—400 to 800 mg every 6 hours, as needed. Do not exceed 3,200 mg/day. Antipyretic—400 mg initially, then 400 mg every 4 to 6 hours, or 100 to 200 mg every 4 hours as needed. Do not exceed 3,200 mg/day.

How Supplied

Solution for injection: 100 mg/mL

Adverse Reactions and Side Effects

CV: Arrhythmias, edema, hypertension

CNS: Headache, dizziness, drowsiness

GI: GI BLEEDING, HEPATITIS, constipation, dyspepsia, nausea, vomiting, abdominal discomfort

EENT: Blurred vision, tinnitus

Derm: EXFOLIATIVE DERMATITIS, STEVENS-JOHNSON SYNDROME, TOXIC EPIDERMAL NECROLYSIS, rashes

Misc: ANAPHYLAXIS

Drug Interactions: Ibuprofen may limit the cardioprotective effects of aspirin. Concurrent use with aspirin may decrease the effectiveness of ibuprofen. There are additive adverse GI side effects with aspirin or other NSAIDs. Ibuprofen may increase the hypoglycemic effects of insulin or oral hypoglycemic agents.

EMS Considerations: Discontinue ibuprofen at the first sign of a rash—this may be life threatening. Treat symptomatically; this may occur once treatment is stopped.

Ketamine (KEE-tuh-meen)

Ketalar

Classifications: Anesthetic, analgesic agent

Pregnancy Class: C

Mechanism of Action: Blocks afferent transmission of impulses associated with pain perception; causes short-acting amnesia without muscular relaxation

Pharmacokinetics

Absorption: Well absorbed

Onset: 30 seconds

Duration: 10 to 15 minutes

Indications: Used as a sedative, for pain control, and as an induction agent for rapid-sequence intubation

Contraindications: Known hypersensitivity; should not be given to hypertensive patients or to patients with increased intracranial pressure

Precautions: Use with caution in the chronic alcoholic and the acutely alcohol-intoxicated patient.

Route and Dosage

IV (Adult): 0.5 to 1 mg/kg over 60 seconds

IM (Adult): 2 to 4 mg/kg

IV (Pediatric over 2 years): 1 to 2 mg over 60 seconds

IM (Pediatric over 2 years): 3 to 5 mg/kg

How Supplied

Vials: 10 mg/mL, 50 mg/mL, 100 mg/mL

Adverse Reactions and Side Effects

Resp: APNEA, SEVERE RESPIRATORY DEPRESSION (following rapid, high-dose IV administration), excess bronchial secretions

CV: Tachycardia or bradycardia, hypotension, arrhythmias

CNS: Hallucinations, explicit dreams

GI: Anorexia, nausea, vomiting

Drug Interactions: Concurrent use of other opioids or barbiturates may prolong recovery time.

EMS Considerations: Monitor vital signs frequently during administration. If possible, keep patients in a quiet environment.

Ketorolac (kee-TOE-role-ak)

Toradol

Classifications: Nonopioid analgesic, nonsteroidal anti-inflammatory

Pregnancy Class: C

Mechanism of Action: Inhibits prostaglandin synthesis, producing peripherally mediated analgesia; also has antipyretic and anti-inflammatory properties

Pharmacokinetics

Absorption: Rapidly and completely absorbed

Onset: IM, IV—10 minutes

Duration: IM, IV—6 hours or longer

Indication: Short-term management of pain. Management is not to exceed 5 days.

Contraindications: Known hypersensitivity; cross-sensitivity with other NSIADs may occur; should not be given to patients with known alcohol intolerance; (!) may inhibit labor and increase maternal bleeding at delivery

Precautions: Use with caution in patients with cardiovascular disease, in patients with a history of GI bleeding, and in patients with renal impairment.

Route and Dosage

IM (Adult under 65 years): Single dose = 60 mg. Multiple dosing = 30 mg every 6 hours, not to exceed 120 mg/day.

IM (Adult over 65 years, under 50 kg, or with renal impairment): Single dose = 30 mg. Multiple dosing = 30 mg every 6 hours, not to exceed 60 mg/day.
IV (Adult under 65 years): Single dose = 30 mg. Multiple dosing = 30 mg every 6 hours, not to exceed 120 mg/day.
IV (Adult over 65 years, under 50 kg, or with renal impairment): Single dose = 15 mg. Multiple dosing = 15 mg every 6 hours, not to exceed 60 mg/day.

effective **Communication**

The duration of ketorolac therapy should not exceed 5 days.

How Supplied
Injection: 15 mg/mL, 30 mg/mL
Adverse Reactions and Side Effects
Resp: Asthma, dyspnea
CV: Edema, pallor, vasodilation
CNS: <u>Drowsiness</u>, abnormal thinking, dizziness, euphoria, headache
GI: GI BLEEDING, abnormal taste, diarrhea, dry mouth, GI pain, nausea
Derm: EXFOLIATIVE DERMATITIS, STEVENS-JOHNSON SYNDROME, TOXIC EPIDERMAL NECROLYSIS, sweating, urticaria
Misc: Anaphylaxis
Drug Interactions: Concurrent use with aspirin may decrease the effectiveness of ketorolac. There is increased risk of GI effects with aspirin or other NSAIDs. Ketorolac may decrease the effectiveness of diuretics or antihypertensives.
EMS Considerations: Patients who have asthma, aspirin-induced allergy, and nasal polyps are at increased risk for hypersensitive reactions.

Lorazepam (lor-AZ-e-pam)

Apo-Lorazepam, Ativan, Novo-Lorazem, Nu-Loraz
Classifications: Anticonvulsant, antianxiety
Pregnancy Class: D
Mechanism of Action: Depresses the CNS by potentiating GABA, an inhibitory neurotransmitter
Pharmacokinetics
Absorption: Rapidly and completely absorbed following IV administration
Onset: 15 to 30 minutes
Duration: 8 to 12 hours
Indications: Used to decrease anxiety and seizure activity (unlabeled)
Contraindications: Known hypersensitivity; should not be given to patients with preexisting CNS depression, uncontrolled severe pain, angle-closure glaucoma, and severe hypotension
Precautions: Use with caution in patients with severe liver, renal, or pulmonary impairment, in patients with a history of suicide attempt or drug abuse, or in patients with COPD.

Route and Dosage (Anticonvulsant)
IV (Adult): 50 mcg (0.05 mg)/kg up to 4 mg; may be repeated after 10 to 15 minutes but not to exceed 8 mg/12 hours

Understand the Numbers

You are ordered to give 50 mcg/kg to your 300-pound patient. Will this dosage exceed the maximum dose of 4 mg? 300 lbs ÷ 2.2 kg = 136 kg. 50 mcg (0.05 mg) × 136 kg = 6800 mcg or 6.8 mg. Therefore, the dose for this patient should be 4,000 mcg or 4 mg, the maximum initial dose.

Check the **Evidence**

Administer lorazepam at a rate not to exceed 2 mg/minute or 0.05 mg/kg over 2 to 5 minutes. Rapid administration may result in apnea, hypotension, bradycardia, or cardiac arrest.

How Supplied
Injection: 2 mg/mL, 4 mg/mL
Adverse Reactions and Side Effects
Resp: Respiratory depression
CV: APNEA, CARDIAC ARREST *(rapid IV only)*
CNS: <u>Dizziness</u>, <u>drowsiness</u>, <u>lethargy</u>, hangover, headache, ataxia, slurred speech, confusion, forgetfulness
GI: Constipation, diarrhea, nausea, vomiting
EENT: Blurred vision
Derm: Rashes
Drug Interactions: Additive CNS depression if used with other CNS depressants
EMS Considerations: Assess patient vital signs continuously. Thoroughly flush the IV line before administering lorazepam if other drugs have already been given.

Midazolam (mid-AY-zoe-lam)

Versed
Classifications: Benzodiazepine, antianxiety, sedative/hypnotic
Pregnancy Class: D
Mechanism of Action: Acts on the CNS to produce generalized CNS depression. The effects are mediated by GABA, an inhibitory neurotransmitter.
Pharmacokinetics
Absorption: Rapidly absorbed by nasal administration; well absorbed followed by IM administration, and IV administration results in complete bioavailability.
Onset: IN—5 minutes
IM—15 minutes
IV—1.5 to 5 minutes
Duration: IN—30 to 60 minutes
IM and IV—2 to 6 hours
Indications: Used as a premedication before painful procedures, such as cardioversion, and can be used for patients experiencing anxiety; can also be used as an anticonvulsant
Contraindications: Known hypersensitivity; should not be given to patients with preexisting CNS depression, uncontrolled severe pain, or angle-closure glaucoma

<u>Underline</u> indicates most frequent; CAPITALS indicates life-threatening; ♣ indicates Canadian drug name. ! Safety and special populations.

Precautions: Use with caution in geriatric patients; in patients with pulmonary disease, CHF, renal impairment, or liver impairment; and in patients who are obese.

Check the Evidence

Patients over 70 years are generally more susceptible to cardiorespiratory depressant effects. Therefore, the dosage of midazolam may have to be reduced.

effective Communication

Patients who are obese should have the midazolam dosage calculated on the basis of ideal body weight.

Route and Dosage (Note: The dosage of midazolam must be individualized. Typically, the initial dosage is given on the basis of ideal body weight and increased as necessary. The average adult dose of midazolam is 5 mg. Many health-care facilities give children midazolam by mouth or intranasally. Check your protocols for the dosing of midazolam.)
IM (Adult): 0.07 to 0.08 mg/kg, initially
IV (Adult): 1 to 2.5 mg initially
How Supplied
Injection: 1 mg/mL, 5 mg/mL
Adverse Reactions and Side Effects
Resp: APNEA, LARYNGOSPASM, RESPIRATORY DEPRESSION, bronchospasm, coughing
CV: CARDIAC ARREST, arrhythmias
CNS: Agitation, drowsiness, excess sedation, headache
EENT: Blurred vision
GI: Hiccups, nausea, vomiting
Derm: Rashes
Local: Phlebitis at the IV site, pain at the IM site
Drug Interactions: Increased CNS depression if used with other CNS depressant drugs; increased risk of hypotension if used with other antihypertensive drugs

effective Communication

If midazolam is used concurrently with other CNS depressant drugs, the dosage of midazolam may have to be reduced by 30 to 50 percent.

EMS Considerations: Monitor blood pressure, pulse, and respirations continuously during administration. Oxygen and resuscitative equipment should be immediately available.

Meperidine (me-PER-i-deen)

Demerol
Classification: Opioid analgesic, opioid agonist
Pregnancy Class: C
Mechanism of Action: Binds to opiate receptors in the CNS, altering the perception of and response to pain
Pharmacokinetics
Absorption: 50 percent from the GI tract, well absorbed from IM. PO doses are about half as effective as parenteral doses.
Onset: PO—15 minutes
SubQ and IM—10 to 15 minutes
IV—Immediate
Duration: PO, IM, SubQ—2 to 4 hours
IV—2 to 3 hours
Indications: Used to treat moderate-to-severe pain, alone or with nonopioid drugs; also used as an analgesic during labor
Contraindications: Known hypersensitivity; should not be given to patients hypersensitive to bisulfites or to patients with recent (2 to 4 weeks) MAO inhibitor therapy
Precautions: Use with caution in patients with head trauma, increased intracranial pressure, or severe renal, liver, or pulmonary disease. ❗ Pediatric patients have an increased risk of seizures when given meperidine.
Route and Dosage
PO, SubQ, IM (Adult): Analgesia—50 mg every 3 to 4 hours. Dosage may be increased as needed (not to exceed 600 mg/24 hours). Analgesia during labor—50 to 100 mg IM or SubQ, when contractions become regular.
PO, SubQ, IM (Pediatric): Analgesia—1 to 1.5 mg/kg every 3 to 4 hours. Do not exceed 100 mg/dose.
IV (Adult): 15 to 35 mg/hour continuous infusion
IV (Pediatric): 0.5 to 1 mg/kg loading dose, followed by continuous infusion of 0.3 mg/kg/hour, titrate to effect up to 0.5 to 0.7 mg/kg/hour
How Supplied
Tablets: 50 mg, 100 mg
Syrup: 50 mg/5 mL
Injection: 🍁 10 mg/mL, 25 mg/0.5 mL, 25 mg/mL, 50 mg/mL, 75 mg/mL, 100 mg/mL
Adverse Reactions and Side Effects
Resp: Respiratory depression
CV: Hypotension, bradycardia
CNS: SEIZURES, confusion, sedation, euphoria, floating feeling, hallucinations, headache, unusual dreams
EENT: Blurred vision, diplopia, miosis
GI: Constipation, nausea, vomiting
Derm: Flushing, sweating
Misc: ANAPHYLAXIS
Drug Interactions: Do not give to patients taking (or have taken within the last 21 days) MAO INHIBITORS or PROCARBAZINE due to the risk of fatal reactions. There is increased CNS depression if given with other CNS depressant drugs.
EMS Considerations: Monitor patient vital signs closely. ❗ Have naloxone available to reverse respiratory depression or overdose.

Morphine (MOR-feen)

Astramorph, Astramorph PF, DepoDur, Duramorph, Embeda, 🍁 Epimorph, Infumorph, 🍁 M-Eslon, 🍁 Morphine HP, 🍁 Morphitec, 🍁 M.O.S., MS Contin, Roxanol, Roxanol Rescudose, 🍁 Statex
Classification: Opioid analgesic, opioid agonist
Pregnancy Class: C

Underline indicates most frequent; CAPITALS indicates life-threatening; 🍁 indicates Canadian drug name. ❗ Safety and special populations.

Mechanism of Action: Binds to the opiate receptors in the CNS, altering the perception of and response to pain

Pharmacokinetics

Absorption: Well absorbed via SubQ, IM, IV, and rectal routes

Onset: SubQ—20 minutes
IM—10 to 30 minutes
IV—Rapid-immediate
Rectal—Unknown

Duration: SubQ, IM, IV—4 to 5 hours
Rectal—3 to 7 hours

Indications: Used in the management of severe pain, pulmonary edema, and pain associated with a myocardial infarction (MI)

Contraindications: Known hypersensitivity; should not be given to patients hypersensitive to tartrazine, bisulfites, or alcohol

Precautions: Use with caution in patients with head trauma, increased intracranial pressure, undiagnosed abdominal pain, severe renal or liver dysfunction, pulmonary disease, or a history of substance abuse. (!) Elderly patients should receive reduced dosages because of increased risk of side effects.

Route and Dosage

Rectal (Adult over 50 kg [over 110 lbs]): 30 mg

Rectal (Adult & Pediatric under 50 kg [under 110 lbs]): 0.3 mg/kg

IM (Adult over 50 kg [over 110 lbs]): 8 to 15 mg

SubQ, IV (Adult over 50 kg [over 110 lbs]): 4 to 10 mg

SubQ, IM, IV (Adult and Pediatric under 50 kg [under 110 lbs]): 0.05 to 0.2 mg/kg. Maximum dose = 15 mg.

Understand the Numbers

You are ordered to give 0.1 mg/kg of morphine to your 85-pound pediatric patient. How many mg will you give? 85 lbs ÷ 2.2 kg = 38.6 or 39 kg. 0.1 mg × 39 kg = 3.9 mg.

How Supplied

Solution for SubQ, IM, and IV injection: 1 mg/mL, 2 mg/mL, 4 mg/mL, 5 mg/mL, 8 mg/mL, 10 mg/mL, 15 mg/mL, 25 mg/mL, 50 mg/mL

Suppositories: 5 mg, 10 mg, 20 mg, 30 mg

Adverse Reactions and Side Effects

Resp: RESPIRATORY DEPRESSION

CV: Hypotension, bradycardia

CNS: Confusion, sedation, dizziness, euphoria, floating feeling, hallucinations, headache, unusual dreams

EENT: Blurred vision, diplopia, miosis

GI: Constipation, nausea, vomiting

Derm: Flushing, itching, sweating

Misc: Physical dependence, psychological dependence, tolerance

Drug Interactions: Use with extreme caution in patients using MAO INHIBITORS within 14 days prior to giving morphine due to unpredictable, severe reactions; initial dose of morphine should be reduced to 25 percent of usual dose. There is increased risk of CNS depression if used with other CNS depressant drugs.

EMS Considerations: Do not confuse morphine with hydromorphone or meperidine—errors have resulted in patient deaths. Assess patient vital signs before and frequently during and after administration. Have naloxone available for administration to reverse respiratory depression and overdose.

Nalbuphine (NAL-byoo-feen)

Nubain

Classification: Opioid analgesic, opioid agonist

Pregnancy Class: C

Mechanism of Action: Binds to opiate receptors in the CNS altering the perception of and the response to pain

Pharmacokinetics

Absorption: Well absorbed from SubQ, IM, and IV routes

Onset: SubQ, IM—less than 15 minutes
IV—2 to 3 minutes

Duration: SubQ, IM, IV—3 to 6 hours

Indications: Used in the management of moderate-to-severe pain; can also be used as analgesia during labor

Contraindications: Known hypersensitivity; should not be given to patients hypersensitive to bisulfites or to patients physically dependent on opioids

Precautions: Use with caution in patients with head trauma; increased intracranial pressure; severe renal, liver, or pulmonary disease; undiagnosed abdominal pain; or alcohol dependence.

Route and Dosage

SubQ, IM, IV (Adult): Usual dose is 10 mg every 3 to 6 hours

effective **Communication**

Higher doses of nalbuphine can be given, but a single dose should not exceed 20 mg; and daily dose is not to exceed 160 mg. Give nalbuphine slowly—each 10 mg over 3 to 5 minutes.

How Supplied

Injection: 10 mg/mL, 20 mg/mL

Adverse Reactions and Side Effects

Resp: Respiratory depression

CV: Orthostatic hypotension, palpitations

CNS: Dizziness, headache, sedation, confusion, euphoria, floating feeling, hallucinations, unusual dreams

EENT: Blurred vision, diplopia, miosis (high doses)

GI: Dry mouth, nausea, vomiting, constipation

Derm: Clammy feeling, sweating

Misc: Physical dependence, psychological dependence, tolerance

Drug Interactions: Use with extreme caution in patients receiving MAO INHIBITORS because of the risk of unpredictable adverse reactions; reduce initial dose of nalbuphine to 25 percent of the usual initial dose. There is additive CNS depression if used with other CNS depressant drugs.

EMS Considerations: Assess patient vital signs before and frequently during and after administration.

Nitrous Oxide-Oxygen Mixture (NYE-trus OX-ide)

Nitronox, Entonox

Classifications: medicinal gas, analgesic
Pregnancy Class: C
Mechanism of Action: Inhalation of a 50 percent mixture of nitrous oxide and oxygen produces CNS depression and rapid pain relief.
Pharmacokinetics
- *Absorption:* Rapid
- *Onset:* 2 minutes
- *Duration:* 2 to 5 minutes

Indications: Used in the management of moderate-to-severe pain
Contraindications: Known hypersensitivity; should not be given to patients with a decreased LOC; to patients with thoracic trauma, respiratory compromise, or abdominal distension; or to patients who cannot follow simple instructions
Precautions: Monitor patients closely during administration. Some patients develop severe nausea and vomiting, and some patients experience syncope.

Route and Dosage

Inhalation (Adult and Pediatric): Self-administration by the patient until pain is relieved

How Supplied

D and E blue and green cylinders: 50 percent nitrous oxide and 50 percent oxygen
🍁 *D and E blue and white cylinders:* 50 percent nitrous oxide and 50 percent oxygen

Adverse Reactions and Side Effects

Resp: Decreased respirations, apnea
CNS: Lightheadedness, drowsiness
GI: Nausea, vomiting
Drug Interactions: Additive CNS depression may occur when other CNS depressants are used.
EMS Considerations: Patients with respiratory compromise should receive 100 percent oxygen to prevent nitrous oxide from collecting in dead air spaces and further aggravating chest injuries. Patients with myocardial pain should receive oxygen when the nitrous oxide-oxygen mixture is not being given. Do not administer a nitrous oxide-oxygen mixture to patients with abdominal pain unless it is certain that intestinal blockage is not present, because nitrous oxide may collect in the obstructed space, aggravating the obstruction.

Promethazine (proe-METH-a-zeen)

🍁 Histantil, Phenergan, Promethacon

Classifications: Sedative/hypnotic
Pregnancy Class: C
Mechanism of Action: Produces CNS depression by indirectly decreased stimulation of the CNS reticular system
Pharmacokinetics
- *Absorption:* Well absorbed by IM and IV. Rectal absorption is less reliable.
- *Onset:* IM, Rectal—20 minutes
  IV—2 to 3 minutes
- *Duration:* Rectal, IM, IV—4 to 12 hours

Indication: Can be given to patients for sedation; can also be given for sedation during labor
Contraindications: Known hypersensitivity; should not be given to comatose patients, patients with prostatic hypertrophy, or patients with bladder neck obstruction
Precautions: Use with caution in patients with hypertension, cardiovascular disease, impaired liver function, glaucoma, asthma, and epilepsy.

Route and Dosage

Sedation
Rectal, IM, IV (Adult): 25 to 50 mg
Rectal, IM (Pediatric over 2 years): 0.5 to 1 mg/kg, not to exceed 50 mg

effective Communication

Promethazine may cause fatal respiratory depression in pediatric patients under 2 years.

Sedation during labor
IM, IV (Adult): 50 mg in early labor; should not exceed 100 mg/24 hours

How Supplied

Injection: 25 mg/mL, 50 mg/mL
Suppositories: 12.5 mg, 25 mg, 50 mg

Adverse Reactions and Side Effects

CV: Bradycardia, hypertension or hypotension, tachycardia
CNS: NEUROLEPTIC MALIGNANT SYNDROME, confusion, disorientation, sedation, dizziness, fatigue, insomnia, nervousness
EENT: Blurred vision, diplopia, tinnitus
GI: Constipation, dry mouth
Derm: Photosensitivity, rashes
Drug Interactions: Additive CNS depression if given with other CNS depressants; may precipitate seizures when used with drugs that lower the seizure threshold
EMS Considerations: IV administration may cause severe injury to tissue if the IV infiltrates. If pain occurs at the IV site, discontinue the IV immediately.

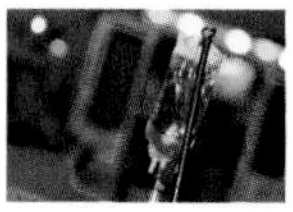

SCENARIO REVISITED

Do you recall the case of Mr. Smyth who dropped a 50-pound weight on his foot?

Mr. Smyth states that he weighs 215 pounds. After stabilizing Mr. Smyth's foot, you are given an order to administer morphine. The appropriate dose of morphine for Mr. Smyth is 4 to 10 mg IV or IM. You may repeat this dose every 3 to 4 hours. During transport, you should continuously monitor Mr. Smyth's vital signs, level of consciousness, and respiratory status. Nausea and vomiting are common with the administration of morphine. You must be prepared should this occur.

Let's Recap

The medications discussed in this chapter are very effective in alleviating pain. It is vital for EMS professionals to understand when it is appropriate to administer analgesics. Analgesics should never be administered if they will preclude the correct diagnosis or assessment of the patient, such as head trauma or abdominal pain. Protocols for pain management vary widely between EMS systems. EMS professionals should be aware of their local protocols.

SCENARIO CONCLUSION

Keeping Mr. Smyth still and lying down decreases his risk of nausea and vomiting. Antiemetic drugs such as promethazine or chlorpromazine are frequently coadministered with morphine to help prevent or treat nausea and vomiting. EMS professionals should have naloxone available to administer if signs or symptoms of opioid overdose occur. This may include loss of consciousness, respiratory depression, or hypotension. The appropriate dose of naloxone is 0.4 mg IV that may be repeated every 2 to 3 minutes, as needed. Some patients may require up to 2 mg. The maximum total dose of naloxone should not exceed 10 mg.

PRACTICE EXERCISES

1. Butorphanol and nalbuphine are opioid analgesics. They should not be administered to patients who are physically dependent on opioids because:
a. Withdrawal may occur
b. Hypotension may occur
c. Loss of consciousness may occur
d. Respiratory depression may occur

2. Patients requiring morphine while on monoamine oxidase inhibitors should:
a. Not receive morphine
b. Receive morphine at the usual dose
c. Receive a dose 25 percent less than the usual dose of morphine
d. Receive a 25 percent increase in the usual dose of morphine

3. A possible life-threatening CNS adverse reaction to meperidine is:
a. Seizures
b. Euphoria
c. Dysphoria
d. Hallucinations

4. Nitrous oxide-oxygen mixture is contraindicated in the following:
a. Pediatric patients
b. Intestinal obstruction
c. Myocardial infarction
d. Chronic obstructive pulmonary disease

5. Which of the following analgesics has the potential adverse effect of GI bleeding?
a. Nalbuphine
b. Morphine
c. Ketorolac
d. Fentanyl

6. The initial adult dose of hydromorphone in a patient who weighs 150 pounds is:
a. 0.015 mg/kg IV
b. 0.15 mg/kg IV
c. 1.5 mg IV
d. 2.5 mg IV

7. Rapid IV administration of lorazepam may result in:
a. Cardiac arrest
b. Hypertension
c. Tachycardia
d. Respiratory depression

8. Which of the following analgesics has the potential adverse effect of GI bleeding?
a. Nalbuphine
b. Morphine
c. Ketorolac
d. Fentanyl

9. You are ordered to administer 0.4 mg/kg of etomidate to your 110-pound, 13-year-old patient. How many milligrams should you administer?
a. 20 mg
b. 22 mg
c. 24 mg
d. 26 mg

10. Rapid or high-dose ketamine may cause:
a. Tachycardia
b. Bradycardia
c. Hypotension
d. Apnea

CASE STUDIES

1. You respond to a motor vehicle crash. The driver is a 40-year-old female. She is complaining of wrist pain. Your assessment reveals obvious deformity of her left wrist. The patient is also complaining of severe head pain. Her head has an obvious abrasion above her left eye, and you also notice that the vehicle's windshield is cracked. The most appropriate analgesic to give to this patient at this time is:
   a. Nitrous oxide-oxygen mixture
   b. Butorphanol
   c. Morphine
   d. Analgesic medication is contraindicated at this time

2. You are transporting a 20-year-old male patient with a femur fracture to the emergency department. Nitrous oxide-oxygen mixture has been ordered to relieve his pain. The patient had been receiving the medication for approximately 20 minutes when he fell asleep, and his hand fell, pulling the mask away from his face. The appropriate action for you to take at this time is:
   a. Attach the mask to the patient's face to continue administering the medication.
   b. Administer morphine 5 mg IM because the patient is no longer able to self-administer nitrous oxide.
   c. Administer naloxone to reverse the effects of the nitrous oxide-oxygen mixture.
   d. Continue to monitor the patient's vital signs, level of consciousness, and respiratory status.

MATH EQUATIONS

1. You are ordered to give 15 mg/kg of acetaminophen rectally to your 90-lb, 7-year-old patient.
   a. How many kg does your patient weigh?
   b. How many mg of the acetaminophen will you give?
2. You are ordered to administer 0.3 mg/kg of etomidate to your 105-lb, 12-year-old patient. The maximum dose of etomidate for this patient is 20 mg.
   a. How many kg does your patient weigh?
   b. How many milligrams of the etomidate should you administer?
3. You are ordered to give a bolus of 1 mcg/kg of fentanyl to your 10-year-old, 90-lb patient. The bolus is to be followed by a 3 mcg/kg/hour infusion of fentanyl.
   a. How many kg does your patient weigh?
   b. What is the dosage (mcg) of the fentanyl bolus?
   c. What is the drip rate using a 60 gtt/mL IV set to deliver 3 mcg/kg/hour?
4. You are ordered to give 0.5 mg/kg of ketamine to your 230-lb adult patient. The ketamine comes as 10 mg/5 mL.
   a. How many kg does your patient weigh?
   b. What is the dosage (mg) of the ketamine?
   c. What volume of the ketamine is required for question b above?
5. You are ordered to give 50 mcg/kg of lorazepam to your 220-lb adult patient. The maximum dose for this patient is 4 mg.
   a. How many kg does your patient weigh?
   b. What is the dosage (mcg) of lorazepam for your patient?
   c. What is the dosage (mg) of lorazepam for your patient?

REFERENCES

Beck, R. K. (2012). Pain management. In *Pharmacology for the EMS provider.* New York: Delmar, Cengage Learning.

Deglin, J. H., Vallerand, A. H., and Sanboski, C.A. (2011). *Davis's drug guide for nurses* (12th ed.). Philadelphia, PA: F. A. Davis Company.

Etomidate. Retrieved February 24, 2014 from www.medscape.com/viewarticle/585288_2

Goodwin, J. (2013). How to manage pain. Retrieved February 22, 2014 from www.emsworld.com/article/11079128/pain-management

Morrow, A. (2009). Death & dying: what is pain? Retrieved March 7, 2014 from www.dying.about.com/od/paincontrol/a/whatispain.htm

Nitrous oxide administration. Retrieved February 20, 2014 from http://emedicine.medscape.com/article/1413427-overview

Venes, D., ed. (2013). *Taber's cyclopedic medical dictionary* (22nd ed.). Philadelphia, PA: F. A. Davis Company.

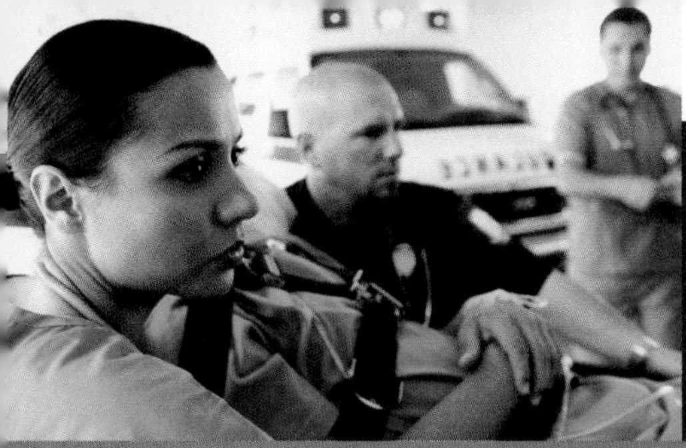

APPENDIX A

Drugs (Generic and Trade Names) and Their Therapeutic Classifications*

Drug Name	Therapeutic Classification(s)
Abeneton (biperiden)	Antiparkinsonian agent
Accolate (zafirlukast)	Antiasthmatic
acebutolol	Antihypertensive, antiarrhythmic
Acephen (acetaminophen)	Non-narcotic analgesic, antipyretic
acetaminophen	Non-narcotic analgesic, antipyretic
acetazolamide	Anticonvulsant, diuretic
acetohexamide	Antidiabetic
acetophenazine	Antipsychotic
acetylcysteine	Antidote (acetaminophen)
Activase (alteplase)	Thrombolytic drug
Adalat (nifedipine)	Antianginal
Adapin (doxepin)	Antidepressant
Adrenalin Chloride (epinephrine hydrochloride)	Bronchodilator, vasopressor, cardiac stimulant, local anesthetic adjunct, topical antihemorrhagic, antiglaucoma agent
Aerolate (theophylline)	Bronchodilator
Akineton (biperiden)	Antiparkinsonian agent
Ak-Zol (acetazolamide)	Anticonvulsant, diuretic
Alazsine Tabs (hydralazine)	Antihypertensive
albuterol	Bronchodilator
albuterol/ipratropium bromide	Combination bronchodilator
Aldactone (spironolactone)	Antihypertensive, diuretic
Alphacaine (lidocaine)	Ventricular antiarrhythmic, local anesthetic
alprazolam	Antianxiety agent—controlled substance, Schedule IV
Altace (ramipril)	Antihypertensive/ACE inhibitor
alteplase	Thrombolytic drug
Alupent (metaproterenol)	Bronchodilator
Alzapam (lorazepam)	Antianxiety agent, sedative/hypnotic—controlled substance, Schedule IV

*Drug names beginning with a capital letter are trade; drug names beginning with a lowercase letter are generic.

Drug Name	Therapeutic Classification(s)
Amcill (ampicillin)	Antibiotic
A-Methapred (methylprednisolone)	Anti-inflammatory
Aminophyllin (aminophylline)	Bronchodilator
aminophylline	Bronchodilator
amiodarone	Ventricular and supraventricular antiarrhythmic
amitriptyline	Antidepressant
amobarbital	Sedative/hypnotic, anticonvulsant—controlled substance, Schedule II
Amodopa Tabs (methyldopa)	Antihypertensive
Amoline (aminophylline)	Bronchodilator
amoxapine	Antidepressant
amoxicillin	Antibiotic
Amoxil (amoxicillin)	Antibiotic
amphotericin B	Antifungal
ampicillin	Antibiotic
amrinone	Inotropic, vasodilator
amyl nitrite	Cyanide poisoning adjunct
Amytal (amobarbital)	Sedative/hypnotic, anticonvulsant—controlled substance, Schedule II
Anacin-3 (acetaminophen)	Non-narcotic analgesic, antipyretic
Anectine (succinylcholine chloride)	Depolarizing neuromuscular blocking drug
Anestacon (lidocaine)	Ventricular antiarrhythmic, local anesthetic
Ang-O-Span (nitroglycerin [oral])	Antianginal, vasodilator
Anspor (cephradine)	Antibiotic
Antilirium (physostigmine)	Antimuscarinic
Apo-Amitriptyline (amitriptyline)	Antidepressant
Apresoline (hydralazine)	Antihypertensive
Aprozide (hydrochlorothiazide)	Diuretic, antihypertensive
Aquachloral (chloral hydrate)	Sedative/hypnotic—controlled substance, Schedule IV
Aquatensen (methyclothiazide)	Diuretic, antihypertensive
Arm-a-Med (isoetharine)	Bronchodilator
Asendin (amoxapine)	Antidepressant
Asthma Nefrin (epinephrine hydrochloride)	Bronchodilator, vasopressor, cardiac stimulant, local anesthetic adjunct, topical antihemorrhagic, antiglaucoma agent
Asthmahaler (epinephrine)	Bronchodilator, vasopressor, cardiac stimulant, local anesthetic adjunct, topical antihemorrhagic, antiglaucoma agent
Astramorph (morphine)	Analgesic—controlled substance, Schedule II
Atarax (hydroxyzine)	Antianxiety agent, sedative
atenolol	Antihypertensive, antianginal
atracurium besylate	Nondepolarizing skeletal muscle relaxant
atropine	Antiarrhythmic
Atrovent (ipratropium)	Bronchodilator
Auto-Injector (lidocaine)	Ventricular antiarrhythmic, local anesthetic
Aventyl (nortriptyline)	Antidepressant
Azmacort (triamcinolone)	Corticosteroid
bacampicillin	Antibiotic

Drug Name	Therapeutic Classification(s)
Barbased (butabarbital)	Sedative/hypnotic—controlled substance, Schedule III
Barbita (phenobarbital)	Anticonvulsant, sedative/hypnotic— controlled substance, Schedule IV
beclomethasone	Anti-inflammatory, antiasthmatic
Beclovent (beclomethasone)	Anti-inflammatory, antiasthmatic
Beconase (beclomethasone)	Anti-inflammatory, antiasthmatic
Beef Regular Iletin II	Antidiabetic agent (insulin [regular])
Beldin (diphenhydramine)	Antihistamine, antiemetic and antivertigo agent, antitussive, sedative/hypnotic, topical anesthetic
Benadryl (diphenhydramine)	Antihistamine, antiemetic and antivertigo agent, antitussive, sedative/hypnotic, topical anesthetic
Benadryl Children's Allergy (diphenhydramine)	Antihistamine, antiemetic and antivertigo agent, antitussive, sedative/hypnotic, topical anesthetic
Benadryl Complete Allergy (diphenhydramine)	Antihistamine, antiemetic and antivertigo agent, antitussive, sedative/hypnotic, topical anesthetic
Bendylate (diphenhydramine)	Antihistamine, antiemetic and antivertigo agent, antitussive, sedative/hypnotic, topical anesthetic
Benylin (diphenhydramine)	Antihistamine, antiemetic and antivertigo agent, antitussive, sedative/hypnotic, topical anesthetic
Benylin DM Cough (dextromethorphan)	Non-narcotic antitussive
benzphetamine	Anorexigenic
$Beta_2$ (isoetharine)	Bronchodilator
biperiden	Antiparkinsonian agent
Bisorine (isoetharine)	Bronchodilator
bitolterol	Bronchodilator
Blocadren (timolol)	Antihypertensive, antiglaucoma agent
Brethine (terbutaline)	Bronchodilator
bretylium tosylate	Antiarrhythmic
Bretylol (bretylium)	Antiarrhythmic
Brevibloc (esmolol)	Antiarrhythmic (class II)/beta-blocker
Bricanyl (terbutaline)	Bronchodilator
Bromo-Seltzer (acetaminophen)	Non-narcotic analgesic, antipyretic
bromocriptine	Antiparkinsonian agent
Bronitin Mist (epinephrine bitartrate)	Bronchodilator, vasopressor, cardiac stimulant, local anesthetic adjunct, topical antihemorrhagic, antiglaucoma agent
Bronkaid Mist (epinephrine)	Bronchodilator, vasopressor, cardiac stimulant, local anesthetic adjunct, topical antihemorrhagic, antiglaucoma agent
Bronkaid Mist Suspension (epinephrine bitartrate)	Bronchodilator, vasopressor, cardiac stimulant, local anesthetic adjunct, topical antihemorrhagic, antiglaucoma agent
Bronkodyl (theophylline)	Bronchodilator
Bronkosol (isoetharine)	Bronchodilator
bumetanide	Antihypertensive, diuretic
Bumex (bumetanide)	Antihypertensive, diuretic
butabarbital	Sedative/hypnotic—controlled substance, Schedule III
Butalan (butabarbital)	Sedative/hypnotic—controlled substance, Schedule III
Butatran (butabarbital)	Sedative/hypnotic—controlled substance, Schedule III
Buticaps (butabarbital)	Sedative/hypnotic—controlled substance, Schedule III

Drug Name	Therapeutic Classification(s)
Butisol (butabarbital)	Sedative/hypnotic—controlled substance, Schedule III
butorphanol	Narcotic agonist-antagonist, opioid partial agonist analgesic
Calan (verapamil)	Antianginal, antiarrhythmic, antihypertensive
calcium chloride	Electrolyte modifier
calcium gluceptate	Electrolyte modifier
calcium gluconate	Electrolyte modifier
Capoten (captopril)	Antihypertensive/ACE inhibitor
captopril	Antihypertensive/ACE inhibitor
carbamazepine	Anticonvulsant, analgesic
carbenicillin	Antibiotic
Cardizem (diltiazem)	Antianginal
Catapres (clonidine)	Antihypertensive
Catapres-TTS (clonidine)	Antihypertensive
Ceclor (cefaclor)	Antibiotic
Cedilanid-D Injections	Antiarrhythmic, inotropic
cefaclor	Antibiotic
Celontin Half Strength Kapseals	Anticonvulsant
Celontin Kapseals (methsuximide)	Anticonvulsant
Centrax (prazepam)	Antianxiety agent—controlled substance, Schedule IV
cephradine	Antibiotic
chloral hydrate	Sedative/hypnotic—controlled substance Schedule IV
Chlordiazepoxide	Antianxiety agent, anticonvulsant, sedative/hypnotic—controlled substance, Schedule IV
Chlorpromazine (prochlorpazine)	Antipsychotic, antiemetic, antianxiety agent
chlorothiazide	Diuretic, antihypertensive
chlorpropamide	Antidiabetic, antidiuretic agent
chlorprothixene	Antipsychotic
chlorthalidone	Diuretic, antihypertensive
Chlorzide (hydrochlorothiazide)	Diuretic, antihypertensive
Chlorzine (chlorpromazine)	Antipsychotic, antiemetic
Choledyl (oxtriphylline)	Bronchodilator
Cin-Quin (quinidine)	Ventricular and supraventricular antiarrhythmic, atrial antiarrythmic
clemastine	Antihistamine
clonazepam	Anticonvulsant—controlled substance, Schedule IV
clonidine	Antihypertensive
clorazepate	Antianxiety agent, anticonvulsant, sedative/hypnotic—controlled substance, Schedule IV
codeine	Analgesic, antitussive—controlled substance, Schedule II
Combivent (albuterol/ipratropium)	Combination bronchodilator
Compazine (prochlorperazine)	Antipsychotic, antiemetic, antianxiety agent
Compazine Spansule (prochlorperazine)	Antipsychotic, antiemetic, antianxiety agent
Compoz (diphenhydramine)	Antihistamine, antiemetic and antivertigo agent, antitussive, sedative/hypnotic, topical anesthetic
Congestrin (dextromethorphan)	Non-narcotic antitussive

Drug Name	Therapeutic Classification(s)
Constant-T (theophylline)	Bronchodilator
Cordarone (amiodarone)	Ventricular and supraventricular antiarrhythmic
Corgard (nadolol)	Antihypertensive, antianginal
Cortef (hydrocortisone)	Anti-inflammatory
Cortisol (hydrocortisone)	Anti-inflammatory
Coumadin (warfarin)	Anticoagulant
Covera-HS (verapamil)	Antianginal, antiarrhythmic, antihypertensive
Cermacoat 1 (dextromethorphan)	Non-narcotic antitussive
cromolyn sodium	Antiasthmatic, antiallergic
Crystodigin (digitoxin)	Antiarrhythmic, inotropic
Dalcaine (lidocaine)	Ventricular antiarrhythmic, local anesthetic
Dalmane (flurazepam)	Sedative/hypnotic—controlled substance, Schedule IV
Darvon (propoxyphene)	Analgesic—controlled substance, Schedule IV
Datril (acetaminophen)	Non-narcotic analgesic, antipyretic
Datril-500 (acetaminophen)	Non-narcotic analgesic, antipyretic
Decadron (dexamethasone)	Anti-inflammatory
Delsym (dextromethorphan)	Non-narcotic antitussive
Demerol (meperidine)	Analgesic—controlled substance, Schedule II
Depakene (valproic acid)	Anticonvulsant
desipramine	Antidepressant, antianxiety agent
deslanoside	Antiarrhythmic, inotropic
dexamethasone	Anti-inflammatory
dextromethorphan	Non-narcotic antitussive
dextrose 50% in water	Hyperglycemic
Dey-Dose (isoetharine)	Bronchodilator
Dey-Lute (isoetharine)	Bronchodilator
DiaBeta (glyburide)	Antidiabetic
Diabinese (chlorpropamide)	Antidiabetic, antidiuretic
Diachlor (chlorothiazide)	Diuretic, antihypertensive
Diahist (diphenhydramine)	Antihistamine, antiemetic, and antivertigo agent, antitussive, sedative/hypnotic, topical anesthetic
Diamox (acetazolamide)	Anticonvulsant, diuretic
Diamox Sequels (acetazolamide)	Anticonvulsant, diuretic
Diaqua (hydrochlorothiazide)	Diuretic, antihypertensive
diazepam	Antianxiety agent, skeletal muscle relaxant, amnesic agent, anticonvulsant, sedative/hypnotic
diazoxide	Antihypertensive
Didrex (benzphetamine)	Anorexigenic
digitoxin	Antiarrhythmic, inotropic
digoxin	Antiarrhythmic, inotropic
Dilantin (phenytoin)	Anticonvulsant, antiarrhythmic
Dilaudid (hydromorphone)	Analgesic, antitussive
Dilocaine (lidocaine)	Ventricular antiarrhythmic, local anesthetic
diltiazem	Antianginal

Drug Name	Therapeutic Classification(s)
Diphen (diphenhydramine)	Antihistamine, antiemetic, and antivertigo agent, antitussive, sedative/hypnotic, topical anesthetic
Diphenadril (diphenhydramine)	Antihistamine, antiemetic, and antivertigo agent, antitussive, sedative/hypnotic, topical anesthetic
diphenhydramine	Antihistamine, antiemetic, and antivertigo agent, antitussive, sedative/hypnotic, topical anesthetic
dipyridamole	Coronary vasodilator, platelet aggregation inhibitor
disopyramide	Ventricular/supraventricular antiarrhythmia, atrial antitachyarrhythmic
Dispos-a-Med (isoetharine)	Bronchodilator
Diuril (chlorothiazide)	Diuretic, antihypertensive
DM Cough (dextromethorphan)	Non-narcotic antitussive
dobutamine	Inotropic
Dobutrex (dobutamine)	Inotropic
Dolene (propoxyphene)	Analgesic—controlled substance, Schedule IV
Dolophine (methadone)	Analgesic, narcotic detoxification adjunct—controlled substance, Schedule II
dopamine	Inotropic, vasopressor
Dopastat (dopamine)	Inotropic, vasopressor
Doriden (glutethimide)	Sedative/hypnotic—controlled substance, Schedule III
Doriglute (glutethimide)	Sedative/hypnotic—controlled substance, Schedule III
Doxaphene (propoxyphene)	Analgesic—controlled substance, Schedule IV
doxepin	Antidepressant
droperidol	Antianxiety, antipsychotic
Duramorph (morphine)	Analgesic—controlled substance, Schedule II
Durapam (flurazepam)	Sedative/hypnotic—controlled substance, Schedule IV
Dymelor (acetohexamide)	Antidiabetic
Edecrin (ethacrynic acid)	Diuretic
edrophonium	Antiarrhythmic, cholinergic agonist
Elavil (amitriptyline)	Antidepressant
Elixophyllin (theophylline)	Bronchodilator
Emitrip (amitriptyline)	Antidepressant
Endep (amitriptyline)	Antidepressant
Enduron (methyclothiazide)	Diuretic, antihypertensive
Enovil (amitriptyline)	Antidepressant
Entonox (nitrous oxide-oxygen mixture)	Analgesic
ephedrine sulfate	Adrenergic
Epifrin (epinephrine hydrochloride)	Bronchodilator, vasopressor, cardiac stimulant, local anesthetic adjunct, topical antihemorrhagic, antiglaucoma agent
epinephrine	Bronchodilator, vasopressor, cardiac stimulant, local anesthetic adjunct, topical antihemorrhagic, antiglaucoma agent
epinephrine bitartrate	Bronchodilator, vasopressor, cardiac stimulant, local anesthetic adjunct, topical antihemorrhagic, antiglaucoma agent
epinephrine hydrochloride	Bronchodilator, vasopressor, cardiac stimulant, local anesthetic adjunct, topical antihemorrhagic, antiglaucoma agent
EpiPen (epinephrine)	Bronchodilator, vasopressor, cardiac stimulant, local anesthetic adjunct, topical antihemorrhagic, antiglaucoma agent

Drug Name	Therapeutic Classification(s)
EpiPen Jr. (epinephrine)	Bronchodilator, vasopressor, cardiac stimulant, local anesthetic adjunct, topical antihemorrhagic, antiglaucoma agent
Epitol (carbamazepine)	Anticonvulsant, analgesic
Epitrate (epinephrine bitartrate)	Bronchodilator, vasopressor, cardiac stimulant, local anesthetic adjunct, topical antihemorrhagic, antiglaucoma agent
Epsom Salts (magnesium sulfate)	Electrolyte
Equanil (meprobamate)	Antianxiety agent—controlled substance, Schedule IV
esmolol	Antiarrhythmic (class II)/beta blocker
Esidrix (hydrochlorothiazide)	Diuretic, antihypertensive
Eskalith (lithium)	Antimanic, antipsychotic
Eskalith CR (lithium)	Antimanic, antipsychotic
ethacrynic acid	Diuretic
ethchlorvynol	Sedative/hypnotic—controlled substance, Schedule IV
ethosuximide	Anticonvulsant
Eutonyl (pargyline)	Antihypertensive
Extentabs (quinidine)	Ventricular and supraventricular antiarrhythmic, atrial antiarrhythmic
fentanyl	Opioid analgesic
Fenylhist (diphenhydramine)	Antihistamine, antiemetic, and antivertigo agent, antitussive, sedative/hypnotic, topical anesthetic
flecainide	Ventricular antiarrhythmic
Flovent (fluticasone propionate)	Corticosteroid
flumazil	Benzodiazepine antagonist
fluphenazine	Antipsychotic
flurazepam	Sedative/hypnotic—controlled substance, Schedule IV
fluticasone propionate	Corticosteroid
Fungizone (amphotericin B)	Antifungal
furosemide	Diuretic, antihypertensive
Fynex (diphenhydramine)	Antihistamine, antiemetic, and antivertigo agent, antitussive, sedative/hypnotic, topical anesthetic
Geopen (carbenicillin)	Antibiotic
Glaucon (epinephrine hydrochloride)	Bronchodilator, vasopressor, cardiac stimulant, local anesthetic adjunct, topical antihemorrhagic, antiglaucoma agent
glipizide	Antidiabetic
Glucamide (chlorpropamide)	Antidiabetic, antidiuretic
Glucotrol (glipizide)	Antidiabetic
Glutethimide	Sedative/hypnotic—controlled substance, Schedule III
glyburide	Antidiabetic
guanabenz	Antihypertensive
guanethidine	Antihypertensive
Halazepam	Antianxiety agent—controlled substance, Schedule IV
Halcion (triazolam)	Sedative/hypnotic—controlled substance, Schedule III
Haldol (haloperidol)	Antipsychotic
haloperidol	Antipsychotic
Hexadrol (dexamethasone)	Anti-inflammatory

Drug Name	Therapeutic Classification(s)
Hold DM (dextromethorphan)	Non-narcotic antitussive
Humulin R (insulin [regular])	Antidiabetic
hydralazine	Antihypertensive
Hydramine (diphenhydramine)	Antihistamine, antiemetic, and antivertigo agent, antitussive, sedative/hypnotic, topical anesthetic
Hydril (diphenhydramine)	Antihistamine, antiemetic, and antivertigo agent, antitussive, sedative/hypnotic, topical anesthetic
HydroDIURIL (hydrochlorothiazide)	Diuretic, antihypertensive
Hydro-Z-50 (hydrochlorothiazide)	Diuretic, antihypertensive
hydrochlorothiazide	Diuretic, antihypertensive
Hydrocortisone	Anti-inflammatory
Hydrocortone (hydrocortisone)	Anti-inflammatory
Hydromal (hydrochlorothiazide)	Diuretic, antihypertensive
hydromorphone	Analgesic, antitussive
hydroxyzine	Antianxiety agent, sedative
Hygroton (chlorthalidone)	Diuretic, antihypertensive
Hyperstat (diazoxide)	Antihypertensive
Hylidone (chlorthalidone)	Diuretic, antihypertensive
Inapsine (droperidol)	Antianxiety, antipsychotic
Inderal (propranolol)	Antihypertensive, antianginal, antiarrhythmic
Inderal LA (propranolol)	Antihypertensive, antianginal, antiarrhythmic
Inocor (amrinone)	Inotropic, vasodilator
insulin (regular)	Antidiabetic
Intal (cromolyn sodium)	Antiasthmatic, antiallergic
Intropin (dopamine)	Inotropic, vasopressor
ipratropium bromide	Bronchodilator
Ismelin (guanethidine)	Antihypertensive
Isosmotic (isosorbide)	Antiglaucoma agent
isocarboxazid	Antidepressant
isoetharine	Bronchodilator
isoproterenol	Antiarrhythmic, bronchodilator, cardiac stimulant
Isoptin (verapamil)	Antianginal, antihypertensive, antiarrhythmic
isosorbide	Antiglaucoma agent
ketorolac	Anti-inflammatory, non-opioid analgesic
Klavikordal (nitroglycerin [oral])	Antianginal, vasodilator
Klonopin (clonazepam)	Anticonvulsant—controlled substance, Schedule IV
L-caine (lidocaine)	Ventricular antiarrhythmic, local anesthetic
labetalol	Antihypertensive
Lanoxicaps (digoxin)	Antiarrhythmic agent, inotropic
Lanoxin (digoxin)	Antiarrhythmic, inotropic
Lasix (furosemide)	Diuretic, antihypertensive
levalbuterol	Bronchodilator
Levoprome (methotrimeprazine)	Sedative, analgesic agent, antipruritic

Drug Name	Therapeutic Classification(s)
Librium (chlordiazepoxide)	Antianxiety agent, anticonvulsant, sedative/hypnotic—controlled substance, Schedule IV
lidocaine	Ventricular antiarrhythmic, local anesthetic
Lidoject (lidocaine)	Ventricular antiarrhythmic, local anesthetic
LidoPen (lidocaine)	Ventricular antiarrhythmic, local anesthetic
Lipoxide (chlordiazepoxide)	Antianxiety agent, anticonvulsant, sedative/hypnotic—controlled substance Schedule IV
lisinopril	Antihypertensive/ACE inhibitor
Lithane (lithium)	Antimanic, antipsychotic
lithium	Antimanic, antipsychotic
Lithobid (lithium)	Antimanic, antipsychotic
Lithonate (lithium)	Antimanic, antipsychotic
Lithotabs (lithium)	Antimanic, antipsychotic
Loniten (minoxidil)	Antihypertensive
Lorax (lorazepam)	Antianxiety agent, sedative/hypnotic—controlled substance, Schedule IV
lorazepam	Antianxiety agent, sedative/hypnotic—controlled substance, Schedule IV
Lopressor (metoprolol)	Antihypertensive
Ludiomil (maprotiline)	Antidepressant
Luminal (phenobarbital)	Anticonvulsant, sedative/hypnotic—controlled substance, Schedule IV
magnesium sulfate	Electrolyte
mannitol	Diuretic
maprotiline	Antidepressant
Marplan (isocarboxazid)	Antidepressant
Mazepine (carbamazepine)	Anticonvulsant, analgesic
Mebaral (mephobarbital)	Anticonvulsant—controlled substance, Schedule IV
Medihaler-Epi (epinephrine bitartrate)	Bronchodilator, vasopressor, cardiac stimulant, local anesthetic adjunct, topical antihemorrhagic, antiglaucoma agent
Mediquell (dextromethorphan)	Non-narcotic antitussive
Medrol (methylprednisolone)	Anti-inflammatory, immunosuppressant
Mellaril-S (thioridazine)	Antipsychotic
meperidine	Analgesic—controlled substance, Schedule II
mephenytoin	Anticonvulsant
mephobarbital	Anticonvulsant—controlled substance, Schedule IV
meprobamate	Antianxiety agent—controlled substance, Schedule IV
Meprospan (meprobamate)	Antianxiety agent—controlled substance, Schedule IV
Mesantoin (mephenytoin)	Anticonvulsant
mesoridazine	Antipsychotic
Metaprel (metaproterenol)	Bronchodilator
metoprolol	Antihypertensive
metaproterenol	Bronchodilator
methadone	Analgesic, narcotic detoxification adjunct—controlled substance, Schedule II
Methadose (methadone)	Analgesic, narcotic detoxification adjunct—controlled substance, Schedule II
Metadate (methylphenidate)	CNS stimulant—controlled substance, Schedule II
methotrimeprazine	Sedative, analgesic agent, antipruritic

Drug Name	Therapeutic Classification(s)
methyclothiazide	Diuretic, antihypertensive
methyldopa	Antihypertensive
methylphenidate	CNS stimulant—controlled substance, Schedule II
methylprednisolone	Anti-inflammatory
methyprylon	Sedative/hypnotic—controlled substance, Schedule III
metoprolol	Antihypertensive
mexiletine	Ventricular antiarrhythmic
Mexitil (mexiletine)	Ventricular antiarrhythmic
Micronase (glyburide)	Antidiabetic
Micronefrin (epinephrine hydrochloride)	Bronchodilator, vasopressor, cardiac stimulant, local anesthetic adjunct, topical antihemorrhagic, anti-glaucoma agent
midazolam	Antianxiety/sedative/hypnotic
Milontin (phensuximide)	Anticonvulsant
milrinone	Inotropic
Miltown (meprobamate)	Antianxiety agent—controlled substance, Schedule IV
Minipress (prazosin)	Antihypertensive
minoxidil	Antihypertensive
morphine	Analgesic—controlled substance, Schedule II
MS Contin (morphine)	Analgesic—controlled substance, Schedule II
Mucomyst (acetylcysteine)	Antidote (acetaminophen)
Murcil (chlordiazepoxide)	Antianxiety agent, anticonvulsant, sedative/hypnotic—controlled substance Schedule IV
Myidone (primidone)	Anticonvulsant
Mysoline (primidone)	Anticonvulsant
N-G-C (nitroglycerin [oral])	Antianginal, vasodilator
nadolol	Antihypertensive, antianginal
nalbuphine	Analgesic
Nalicaine (lidocaine)	Ventricular antiarrhythmic, local anesthetic
nalmefene	Narcotic antagonist
naloxone	Narcotic antagonist
Napamide (disopyramide)	Ventricular/supraventricular antiarrhythmia, atrial antitachyarrhythmic
Narcan (naloxone)	Narcotic antagonist
Nardil (phenelzine)	Antidepressant
Navane (thiothixene)	Antipsychotic
Nembutal (pentobarbital)	Anticonvulsant, sedative/hypnotic—controlled substance, Schedule II; suppositories under Schedule III
Nervine (diphenhydramine)	Antihistamine, antiemetic, and antivertigo agent, antitussive, sedative/hypnotic, topical anesthetic
Nervocaine (lidocaine)	Ventricular antiarrhythmic, local anesthetic
Neuramate (meprobamate)	Antianxiety agent—controlled substance, Schedule IV
Neurate (meprobamate)	Antianxiety agent—controlled substance, Schedule IV
nifedipine	Antianginal
NightTime Sleep Aid (diphenhydramine)	Antihistamine, antiemetic, and antivertigo agent, antitussive, sedative/hypnotic, topical anesthetic

Drug Name	Therapeutic Classification(s)
Niong (nitroglycerin [oral])	Antianginal, vasodilator
Nitro-Bid (nitroglycerin [oral])	Antianginal, vasodilator
Nitro-Bid (nitroglycerin [topical])	Antianginal, vasodilator
Nitrocap (nitroglycerin [oral])	Antianginal, vasodilator
Nitrocap T.D. (nitroglycerin [oral])	Antianginal, vasodilator
nitroglycerin (oral)	Antianginal, vasodilator
nitroglycerin (sublingual)	Antianginal, vasodilator
nitroglycerin (topical)	Antianginal, vasodilator
Nitroglyn (nitroglycerin [oral])	Antianginal, vasodilator
Nitrol (nitroglycerin [topical])	Antianginal, vasodilator
Nitrolin (nitroglycerin [oral])	Antianginal, vasodilator
Nitronet (nitroglycerin [oral])	Antianginal, vasodilator
Nitrong (nitroglycerin [oral])	Antianginal, vasodilator
Nitrong (nitroglycerin [topical])	Antianginal, vasodilator
Nitronox (nitrous oxide-oxygen	Analgesic
Nitropress (nitroprusside)	Antihypertensive
nitroprusside	Antihypertensive
Nitrospan (nitroglycerin [oral])	Antianginal, vasodilator
Nitrostat (nitroglycerin)	Antianginal, vasodilator
Nitrostat (nitroglycerin [topical])	Antianginal, vasodilator
Nitrostat SR (nitroglycerin [oral])	Antianginal, vasodilator
nitrous oxide-oxygen mixture	Analgesic
Noctec (chloral hydrate)	Sedative/hypnotic—controlled substance, Schedule IV
Noludar (methyprylon)	Sedative/hypnotic—controlled substance, Schedule III
Norcuron (vecuronium bromide)	Nondepolarizing neuromuscular blocking drug
Nordryl (diphenhydramine)	Antihistamine, antiemetic, and antivertigo agent, antitussive, sedative/hypnotic, topical anesthetic
Normodyne (labetalol)	Antihypertensive
Norpace (disopyramide)	Ventricular/supraventricular antiarrhythmic, atrial antitachyarrhythmic
Norpace CR (disopyramide)	Ventricular/supraventricular antiarrhythmic, atrial antitachyarrhythmic
Norpramin (desipramine)	Antidepressant, antianxiety agent
nortriptyline	Antidepressant
Novo-chlorhydrate (chloral hydrate)	Sedative/hypnotic—controlled substance, Schedule IV
Novolin (insulin [regular])	Antidiabetic agent
Nubain (nalbuphine)	Analgesic
Numorphan (oxymorphone)	Analgesic—controlled substance, Schedule II
Nytol with DPH (diphenhydramine)	Antihistamine, antiemetic, and antivertigo agent, antitussive, sedative/hypnotic, topical anesthetic
Omnipen (ampicillin)	Antibiotic
Oramide (tolbutamide)	Antidiabetic agent
Oretic (hydrochlorothiazide)	Diuretic, antihypertensive
Orinase (tolbutamide)	Antidiabetic agent
Osmitrol (mannitol)	Diuretic

Drug Name	Therapeutic Classification(s)
oxazepam	Antianxiety, sedative/hypnotic—controlled substance, Schedule IV
oxtriphylline	Bronchodilator
oxymorphone	Analgesic—controlled substance, Schedule II
oxytocin	Oxytocic
Pamelor (nortriptyline)	Antidepressant
pancuronium	Neuromuscular blocking drug
Panwarfin (warfarin)	Anticoagulant
Parlodel (bromocriptine)	Antiparkinsonian agent
Parnate (tranylcypromine)	Antidepressant
Pavulon (pancuronium bromide)	Neuromuscular blocking drug
Paxipam (halazepam)	Antianxiety agent—controlled substance, Schedule IV
PediaCare (dextromethorphan)	Non-narcotic antitussive
pentazocine	Analgesic—controlled substance, Schedule IV
pentobarbital	Anticonvulsant, sedative/hypnotic—controlled substance, Schedule II; suppositories under Schedule III
Perphenazine (perphenazine)	Antipsychotic, antiemetic
Persantine (dipyridamole)	Coronary vasodilator, platelet aggregation inhibitor
Pertofrane (desipramine)	Antidepressant, antianxiety agent
Pertussin 8 Hour Cough Formula	Non-narcotic antitussive
phenelzine	Antidepressant
Phenergan (promethazine)	Antihistamine
phenobarbital	Anticonvulsant, sedative/hypnotic—controlled substance, Schedule IV
phensuximide	Anticonvulsant
phentolamine	Agent for pheochromocytoma (alpha-adrenergic blocker)
phenytoin	Anticonvulsant, antiarrhythmic
Phyllocontin (aminophylline)	Bronchodilator
physostigmine	Antimuscarinic
pindolol	Antihypertensive
Pitocin (oxytocin)	Oxytocic
Placidyl (ethchlorvynol)	Sedative/hypnotic—controlled substance, Schedule IV
Polycillin (ampicillin)	Antibiotic
Polymox (amoxicillin)	Antibiotic
Pork Regular Iletin II (insulin)	Antidiabetic agent
pralidoxime	Anticholinesterase inhibitor
prazepam	Antianxiety agent—controlled substance, Schedule IV
prazosin	Antihypertensive
Primacor (milrinone)	Inotropic
Primatene Mist Solution (epinephrine)	Bronchodilator, vasopressor, cardiac stimulant, local anesthetic adjunct, topical antihemorrhagic, antiglaucoma agent
Primatene Mist Suspension (epinephrine bitartrate)	Bronchodilator, vasopressor, cardiac stimulant, local anesthetic adjunct, topical antihemorrhagic, antiglaucoma agent
primidone	Anticonvulsant
Principen (ampicillin)	Antibiotic
Prinivil (lisinopril)	Antihypertensive/ACE inhibitor

Drug Name	Therapeutic Classification(s)
procainamide	Ventricular and supraventricular antiarrhythmic, atrial antitachyarrhythmic
Procan SR (procainamide)	Ventricular and supraventricular antiarrhythmic, atrial antitachyarrhythmic
Procardia (nifedipine)	Antianginal
prochlorperazine	Antipsychotic, antiemetic, antianxiety agent
Profene (propoxyphene)	Analgesic—controlled substance, Schedule IV
Proglycem (diazoxide)	Antihypertensive
Prolixin (fluphenazine)	Antipsychotic
Promapar (chlorpromazine)	Antipsychotic, antiemetic
promazine	Antipsychotic, antiemetic, analgesic—controlled substance, Schedule IV
promethazine	Antihistamine
Promine (procainamide)	Ventricular and supraventricular antiarrhythmic, atrial antitachyarrhythmic
Pronestyl (procainamide)	Ventricular and supraventricular antiarrhythmic, atrial antitachyarrhythmic
Pronestyl-SR (procainamide)	Ventricular and supraventricular antiarrhythmic, atrial antitachyarrhythmic
propoxyphene	Analgesic—controlled substance, Schedule IV
propranolol	Antihypertensive, antianginal, antiarrhythmic
Protopam (pralidoxime)	Anticholinesterase inhibitor
protriptyline	Antidepressant
Proventil (albuterol)	Bronchodilator
Proventil Syrup (albuterol)	Bronchodilator
Prozine (promazine)	Antipsychotic, antiemetic, analgesic—controlled substance, Schedule IV
Purodigin (digitoxin)	Antiarrhythmic agent, inotropic agent
Pyopen (carbenicillin)	Antibiotic
Pyridamole (dipyridamole)	Coronary vasodilator, platelet aggregation inhibitor
Quinidex (quinidine)	Ventricular and supraventricular antiarrhythmic, atrial antiarrhythmic
quinidine	Ventricular and supraventricular antiarrhythmic, atrial antiarrhythmic
Quinora (quinidine)	Ventricular and supraventricular antiarrhythmic, atrial antiarrhythmic
ramipril	Antihypertensive/ACE inhibitor
Razepam (temazepam)	Sedative/hypnotic—controlled substance, Schedule IV
Regitine (phentolamine)	Agent for pheochromocytoma (alpha-adrenergic blocker)
Regular Iletin I (insulin [regular])	Antidiabetic agent
Regular Iletin II (insulin [regular])	Antidiabetic agent
Regular Pork Insulin (insulin)	Antidiabetic agent
Reposans-10 (chlordiazepoxide)	Antianxiety agent, anticonvulsant, sedative/hypnotic—controlled substance, Schedule IV
reserpine	Antihypertensive, antipsychotic
Restoril (temazepam)	Sedative/hypnotic—controlled substance, Schedule IV
Revex (nalmefene)	Narcotic antagonist
Rhythmin (procainamide)	Ventricular and supraventricular antiarrhythmic, atrial antitachyarrhythmic
Ritalin (methylphenidate)	CNS stimulant—controlled substance, Schedule II
Ritalin SR (methylphenidate)	CNS stimulant—controlled substance, Schedule II
Rivotril (clonazepam)	Anticonvulsant—controlled substance, Schedule IV
RMS Uniserts (morphine)	Analgesic—controlled substance, Schedule II
Ro-Chlorozide (chlorothiazide)	Diuretic, antihypertensive

Drug Name	Therapeutic Classification(s)
Ro-Hydrazide (hydrochlorothiazide)	Diuretic, antihypertensive
Robalyn (diphenhydramine)	Antihistamine, antiemetic and antivertigo agent, antitussive, sedative/hypnotic, topical anesthetic
rocuronium bromide	Neuromuscular blocking drug
Romazicon (flumazenil)	Benzodiazepine antagonist
Ronase (tolazamide)	Antidiabetic agent
Roxanol (morphine)	Analgesic—controlled substance, Schedule II
S2 Inhalant (epinephrine hydrochloride)	Bronchodilator, vasopressor, cardiac stimulant, local anesthetic adjunct, topical antihemorrhagic, antiglaucoma agent
Sandril (reserpine)	Antihypertensive, antipsychotic
salmeterol xinafoate	$Beta_2$-adrenergic agonist
Sarisol No. 2 (butabarbital)	Sedative/hypnotic—controlled substance, Schedule III
secobarbital	Sedative/hypnotic, anticonvulsant—controlled substance, Schedule II; suppositories are under Schedule III
Seconal (secobarbital)	Sedative/hypnotic, anticonvulsant—controlled substance, Schedule II; suppositories are under Schedule III
Sectral (acebutolol)	Antihypertensive, antiarrhythmic
Sedabamate (meprobamate)	Antianxiety agent—controlled substance, Schedule IV
Serax (oxazepam)	Antianxiety, sedative/hypnotic—controlled substance, Schedule IV
Sereen (chlordiazepoxide)	Antianxiety agent, anticonvulsant, sedative/hypnotic—controlled substance, Schedule IV
Serentil (mesoridazine)	Antipsychotic
Serevent (salmeterol xinafoate)	$Beta_2$-adrenergic agonist
Serpanray (reserpine)	Antihypertensive, antipsychotic
Serpasil (reserpine)	Antihypertensive, antipsychotic
Serpate (reserpine)	Antihypertensive, antipsychotic
Sertan (primidone)	Anticonvulsant
Sinequan (doxepin)	Antidepressant
Sintocinon (oxytocin)	Oxytocic
Sk-Amitriptyline (amitriptyline)	Antidepressant
SK-Bamate (meprobamate)	Antianxiety agent—controlled substance, Schedule IV
SK-Chlorozide (chlorothiazide)	Diuretic, antihypertensive
Sk-Hydrochlorothiazide (hydrochlorothiazide)	Diuretic, antihypertensive
Sk-Lygen (chlordiazepoxide)	Antianxiety agent, anticonvulsant, sedative/hypnotic—controlled substance, Schedule IV
Sk-Quinidine Sulfate (quinidine)	Ventricular and supraventricular antiarrhythmic, atrial antiarrhythmic
Sk-Tolbutamide (tolbutamide)	Antidiabetic agent
Sleep-Eye 3 (diphenhydramine)	Antihistamine, antiemetic and antivertigo agent, antitussive, sedative/hypnotic, topical anesthetic
Slo-Bid (theophylline)	Bronchodilator
Slo-Phyllin (theophylline)	Bronchodilator
sodium thiosulfate	Cyanide poisoning adjunct
Sofarin (warfarin)	Anticoagulant
Solfoton (phenobarbital)	Anticonvulsant, sedative/hypnotic—controlled substance, Schedule IV
Solu-Medrol (methylprednisolone sodium succinate)	Anti-inflammatory, immunosuppressant

Drug Name	Therapeutic Classification(s)
Sominex Formula 2 (diphenhydramine)	Antihistamine, antiemetic and antivertigo agent, antitussive, sedative/hypnotic, topical anesthetic
Somophyllin-T (theophylline)	Bronchodilator
Somophyllin (aminophylline)	Bronchodilator
Sonayine (chlorpromazine)	Antipsychotic, antiemetic
Sparine (promazine)	Antipsychotic, antiemetic, analgesic—controlled substance, Schedule IV
Spectrobid (bacampicillin)	Antibiotic
spironolactone	Antihypertensive, diuretic
St. Joseph for Children (dextromethorphan)	Non-narcotic antitussive
Stadol (butorphanol)	Narcotic agonist-antagonist, opioid partial agonist
Stelazine (trifluoperazine)	Antipsychotic, antiemetic
streptokinase	Thrombolytic
Sublimaze (fentanyl)	Opioid analgesic
succinylcholine	Depolarizing neuromuscular blocking drug
Sucrets Cough Control	Non-narcotic antitussive
Super Totacillian (ampicillin)	Antibiotic
Suprazine (trifluoperazine)	Antipsychotic, antiemetic
Sus-Phrine (epinephrine)	Bronchodilator, vasopressor, cardiac stimulant, local anesthetic adjunct, topical antihemorrhagic, antiglaucoma agent
Sustaire (theophylline)	Bronchodilator
Talwin NX (pentazocine)	Analgesic—controlled substance, Schedule IV
Tambocor (flecainide)	Ventricular antiarrhythmic
Taractan (chlorprothixene)	Antipsychotic
Tavist-1 (clemastine)	Antihistamine
Tavist (clemastine)	Antihistamine
Tegretol (carbamazepine)	Anticonvulsant, analgesic
temazepam	Sedative/hypnotic—controlled substance, Schedule IV
Tempay (temazepam)	Sedative/hypnotic—controlled substance, Schedule IV
Tempra (acetaminophen)	Non-narcotic analgesic, antipyretic
Tenormin (atenolol)	Antihypertensive, antianginal
Tensilon (edrophonium)	Antiarrhythmic, cholinergic agonist
terbutaline	Bronchodilator
Thalitone (chlorthalidone)	Diuretic, antihypertensive
Theo-24 (theophylline)	Bronchodilator
Theo-Dur (theophylline)	Bronchodilator
Theobid (theophylline)	Bronchodilator
Theoclear (theophylline)	Bronchodilator
Theophyl (theophylline)	Bronchodilator
theophylline	Bronchodilator
Theospan-SR (theophylline)	Bronchodilator
Theovent (theophylline)	Bronchodilator
thioridazine	Antipsychotic
thiothixene	Antipsychotic
Thor-Prom (chlorpromazine)	Antipsychotic, antiemetic

Drug Name	Therapeutic Classification(s)
Thorazine (chlorpromazine)	Antipsychotic, antiemetic
timolol	Antihypertensive, antiglaucoma agent
Timoptic (timolol)	Antihypertensive, antiglaucoma agent
Tindal (acetophenazine)	Antipsychotic
tocainide	Ventricular antiarrhythmic
tolazamide	Antidiabetic agent
tolbutamide	Antidiabetic agent
Tolinase (tolazamide)	Antidiabetic agent
Tonocard (tocainide)	Ventricular antiarrhythmic
Toradol (ketorolac)	Anti-inflammatory, non-opioid analgesic
Tornalate (bitolterol)	Bronchodilator
Tracrium (atracurium)	Nondepolarizing skeletal muscle relaxant
Trandate (labetalol)	Antihypertensive
Tranmep (meprobamate)	Antianxiety agent—controlled substance, Schedule IV
Tranxene SD (clorazepate)	Antianxiety agent, anticonvulsant, sedative/hypnotic—controlled substance Schedule IV
Tranxene SD Half Strength (clorazepate)	Antianxiety agent, anticonvulsant, sedative/hypnotic—controlled substance, Schedule IV
tranylcypromine	Antidepressant
triamcinolone	Corticosteroid
triazolam	Sedative/hypnotic—controlled substance, Schedule III
Tridione (trimethadione)	Anticonvulsant
trifluoperazine	Antipsychotic, antiemetic
Trilafon (perphenazine)	Antipsychotic, antiemetic
trimethadione	Anticonvulsant
Trimox (amoxicillin)	Antibiotic
Triptil (protriptyline)	Antidepressant
Truphylline (aminophylline)	Bronchodilator
Tubocurarine chloride	Nondepolarizing neuromuscular blocking drug
Tusstat (diphenhydramine)	Antihistamine, antiemetic and antivertigo agent, antitussive, sedative/hypnotic, topical anesthetic
Twilite (diphenhydramine)	Antihistamine, antiemetic and antivertigo agent, antitussive, sedative/hypnotic, topical anesthetic
Tylenol (acetaminophen)	Non-narcotic analgesic, antipyretic
Uniphyl (theophylline)	Bronchodilator
Utimox (amoxicillin)	Antibiotic
Validol (acetaminophen)	Non-narcotic analgesic, antipyretic
Valdrene (diphenhydramine)	Antihistamine, antiemetic and antivertigo agent, antitussive, sedative/hypnotic, topical anesthetic
Valium (diazepam)	Antianxiety agent, skeletal muscle relaxant, amnesic, anticonvulsant, sedative/hypnotic—controlled substance, Schedule IV
Valorin (acetaminophen)	Non-narcotic analgesic, antipyretic
valproic acid	Anticonvulsant
Valrelease (diazepam)	Antianxiety agent, skeletal muscle relaxant, amnesic agent, anticonvulsant, sedative/hypnotic

Drug Name	Therapeutic Classification(s)
Vancerase (beclomethasone)	Anti-inflammatory, antiasthmatic
Vanceril (beclomethasone)	Anti-inflammatory, antiasthmatic
Vaponefrin (epinephrine hydrochloride)	Bronchodilator, vasopressor, cardiac stimulant, local anesthetic adjunct, topical antihemorrhagic, antiglaucoma agent
vecuronium bromide	Nondepolarizing neuromuscular blocking drug
Velosef (cephradine)	Antibiotic
Velosulin (insulin [regular])	Antidiabetic agent
Velosulin Human (insulin [regular])	Antidiabetic agent
Ventolin (albuterol)	Bronchodilator
Ventolin Syrup (albuterol)	Bronchodilator
verapamil	Antianginal, antihypertensive, antiarrhythmic
Versed (midazolam)	Antianxiety/sedative/hypnotic
Viscous (lidocaine)	Ventricular antiarrhythmic, local anesthetic
Visken (pindolol)	Antihypertensive
Vistaril (hydroxyzine)	Antianxiety agent, sedative
Vivactil (protriptyline)	Antidepressant
Volmax (albuterol)	Bronchodilator
warfarin	Anticoagulant
Wymox (amoxicillin)	Antibiotic
Wytensin (guanabenz)	Antihypertensive
Xanax (alprazolam)	Antianxiety agent—controlled substance, Schedule IV
Xopenex (levalbuterol)	Bronchodilator
Xylocaine (lidocaine)	Ventricular antiarrhythmic, local anesthetic
zafirlukast	Antiasthmatic
Zarontin (ethosuximide)	Anticonvulsant
Zemuron (rocuronium bromide)	Neuromuscular blocking drug
Zepine (reserpine)	Antihypertensive, antipsychotic
Zestril (lisinopril)	Antihypertensive/ACE inhibitor
zileuton	Antiasthmatic
Zyflo (zileuton)	Antiasthmatic

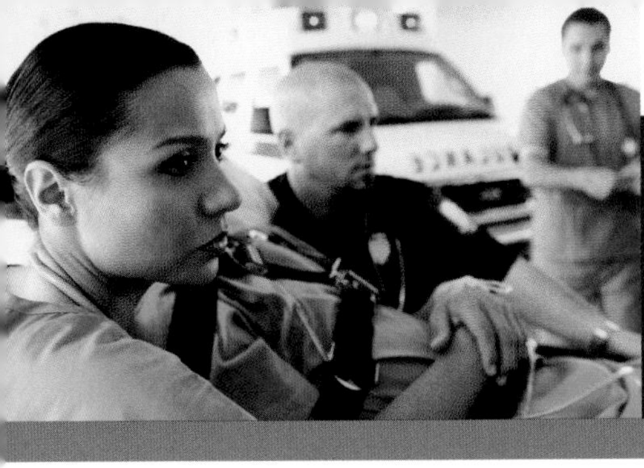

APPENDIX **B**

Pediatric Normal Values, Dosages, and Infusion Rates

Statistically Common Pediatric Normal Values

Age	**Average Weight***	**Respiratory Rate**	**Pulse Rate**	**Blood Pressure**†
Birth–6 wk	4–5 kg (9–11 lb)	30–50 breaths/min	120–160 beats/min	74–100 mm Hg 50–68 mm Hg
7 wk–1 yr	4–11 kg (9–24 lb)	20–30 breaths/min	80–140 beats/min	84–106 mm Hg 45–70 mm Hg
1–2 yr	11–14 kg (24–31 lb)	20–30 breaths/min	80–130 beats/min	98–106 mm Hg 58–70 mm Hg
2–6 yr	14–25 kg (31–55 lb)	20–30 breaths/min	80–120 beats/min	98–112 mm Hg 64–70 mm Hg
6–13 yr	25–63 kg (55–139 lb)	12–20 breaths/min	60–100 beats/min	104–124 mm Hg 64–80 mm Hg
13–16 yr	62–80 kg (136–176 lb)	12–20 breaths/min	60–100 beats/min	118–132 mm Hg 70–82 mm Hg

*Weight estimation: 8 + (12 ∞ age [y]) = weight in kg.
†Systolic blood pressure estimation: 80 + (2 ∞ age [y]) = approx systolic B/P.

Pediatric Drug Dosages

	Body Weight (kg/lb)†				
Drug	**1 kg/2 lb**	**2 kg/4 lb**	**3 kg/7 lb**	**4 kg/9 lb**	**5 kg/11 lb**
Adenosine	0.1 mg	0.2 mg	0.3 mg	0.4 mg	0.5 mg
Aminophylline*	6 mg	12 mg	18 mg	24 mg	30 mg
Amiodarone	5 mg	10 mg	15 mg	20 mg	25 mg
Atropine	0.02 mg	0.04 mg	0.06 mg	0.08 mg	0.10 mg
Calcium chloride	20 mg	40 mg	60 mg	80 mg	100 mg
Calcium gluconate	60–100 mg	120–200 mg	180–300 mg	240–400 mg	300–500 mg
Dextrose 50% in water	0.5–1 mg	1–2 mg	1.5–3 mg	2–4 mg	2.5–5 mg
Diazoxide	1–3 mg	2–6 mg	3–9 mg	4–12 mg	5–15 mg
Diphenhydramine	2–5 mg	4–10 mg	6–15 mg	8–20 mg	10–25 mg
Dopamine	2–20 mcg/min	4–40 mcg/min	6–60 mcg/min	8–80 mcg/min	10–100 mcg/min
Epinephrine (1:10000)	0.01 mg	0.02 mg	0.03 mg	0.04 mg	0.05 mg

*Doses are the usual initial single dose.
†Pounds have been rounded to the nearest pound.

	Body Weight (kg/lb)[†]				
Drug	**1 kg/2 lb**	**2 kg/4 lb**	**3 kg/7 lb**	**4 kg/9 lb**	**5 kg/11 lb**
Etomidate	0.2–0.4 mg	0.4–0.8 mg	0.6–1.2 mg	0.8–1.6 mg	1.0–2.0 mg
Furosemide	1 mg	2 mg	3 mg	4 mg	5 mg
Isoproterenol	0.1–0.2 mcg/min	0.2–0.4 mcg/min	0.3–0.6 mcg/min	0.4–0.8 mcg/min	0.5–1 mcg/min
Lidocaine	1 mg	2 mg	3 mg	4 mg	5 mg
Naloxone	0.1 mg	0.2 mg	0.3 mg	0.4 mg	0.5 mg
Propranolol	0.01 mg	0.02 mg	0.03 mg	0.04 mg	0.05 mg
Sodium bicarbonate	1 mEq	2 mEq	3 mEq	4 mEq	5 mEq
Verapamil	0.1–0.3 mg	0.2–0.6 mg	0.3–0.9 mg	0.4–1.2 mg	0.5–1.5 mg
	6 kg/13 lb	**7 kg/15 lb**	**8 kg/18 lb**	**9 kg/20 lb**	**10 kg/22 lb**
Adenosine	0.6 mg	0.7 mg	0.8 mg	0.9 mg	1.0 mg
Aminophylline	36 mg	42 mg	48 mg	54 mg	60 mg
Amiodarone	30 mg	35 mg	40 mg	45 mg	50 mg
Atropine	0.12 mg	0.14 mg	0.16 mg	0.18 mg	0.2 mg
Calcium chloride	120 mg	140 mg	160 mg	180 mg	200 mg
Calcium gluconate	360–600 mg	420–700 mg	480–800 mg	540–900 mg	600–1000 mg
Dextrose 50% in water	3–6 mg	3.5–7 mg	4–8 mg	4.6–9 mg	5–10 mg
Diazoxide	6–18 mg	7–21 mg	8–24 mg	9–27 mg	10–30 mg
Diphenhydramine	12–30 mg	14–35 mg	16–40 mg	18–45 mg	20–50 mg
Dopamine	12–120 mcg/min	14–140 mcg/min	16–160 mcg/min	18–180 mcg/min	20–200 mcg/min
Epinephrine (1:10000)	0.06 mg	0.07 mg	0.08 mg	0.09 mg	0.1 mg
Etomidate	1.2–2.4 mg	1.4–2.8 mg	1.6–3.2 mg	1.8–3.6 mg	2.0–4.0 mg
Furosemide	6 mg	7 mg	8 mg	9 mg	10 mg
Isoproterenol	0.6–1.2 mcg/min	0.7–1.4 mcg/min	0.8–1.6 mcg/min	0.9–1.8 mcg/min	1.0–2 mcg/min
Lidocaine	6 mg	7 mg	8 mg	9 mg	10 mg
Naloxone	0.6 mg	0.7 mg	0.8 mg	0.9 mg	1.0 mg
Propranolol	0.06 mg	0.07 mg	0.08 mg	0.09 mg	0.1 mg
Sodium bicarbonate	6 mEq	7 mEq	8 mEq	9 mEq	10 mEq
Verapamil	0.6–1.8 mg	0.7–2.1 mg	0.8–2.4 mg	0.9–2.7 mg	1–3 mg
	12.5 kg/28 lb	**15 kg/33 lb**	**17.5 kg/39 lb**	**20 kg/44 lb**	**20.5 kg/50 lb**
Adenosine	1.25 mg	1.5 mg	1.75 mg	2.0 mg	2.05 mg
Aminophylline	75 mg	90 mg	105 mg	120 mg	135 mg
Amiodarone	62.5 mg	75 mg	87.5 mg	100 mg	102.5 mg
Atropine	0.25 mg	0.30 mg	0.35 mg	0.4 mg	0.45 mg
Calcium chloride	250 mg	300 mg	350 mg	400 mg	410 mg
Calcium gluconate	750–1250 mg	900–1500 mg	1.05–1.75 mg	1.2–2.0 mg	1.23–2.05 mg
Dextrose 50% in water	6.25–12.5 g	7.5–15 g	8.75–17.5 g	10–20 g	11.25–22.5 g
Diazoxide	12.5–37.5 mg	15–45 mg	17.5–52.5 mg	20–60 mg	22.5–67.5 mg
Diphenhydramine	25–62.5 mg	30–75 mg	35–87.5 mg	40–100 mg	45–112.5 mg
Dopamine	25–250 mcg/min	30–300 mcg/min	35–350 mcg/min	40–400 mcg/min	41–410 mcg/min

*Doses are the usual initial single dose.
[†]Pounds have been rounded to the nearest pound.

	Body Weight (kg/lb)†				
Drug	**12.5 kg/28 lb**	**15 kg/33 lb**	**17.5 kg/39 lb**	**20 kg/44 lb**	**20.5 kg/50 lb**
Epinephrine (1:10000)	0.125 mg	0.15 mg	0.175 mg	0.2 mg	0.225 mg
Etomidate	2.5–5.0 mg	3.0–6.0 mg	3.5–7.0 mg	4.0–8.0 mg	4.1–8.2 mg
Furosemide	12.5 mg	15 mg	17.5 mg	20 mg	22.5 mg
Isoproterenol	1.25–2.5 mcg/min	1.5–3 mcg/min	1.75–3.5 mcg/min	2–4 mcg/min	2.25–4.5 mcg/min
Lidocaine	12.5 mg	15 mg	17.5 mg	20 mg	22.5 mg
Naloxone	1.25 mg	1.5 mg	2.0 mg	2.0 mg	2.0 mg
Propranolol	0.125 mg	0.15 mg	0.175 mg	0.2 mg	0.225 mg
Sodium bicarbonate	12.5 mEq	15 mEq	17.5 mEq	20 mEq	22.5 mEq
Verapamil	1.25–3.75 mg	1.5–4.5 mg	1.75–5 mg	2–5 mg	2–5 mg
	25 kg/55 lb	**30 kg/66 lb**	**35 kg/77 lb**	**40 kg/88 lb**	**45 kg/99 lb**
Adenosine	2.5 mg	3.0 mg	3.5 mg	4.0 mg	4.5 mg
Aminophylline	150 mg	180 mg	210 mg	240 mg	270 mg
Amiodarone	125 mg	150 mg	175 mg	200 mg	225 mg
Atropine	0.5 mg	0.5 mg	0.5 mg	0.5 mg	0.5 mg
Calcium chloride	500 mg	600 mg	700 mg	800 mg	900 mg
Calcium gluconate	1.5–2.5 mg	1.8–3.0 mg	2.1–3.5 mg	2.4–4.0 mg	2.7–4.5 mg
Dextrose 50% in water	12.5–25 g	15–30 g	17.5–35 g	20–40 g	22.5–45 g
Diazoxide	25–75 mg	30–90 mg	35–105 mg	40–120 mg	45–135 mg
Diphenhydramine	50–125 mg	60–150 mg	70–176 mg	80–200 mg	90–225 mg
Dopamine	50–500 mcg/min	60–600 mcg/min	70–700 mcg/min	80–800 mcg/min	90–900 mcg/min
Epinephrine (1:10000)	0.25 mg	0.3 mg	0.35 mg	0.4 mg	0.45 mg
Etomidate	5.0–10.0 mg	6.0–12.0 mg	7.0–14.0 mg	8.0–16.0 mg	9.0–18.0 mg
Furosemide	25 mg	30 mg	35 mg	40 mg	45 mg
Isoproterenol	2.5–5 mcg/min	3–6 mcg/min	3.5–7 mcg/min	4–8 mcg/min	4.5–9 mcg/min
Lidocaine	25 mg	30 mg	35 mg	40 mg	45 mg
Naloxone	2.0 mg	2.0 mg	2.0 mg	2.0 mg	2.0 mg
Propranolol	0.25 mg	0.3 mg	0.35 mg	0.4 mg	0.45 mg
Sodium bicarbonate	25 mEq	30 mEq	35 mEq	40 mEq	45 mEq
Verapamil	2.5–7.5 mg	3–9 mg	3.5–10.5 mg	4–12 mg	4.5–13.5 mg
	50 kg/110 lb	**55 kg/121 lb**	**60 kg/132 lb**	**65 kg/143 lb**	**70 kg/154 lb**
Adenosine	5.0 mg	5.5 mg	6.0 mg	6.5 mg	7.0 mg
Aminophylline	300 mg	330 mg	360 mg	390 mg	420 mg
Amiodarone	250 mg	275 mg	300 mg	325 mg	350 mg
Atropine	0. 5 mg	0.5 mg	0.5 mg	0.5 mg	0.5 mg
Calcium chloride	1 g	1.1 g	1.2 g	1.3 g	1.4 g
Calcium gluconate	3.0–5.0 mg	3.3–5.5 mg	3.6–6.0 mg	3.9–6.5 mg	4.2–7.0 mg
Dextrose 50% in water	25–50 g	27.5–55 g	30–60 g	32.5–65 g	35–70 g
Diazoxide	50–150 mg	55–150 mg	60–150 mg	65–150 mg	70–150 mg
Diphenhydramine	100–250 mg	110–275 mg	120–300 mg	130–325 mg	140–350 mg

*Doses are the usual initial single dose.
†Pounds have been rounded to the nearest pound.

	Body Weight (kg/lb)†				
Drug	**50 kg/110 lb**	**55 kg/121 lb**	**60 kg/132 lb**	**65 kg/143 lb**	**70 kg/154 lb**
Dopamine	100–1,000 mcg/min	110–1,100 mcg/min	120–1,200 mcg/min	130–1,300 mcg/min	140–1,400 mcg/min
Epinephrine (1:10000)	0.5 mg	0.55 mg	0.6 mg	0.65 mg	0.7 mg
Etomidate	10–20 mg	11–22 mg	12–24 mg	13–26 mg	14–28 mg
Furosemide	50 mg	55 mg	60 mg	65 mg	70 mg
Isoproterenol	5–10 mcg/min	5.5–11 mcg/min	6–12 mcg/min	6.5–13 mcg/min	7–14 mcg/min
Lidocaine	50 mg	55 mg	60 mg	65 mg	70 mg
Naloxone	2.0 mg	2.0 mg	2.0 mg	2.0 mg	2.0 mg
Propranolol	0.5 mg	0.55 mg	0.6 mg	0.65 mg	0.7 mg
Sodium bicarbonate	50 mEq	55 mEq	60 mEq	65 mEq	70 mEq
Verapamil	2–5 mg	2–5 mg	2–5 mg	2–5 mg	2–5 mg

*Doses are the usual initial single dose.
†Pounds have been rounded to the nearest pound.

Calculating Drug Concentrations and Infusion Rates for Common Pediatric Medications

Drug	Commonly Found Drug Concentration	Desired Rate of Administration	Amount of Drug Solution to Add to 100 mL of D_5W
Isoproterenol	0.2 mg/mL	0.1 mcg/kg/min	3 mL
Epinephrine	1:1000 (1 mg/mL)	0.1 mcg/kg/min	0.6 mL
Dopamine	40 mg/mL	10 mcg/kg/min	1.5 mL
Dobutamine	25 mg/mL	10 mcg/kg/min	2.4 mL
Lidocaine	1% (10 mg/mL)	20 mcg/kg/min	12 mL

Shown in the previous chart are five out-of-hospital pediatric drugs. For each drug, the chart shows the drug's concentration in its most common preparation and the rate of administration that medical control usually orders for the drug. The last column shows the amount of drug preparation to add to 100 mL of D_5W. By infusing the resulting solution at the rate of administration indicated on the body weight chart below, you will achieve the desired rate of drug administration.

Weight

kg	lb	Infusion Rate (mL/h)	kg	lb	Infusion Rate (mL/h)
3	6.6	3	30	66	30
7	15.4	7	35	77	35
10	22	10	40	88	40
12.5	27.5	12.5	45	99	45
15	33	15	55	110	50
17.5	38.5	17.5	55	121	55
20	44	20	60	132	60
22.5	49.5	22.5	65	143	65
25	55	25	70	154	70

Drugs Used in Pediatric Advanced Life Support*

Drug	Dose	Remarks
Adenosine	0.1 mg/kg Maximum 1st dose: 6 mg Maximum 2nd dose: 12 mg Maximum single dose: 12 mg	Rapid IV push
Amiodarone	5 mg/kg (VF) 5 mg/kg (SVT)	Rapid IV/IO bolus IV/IO over 20–60 minutes
Amrinone	0.75–1.0 mg/kg	IV/IO over 5 minutes
Atropine sulfate	0.02 mg/kg per dose	Minimum dose: 0.1 mg Maximum single dose: 0.5 mg in child, 1.0 mg in adolescent
Calcium chloride 10%	20 mg/kg per dose	Give slowly
Calcium gluconate	60–100 mg/kg	Slow IV/IO push
Dopamine hydrochloride	2–20 mcg/kg/min	α-Adrenergic action dominates at 15–20 mcg/kg/min
Dobutamine hydrochloride	2–20 μg/kg/min	Titrate to desired effect
Epinephrine for bradycardia	IV/IO: 0.01 mg/kg (1:10000) ET: 0.1 mg/kg (1:1000)	Be aware of effective dose of preservatives administered (if preservatives are present in epinephrine preparation) when high doses are used
Epinephrine for asystolic or pulseless arrest	First dose: IV/IO: 0.01 mg/kg (1:10000) ET: 0.1 mg/kg (1:1000). Doses as high as 0.2 mg/kg may be effective. Subsequent doses: IV/IO/ET: 0.1 mg/kg (1:1000). Doses as high as 0.2 mg/kg may be effective.	Be aware of effective dose of preservative administered (if preservatives present in epinephrine preparation) when high doses are used
Epinephrine infusion	Initial at 0.1 mcg/kg/min. Higher infusion dose used if asystole present	Titrate to desired effect (0.1–1.0 mcg/kg/min)
Etomidate	0.2–0.4 mg/kg	Infused over 30–60 seconds
Glucose	0.5–1.0 g/kg	Maximum concentration: 25%, 2–4 mL/kg
Lidocaine	1 mg/kg per dose	
Lidocaine infusion	20–50 mcg/kg/min	
Magnesium sulfate	25–50 mg/kg	Maximum: 2 g over 10–20 minutes
Naloxone	0.1 mg/kg 2.0 mg	Up to 20 kg Over 20 kg
Nitroprusside	1 mcg/kg/min	Titrate up to 8 mcg/kg/min if needed
Norepinephrine	0.1–2.0 mcg/kg/min	Adjust infusion rate to achieve desired blood pressure
Procainamide	15 mg/kg	IV/IO over 30–60 minutes
Sodium bicarbonate	1 mEq/kg per dose or 0.3 × kg × base deficit	Infuse slowly and only if ventilation is adequate

*IV indicates intravenous route; IO, intraosseous route; and ET, endotracheal route.

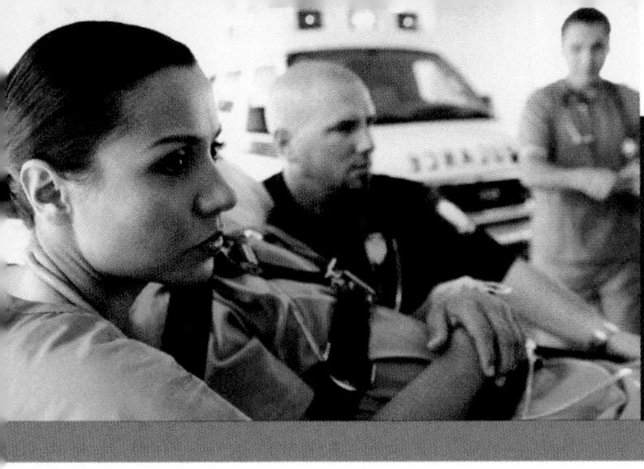

APPENDIX C

Herbal Remedies

Herb	Possible Uses	Possible Side Effects	Cautions	Drug Interactions
Alfalfa	Used to reduce LDL cholesterol levels; may reduce blood sugar levels in diabetic patients	Stomach discomfort, diarrhea, dermatitis	Caution is advised in patients with hypoglycemia due to a possible reduction in blood sugar levels.	May reduce the blood-thinning effects of warfarin; may add to the effects of atorvastatin or simvastatin
Aloe	Used topically to assist in healing of minor wounds, burns, and other skin irritations; used orally as a laxative and to treat colic	Cramps, diarrhea, allergic reactions	Some wound healing may be delayed when using topical gel. Patients with allergies to plants should use caution.	With oral use: digoxin, diuretics, corticosteroids, antiarrhythmics, AZT
Arginine (L-arginine)	May improve exercise tolerance and blood flow in arteries of the heart. Adding arginine to ibuprofen may decrease migraine headache pain. Arginine may decrease the severity of diabetes.	Nausea, stomach cramps	May increase blood sugar levels	May reduce the effectiveness of ranitidine or esomeprazole; may increase the risk of bleeding when used with anticoagulants
Ashwagandha	Enhances mental and physical performance; improves learning ability; decreases stress and fatigue; provides chemotherapy and radiation protection	Nausea, vomiting, GI distress	Do not use during pregnancy or lactation. Use with caution in patients receiving narcotic analgesics.	CNS depressants
Astragalus (Milk Vetch)	Increases stamina and energy; supports chemotherapy and radiation; improves immune function; improves tissue oxygenation	Nausea, vomiting, GI distress	Use with caution in patients with acute infections, especially when accompanied by fever.	Immunosuppressants
Bacopa	Enhances memory; improves cognitive function	CNS depression, seizures	Not for chronic use. Do not use in patients with seizure disorders.	CNS depressants, tricyclic antidepressants, antipsychotics
Bearberry	Diuretic; may be used in the short term for kidney stones and cystitis	CNS depression, hypotension	Do not use in kidney disease or digestive disorders. Long-term use is not recommended as it may lead to GI distress.	Antihypertensives
Belladonna	Can cause relaxation of the airway and reduce the amount of mucus produced; used for the treatment of irritable bowel	Dry mouth, rapid heartbeat, nervousness. Small amounts may cause death in children. Large amounts may cause death in adults.	Older adults and children should avoid belladonna. Not recommended during pregnancy or while breastfeeding.	May interact with alkaloids, atropine, ergot derivatives, hormonal drugs, drugs that increase sun sensitivity, and drugs cleared by the kidneys

Herb	Possible Uses	Possible Side Effects	Cautions	Drug Interactions
Bilberry	Used to treat eye disorders: myopia, decreased visual acuity, macular degeneration, night blindness, diabetic retinopathy, and cataracts; also used to treat vascular disorders: varicose veins, capillary permeability/stability, phlebitis	Bleeding, impaired glucose control in diabetics	Use with caution during pregnancy and lactation. Diabetics should use with caution because of potential to alter glucose regulation. Discontinue use at least 14 days prior to dental or surgical procedures.	Insulin, oral hypoglycemics, hormone-replacement therapy
Black Alder	Used as a cathartic	Diarrhea, vomiting, hypokalemia, abdominal cramping	Do not use in patients with intestinal obstruction or inflammatory bowel disease. Do not use in children. Do not use for more than 8 to 10 days.	Antiarrhythmics, digoxin, corticosteroids, diuretics; may alter absorption of oral medications
Black Cohosh	Used to treat menopausal disorders, PMS, mild depression, and arthritis	Nausea, vomiting, headache, hypotension, vertigo, impaired vision	Do not use during pregnancy or lactation. Do not use for more than 6 months. Use with caution in patients with a history of breast or endometrial cancer, thromboembolic disease, or CVA. Use with caution in patients allergic to salicylates.	Oral contraceptives, hormone-replacement therapy
Blessed Thistle	May have activity against several types of bacteria	Stomach irritation and vomiting	May increase the risk of bleeding; caution advised in patients with bleeding disorders or those taking drugs that may increase the risk of bleeding	None
Bromelain	Used to treat inflammation and sports injuries; aids in digestion; also used to treat respiratory tract infections; aids in vision and circulation	Nausea, vomiting, diarrhea, menstrual irregularities, hypotension	Use with caution in patients with peptic ulcer disease, hypertension, and cardiovascular active bleeding. Stop use at least 14 days prior to dental or surgical procedures.	Anticoagulants, antiplatelet agents, aspirin, NSAIDs
Buckthorn	Used as a cathartic	Diarrhea, vomiting, hypokalemia, abdominal cramping	Should not be used for more than 8 to 10 days. Do not use in patients with intestinal obstruction or inflammatory bowel disease or in children.	Antiarrhythmics, digoxin, diuretics, corticosteroids; may alter absorption of oral medications
Burdock	Used in diabetes treatment due to its possible blood sugar-lowering effects	Dry mouth and bradycardia	Use with caution during pregnancy due to uterine stimulation.	May increase the risk of bleeding when taken with other drugs that increase the risk of bleeding. Patients taking drugs for diabetes should be monitored closely.
Bupleurum	Used to treat chronic inflammatory disease; hepatoprotective against liver toxins	Hypertension, tachycardia, sweating, hyperglycemia, edema	Use with caution in patients with diabetes, hypertension, or edema.	Corticosteroids, diuretics, antihypertensives

Herb	Possible Uses	Possible Side Effects	Cautions	Drug Interactions
Calendula	Used topically to treat minor wounds and burns	Contact dermatitis	Use with caution in patients with allergies to plants.	None
Cascara	Used as a laxative	Hypokalemia, diarrhea, abdominal cramping	Avoid use in children less than 12 years of age. Do not use in patients with bowel obstruction, diarrhea, or dehydration. Use with caution in patients with bowel disorders, inflammatory bowel disease, or appendicitis. Use with caution in those with cardiovascular disease.	Antiarrhythmics, digoxin, phenytoin, laxatives, lithium, theophylline, diuretics; may alter the absorption of oral medications
Cat's Claw	Stimulates the immune system; used as an adjunct therapy for AIDS and cancer therapy and post-radiation therapy; has anti-inflammatory activity in the treatment of allergies and arthritis; used to treat bacterial, fungal, and viral infections	Bleeding, diarrhea, changes in bowel movements	Do not take during pregnancy or lactation. Use with caution in transplant patients and patients on immunosuppressants or IV immunoglobulin.	IV immunoglobulin, immunosuppressants, anticoagulants, aspirin, NSAIDs, antiplatelet agents
Cayenne	Used topically to relieve pain associated with arthritis, rheumatism, and cold injuries; taken orally to increase peripheral circulation and improve digestion	Burning sensation when used topically. Oral use may cause GI distress, nausea, and vomiting.	Use with caution in patients with peptic ulcer disease.	Monoamine oxidase inhibitors, aspirin, antihypertensives
Chamomile	Used to treat anxiety and insomnia; also used to treat GI disturbances: indigestion, heartburn, and flatulence; used as a mouthwash for the treatment of gingivitis and pharyngitis; used topically for the treatment of acne, superficial infections, minor wounds, and burns	Allergic reactions, vomiting. Large doses may cause depression and drowsiness.	Avoid use in patients with allergies to plants in the chrysanthemum or daisy family or to ragweed pollens. Do not use during pregnancy or lactation. Large doses may cause drowsiness—use caution when driving or operating machinery. Not for chronic use.	CNS depressants
Chasteberry	Progesterone-like agent used to treat PMS, menopausal symptoms, endometriosis, menstrual cycle irregularities, corpus luteum insufficiency, insufficient lactation, hyperprolactinemia, and acne vulgaris	Heavy menstrual flow	Do not use during pregnancy.	Hormone-replacement therapy, oral contraceptives, metoclopramide, levodopa, bromocriptine, pramipexole, antipsychotics
Clove	Used topically to relieve toothache and teething problems	Use for more than 48 hours may cause gingival damage.	Not for internal use. Use cautiously in patients allergic to plants.	None

Herb	Possible Uses	Possible Side Effects	Cautions	Drug Interactions
Coleus	Used to treat allergies, asthma, hypertension, congestive heart failure, eczema, and psoriasis	Hypotension, bleeding	Use with caution in patients at risk of hypotension, those who are elderly, or those who would not tolerate hypotension. Do not use in patients with active bleeding. Use with caution in patients with a history of bleeding or hematologic disorders. Discontinue use at least 14 days prior to dental or surgical procedures.	Anticoagulants, antiplatelet agents, aspirin, NSAIDs, antihistamines, decongestants, antihypertensives
Cordyceps	Enhances endurance and stamina; improves energy in patients with fatigue; used as an adjunctive treatment for chemotherapy and radiation; protects liver from toxins; enhances sexual vitality; used to treat lung and kidney disorders	Bleeding, hypertension	Use with caution in patients allergic to molds or fungi. Do not use in patients taking monoamine oxidase inhibitors. Do not use in patients with active bleeding. Use with caution in patients with a history of bleeding or hematologic disorders. Discontinue use at least 14 days prior to dental or surgical procedures.	Monoamine oxidase inhibitors, anticoagulants, antiplatelet agents
Cranberry	Used to prevent kidney stones; also used to treat urinary tract infections	Large doses may cause GI symptoms.	None	Drugs that increase uric acid levels
Creatine	May increase muscle mass; may also improve heart muscle strength; has potential benefit in the treatment of depression; may improve cognition	Stomach discomfort, diarrhea, nausea; may cause muscle cramps; patients with kidney disease should avoid creatine.	Long-term use of large amounts of creatine may increase the production of formaldehyde, which may cause serious side effects. Creatine use is not recommended during pregnancy.	May interact with stimulants such as caffeine; may alter the effectiveness of insulin
Dandelion	Used in digestive disorders to increase bile secretion, increase appetite, and treat dyspepsia; diuretic	Electrolyte disturbances, allergic reactions	Avoid use in patients with biliary obstruction or if gallstones are present.	Diuretics, lithium, digoxin
Devil's Claw	Used as an analgesic in the treatment of arthritis, tendonitis, gout, myalgia, and other inflammatory conditions	Bleeding, GI distress	Do not use during pregnancy or lactation. Use with caution in patients with GI disorders. Do not use in patients with active bleeding. Use with caution in patients with a history of bleeding or hematologic disorders. Discontinue use at least 14 days prior to dental or surgical procedures.	Antiarrhythmics, digoxin, aspirin, NSAIDs, anticoagulants, antiplatelet agents
DHEA	May improve quality of life in patients with Addison's disease; may be beneficial as a supplement in lowering cholesterol levels	Fatigue, nasal congestion, headache, irregular heartbeats	Risk for developing prostate, breast, or ovarian cancer; not recommended during pregnancy or while breastfeeding	Should be used with caution with medications that affect heart rhythm. Alcohol may increase the effects of DHEA.

Herb	Possible Uses	Possible Side Effects	Cautions	Drug Interactions
Dong Quai	Used to improve energy, especially in women; used to treat anemia, menopausal symptoms, dysmenorrhea, PMS, and amenorrhea; used to treat hypertension	Hypotension, bleeding, photosensitivity	Do not use during the first trimester of pregnancy or in patients with excessive menses, hematologic disorders, or severe flu. Use with caution in patients with GI distress, patients at risk of hypotension, or those who would not tolerate a hypotensive episode. May cause photosensitivity, so prolonged exposure to sunlight or UV radiation should be avoided. Use with caution in patients with a history of breast or endometrial cancer, thromboembolism, or CVA.	Antihypertensives, hormone-replacement therapy, oral contraceptives, tamoxifen, anticoagulants, antiplatelet agents
Echinacea	Used to stimulate the immune system; also used for prevention and treatment of colds, flus, allergies, and other upper-respiratory infections; used topically to treat boils, abscesses, tonsillitis, eczema, mild burns, canker sores, herpes, and minor wounds	Immunosuppression with prolonged use, allergic reactions	Should not take for more than 8 weeks because of potential immunosuppressive effects; should not be used for more than 10 days in patients with acute infection or immunosuppression. Use with caution in patients allergic to ragweed, daisies, asters, chrysanthemums, and other pollen.	Immunosuppressants, corticosteroids
Elder	Used to prevent or treat colds, flu, or other respiratory infections; diuretic; promotes sweating	Hypokalemia with prolonged use or high doses	Use caution with drugs that cause hypokalemia or drugs whose toxicity is increased by hypokalemia.	Diuretics, digoxin, lithium
Ephedra (Ma Huang)	Used as a bronchodilator in the treatment of asthma; used as a decongestant in allergies, colds, sinusitis, and hay fever; used to suppress appetite for weight loss	CNS stimulation, nervousness, insomnia, headache, dizziness, skin flushing, palpitations, MI, hypertension, CVA	Should only be used under medical supervision. Do not use in patients who are pregnant, lactating, or taking monoamine oxidase inhibitors. Use with extreme caution in patients with renal impairment, hypertension, cardiovascular disease, thyroid disease, diabetes, prostate disorder, glaucoma, and seizure disorders. Ephedra has been used as a drug of abuse.	Caffeine, oxytocin, decongestants, methyldopa, beta blockers, calcium channel blockers, thyroid medications, antiarrhythmics, digoxin, halothane, theophylline

Herb	Possible Uses	Possible Side Effects	Cautions	Drug Interactions
Evening Primrose	Used as a digestive aid in irritable bowel syndrome; used in the treatment of eczema, dermatitis, and psoriasis; used in the treatment of endometriosis, PMS, and menopausal symptoms; also used for the treatment of diabetic neuropathy, rheumatoid arthritis, and multiple sclerosis; a source of omega-6 fatty acids	Seizures, bleeding	Do not use in patients with seizure disorders, schizophrenia, or active bleeding. Use with caution in patients with a history of bleeding or hematologic disorders. Discontinue use at least 14 days prior to dental or surgical procedures.	Anticoagulants, anticonvulsants, antiplatelet agents, phenothiazines, antipsychotics
Fenugreek	Used to regulate blood glucose	Hypoglycemia	Blood glucose levels should be monitored closely; may alter insulin or oral hypoglycemic requirements in diabetics	Insulin, oral hypoglycemic agents
Feverfew	Used to prevent migraine headaches; also used to treat rheumatoid arthritis	Mouth ulcers, unpleasant taste, abdominal pain, indigestion, tachycardia, bleeding. Post-feverfew syndrome may occur with abrupt discontinuation, causing nervousness, insomnia, joint stiffness, and pain. Abrupt discontinuation may increase migraine frequency.	Do not use during pregnancy or lactation, in children under 2 years, or in patients with allergies to chrysanthemums or daisies. The onset of effect may take weeks; patients should be advised to take it for 1 month before deciding it is not effective. Do not use in patients with active bleeding. Use with caution in patients with a history of bleeding or hematologic disorders. Discontinue use at least 14 days prior to dental or surgical procedures.	Anticoagulants, antiplatelet agents, aspirin, NSAIDs
Flaxseed Oil	Omega-3 fatty acid supplement	None	Must be refrigerated	May delay absorption of oral medications. Do not take within 2 hours of medications.
Garcinia	Used for glucose regulation in diabetes and for weight loss	Hypoglycemia	Blood glucose should be closely monitored if patients are taking insulin or oral hypoglycemics. Dosages of these drugs may need to be adjusted. Use with caution in patients with diabetes or those predisposed to hypoglycemia.	Insulin, oral hypoglycemics, hypolipidemic agents

Herb	Possible Uses	Possible Side Effects	Cautions	Drug Interactions
Garlic	Aids in digestion; lowers cholesterol and blood pressure; protects against heart disease by antiplatelet activity; stimulates immune system; prevents infection, including bacterial and fungal; protects against cancer and liver toxicity	GI distress at beginning of therapy, bleeding, sweating, hypoglycemia, hypotension	Do not use in patients with active bleeding. Use with caution in patients with a history of bleeding or hematologic disorders. Discontinue use at least 14 days prior to dental or surgical procedures. Use caution in patients at risk of hypotension, those who are elderly, or patients who would not tolerate hypotensive episodes. Garlic may alter glucose regulation. Use with caution in patients with diabetes or those predisposed to hypoglycemia. Monitor blood glucose closely.	Anticoagulants, aspirin, antiplatelet agents, NSAIDs, antihypertensives, insulin, oral hypoglycemics
Ginger	Used for treatment of motion sickness, dyspepsia, and nausea; anticoagulant activity; also used to treat arthritis, cough, colds, and flu	High doses (over 6 g) may cause a burning sensation and nausea; bleeding	Do not use in patients with active bleeding or hematologic disorders. Discontinue use at least 14 days prior to dental or surgical procedures.	Anticoagulants, antiplatelet agents, aspirin, NSAIDs
Ginkgo	Improves cerebral vascular and peripheral blood flow and oxygen delivery; improves cognitive function in Alzheimer disease; treats peripheral vascular disease, Raynaud disease, and coronary artery disease; treats impotence, tinnitus, depression, macular degeneration, and asthma	GI distress, headache, dizziness, bleeding (including hyphema and subdural hematoma), palpitations, dermatitis	Do not use in patients with active bleeding or hematologic disorders. Discontinue use at least 14 days prior to dental or surgical procedures.	Monoamine oxidase inhibitors, acetylcholinesterase inhibitors, aspirin, NSAIDs, antiplatelet agents, anticoagulants
Ginseng	Enhances mental and physical performance; increases energy; decreases stress; improves immune function; provides adjunct support for chemotherapy and radiation	Nervousness, depression, insomnia, hypertension at low doses; tachycardia and hypotension at high doses; dermatitis, fever, bleeding, diarrhea, and gynecomastia with prolonged use or high doses	Do not use in patients with renal failure, acute infection, pregnancy, lactation, or active bleeding. Use with caution in patients with hypertension and those at risk of hypotension, those who are elderly, those who would not tolerate hypotensive episodes, or patients with hematologic disorders.	Anticoagulants, antiplatelet agents, aspirin, NSAIDs, antihypertensives, monoamine oxidase inhibitors, CNS stimulants, caffeine, decongestants, hormonal therapies, and drugs that cause gynecomastia: calcium channel blockers, digoxin, methyldopa, phenothiazines, and spironolactone
Glucosamine	Has possible benefits in the treatment of general osteoarthritis of various joints of the body; may also benefit patients with rheumatoid arthritis	Stomach upset, drowsiness, insomnia, headache, sun sensitivity	Use cautiously in patients with bleeding disorders or those taking drugs that may increase the risk of bleeding.	May decrease the effectiveness of insulin; may cause an increased risk of side effects when used in combination with diuretics

Herb	Possible Uses	Possible Side Effects	Cautions	Drug Interactions
Goldenseal	Used to treat inflamed mucous membranes, gastritis, bronchitis, cystitis, and infectious diarrhea	Doses of 2 to 3 g may decrease heart rate and cause GI distress and hypotension. High doses of 18 g may cause CNS depression, hypertension, paralysis, and seizures. Extended use of high doses may cause CNS stimulation, hallucinations, delirium, and GI disorders.	Do not use during pregnancy or lactation. Use with caution in patients with cardiovascular disease or hypertension. Should not be taken for an extended period of time.	Antihypertensives, anticoagulants
Gotu Kola	Used topically to promote healing of wounds from trauma, inflammation, or infection; also used topically to treat hemorrhoids; used orally to treat scleroderma	Topical use may cause contact dermatitis. Large oral doses may cause sedation and elevated cholesterol levels.	Do not use during pregnancy. Use caution when driving or operating machinery as it may cause drowsiness.	CNS depressants
Grape Seed	Used to treat allergies and asthma; improves circulation by antiplatelet activity and improvement of capillary fragility; used to treat intermittent claudication, varicose veins, and arterial and venous insufficiency	Bleeding	Do not use in patients with active bleeding. Use with caution in patients with hematologic disorders. Discontinue use at least 14 days prior to dental or surgical procedures.	Anticoagulants, aspirin, NSAIDs, antiplatelet agents, xanthine oxidase inhibitors, methotrexate
Green Tea	Used as a preventative for cancer and cardiovascular disease; also used as adjunctive treatment for chemotherapy and radiation; lowers cholesterol and inhibits platelet aggregation	Contains caffeine: may cause GI irritation, decreased appetite, insomnia, tachycardia, palpitations, nervousness, or bleeding	Use with caution in patients with peptic ulcer disease, cardiovascular disease, and hematologic disorders. Do not use in patients with active bleeding. Discontinue use at least 14 days prior to dental or surgical procedures.	Monoamine oxidase inhibitors, CNS stimulants, caffeine, decongestants, aspirin, NSAIDs, antihypertensives, anticoagulants, antiplatelet agents, theophylline
Gymnema	Used in diabetes to regulate blood glucose levels	Hypoglycemia	Monitor blood glucose closely. Dosage of insulin or oral hypoglycemics may require adjustments. Patients should take only under medical supervision.	Insulin, oral hypoglycemic
Hawthorn	Used to treat angina, arrhythmias, tachycardia, hypotension or hypertension, peripheral vascular disease, and mild congestive heart failure	Hypotension, dizziness, headache	Do not use during pregnancy. Use with caution in patients at risk of hypotension, those who are elderly, or those who would not tolerate hypotensive episodes.	Antihypertensives, digoxin, antiarrhythmics
Horse Chestnut	Used orally and topically for the treatment of varicose veins, hemorrhoids, deep venous thrombosis, lower extremity edema, and other venous insufficiencies	Gastroenteritis, bleeding	Use with caution in patients with hepatic or renal impairment or hematologic disorders. Do not use in patients with digestive disorders or active bleeding. Discontinue use at least 14 days prior to dental or surgical procedures.	Anticoagulants, aspirin, NSAIDs, antiplatelet agents

Herb	Possible Uses	Possible Side Effects	Cautions	Drug Interactions
Horsetail	Used as a diuretic; used in osteoporosis to strengthen bone and connective tissue	Electrolyte disorders, thiamine (vitamin B_1) deficiency	Do not use in patients with hypotension or hypokalemia.	Antiarrhythmics, digoxin, phenytoin, diuretics, lithium, theophylline
Isoflavones (Soy)	Used in the prevention of cancer; also used as an adjunctive treatment for chemotherapy decreases bone loss; used to treat hypercholesterolemia and menopausal symptoms	None	Use with caution in patients with a history of breast or endometrial cancer.	Oral contraceptives, hormone-replacement therapy
Kava Kava	Relieves anxiety and treats insomnia; protects against CNS ischemia; provides skeletal muscle relaxation; used in children to treat ADD and ADHD	Long-term use may cause rash, drowsiness, or hallucinations.	Do not use during pregnancy or lactation or in patients with Parkinson disease. Use with caution when driving or operating machinery as it may cause drowsiness.	CNS depression, antipsychotics, levodopa
Lavender	Used topically as a wound-healing agent and on minor burns	None	For topical use only	None
Lemon Balm	Used topically for cold sores and fever blisters; used orally in pediatrics for teething	None	None	None
Licorice	Used to treat gastric and duodenal ulcers, adrenal insufficiency, and cough	Pseudohyperaldosteronism: hypokalemia, sodium retention, edema, and hypertension; hepatotoxicity	Do not use in patients who are pregnant or those with diabetes, severe renal insufficiency, hypertension, cardiac disease, hypokalemia, or liver disease. Prolonged use (more than 4 to 6 weeks) is not recommended.	Laxatives, diuretics, corticosteroids, nitrofurantoin
Marshmallow	Used to treat peptic ulcers; also used as a cough suppressant and expectorant	Hypoglycemia	Blood glucose should be monitored closely in patients receiving insulin or oral hypoglycemics.	Insulin, oral hypoglycemic
Milk Thistle	Used as an antidote in death cap mushroom poisoning; promotes bile flow; protects the liver when damaged by chronic drug abuse or drugs that are hepatotoxic; relieves symptoms of jaundice and hepatitis	Diarrhea, gastroenteritis, thrombocytopenia	Do not use in patients with hematologic or digestive disorders.	None
Passion Flower (Maypop)	Used to treat anxiety and insomnia	Drowsiness, vasculitis	Use caution when driving or operating machinery as it may cause drowsiness. Not for chronic use	CNS depressants
Peppermint	Used as a digestive aid to treat abdominal cramps, nausea, flatulence, heartburn, and irritable bowel syndrome	None	Do not use in patients with biliary tract obstruction, cholecystitis, gallstones, hiatal hernia, or severe liver damage.	Calcium channel blockers

Herb	Possible Uses	Possible Side Effects	Cautions	Drug Interactions
Propolis	Used to treat minor burns; also has antiviral and anti-inflammatory effects	Generalized allergic reactions	Contains high levels of alcohol and should be avoided during pregnancy and while breastfeeding	May interact with anticoagulants, antibiotics, antineoplastics, antifungals, and immunosuppressants
Pycnogenol	Used in treating asthma; also used in the treatment of attention deficit hyperactivity disorder (ADHD) to improve cognition; may decrease systolic blood pressure and reduce LDL cholesterol	Minor stomach discomfort	Use with caution in patients with diabetes or hypoglycemia.	May interact with angiotensin-converting enzyme (ACE) inhibitors
Psyllium	Used as a bulk-forming laxative	Abdominal cramps, diarrhea, constipation	Avoid use in patients with bowel obstruction.	May decrease absorption of oral medications. Do not take within 2 hours of medications.
Pygeum	Used to improve urinary symptoms associated with benign prostatic hypertrophy (BPH)	Stomach pain, diarrhea, nausea, constipation	Use beyond 1 year has not been studied.	None
Saw Palmetto	Used to treat benign prostatic hypertrophy	Rarely—headache, nausea; hypokalemia and other electrolyte disorders	Prostatic cancer should be ruled out by prostatic exam and PSA prior to taking saw palmetto.	Finasteride, alpha-adrenergic blockers
Senna	Used as a laxative	Overuse may cause bowel atony.	Avoid use in children less than 12 years of age and in patients with bowel obstruction, diarrhea, or dehydration. Use with caution in patients with bowel disorders, inflammatory bowel disease, appendicitis, or cardiovascular disease.	Antiarrhythmics, diuretics, digoxin, phenytoin, laxatives, lithium, theophylline; may decrease absorption of oral medications
St. John's Wort	Used in the treatment of depression and anxiety; used topically for minor wounds, burns, and infections, neuralgia, bruises, muscle soreness, and sprains	Drowsiness, GI distress, fatigue, restlessness, photosensitivity, hypertension, hypomania, serotonin syndrome	Do not use in patients who are pregnant or hypertensive or in those who are bipolar, suicidal, psychotic, or severely depressed. Use with caution when driving or operating machinery as it may cause drowsiness. Avoid prolonged exposure to sunlight or UV radiation since it may cause photosensitivity.	Pseudoephedrine, CNS depressants, meperidine, dextromethorphan, lithium, selegiline, monoamine oxidase inhibitors, antidepressants, yohimbine, serotonergic drugs, cyclosporin, digoxin, oral contraceptives, theophylline, anticoagulants
Schisandra	Used for hepatic protection and detoxification; also used as adjunct support for chemotherapy and radiation; increases endurance, stamina, and work performance	None	Do not use during pregnancy. Use with caution in patients with liver damage, acute infections, and fever.	Calcium channel blockers, warfarin, phenytoin, cimetidine, theophylline

Herb	Possible Uses	Possible Side Effects	Cautions	Drug Interactions
Soy	Adding soy to a diet can moderately decrease total cholesterol. Soy can treat diarrhea in infants and young children (2 to 38 months old).	GI bloating, nausea, constipation	Use of soy is safe during pregnancy and while breastfeeding. High doses of soy at any age are not recommended.	Soy may interact with warfarin.
Spirulina	Used to treat nasal allergies due to its anti-inflammatory properties; may lower cholesterol and triglyceride levels	Headache, muscle pain, flushing of the face	Not recommended during pregnancy or while breastfeeding	May react with ACE inhibitors
Tea Tree	Used as a mouthwash for dental and oral health; also used topically for burns, cuts, scrapes, and insect bites	Allergic dermatitis	For external use only	None
Valerian	Used as a sedative/hypnotic to treat anxiety and insomnia; also used to treat nervous tension during PMS and menopause; used to treat restless motor syndromes and muscle spasms	Drowsiness, increased muscle relaxation, ataxia, hallucinations, headache, hepatotoxicity	Use with caution when driving or operating machinery as it may cause drowsiness. Use with caution during pregnancy. Do not use in children less than 3 years of age.	CNS depressants
White Oak	Used as a mouthwash in the treatment of mild inflammation of the throat and mouth	None	Should not be swallowed	None
White Willow Yohimbe	Used to reduce fever and treat arthritis; increases sexual vitality in men and women; used to treat male erectile dysfunction	GI distress or ulceration, hypertension, tachycardia, palpitations, anxiety, insomnia	Do not use in children or patients allergic to salicylates. Use with caution in patients with renal or hepatic dysfunction. Do not use during pregnancy or in patients with hypertension or cardiovascular disease.	Aspirin, NSAIDs, methotrexate, warfarin, metoclopramide, phenytoin, probenecid, spironolactone, valproic acid monoamine oxidase inhibitors, antihypertensives, naloxone, tricyclic antidepressants, $alpha_2$-adrenergic blockers, caffeine, sympathomimetics

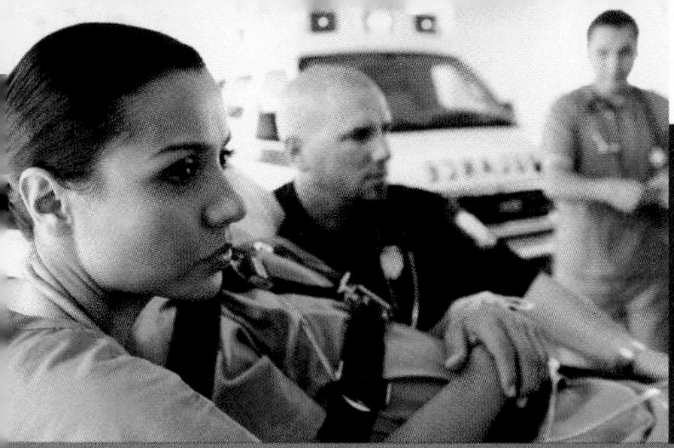

APPENDIX D

Street Drugs

Cannabinoids

Hashish

Broom
Chronic
Gangster
Hash
Hash oil
Hemp

Marijuana

A-bomb (with heroin or opium)
Acapulco gold
Acapulco red
Ace (with PCP)
African
Angola
Ashes
Assassin of Youth
Astro turf
Atshitshi
Aunt Mary
Baby bhang
Blunt
Dope
Ganja
Grass
Happy sticks (with PCP)
Herb
Joints
Kif
Love boat (with PCP)
Mary Jane
Maui Wowie
Pot
Primos (with crack)
Reefer
Sinsemilla
Skunk
Texas tea
Tical (with PCP)
Weed
Woolies (with crack)

Clinical Effects of Cannabinoids

Euphoria
Slowed thinking and reaction time
Confusion
Impaired balance and coordination
Cough
Frequent respiratory infections
Impaired memory and learning
Tachycardia
Anxiety
Panic attacks
Hypertension
Increased thirst and appetite
Tolerance
Addiction

Club Drugs

Flunitrazepam (Rohypnol)

Circles
Forget me drug
Forget pill
La Roche
Mexican valium
Pappas
Pastas
Peanuts
R-2
Reynol
Rib
Roaches
Robinol
Roches
Rohibinol
Roofenol
Roofies
Roopies
Ropanyl
Rope
Rophies
Ro-shays
Rubies
Ruffiew
Whiteys

Club Drugs Used for

Incapacitation of women/sexual assault

Clinical Effects of Club Drugs

Sedation (onset within 15 to 20 minutes)
CNS depressant
Disinhibitory
Dizziness
Disorientation
Slurred speech
Loss of muscle control/coordination
Unconsciousness
Amnesia
Respiratory depression
Hot and cold flashes in rapid alteration
Nausea
Effects last 4 to 6 hours and up to 12 hours

Gamma-hydroxybutyrate (GHB)

Easy lay
Georgia home boy
Great hormones at bedtime
Grievous bodily harm
G-riffic
Jolt
Liquid
Liquid E
Liquid X
Max
Natural sleep-500
Organic quaalude
Salty water
Scoop
Soap
Somatomax

GHB Used for

Incapacitation of women/sexual assault
Anabolic effects/increased muscle mass

Clinical Effects of GHB (onset within 15–30 minutes)

CNS depressant
Drowsiness
Dizziness
Euphoria
Asymptomatic bradycardia
Nausea/vomiting
Unconsciousness
Hallucinations
Seizures
Respiratory depression
Respiratory acidosis
Delirium
Amnesia
Hypotonia
Mild hypothermia
Coma

Ketamine hydrochloride

Bump
Cat Valium
Green
Honey oil
Jet
K
Kay
Keets
Kit-kat
Mauve
Purple
Special "K"
Special LA coke
Super acid
Super C
Vitamin K

Clinical Effects of Ketamine Hydrochloride (onset of effects 15 to 30 minutes)

Sedation
Hallucinations (duration: about 1 hour)
Impaired judgment
Impaired coordination
Hypertension
Vomiting
Hypersalivation
Rapid movements
Dizziness
Disorientation
Vivid dreams
Delirium
Nystagmus
Blurred or temporary loss of vision
Duration of effects 18 to 24 hours

Methylenedioxymethamphetamine (MDMA)

Adam
B-bombs
Bens
Blue kisses
Blue lips
Cristal
Disco biscuit
Ecstasy
Go
Hug drug
XTC

MDMA Used for

CNS stimulant
Psychedelic

Clinical Effects of MDMA

Confusion
Depression
Anxiety
Paranoia
Nausea
Syncope
Hypertension
Tachycardia
Rhabdomyolysis
Renal failure
Cardiovascular failure

CNS Depressants

Barbiturates (Amytal, Nembutal, Phenobarbital, Seconal)

Barb
Barbies
Barbs
Phennies
Red birds
Reds
Seccy
Tooies
Yellow Jackets
Yellows

Benzodiazepines (Ativan, Halcion, Librium, Valium, Xanax)

Candy
Downers
Green and whites
Sleeping pills
Tranks

Clinical Effects of CNS Depressants

Sedation/drowsiness
Reduced pain
Reduced anxiety
Feeling of well-being
Dizziness
Disinhibition
Bradycardia
Respiratory depression
Poor concentration
Confusion
Impaired coordination
Impaired memory
Impaired judgment
Depression
Paradoxical excitation
Fever
Irritability
Slurred speech
Addiction

CNS Stimulants

Amphetamine

A
Aimies
Amp
B-bombs
Back dex
Bam
Bambita
Beans
Bennie
Bens
Benz
Benzedrine
Candy
Chalk
Christina
Christmas tree
Coasts to coasts
Crisscross
Crystal methedrine
Dex
Dexedrine
Dexies
Diet pills
Drivers
Eye opener
Fastin
Glass
Go
Head drugs
Hearts
Iboga
Jolly bean
L.A.
Lid poppers
Marathons
Methedrine
Mini beans
Minibennies
Oranges
Peaches
Pep pills
Pink hearts
Pixies
Powder
Purple hearts

Red phosphorus
Snow
Speed
Speedball
Tens
Truck drivers
Uppers
Uppies

Alpha-ethyltryptamine

Alpha-ET
ET
Love pearls
Love pills
Trip

Cocaine

All-American drug
Angie
Aunt Nora
Bazooka
Beam-me-up Scotty (w/PCP)
Belushi (with heroin)
Bernie
Big C
Big flake
Big rush
Blanco
Blast
Blow
C
C&M (with morphine)
C-dust
Cadillac
Caine
California cornflakes
Came
Candy
Candy C
Candy flipping on a string (with LSD/MDMA)
Caviar (with marijuana)
Champagne (with marijuana)
Charlie
Coca
Coke
Cola
Crystal
Dust
El diablito (with marijuana/heroin/PCP)
El diablo (with marijuana/heroin)
Flake
Florida snow
Freebase
Girlfriend
Glad stuff
Gold dust
Half piece (1/2 ounce)
Happy dust
Happy powder
Ice
Love affair
Marching dust
Movie star drug
Murder one (with heroin)
Nose
Nose candy
Nose powder
Nose stuff
Paradise white
Peruvian flake
Powder
Rock(s)
Rush
Snow
Snowball (with heroin)
Speedball (with heroin)
Stardust
Sugar
Toot
White dragon
White horse
White mosquito
White powder

2-(4-Bromo-2,5 dimethoxyphenethylamine)

2-CB
Nexus
Spectrum
Toonies
Venus

Crack

24-7
Apple Jacks
B.J.'s
Baby T
Bad
Badrock
Ball
Base
Baseball
Basing
Beamers
Beans
Beautiful boulders
Bill Blass
Biscuit (50 rocks)
Blanca
Blowcaine (with procaine)
Blowout
Bollo
Bomb
Boulder
Brick

Bubble gum
Butter
Caine
Cakes
Candy
Casper
Chalk
Chasing the dragon (with heroin)
Cheap basing
Climax
Cloud nine
Coke
Cookies
Crank
Crib
Crumbs
Crunch & munch
Cubes
Devil drug
Hard ball
Hard rock
Hot cakes
Ice
Ice cube
Kryptonite
Liprimo (with marijuana)
Moonrock (with heroin)
Nuggets
One tissue box (1 ounce)
Outerlimits (with LSD)
Pebbles
Pee Wee ($5 worth)
Piles
Pony
Primo
Rock(s)
Smoke
Snow coke
Space base (with PCP)
Space cadet (with PCP)
Space dust (with PCP)
Spaceball (with PCP)
Stones
Sugar block
White ghost

Dimethyltryptamine

45-minute psychosis
AMT
Businessman's LSD
Businessman's special
Businessman's trip
DET
DMT
Fantasia

Methamphetamine

Bathtub crank
Batu
Blue meth
Crink
Cris
Cristina
Cristy
Croak (with crack)
Crypto
Crystal
Crystal meth
Fire (with crack)
Hanyak
Hironpon
Hot ice
Ice
L.A. glass
L.A. ice
Meth
Meth speedball (with heroin)
Methlies Quik
Mexican crack
Mexican speedballs (with crack)
Quartz
Redneck cocaine
Super ice
Trash
White cross
Working man's cocaine
Yellow powder

Methcathinone

Bathtub speed
Cadillac express
Cat
Ephedrone
Gaggers
Go-fast
Khat
Qat
Slick superspeed
Somali tea
Stat
Wild cat (with cocaine)
Wonder star

Methylphenidate (Ritalin®)

Crackers (with Talwin)
One and ones (with Talwin)
Poor man's heroin (with Talwin)
Ritz and T's (with Talwin)
Speedball (with heroin)
Ts and Rits (with Talwin)
Ts and Rs (with Talwin)
West Coast

4-Methylthioamphetamine

Flatliners
Golden eagle

Clinical Effects of CNS Stimulants

Hypertension
Decreased appetite
Tremors
Hyperreflexia
Irritability
Insomnia
Diaphoresis
Aggressive behavior
Anxiety
Delirium
Suicidal/homicidal tendencies
Violent behavior
Palpitations
Arrhythmias
Nausea
Abdominal cramps
Agitation
Temporary illusion of enhanced power and energy
Myocardial infarction
CVAs
Seizures
Paranoia
Cocaine: necrosis of the septum of the nose
Withdrawal: severe depression

Hallucinogens

Lysergic acid diethylamide (LSD)

Acid
Acid cube
Back breakers (with strychnine)
Beavis & Butthead
Big D
Blotter
Blotter acid
Blue dots
Boomers
D
Dots
Microdot
Owsleys
Pane
Paper acid
Sugar
Sugar cubes
Window glass
Window pane
Yellow sunshines

Mescaline

Beans
Buttons
Cactus
Mesc

Morning glory seeds

Pearly gates
Psilocybin:
- Magic mushroom
- Mexico mushroom
- Purple passion
- Shrooms

Clinical Effects of Hallucinogens

Hallucinations
Hyperthermia
Tachycardia
Dilated pupils
"Bad trip": 24-hour period of pain or loss of control
Hypertension
Decreased perception of pain
Insomnia
Alternating agitation and depression
Tremors
Numbness/weakness
Persisting perception disorder (flashbacks)
Cardiovascular collapse
Death

Inhalants

Air blast
Aimes (amyl nitrate)
Aimies (amyl nitrate)
Ames (amyl nitrate)
Aroma of men (isobutyl nitrite)
Bagging (using inhalants)
Bolt (isobutyl nitrite)
Boppers (amyl nitrite)
Bullet (isobutyl nitrite)
Buzz bomb (nitrous oxide)
Climax (isobutyl nitrite)
Gluey (one who sniffs or inhales glue)
Huffing (sniffing an inhalant)
Laughing gas (nitrous oxide)
Locker room (isobutyl nitrite)
Pearls (amyl nitrite)
Poppers (isobutyl nitrite, amyl nitrite)
Quicksilver (isobutyl nitrite)
Rush (isobutyl nitrite)
Rush snappers (isobutyl nitrite)
Shoot the breeze (nitrous oxide)
Snappers (isobutyl nitrite)

- Snorting (using inhalants)
- Snotballs (rubber cement)
- Thrust (isobutyl nitrite)
- Toncho (octane booster)
- Whippets (nitrous oxide)
- Whiteout

Commercial Products

- Adhesives
- Aerosols
- Anesthetics
- Cleaning agents
- Food products (vegetable cooking spray, dessert spray)
- Gases
- Solvents

Indicators of Inhalant Abuse

- Paint or stains on the body or clothing
- Spots or sores around the mouth
- Red or runny eyes and nose
- Chemical odor on the breath
- Intoxicated, dazed, or dizzy appearance
- Loss of appetite
- Excitability or irritability

Clinical Effects of Inhalants

- Initially:
  - CNS stimulation
  - Disinhibition
  - Distorted perception
- Followed by:
  - CNS depression
  - Lethargy
  - Headache
  - Nausea or vomiting
  - Slurred speech
  - Loss of motor coordination
  - Wheezing
  - Acoustic nerve damage may cause deafness
  - Inhibition of oxygen-carrying capacity of the blood
  - Benzene may cause leukemias
- Damage to the cerebral cortex and cerebellum:
  - Personality changes
  - Memory impairment
  - Hallucinations
  - Loss of coordination
  - Slurred speech
- Sudden sniffing death syndrome (SSD):
  - Fatal cardiac arrhythmias
  - Kidney stones
  - Metabolic acidosis
  - Hepatotoxicity
  - Muscle wasting
- Peripheral nerve damage:
  - Numbness
  - Tingling
  - Paralysis
  - "Glue sniffers rash" around nose and mouth
- Withdrawal symptoms:
  - Diaphoresis
  - Tachycardia
  - Hand tremors
  - Insomnia
  - Nausea or vomiting
  - Agitation
  - Anxiety
  - Hallucinations
  - Generalized motor seizures

Opium Derivatives

Codeine

- AC/DC
- Captain Cody
- Cody
- Doors & fours (with glutethimide)
- Lean
- Loads (with glutethimide)
- Nods
- Pancakes & syrup (with glutethimide)
- Schoolboy
- Terp (with terpin hydrate)

Dextromethorphan

- DXM
- Robo

Fentanyl

- Apache
- China girl
- China white
- Dance fever
- Friend
- Goodfella
- Jackpot
- King ivory
- Murder 8
- TNT
- Tango and Cash

Heroin

- AIP
- Al Capone
- Antifreeze
- Aunt Hazel
- Bart Simpson
- Black tar
- Brown sugar
- Chinese white

Dope
H
H and stuff
Horse
Junk
Mexican mud
Scat
Skag
Skunk
Smack
Snow
White horse

Hydromorphone (Dilaudid®)

Hospital heroin

Methadone

Amidone
Dollies

Morphine

M
Microdots
Miss Emma
Mister blue
Monkey
Morf
M.S.
White stuff

Opium

Ah-pen-yen
Auntie
Aunti Emma
Big O
Black stuff
Block
Gum
Hop
Pingon
Pin yen
Poppy
Tar

Oxycontin

Hillbilly heroin
OC
Oxi cotton
Oxy 80's
Oxy
Oxycet
Oxycotton

Paregoric

Blue velvet (with amphetamine)
PG or PO
Propoxyphene hydrochloride
Pinks and grays

Clinical Effects of Opium Derivatives

Pain relief
Euphoria
Respiratory depression/arrest
Nausea/vomiting
Confusion
Constipation
Sedation
Unconsciousness
Coma
Tolerance
Addiction
Withdrawal symptoms:
- Chills
- Diaphoresis
- Rhinitis
- Tearing
- Abdominal cramps

Muscle pain
Insomnia
Nausea/vomiting/diarrhea
Dextromethorphan (effects similar to PCP and ketamine)

Phencyclidine (PCP)

Ace
Amoeba
Angel
Angel dust
Angel hair
Angel mist
Animal trank
Animal tranquilizer
Aurora borealis
Black acid (with LSD)
Boat
Bush
Cheap cocaine
Cosmos
Devil's dust
DOA
Domex (with MDMA)
Dummy dust
Dummy mist
Hog
Jet
K
Kools (with marijuana)
Lemon 714
Love boat
Magic dust
Mauve
Monkey tranquilizer
Octane (with gasoline)
Ozone
Peace
Rocket fuel

Special LA coke
Superacid
Supercoke
Supergrass
Superjoint
Superweed
Trangs
Wack
Zombie

Clinical Effects of PCP

Acute onset of unusual behavior

Agitation
Excitement
Euphoria
Hallucinations
Incoordination
Slurred speech
Catatonic rigidity
Hostility
Apathy
Amnesia
Nystagmus
Constricted pupils
Decreased pain perception
Seizures
Tremors
Weakness
Coma
Death
Involuntary muscle contractions
Hypertension
Arrhythmias
Flushing
Nausea/vomiting
Hypersalivation
Fever/hyperthermia
Diaphoresis
Psychosis
Violent or suicidal behavior
Rhadomyolysis/renal failure

Steroids

Oral

Anadrol (oxymetholone)
Oxandrin (Oxandrolone)
Dianabol (methandrostenolone)
Winstrol (stanozolol)

Injectable

Deca-Durabolin® (nandrolone decanoate)
Durabolin (nandrolone phenylpropionate)
Depo-Testosterone (testosterone cypionate)
Equipoise (boldenone undecylenate)

Desired Effects of Steroids

Growth of skeletal muscle

Adverse Side Effects of Steroids

Acne
Tendon rupture
Irritability
Delusions
Mania
Aggression or homicidal rage
Liver cancer
MIs
CVAs
Left ventricular hypertrophy
Hypercholesterolemia
Adolescent use:
- Stunted growth

Men:
- Gynecomastia
- Infertility
- Testicular atrophy

Women:
- Masculinization
- Decreased breast size
- Decreased body fat
- Coarsening of skin
- Deepening of voice
- Excessive growth of body hair
- Menstrual irregularities

NOTE: Slang terminology for street drugs changes regularly. Appendix D covers some of the more common street drug names. Included here are two websites that are comprehensive for slang terminology worldwide:
- https://www15.uta.fi/FAST/GC/drugslan.html (Glossary of Drug-Related Slang (Street Language)
- http://www.spraakservice.net/slangportal/drug.htm (Street Drug Names Around the World)

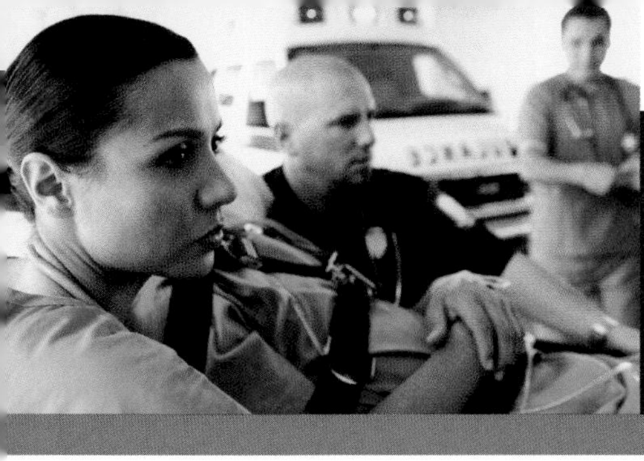

APPENDIX E

Commonly Used Abbreviations and Symbols

a	before
aa	of each; arteries
abd	abdominal/abdomen
ABG	arterial blood gas
a.c., ac	before meals
ACE	angiotensin-converting enzyme
ACH	acetylcholine
ACLS	advanced cardiac life support
ACS	acute coronary syndrome
ACTH	adrenocorticotropic hormone
ad	to, up to
a.d.	right ear
add.	add
ADD	attention deficit disorder
ad lib	as desired, at pleasure
ADP	adenosine diphosphate
ADA	adenosine deaminase
ADH	antidiuretic hormone
ADL	activities of daily living
AFB	acid-fast bacillus
AHF	antihemophilic factor
AIDS	acquired immune deficiency syndrome
a.l.	left ear
ALT	alanine aminotransferase
a.m., A.M.	morning
AMI	acute myocardial infarction
AML	acute myeloid leukemia
AMP	adenosine monophosphate
ANA	antinuclear antibody
ANC	active neutrophil count
ANS	autonomic nervous system
APLS	advanced pediatric life support
APTT	activated partial thromboplastin time
aq	water
aq dist.	distilled water
ARC	AIDS-related complex
ARDS	acute respiratory distress syndrome
ASA	aspirin
ASAP	as soon as possible
ASCVD	atherosclerotic cardiovascular disease
ASD	atrial septal defect
ASHD	arteriosclerotic heart disease
AST	aspartate aminotransferase
ATC	around the clock
ATP	adenosine triphosphate
ATS	American Thoracic Society
ATU	antithrombin unit
ATX	antibiotics
a.u.	each ear, both ears
AV	atrioventricular
BCLS	basic cardiac life support
b.i.d.	two times per day
b.i.n.	two times per night
BMR	basal metabolic rate
BP	blood pressure
BPD	bronchopulmonary dysplasia
BPH	benign prostatic hypertrophy
bpm	beats per minute
BS	blood sugar/bowel sounds
BSA	body surface area
BSE	breast self-exam
BSP	Bromsulphalein

BTLS	basic trauma life support
BUN	blood urea nitrogen
C	Celsius/Centigrade
c̄	with
CABG	coronary artery bypass graft
C&DB	cough and deep breath
CAD	coronary artery disease
caps, Caps	capsule(s)
CBC	complete blood count
CCB	calcium channel blocker
Ccr	creatinine clearance
CD_4	helper T_4 lymphocyte cells
CDC	Centers for Disease Control and Prevention
CF	cystic fibrosis
CHD	congenital heart disease/coronary heart disease
CHF	congestive heart failure
CHO	carbohydrate
CLL	chronic lymphocytic leukemia
cm	centimeter
CML	chronic myeloid leukemia
CMV	cytomegalovirus
CN	cranial nerve
c.n.	tomorrow night
CNS	central nervous system
CO	cardiac output
COMT	catechol-o-methyltransferase
COPD	chronic obstructive pulmonary disease
CP	cardiopulmonary
CPAP	continuous positive airway pressure
CPB	cardiopulmonary bypass
CPK	creatine phosphokinase
CPR	cardiopulmonary resuscitation
CRF	chronic renal failure
C&S	culture and sensitivity
CSF	cerebrospinal fluid
CSID	congenital sucrase-isomaltase deficiency
CT	computerized tomography
CTS	carpal tunnel syndrome
CTZ	chemoreceptor trigger zone
CV	cardiovascular
CVA	cerebrovascular accident
CVP	central venous pressure
CXR	chest x-ray
/d	per day
dATP	deoxy ATP
DBP	diastolic BP
dc	discontinue
DEA	Drug Enforcement Agency
DI	diabetes insipidus
DIC	disseminated intravascular coagulation
dil.	dilute
dL	deciliter (one-tenth of a liter)
DM	diabetes mellitus
DNA	deoxyribonucleic acid
DNR	do not resuscitate
DOA	dead on arrival
DOB	date of birth
DOE	dyspnea on exertion
dr.	dram (0.0625 ounce)
DTR	deep tendon reflex
DVT	deep vein thrombosis
EC	enteric-coated
ECB	extracorporeal cardiopulmonary bypass
ECG, EKG	electrocardiogram, electrocardiograph
ED	emergency department/effective dose
EDTA	ethylenediaminetetraacetic acid
EEG	electroencephalogram
EENT	eye, ear, nose, and throat
EF	ejection fraction
e.g.	for example
elix	elixir
EMS	emergency medical services
emuls.	emulsion
ENL	erythema nodosum leprosum
ENT	ear, nose, and throat
EPS	electrophysiology studies/extrapyramidal symptoms
ER	extended release/emergency room
ESR	erythrocyte sedimentation rate
ESRD	end-stage renal disease
ET	endotracheal
ETOH	alcohol
ext.	extract
F	Fahrenheit, fluoride
f	female
FBS	fasting blood sugar
FD	fatal dose

FDA	Food and Drug Administration
FEV	forced expiratory volume
FFP	fresh frozen plasma
FOB	fecal occult blood
FS	finger stick
FSH	follicle-stimulating hormone
F/U	follow-up
FUO	fever of unknown origin
FVC	forced vital capacity
g, gm	gram (1,000 mg)
GABA	gamma-aminobutyric acid
GERD	gastroesophageal reflux disease
GFR	glomerular filtration rate
GGT	gamma-glutamyl transferase: *syn.* gamma-glutamyl transpeptidase
gi, GI	gastrointestinal
GnRH	gonadotropin-releasing hormone
GP	glycoprotein
G6PD	glucose-6-phosphate dehydrogenase
gr	grain
Gtt/gtt	a drop, drops
GU	genitourinary
GYN	gynecology
H^+	hydrogen ion
h, hr	hour
HA, HAL	hyperalimentation
HCG	human chorionic gonadotropin
HCP	health-care provider
HCV	hepatitis C virus
HDL	high-density lipoprotein
HFN	high-flow nebulizer
H&H	hematocrit and hemoglobin
HIT	heparin-induced thrombocytopenia
HIV	human immunodeficiency virus
HMG-CoA	3-hydroxy-3-methyl-glutaryl-coenzyme A
h/o	history of
HOB	head of bed
HR	heart rate
h.s.	at bedtime
HSE	herpes simplex encephalitis
HSV	herpes simplex virus
5-HT	5-hydroxytryptamine
HTN	hypertension
Hx, hx	history
IA	intra-arterial
IBD	inflammatory bowel disease
ICP	intracranial pressure
ICU	intensive care unit
IDDM	insulin-dependent diabetes mellitus
Ig	immunoglobulin
im, IM	intramuscular
IMV	intermittent mandatory ventilation
in d.	daily
inj.	injection
INR	international normalized ratio
I&O	intake and output
IOP	intraocular pressure
IPPB	intermittent positive pressure breathing
ITP	idiopathic thrombocytopenic purpura
IU	international unit
iv, IV	intravenous
IVPB	IV piggyback, a secondary IV line
J	joule
JVD	jugular venous distention
kg	kilogram (2.2 lb)
KVO	keep vein open
L	liter (1,000 mL)
L	left
L&D	labor and delivery
LDH	lactate dehydrogenase
LDL	low-density lipoprotein
LFTs	liver function tests
LH	luteinizing hormone
LHRH	luteinizing hormone-releasing hormone
LLL	left lower lobe
LLQ	left lower quadrant
LOC	level of consciousness
LR	lactated Ringer's
LTD	lowest tolerated dose
LV	left ventricular
LVFP	left ventricular function pressure
M	mix
m^2, M^2	square meter
m	meter or male
MAC	*Mycobacterium avium* complex
MAO	monoamine oxidase
MAP	mean arterial pressure

max	maximum
mcg	microgram
mCi	millicurie
MDI	metered-dose inhaler
MED	minimum effective dose
mEq	milliequivalent
mg	milligram
MI	myocardial infarction
MIC	minimum inhibitory concentration
min	minute or minim
mist, mixt	mixture
mL	milliliter
MLD	minimum lethal dose
mm	millimeter
MRI	magnetic resonance imaging
MS	multiple sclerosis or mitral stenosis
μg	microgram
NaCl	sodium chloride
ng	nanogram
NG	nasogastric
NGT	nasogastric tube
NICU	neonatal intensive care unit
NIDDM	noninsulin-dependent diabetes mellitus
NKA	no known allergies
NKDA	no known drug allergies
noct	at night or during the night
non rep	do not repeat
NPN	nonprotein nitrogen
NPO	nothing by mouth
NR	do not refill (for example, a prescription)
NS	normal saline
NSAID	nonsteroidal anti-inflammatory drug
NSR	normal sinus rhythm
NSS	normal saline solution
N&V, N/V	nausea and vomiting
O_2	oxygen
OB	obstetrics
o.d.	once a day
O.D.	right eye
OH	orthostatic hypotension
OOB	out of bed
OR	operating room
os	mouth
O.S.	left eye
O_2 sat	oxygen saturation
OTC	over the counter
OU	each eye or both eyes
oz	ounce
PA	pulmonary artery
PABA	para-aminobenzoic acid
PALS	pediatric advanced life support
PAWP	pulmonary artery wedge pressure
PBI	protein-bound iodine
p.c.	after meals
PCA	patient-controlled analgesia
PCI	percutaneous coronary intervention
PCN	penicillin
PCP	*Pneumocystis carinii* pneumonia
PCWP	pulmonary capillary wedge pressure
PDR	*Physician's Desk Reference*
PE	pulmonary embolus
PEEP	positive end expiratory pressure
per	by or through
PFT	pulmonary function test
pH	hydrogen ion concentration
Pharm	pharmacy
PHTLS	prehospital trauma life support
PID	pelvic inflammatory disease
PMH	past medical history
PMI	point of maximal impulse
PMS	premenstrual syndrome
PND	paroxysmal nocturnal dyspnea
po, p.o., PO	by mouth
PPD	purified protein derivative
p.r.	through the rectum
p.r.n.	as needed
PSA	prostatic-specific antigen
PSP	phenolsulfonphthalein
PT	prothrombin time or physical therapy
PTCA	percutaneous transluminal coronary angioplasty
PTH	parathyroid hormone
PTSD	post-traumatic stress disorder
PTT	partial thromboplastin time
PUD	peptic ulcer disease
PVC	premature ventricular contraction/polyvinyl chloride
PVD	peripheral vascular disease
q	every

q.d.	every day
q.h.	every hour
q.2h.	every two hours
q.3h.	every three hours
q.4h.	every four hours
q.6h.	every six hours
q.8h.	every eight hours
qhs	every night
q.i.d.	four times a day
q.m.o.	every month
q.o.d.	every other day
q.s.	as much as needed/quantity sufficient
RA	right atrium/rheumatoid arthritis
RBC	red blood cell
RDA	recommended daily allowance
REM	rapid eye movement
Rept.	let it be repeated
RNA	ribonucleic acid
ROM	range of motion
ROS	review of systems
RRMS	relapsing-remitting multiple sclerosis
R/T	related to
RV	right ventricular
RUQ	right upper quadrant
Rx	symbol for a prescription
s̄	without
SA	sinoatrial or sustained action
SAH	subarachnoid hemorrhage
SBE	subacute bacterial endocarditis
SBP	systolic BP
sc, SC, SQ	subcutaneous
SCID	severe combined immunodeficiency disease
S.D.	standard deviation
SGOT	serum glutamic-oxaloacetic transaminase
SGPT	serum glutamic-pyruvic transaminase
S., Sig.	mark on the label
SI	sacroiliac
SIADH	syndrome inappropriate antidiuretic hormone
SIMV	synchronized intermittent mandatory ventilation
SL	sublingual
SLE	systemic lupus erythematosus
SOB	shortness of breath
sol	solution
sp	spirits
S/P	no change after
SR	sustained-release
ss	one-half
S&S	signs and symptoms
SSS	sick sinus syndrome
stat.	immediately
STD	sexually transmitted disease
SV	stroke volume
SVT	supraventricular tachycardia
syr	syrup
tab	tablet
TB	tuberculosis
TCA	tricyclic antidepressant
TENS	transcutaneous electrical nerve stimulation
TIA	transient ischemic attack
TIBC	total iron binding capacity
t.i.d.	three times per day
t.i.n.	three times per night
TKR	total knee replacement
TNF	tumor necrosis factor
T.O.	telephone order
TPN	total parenteral nutrition
TSH	thyroid-stimulating hormone
U	unit
m	micron
mCi	millicurie
μg or mcg	microgram
μm	micrometer
UGI	upper gastrointestinal
ULN	upper limit of normal
ung.	ointment
UO	urine output
URI, URTI	upper respiratory infection
US	ultrasonic
USP	United States Pharmacopeia
ut. dict.	as directed
UTI	urinary tract infection
UV	ultraviolet
v	vein
VAD	venous access device
VF	ventricular fibrillation
vin	wine
vit	vitamin
VLDL	very low density lipoprotein

VMA	vanillylmandelic acid
vol.	volume
V.O.	verbal order
VS	vital signs or volumetric solution
VT	ventricular tachycardia
WBC	white blood cell or white blood count
XRT	radiation therapy
&	and
>	greater than
<	less than
↑	increased, higher
↓	decreased, lower
–	negative
/	per
%	percent
+	positive
X	times, frequency

Glossary

Absorption: Passage of a substance through a body surface into body fluids and tissues

Acetylcholine: Naturally occurring body substance necessary for the functioning of the parasympathetic nervous system

Acidosis: Condition resulting from an excess of acid or a deficit of alkaline (bicarbonate) in body fluid

Active transport: Mechanism for moving substances across cell membranes from a dilute solution to a concentrated solution

Adams-Stokes syndrome: Also referred to as Stokes-Adams syndrome, a loss of consciousness caused by decreased flow of blood to the brain

Adrenergic: Term for (sympathetic) nerve fibers that, when stimulated, release epinephrine; also, a class of drugs that produce the effect of epinephrine

Affinity: In pharmacology, the attraction between a receptor and a drug

Afterload: Arterial pressure that the heart must push against to eject blood; tension in the ventricular wall during systole

Agglutination: A type of antigen-antibody reaction

Agglutinin: An antibody present in the blood that causes antigens to bind together

Agglutinogen: A specific antigen that stimulates the recognition of an antibody

Agonist: Substance that activates a receptor

Alimentary route: Route of drug administration via the alimentary canal

Alkalosis: Condition resulting from an excess of alkaline or a deficit of acid in the body fluid

Alpha$_1$-adrenergic receptor: A site on the post-synaptic adrenergic nerve pathway that responds when norepinephrine is released

Alpha$_2$-adrenergic receptor: A site on the presynaptic adrenergic nerve pathway that responds when norepinephrine is released

Analgesic: Drug that relieves pain

Angina pectoris: Chest pain possibly spreading to the jaws and arms. Anginal attacks occur when the demand for blood by the heart exceeds the supply of the coronary arteries.

Angiotensin-converting enzyme (ACE) inhibitor: Drug that prevents the conversion of angiotensin I to angiotensin II. This action results in a decrease in peripheral resistance and decreased aldosterone secretion (leading to fluid loss) and, therefore, a decrease in blood pressure.

Anion: See *ion.*

Antagonist: Drug that interferes with the action of an agonist

Antianginal: Drug that relieves the pain of angina pectoris

Antianxiety agent: Drug that is used to treat anxiety

Antiarrhythmic: Drug that controls or prevents cardiac arrhythmias

Antiasthmatic: Drug that is used to treat asthma

Antibody: Substance produced by the body in response to an *antigen*; each antibody reacts only with its specific antigen.

Anticholinergic: Drug that inhibits the action of acetylcholine

Anticholinesterase agent: Drug that opposes the action of cholinesterase

Anticoagulant: Drug that prevents or dissolves blood clots

Anticonvulsant: Drug that prevents, terminates, or reduces seizures

Antidote: Substance that neutralizes a poison or the toxic effects of a drug

Antiemetic: Drug to prevent or relieve nausea and vomiting

Antigen: Foreign particle or substance whose presence in the body causes *antibody* production

Antihistamine: Drug that blocks the effects of histamine

Antihypertensive: Drug that lowers blood pressure

Anti-inflammatory agent: Drug that reduces inflammation

Antimuscarinic agent: Drug that opposes the action of muscarine

Antiplatelet: Drug used to prevent platelet aggregation; used in the treatment of angina and the prophylaxis of myocardial infarction

Antipsychotic: Drug used to treat psychosis

Antitussive: Drug used to prevent or relieve coughing

Anxiety: A vague feeling of discomfort accompanied by an autonomic response

Apothecaries' system: A system of weight and measure used mostly by pharmacists

Asepsis: A condition free from any form of life

Assay: Chemical processing that determines the ingredients present in a drug and their amounts

Asthma: A disease caused by a narrowing and inflammation of the tracheobronchial tree by various stimuli

Autonomic nervous system: The component of the peripheral nervous system that controls automatic functions

Beta$_1$-adrenergic receptor: A site within the autonomic nervous system that, when stimulated, causes an excitatory response to the heart

Beta$_2$-adrenergic receptor: A site located within the autonomic nervous system that, when stimulated, produces bronchial dilation

Beta-blocker: A beta-adrenergic blocking agent; a substance that blocks the inhibitory effects of sympathetic nervous system agents, such as epinephrine

Bioassay: Biological method that determines the amount of preparation to produce a predetermined effect on a laboratory animal

Bioavailability: The rate at which a drug enters the general circulation, permitting access to the site of action

Biotransformation: Changes in chemical makeup resulting from metabolism

Blood-brain barrier: membrane that separates the brain and spinal fluid from circulating blood and prevents certain substances in blood (such as drugs) from reaching brain tissue or spinal fluid; also called the blood-cerebro spinal fluid barrier

Blood typing: Test run to determine the patient's blood type

Body substance isolation: See *Standard Precautions.*

Bolus: A concentrated mass of a substance; pharmacologically, a rounded preparation for oral ingestion or a single dose, injected all at once

Bound drug: Portion of a drug dose that chemically binds with blood proteins or becomes stored in fatty tissue and is unavailable for therapeutic action; see *free drug.*

Bronchodilator: Drug used to relieve airway obstruction caused by constriction of the bronchi

Calcium channel blocker: Drug that inhibits the influx of calcium through the cell membrane, resulting in depression of automaticity and conduction velocity in smooth and cardiac muscle

Capnography: The continuous monitoring of CO_2 levels in the expired air of mechanically ventilated patients

Cardiogenic shock: A state of shock caused by failure of the heart to pump an adequate amount of blood to body tissues

Cation: See *ion.*

Celsius: System of temperature measurement; the freezing and boiling points of water are 0 and 100 degrees, respectively.

Central nervous system (CNS): The brain and spinal cord

Cerebrovascular accident (CVA): The sudden cessation of blood flow to a region of the brain, caused by a thrombus, embolus, or hemorrhage

Chemical name: Description, in the specialized language of chemistry, of the structure of a drug; see *generic name, official name,* and *trade name.*

Chemoreceptor: A nerve ending that is stimulated by certain chemical stimuli and located outside the central nervous system (CNS)

Cholinergic: Term for (parasympathetic) nerve fibers that, when stimulated, release acetylcholine; class of drugs that mimic the action of acetylcholine

Chronotropic: Having an influence on the rate of occurrence of an event, such as a heartbeat

Colloid: Substance that forms a suspension instead of a true solution; the molecules of a colloid do not cross body membranes.

Concentration: The amount of an ingredient relative to the whole compound; in pharmacology, the *strength* of a drug

Congestive heart failure (CHF): A condition that reflects abnormal cardiac pumping, including alterations in rate, rhythm, and electrical conduction

Contraindication: Symptom or circumstance that makes an otherwise-desirable action or treatment unadvisable

Corticosteroids: Any of several steroid hormones secreted by the adrenal gland

Crossmatching: Process that determines the compatibility between blood donor and patient (recipient)

Crystalloid: Crystal-forming substance that can dissolve and cross body membranes in solution

Cumulative drug effects: Effects of repeated doses of a drug that the body does not completely or immediately eliminate; such drugs accumulate in the system, and their effects can be greater than the sum of the effects of individual doses.

Depressant: Agent that depresses a body function

Diabetes mellitus: A chronic metabolic disorder marked by hyperglycemia

Diabetic ketoacidosis: Acidosis caused by an accumulation of ketone bodies, in advanced stages of uncontrolled diabetes mellitus

Diffusion: The tendency of particles of substances in solution to move about until the concentration of the substance is the same throughout the solution

Distribution: The dividing and spreading; the presence of entities throughout the body

Diuretic: Drug that increases the volume of urine produced by increasing the excretion of sodium and water from the kidney

Dopaminergic: Describes receptors that are stimulated by dopamine. Stimulation results in renal and mesenteric vasodilation to improve blood flow to these regions.

Dose-dependent: Drug effects that vary with changes in the amount administered

Drug: Substance that, when introduced into the body, causes a change in the way the body functions

Eclampsia: Coma and convulsive seizures between the 20th week of pregnancy and the first week after delivery, occurring in 1 out of 200 patients with *preeclampsia*

Effector organ: Muscle or gland that, when stimulated by the nervous system, produces an effect

Efficacy: Power to produce a therapeutic effect

Electrolyte: A substance that, in solution, separates into *ions* and, thus, becomes capable of conducting electricity. In the body fluid, the electrolytes (sodium, potassium, calcium, magnesium, and chloride) are necessary for cell function and *acid-base balance.*

End-tidal carbon dioxide ($ETCO_2$) detector: Device used in capnography

Endotracheal (ET): Through the throat, also called transtracheal; a method of introducing medication into the airway through a tube down the throat (endotracheal tube)

Epitope: Portion of the antigen with which an antibody combines

Excretion: Elimination of waste products, including drug metabolites, from the body

Facilitated diffusion: When active transport is required for diffusion to take place

Fahrenheit: System of temperature measurement; the freezing and boiling points of water are 32 and 212 degrees, respectively.

Filtration: The movement of fluid through a membrane, caused by differences in hydrostatic pressure

Fluid, body: The nonsolid, liquid portion of the body, consisting of:

Intracellular fluid—the liquid content of body cells

Extracellular fluid—all other body fluid, consisting of:

Interstitial fluid—the liquid in the spaces between cells, and

Intravascular fluid—the nonsolid portion of the blood, or *plasma*

Food and Drug Administration (FDA): The official United States regulatory agency for food, drugs, cosmetics, and medical devices. The FDA is part of the Department of Health and Human Services.

Free drug: Portion of a drug dose not bound to blood protein or stored in fatty tissue and thereby available for therapeutic action; See *bound drug.*

Ganglia: Nervous tissue composed mainly of neuron cell bodies outside the brain and spinal cord

Generalized motor seizure: A type of seizure that has no definable focus in the brain. This class includes petit mal and grand mal seizures.

Generic name (nonproprietary name): Name, usually the shortened form of the chemical name by which a drug is identified; see *chemical name, official name,* and *trade name.*

Genotype: Special combination of genes unique to each person

Glucocorticoid: A steroid hormone produced by the adrenal gland with very potent anti-inflammatory effects

Glycogen: Starch, the form in which carbohydrates are stored in the body; when needed for metabolism, it is converted to glucose.

Gram: Basic unit of mass (weight) in the metric system

Homeostasis: State of equilibrium in which the internal environment of the body is kept

Hydrogen ion buffer: A substance in a fluid that minimizes changes in the hydrogen ion concentration (pH) in the body fluids that would otherwise result from the addition of acid or base to the fluid

Hydrostatic pressure: The force exerted by the weight of a solution

Hypersensitivity: Above-normal susceptibility to a foreign substance, such as pollen

Hypertensive crisis: Any severe elevation in blood pressure (generally greater than 130 mm Hg diastolic)

Hypertonic: Having higher osmotic pressure than another solution

Hypnotic: Drug that induces sleep

Hypotonic: Having lower osmotic pressure than another solution

Hypoxic drive: Stimulus for respiration triggered by a deficiency of oxygen

Immune response: Ability of the immune system to recognize and respond to foreign invaders

Immunity: Condition in which a person is protected from disease

Inhalation: Act of drawing air or gas into the lungs; a route of drug administration

Inhaler: Small handheld device, usually an aerosol unit, containing a microcrystalline suspension of a drug

Innervate: To stimulate

Inotropic: Influencing the force of muscle contraction

Intradermal: Into the upper layers of the skin; route of drug administration

Intramuscular (IM): Into the muscle; route of drug administration

Intraosseous (IO): Into the bone; route of drug administration

Intravenous (IV): Into the vein; route of drug administration

Intravenous infusion (IV infusion): Controlled introduction of a drug into the bloodstream over a period of time

Ion: An atom with an excess or shortage of electrons, which gives it a charge of negative *(anion)* or positive *(cation)* electrical energy. See *electrolyte.*

Isoantigen: Substance that can stimulate production of antibodies when introduced into the body

Isotonic: Having the same osmotic pressure

Ketone: Compound produced during the oxidation of fatty acids

Korsakoff syndrome: A neurological disorder caused by the lack of thiamine (vitamin B_1) in the brain

Kussmaul breathing: Very deep, gasping breaths associated with diabetic acidosis and coma

Length: The distance between two points

Leukotriene: Substance that induces smooth muscle contraction

Liter: Basic unit of volume in the metric system

Local: Limited area of effect; topical, not systemic

Mass: Weight; how much matter is in an object or substance

Mechanism of action: Explanation of what a drug does to achieve its therapeutic effect

Metabolism: All the physical and chemical changes within an organism resulting in the transformation of ingested substances (food, oxygen, and so on) into cell material of energy

Metabolite: Any substance that results from metabolism

Meter: Basic unit of length in the metric system

Metered-dose inhaler: An inhaler designed to administer a specific amount (dose) of a drug

Metric system: Decimal system for weights and measures used in all scientific disciplines

Minimum therapeutic concentration: Minimum concentration necessary for a drug to produce the desired therapeutic response

Motoneuron: A neuron that stimulates a muscle or gland

Myocardial infarction (MI): Death of heart muscle caused by blockage of blood flow through a coronary artery

Narcotic: A drug that depresses the central nervous system

Narrow-angle glaucoma: Disease in which the pressure inside the eye is higher than normal because of structural abnormality

Neurogenic shock: Shock caused by vasodilation and pooling of the blood in the peripheral vessels so that adequate perfusion of tissues cannot be maintained

Neuromuscular blocking agents: Compete with acetylcholine for receptor sites in muscle cells and cause paralysis

Neurotransmitter: Substance (for example, acetylcholine, norepinephrine) that allows the transmission of impulses between synapses in a neural pathway

Nitrates: A classification of drugs that cause arteriovenous dilation; used to treat angina pectoris, hypertension, and congestive heart failure (CHF)

Nonelectrolytes: Compounds with no electrical charges

Norepinephrine: A hormone produced by the adrenal medulla that chiefly causes vasoconstriction

Official name: The name of a drug given to it by the U.S. Pharmacopeial Convention; usually, it is the generic name, followed by the letters USP. See *chemical name, generic name,* and *trade name.*

Onset of drug action: The time required for a drug preparation to reach an effective concentration at the desired site

Opioid: A synthetic narcotic that is not derived from opium

Organophosphate: Chemical compound, common in pesticides, that inhibits *cholinesterase*

Osmosis: The movement of a solvent through a semipermeable membrane (such as a cell wall) into a solution with a higher solute concentration, so as to equalize the concentration of solute on both sides of the membrane

Osmotic diuretic: Drug or agent that causes increased excretion of water and electrolytes (diuresis) by increasing the osmotic pressure of the glomerular filtrate

Osmotic pressure: The pressure produced by the difference in solute concentration between two solutions separated by a semipermeable membrane

Overdose: Dose of a drug sufficient to cause an acute reaction

Oxytocic: An agent that stimulates uterine contractions

Pain: An unpleasant sensory and emotional experience that occurs from actual or potential tissue damage

Parasympathetic nervous system: A division of the autonomic nervous system

Parasympatholytic: Having the ability to block parasympathetic nerves

Parasympathomimetic: Having the ability to produce effects similar to those resulting from stimulation of the parasympathetic nervous system

Parenteral: Describing any route of administration other than the alimentary canal, including intravenous and intramuscular

Passive transport: The mechanisms for moving substances across cell membranes from a solution with a higher concentration of the substance to a solution with a lower concentration

Peripheral nervous system (PNS): All nervous tissue found outside the central nervous system

pH (potential of hydrogen): A number on a scale of 0 to 14 that expresses the acidity or alkalinity of a substance. A substance with a pH of 7 is neutral, one with a pH of less than 7 is acidic, and one with a pH of more than 7 is alkaline.

Pharmacodynamics: The study of the actions of drugs on the body

Pharmacogenetics: Study of the influence of hereditary factors on the response to drugs

Pharmacokinetics: The study of the movement of drugs through the systems of the body

Pharmacology: The study of drugs and their sources, characteristics, and effects

Pharmacotherapy: The use of drugs in the treatment of disease

Physical dependence: A physiological state that occurs after prolonged use of drugs

Physicians' Desk Reference (PDR): A book, published annually, that describes all currently used drugs

Piggyback: Attaching an additional IV bag (different medication) to an already established IV infusion

Plasma: The liquid part of blood and lymph that forms 52 to 62 percent of the total blood volume

Poison: Any substance taken into the body that interferes with normal physiological function

Postpartum hemorrhage: In a woman who has given birth, the loss of more than 500 mL of blood within 24 hours of delivery

Preeclampsia: Hypertension and other abnormalities resulting from toxemia of pregnancy and, in some cases, leading to eclampsia

Preload: The degree of stretch of the heart muscle fibers at the beginning of a contraction; the volume or pressure within the ventricle at the end of diastole

Preterm labor: Occurs between the beginning of the 21st and end of the 37th week of pregnancy

Prodrug: Drug that becomes therapeutically active as a result of biotransformation

Prophylactic: An agent, device, or process designed to prevent an unhealthy outcome

Proportion: Formed by using two ratios that are equal

Proprietary name: Trade name

Psychosis: Mental disorder characterized by loss of contact with reality

Pulmonary embolus: An embolus (occlusion) in the pulmonary artery or one of its branches

Pulse oximetry: Tool used to determine the oxygenation status of patients

Ratio: The relationship of two quantities

Receptor: In pharmacology, a part of a cell that combines with a drug or body substance to alter the cell's function

Rectal: Into the rectum; route of drug administration

Reflex arc: The neural pathway of a reflex action

Sedative: A drug that has a soothing or tranquilizing effect

Seizure: A sudden attack of pain or other symptoms. Seizures associated with epilepsy include tonic-clonic (grand-mal) and partial or absence (petit mal).

Seizure threshold: Level of stimulus intensity sufficient to set off a seizure

Semipermeable membrane: A membrane that allows passage of water, but not substances in solution (see *osmosis*)

Sick sinus syndrome: An abnormality caused by a malfunction of the sinoatrial (SA) node of the heart

Skeletal muscle relaxant: A drug that causes relaxation of voluntary muscles

Small-volume nebulizer: Device that allows both a drug and oxygen to be inhaled simultaneously

Solubility: The ability to dissolve in a substance

Solute: See *solution.*

Solution: A mixture of a liquid (solvent) and a solid (solute) in which the particles of the solid are so well mixed that they cannot be distinguished from the resulting fluid; see *suspension*

Solvent: See *solution.*

Somatic nervous system: That part of the nervous system that controls the skeletal muscles of the body

Standard Precautions (body substance isolation precautions): Uniform procedures of infection control through the use of barrier precautions; determined by the degree of risk of exposure to body substance and not by the diagnosis of infectious disease

Status asthmaticus: Continuous asthma attacks; may be fatal

Status epilipticus: The occurrence of two or more seizures without a period of consciousness between them

Steroid: Any of a class of complex compounds important in body chemistry, including sex and other hormones and vitamins

Stevens-Johnson syndrome: A rare but serious adverse effect of phenytoin that is characterized by inflammation of the mucous membranes and skin. Blistering occurs. Skin sloughing, high fever, and possibly infection occur as the disorder progresses.

Subcutaneous (SC or SQ or SubQ): Under the skin; a route of drug administration

Sublingual (SL): Under the tongue; a route of drug administration

Suppository: A semisolid drug preparation in the form of a cone or cylinder that is inserted into the rectum, vagina, or urethra

Suspension: A mixture of a solid and a fluid in which the particles of the solid are mixed with, but not dissolved in, the fluid; see *solution.*

Sympathetic nervous system: Division of the autonomic nervous system

Sympatholytic: Drug or agent that produces effects like those produced by inhibiting the sympathetic nervous system

Sympathomimetic: Drug or agent that produces effects like those produced by stimulating the sympathetic nervous system

Synapse: The connecting space between two neurons in a neural pathway

Synergism: The acting together of two substances (drugs, hormones, or other body chemicals) whose combined effect is different from, and perhaps greater than, the individual effect of each substance

Systemic: Effective throughout the body via the circulation

Therapeutic index: A number representing the ratio of the lethal or toxic dose of a drug to its therapeutic dose; an expression of the relative safety of a drug—the higher the number, the wider the margin of safety

Therapeutics: The study of the effects of remedies, such as drugs, and the treatment of disease

Tocolytic: Drug used to decrease or inhibit uterine contraction

Toxemia of pregnancy: Pathological condition resulting from metabolic disturbances in pregnant women, manifested in preeclampsia and, less often, in eclampsia

Toxicity: The quality of being poisonous

Toxicology: The study of poisons

Trade name: The name of a drug given to it by a manufacturer and registered as a trademark; see *chemical name, generic name,* and *official name.*

Unit: One of anything

United States Pharmacopeia (USP): A book, published every 5 years by the U.S. Pharmacopeial Convention, which sets forth the official formulas for all drugs used in the United States and the specifications and standards for preparing and administering them. Since 1975, a similar publication, the *National Formulary,* has been included in the *Pharmacopeia.*

Universal donor: A person who has type O blood

Universal recipient: A person who has type AB blood

U.S.P. unit: A standard of measurement determined by the *United States Pharmacopeia* for a "biologic" (derived from living substance) drug, such as a vaccine, penicillin, and so forth; the amount of such a drug that produces a determined therapeutic effect under controlled conditions

U.S. system: System for weights and measures used in the United States

Vagus nerve: One of a pair of cranial nerves, the major sensory and motor nerve of the parasympathetic nervous system

Vasoconstrictor: A drug used to decrease the diameter of blood vessels

Vasodilator: A drug used to increase the diameter of blood vessels

Vasopressor: A drug that causes the muscles of the arteries and capillaries to contract

Volatile: Easily evaporated

Volume: Amount of space occupied by an object or substance

Volume of distribution: The amount of fluid (body water or plasma) necessary to achieve the desired concentration of a drug in the body

Wernicke encephalopathy: A neurological disorder caused by the lack of thiamine (vitamin B_1) in the brain

Withdrawal syndrome: Partial collapse resulting from withdrawal of alcohol, stimulants, or some opiates

Wolff-Parkinson-White syndrome: Abnormality of cardiac rhythm characterized by an initial slurring of the R wave (called the delta wave), a shortened P-R interval, and a widened QRS complex

Drug Index

Page numbers followed by b indicate boxed material and by t indicate tables. Therapeutic fluids and gases such as Dextrose, Oxygen, Saline, etc. can be found in General Subject Index.

A

E

F

G

H

I

J

K

L

M

N

O

P

Q

R

S

Index

Page numbers followed by b indicate boxed material; f, figures; t, tables. For specific drugs, refer to Drug Index.

A

B

D

E

I

O

P

Q

R

S

T

U

V

W

X